High Praise for *Conducting Clinical Research*

"A valuable guide for practicing physicians interested in becoming involved in clinical trials, written by a talented physician investigator who has 'been there' and 'done this' successfully."

Robert Moellering, MD, Professor of Medicine, Harvard Medical School, Physician-in-Chief and Chairman of the Department of Medicine, Beth Israel Deaconess Medical Center

"A readable, insightful overview of research conduct for healthcare workers."

Henry Masur, MD, Chief, Critical Care Medicine, Clinical Center, National Institutes of Health

"A lucid, user-friendly guide that should encourage even the most hesitant among us to forge ahead."

Thomas Brushart, MD, Director of Hand Surgery Service, Johns Hopkins University, Vice Chairman for Research, Department of Orthopedics

"An invaluable how-to manual for clinical investigators . . . a wealth of useful information . . . provides answers to myriad questions encountered at different stages in clinical research . . . for investigators in academic as well as nonacademic settings."

Prakash Pande, MD, FACC, FACP, FAHA, FSCAI, Professor of Clinical Medicine (Cardiology), Indiana University School of Medicine, former head of Cardiology Unit, Rochester General Hospital, Clinical Professor, University of Rochester

"Everything you need to know about clinical research. A step-by-step tutor."

Tracy Zivin-Tutela, MD

"An enjoyable and comprehensive guide to the world of clinical trials. It is just what my fellows need—as part of their clinical research training and in their future roles as clinical investigators."

Gail Skowron, MD, clinical investigator, Infectious Disease Fellowship Program Director, Roger Williams Medical Center and Boston University School of Medicine

"Excellent practical, down-to-earth guide for the novice and a great review for those who regularly do clinical trials . . . hits all the important points from do you really want to do clinical trials all the way to regulatory checklists. A must for those contemplating involvement in clinical trials."

Robert M. D'Alessandri, MD, Dean, The Commonwealth Medical College, Scranton, Pennsylvania

"A good . . . resource for anyone interested in adding clinical research to their practice."

Bruce S. Bochner, MD, Professor of Medicine and Director, Division of Allergy and Clinical Immunology, Johns Hopkins University

"A compelling look at the practical and ethical challenges of clinical research. Dr. Stone's 'from the trenches' reporting offers a warmth and wisdom missing from most texts. A must-read for those considering entering into this type of research."

Deborah Rudacille, science writer, Johns Hopkins University, author of The Scalpel and the Butterfly *and* The Riddle of Gender

"A fascinating journey through the difficult maze of clinical research. Dr. Stone whimsically shares her 'View from the Trenches,' which makes this several steps beyond your usual 'how to' experience. The book is well written and should be a must for anyone involved in clinical research . . . required reading for all NIH grant programs designed to prepare clinical investigators."

Patricia Lund, EdD, RN, President, Lund Associates, nurse executive, educator, and international consultant to healthcare organizations

"For the community physician, or even the uninitiated academician contemplating a venture into clinical research, this book is an invaluable resource. I highly recommend it. It is truly a 'view from the trenches' with expert advice on what to do and what not to do. The appendices are particularly valuable as a source of regulatory information and contain useful documents that all researchers can adapt for their needs."

Michael F. Parry, MD, Chair of Infectious Diseases and IRB and Director of Microbiology, Stamford Hospital, Professor of Clinical Medicine, Columbia University College of Physicians & Surgeons

"A comprehensive, readable guide for the physician who wants to become involved in clinical research! . . . an exceptional review of the clinical trials process . . . a perfect resource for orienting subinvestigators, aspiring coordinators, and clinical trial administrators new to clinical research. As an experienced investigator, I thoroughly enjoyed this book!"

Herb Baraf, Director, Center for Rheumatology and Bone Research, Clinical Professor of Medicine (Rheumatology), George Washington University

"Offers clear discussions of the regulations that affect clinical research and explains how to make sure your site is compliant with them."

Jean Helz, MD, former IRB member, Memorial Hospital of Cumberland

"Takes the covers off community-based clinical trials and shows how excellent community-based research can be accomplished . . . well written and easy to understand and highlights the challenges and obstacles but also gives a great road map for success . . . Entertaining and informative—this book is what you need to get started in clinical trials."

Stephen Sears, MD, Maine State Epidemiologist

"Should become required reading for all those who contemplate participating in a freestanding clinical research program."

Stuart F. Seides, MD, Vice Chairman of Cardiology, Washington Hospital Center, Clinical Professor of Medicine, George Washington University

"An excellent introduction to clinical research in the modern era . . . for all those beginning to do clinical research."

Gerald R. Donowitz, MD, Professor, Internal Medicine and Infectious Diseases, Director, Residency Programs, Medical Director, General Medicine Services, University of Virginia Health System

"Very well organized, clearly written, and comprehensive . . . a much-needed guide for clinicians who want practical and up-to-date information. Written from the heart, with compassion and experience, Stone focuses on the basic principles of conducting clinical research with an engaging and entertaining approach."

Isabel Pande, PharmD, Intermountain Healthcare, Salt Lake City

"The most practical and comprehensive 'how-to' guide for conducting clinical trials. University programs, community practices, and pharmaceutical investigators will all find this book an invaluable road map to the pitfalls and joys of clinical research. Fascinating personal anecdotes enliven the advice and wealth of experience detailed in this primer."

Eric J. Seifter, MD, FACP, Associate Professor of Medicine and Oncology, Johns Hopkins University

"Leads those interested in medical research through the ethical and even political dilemmas that can interpose themselves when participants are treated as merely the objects of research rather than people deserving of respect for their humanity. Real-life examples bring a real poignancy to the discussion."

The Reverend Lance Beizer, Episcopal priest and retired deputy district attorney specializing in the representation of abused and neglected children

"Provides an informative overview of this field of inquiry and explains the challenges and rewards of careers in clinical research . . . a welcome addition to any career library."

Nancy Burkett, Director of Career Services, Swarthmore College

"A great learning tool . . . Your commentary on the ethical implications [of overseas trials] was very useful, insightful, and timely."

Sarah Noonberg, MD, PhD, Senior Director, Clinical Development, Medivation

"Provides essential information and tools that will help all members of the clinical research team follow the rules, safely navigate the regulatory mine field, and conduct trials successfully."

Glenn Kashurba, MD, Distinguished Fellow, American Academy of Child and Adolescent Psychiatry, author, Courage after the Crash

"All of the essential knowledge to get started in clinical research is here. How I wish I had this book at the beginning of my research career! Captures the humor and excitement in the process of clinical research, while guiding us through the daunting details of setting up and maintaining a successful research program."

David Willms, MD, Co-director, Pulmonary/Critical Care, Sharp Memorial Hospital

Updated, revised, and expanded
SECOND EDITION

Conducting Clinical Research

A PRACTICAL GUIDE
for PHYSICIANS, NURSES, STUDY COORDINATORS, *and* INVESTIGATORS

JUDY STONE, M.D.

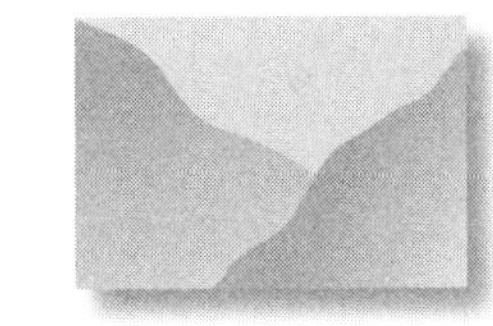

MOUNTAINSIDE MD PRESS
CUMBERLAND, MARYLAND

Mountainside MD Press
725 Park Street, Suite 400
Cumberland, MD 21502
Tel: (240) 362-7245 Fax: (240) 362-7697
www.ConductingClinicalResearch.com

Ordering Information

Quantity sales. Special discounts are available on quantity purchases by corporations, associations, and others. For details, contact the Special Sales Department at the address above.

Orders for college textbook/course adoption use. Please contact Mountainside MD Press at Tel: (240) 362-7245; Fax: (240) 362-7697.

Orders by U.S. trade bookstores and wholesalers. Please contact Cardinal Publishers Group. Tel: (800) 296-0481; Fax: (317) 879-0872, www.cardinalpub.com.

Cataloging-in-Publication Data

Stone, Judy Ann.
Conducting clinical research: a practical guide for physicians, nurses, study coordinators, and investigators, 2nd edition / Judy Stone, M.D.
p. cm.
"Updated, revised, and expanded 2nd edition."
ISBN 978-0-9749178-1-8
Includes bibliographical references and index.

1. Medicine—Research—Methodology. 2. Research design. 3. Medical sciences— Research—Methodology—Handbooks, manuals, etc. 4. Clinical trials—Technique.
5. Drugs—Research—Standards. 6. Medicine—Research—Moral and ethical aspects.
7. Medical ethics. 8. Pharmaceutical ethics. 8. Pharmaceutical ethics. 9. Nursing—Research—Study and teaching. 10. Nursing Research. I. Title.

R852 .S75 2010
610.7220—dc22

15 14 13 12 11 10 1 2 3 4 5 6 7 8 9 10

DISCLAIMER: This manual is intended to provide the reader with an overview, from the perspective of the investigator and coordinator, of what is involved in conducting a clinical trial. It covers the major aspects of clinical research, but it is not intended to be all-inclusive or to provide legal or medical advice or assurances. Regulations affecting clinical research change rapidly, and the reader must assume responsibility for checking the most current requirements and for obtaining appropriate legal and other professional advice and expertise.

Cover design: Bookwrights

Interior design: Graffolio

Editing and proofreading: PeopleSpeak

For my family, my aunt, Klari,
Mrs. G., and for my mother, Magdus,
whose love of reading made
seeing both her children become authors
her proudest moment

Contents

Preface | ix

How Not to Kill the Patient—or the Investigator . . . ix

Why Read This Book? A View from the Trenches . . . ix

Acknowledgments | xiii

Introduction | xv

Chapter 1: Overview | 3

Why Do Studies? . . . 3

Liability? . . . 4

Jargon . . . 5

Who's Who . . . 5

Study Activities . . . 10

Phases of Drug Development . . . 10

Protocol Design Part 1: Parts of a Protocol . . . 16

Protocol Design Part 2: Patient Mix . . . 18

Product Quality: Seals of Approval . . . 19

Protocol Design Part 3: Mixing the Ingredients . . . 20

Medical Device Trials . . . 22

Vaccines and Other Biologics . . . 28

The Evolution of U.S. Drug Law . . . 38

Problems with Antibiotics . . . 41

Conclusion . . . 43

Chapter 2: Scrounging Your First Study | 45

What Do You Need to Get Started? . . . 45

Navigating Site Selection: Landing Your First Study . . . 48

Newer Methods for Landing a Study . . . 49

Why It's So Difficult to Get Studies . . . 53

Site Selection: Be Careful What You Wish for—You Might Get It . . . 55

Site Selection: Why a Site Is Chosen, or a Marriage of Convenience . . . 57

Site Qualification Visit, or "Shall We Dance?" 59
Do Size and Setting Matter? 62
Conclusion 65

Chapter 3: Reality Testing: Feasibility, Budgets, and Contracts | 67

Feasibility Overview 67
Protocol Feasibility 68
Patient Pool 72
Staffing 73
Regulatory Considerations: IRBs 76
Managing the IRB Submission Process 78
Regulatory Considerations: Billing for Clinical Trials 80
Antikickback, False Claims, and Stark Laws 82
Budget Feasibility 83
CROs and SMOs—Dealing with the Middleman 97
Contract Basics 100
The Dark Side of Contracts, or Things Your Mother Never Told You 109
Win-Win Relationships 110
Conclusion 112

Chapter 4: Regulatory Issues | 113

New Regulations 115
Form FDA 1572—What Are You Really Signing? 121
IRBs 123
HIPAA 125
Drug Accountability 129
Financial Disclosure, or Whose Business Is It Anyway? 130
Audits 132
How to Prepare for an Audit 143
Conclusion 145

Chapter 5: Study Start-Up | 147

Informed Consent: Safe, Sane, and Consensual 147
Start-Up in Theory 157
Start-Up in Practice: The Paper Trail—Implementing Regulatory Details 159
Initiation Visit 160
Electronic Medical Records 161
Volunteer Recruitment Strategies 164
Advertising 170
Web Advertising and Social Networking 175

Approaching the Patient, or "You Want Me to Do What?" 178
Conclusion 180

Chapter 6: Study Activities: Strategies and Tools | 181

SOPS—Why Bother? 181
Study Tracking: What Day Is Today? 185
General Tracking Procedures 185
Worksheets, Forms, and Study Folders: Getting in Touch with Your Inner OCD 186
Project Management Techniques 189
Software Programs 189
Coping with Minutiae 190
Billing Compliance—Practicalities 191
Drug Storage and Accountability 192
Maintaining Drug and Supply Inventories 193
Monitoring Visits 194
Volunteer Retention and Satisfaction 195
Patient Instructions 198
The Paper Trail Continues 202
Study Closing 213
Conclusion 216

Chapter 7: Perspective on the State of the Industry | 217

Costs of Clinical Trials 217
"Breaking the Scientific Bottleneck" 225
Where Have All the Trials Gone? 237
Overseas Drug Manufacturing 241
Conclusion 242

Chapter 8: Ethical Issues in Human Subjects Research | 243

Historical Context 244
Ethical Principles (the Belmont Report) 248
Special Populations 255
Individual Research Practice: The Nature of the Beast 258
Financial Pressure and Conflict of Interest 258
Whose Body Is It? Tissue Ownership 265
Patient-Prompted Ethical Issues 270
Adverse Events: Related Ethical Issues 271
Publication Ethics 275
Practice Guidelines 277
Off-Label Uses 278

IRB-Related Ethical Issues . . . 279
Unanticipated Risk in Clinical Trials . . . 281
Who's Minding the Store? A Case Study . . . 286
Conclusion . . . 290

Chapter 9: Society and Politics | 293

Politics of Research: The FDA . . . 293
Politics of Research: Women . . . 300
Politics of Research: Religion . . . 307
Politics of Research: Race . . . 311
Politics of Research: Race and Gender Overlap . . . 313
Politics of Research: Shifting Studies to Developing Countries . . . 315
Justice and Societal Needs . . . 324
Conclusion . . . 336

Chapter 10: Opportunities and Training in Clinical Research | 337

Enhancing Your Practice . . . 338
Brief Training Options . . . 339
Formal Training Programs . . . 341
Conclusion . . . 344

Epilogue | 345

Appendix A: Background Resource Information | 349

Appendix B: Suggested Resources | 387

Appendix C: Career Information and Training Programs | 401

Notes | 443

Glossary and Acronym Guide | 511

Bibliography | 525

Index | 579

About the Author | 601

Preface

Readers might wonder how this book came to be and what is in store. Let me begin by sharing my unusual orientation toward teaching.

How Not to Kill the Patient—or the Investigator

When I was a medical resident with the responsibility of training medical students and physicians less experienced than I was, the most difficult task was helping them identify what was important versus what was "interesting." I had to teach them how to prioritize in diagnosing and treating a patient's illness and how to wade through seemingly overwhelming amounts of information. I developed a series of minilectures called "How Not to Kill Your Patient" that focused on recognizing, defining, and responding to symptoms, signs, or lab results that were medical emergencies. Only later could my trainees address more esoteric points.

I have tried to do the same in this guide to clinical trials, emphasizing the elements that are critical for patient safety as well as for investigator survival. These points are marked by an icon.

Why Read This Book? A View from the Trenches

I offer a unique perspective, having experienced research from a variety of angles. I have participated in clinical trials since college and have been a patient in a clinical research center. I conducted bench and clinical research during my infectious disease fellowship, for which I designed and oversaw my first clinical trial (with mentoring, of course). In all, I have had over 25 years experience in conducting clinical trials.

As background, I am a physician specializing in internal medicine with a subspecialty in infectious diseases. My initial medical training was at the University of Maryland, where the caliber of the infectious disease faculty was topnotch and the enthusiasm contagious. Infectious diseases, a specialty that spans all ages of patients and that involves being a sleuth and puzzling things out, fascinated me. When Memorial Hospital recruited me to practice in Cumberland, Maryland, there was no infectious disease specialist on the eastern side of the Appalachian Mountains within almost 150 miles.

I chose infectious diseases as my niche, initially thinking that this would be a relatively cheery and gratifying specialty—that I would be able to sprinkle antibiotics on patients and have them rapidly recover from their grave illnesses. Instead, the specialty has increasingly evolved to caring for critically ill patients, many of whom are immunocompromised by cancer, organ transplantation, kidney failure, or trauma or by treatments for same. Additionally, we are seeing the rapid emergence of "superbugs," bacteria that are resistant to most, if not all, antibiotics. The press speaks of our returning to the "preantibiotic era." This is due to the widespread misuse of antibiotics—to our squandering of them. For example, antibiotics are widely used in agriculture to boost animal productivity. Similarly, uncontrolled and irrational use occurs to appease public demand for instant gratification and the relief of uncomfortable symptoms, such as from flu or colds, even though many of these illnesses are obviously viral and are not going to respond to antibiotics.

Over the past 25 years, the specialty of infectious diseases has also changed. We have identified many new illnesses, such as AIDS, legionnaires' disease, and hantavirus. Many other diseases are increasingly thought to be due to infectious agents, such as in the potential links between chlamydia and coronary artery disease or juvenile diabetes and viral infections. Discovery of new infectious diseases occurs regularly. Attempts to develop effective therapies soon follow.

Different specialties attract different kinds of people. Patience, the desire to puzzle things out, and obsessive-compulsive traits are characteristic of infectious disease specialists and are a natural fit with the requirements of carrying out clinical research.* I thrive on conducting clinical trials as these

---

* See "Laments of a Clinical Clerk" in the epilogue.

studies provide a stimulating balance with and break from the rest of my practice, especially from what I call "antibiotic last rites," or "coma rounds," in the ICU. Instead of complete burnout from attending the seemingly unending stream of dying patients, I feel passionately that I am making a broader contribution to humankind by helping to develop new medicines. Families of my critically ill patients often feel it helpful to learn something and to see something positive come out of their loved ones' deaths that will help future generations.

I love the challenge—and ability—to outshine the big medical centers in the number of patients I enroll in research trials. I have been very successful in enrolling "quality" patients, who are highly compliant, reliable, and evaluable. I delight in attracting drug companies to place studies at my site in a small rural town, rather than in a large metropolitan area. This "we try harder" attitude provides me with a competitive advantage.

Except for my initial foray, all has been learned the hard way, as I am one of the last of a dying breed, the successful rural solo practitioner of internal medicine and infectious diseases.

I know where the pitfalls are as I've survived them all: attracting studies, negotiating contracts, dealing with all the administrative aspects, and performing all the activities that a study coordinator must do.

This book is intended to provide an overview of how research is conducted for drug companies and how you might become involved. It introduces career opportunities in medical research and describes how you can pursue them. It is primarily directed toward physicians interested in running research studies at their practices, though other healthcare workers and the curious will find the considerable background information of interest. My premise is that most people are ill prepared to explore this field. My intent is to give you a good idea of what you might be getting into, both the warts and the gratifying aspects, and teach you how to thrive in these endeavors.

You, too, can conduct clinical studies successfully. I'll show you how.

Acknowledgments

Many people have contributed to this book in one form or another, and I would like to express my thanks. If I have inadvertently omitted anyone, my apologies for my transient synapse failure.

Particular thanks go to Ron Montgomery, for taking the chance to give me my first study, more than 20 years of OCD (obsessive-compulsive disorder) guidance, and continued friendship; Dr. Glenn Kashurba, for his friendship and encouragement; Dr. Bennett Lorber, for his direction and kindness to strangers; Larry Ceppos, for his thoughtful comments and healthy perspective; Hassan Movahhed, for his decency and generosity to me; Dr. David Ross, for patience in answering regulatory questions and for valuing my different perspective; Dr. Harold Glass, for background information and perspective; Dr. Arthur Anderson, for providing the IRB Follies and permissions; and to the authors of the follies for their much needed comic relief: Jeff Cooper, Kathy Schulz, Jon Hart, and Jeff Cohen. In addition, thanks go to Buddy West, for providing resources and advocacy; Alicia Pouncey, William Tobia, and Henry Masur, for suggestions on topics; Drs. Charlotte Dalton and Fern Hauck, for generously sharing their course materials on health literacy and cultural competency; and Medidata and Cutting Edge, for providing valuable background material.

Much thanks also to the staff of Memorial Hospital, Cumberland, Maryland, without whom none of this would have been possible; Dr. Robert Manasse, for his meticulous attention to detail and perspective and for his excellence as a microbiologist, which has enabled me to conduct clinical trials and provide better care for my patients; Jeannie Spataro, my "secret weapon"; and Barry, for creating conditions that forced me to look beyond and expand my horizons.

And thanks to April Corley, my secretary, coordinator, and worksheet designer; Sasha Beyer, for her careful review and astute comments; Joe Neil and Drs. Art Jacknowitz and Leonard Frank, for providing materials, perspective, longstanding friendship, and humor; Liz Jonsson and Drs. Kari Anderson, Drew Lewis, and Barry Hafkin, for insights into the drug industry; Joel Remmer, for understanding and support; Deborah Rudacille, for her advice; Jean Hathaway, for generously helping me learn the ropes early in the game; and Dr. Harold Tubbs, the master of creative solutions, for showing me another way.

I am also grateful to Mark, for patient critiquing and rereading countless revisions, for tolerating my inexplicable need to write, and for supporting me in this endeavor, despite the toll of having me unavailable for far too long; Michael, for his pointed and perceptive comments, cogent arguments, and efforts to teach me computer speak; Heather, my charming source of inspiration, for her continued encouragement; Uncle Grease, for leading the way and for his wry reviews of drafts; and Sharon Goldinger, my excellent editor, who has expertly guided and cajoled me through the editorial process.

And thanks especially to my family—husband Mark Skinner, Michael, Heather, and Cuddles, for love, hugs, and companionship through years of writing and life.

Introduction

Clinical research is a rapidly changing field of study because of the promises from new technologies and the challenges of using these resources wisely. The field is receiving considerable attention, and many people wish to explore the excitement of the biotechnology and pharmaceutical industries. A variety of positions offer many opportunities to participate in these sectors.

This is a guidebook with several parts that may be read sequentially as a detailed look at how drugs are developed or referred to as independent topics that can serve as resources when needed. Although I refer to drug development, you should note that biologic agents and medical devices go through similar evaluation procedures, as will be discussed in chapter 1.

When asked to consider revising and updating my book, I anticipated the task to be relatively straightforward. After all, I have enjoyed and worked in this field for many years. As I stopped to further reflect, I realized that an astonishing number of changes have happened just over the past 5 years. As a result, the book has been largely rewritten to incorporate changes in the global drug development industry, and many new topics have been added.

Chapter 1 provides the framework for deciding whether you might want to go into clinical research, either full time or as a part-time supplement to your practice as I have done. You will also find an overview of the drug development process in chapter 1.

Entirely new sections have been added, devoted to the differences between drug development and the unique needs of device trials and vaccine trials.

Chapter 2 focuses on how sites attract studies, which is particularly difficult for inexperienced investigators to achieve in this highly competitive field. Additional insights are given about what sponsors are looking for in a site and how you might best position your site for successful selection.

Chapter 3 tackles some of the more difficult preparatory logistics you might encounter. You also will learn in chapter 3 how to determine if a particular drug company or protocol is a good match for you. Because the pharmaceutical industry has downsized, it is more important than ever to learn how to make an accurate budget. Chapter 3 explores this topic, with particular attention to hidden costs and several approaches to budgeting are detailed. Similarly, contracts have become more complex, and companies are inserting more unfriendly language, particularly regarding subject injury. These hazards to your financial and professional health are examined.

New topics include regulatory considerations about billing for clinical trials, warnings regarding the legal land mines of antikickback or false claims clauses, insurance for clinical trials, and subject injury clauses.

Skills for handling the bureaucratic aspects of studies, including audits and regulatory requirements, are handled in chapter 4. The number of new regulations affecting research is enough to make your head spin. Expanded sections in this chapter guide you through the flurry of paper and better prepare you for a possible audit. Being proactive in your quality practices will hold you in good stead. The impact of HIPAA (Health Insurance Portability and Accountability Act) on research in the United States is also discussed. Throughout this and other chapters, you will find icons highlighting legal dangers for investigators.

Chapter 5 explores how to recruit volunteers for a study, including information on social networking and electronic media tools, and how to begin to implement the protocol. Important new sections discuss cultural competency and health literacy, both vitally important to successfully recruiting and enrolling volunteers.

Chapter 6 gives tips for tackling the myriad details in conducting a study successfully. It includes updated tips on billing compliance practices to keep you out of trouble, electronic data capture, and lessons from Hurricane Katrina. New sections cover standard operating procedures and access to electronic medical records.

Chapter 7 provides a broad perspective on the state of the drug development industry, beginning with an overview of the costs of conducting clinical trials. Some of the difficulties facing the clinical research industry—especially the causes of the scientific bottleneck—are explored.

An enormous shift in clinical trials from the United States to developing countries has occurred in recent years. Chapter 7 explores the reasons behind the outsourcing, the soaring costs of trials, and the bottlenecks in research in greater detail than before. Additions have been made regarding phase 0 and microdosing studies, use of surrogate biomarkers, adaptive trials, postmarketing trials, and drug safety and surveillance, among other topics.

Basic ethical issues in research are introduced in chapter 8—topics that should be required study for anyone working in this area. New topics include conflicts of interest related to Data Safety Monitoring Boards, as well as to the investigator and institutional review board, and tips for avoiding pitfalls in publication that might harm the unwary.

Controversies surrounding research ethics, politics, and social issues are presented in chapter 9. This supplementary chapter is not for the faint of heart; it might be considered optional for new investigators. I find these topics both distressing and intriguing. They have no clear-cut answers, and these areas unfortunately receive little attention or discussion in traditional curricula and warrant greater public debate. New additions explore the politicization of research at the Food and Drug Administration and its consequences.

Finally, chapter 10 concludes by providing some information about career development, including training programs geared toward students with varying levels of experience in clinical research.

Supplementary information can be found in appendices A, B, and C. Pertinent worksheets and forms are available on my Web site: http://conductingclinicalresearch.com.

I have experienced clinical trials from a volunteer's perspective, done bench research, been in solo practice, and conducted clinical research trials for pharmaceutical companies. I'm like a member of an endangered species, about to become extinct—a rare creature who has not only witnessed but experienced the changes in drug development over more than 25 years, at a time when only 10 percent of investigators stay in the business for 5 years or longer.

And I have been gratified to see, over the years, how participating in clinical trials has made me a better physician and improved care at our institution. I learned a great deal from investigator meetings and by more closely assessing and managing many of my patients. A 2008 study confirmed my experience: "Patients treated at hospitals that participated in trials had significantly lower mortality than patients treated at nonparticipating hospitals."[1]

This guidebook distills a wealth of hard-earned lessons into a practical, clinically oriented series of topics for you. It should enable you to reap important rewards from your practice professionally, financially, and personally and to derive satisfaction from knowing you are providing the best care you can for your patients.

Conducting Clinical Research

CHAPTER 1

Overview

The desire to take medicine
is perhaps the greatest feature
which distinguishes man from animals.
—VOLTAIRE

Before you undertake a clinical study, you must consider a number of issues. This overview is presented to help you better understand what is involved. This chapter introduces some of the advantages and disadvantages to entering this field, describes the people who conduct trials, and summarizes the drug development process.

Why Do Studies?

As in any endeavor, there are many reasons why one may choose to conduct clinical trials. Some of these reasons may be thought of as fitting into Maslow's Hierarchy of Needs, by which one can pursue more idealistic goals only after basic needs of food, shelter, and security have been met.[1] Each of Maslow's needs is similarly met by some aspect of clinical research:

- Basic physiologic and safety needs can be satisfied as studies provide income to support your family and practice. Publications resulting from studies can also ease the pressure to gain tenure, providing further security.
- The need for love or a sense of belonging can be met by the acceptance of membership in a research group or department.

- The need for esteem may be fulfilled by publication and recognition and the accompanying boosts to the ego.
- The higher needs of self-actualization and transcendence may be attained through altruism, wanting to develop a medicine or device that will help other people, and by the sense of personal satisfaction that comes from meeting the intellectual challenges of a well-designed clinical trial.

For many, the attraction of conducting clinical studies includes fulfillment of most of these needs.

Liability?

Many readers probably wonder if they are risking everything by participating in research, given some of the recent adverse publicity particularly regarding unexpected volunteer deaths and lack of adequate oversight at major universities. This is further discussed in chapters 8 and 9. Although you may be surprised, I have much *less concern about liability* with my study patients than I do with many of my other patients! "Why is this?" you may be wondering as you breathe a sigh of relief. If you are a responsible investigator, your volunteers have a very good understanding of what they have agreed to do. You will have done careful histories and physical examinations, explained to them that they have no underlying health problems that raise concerns about their participation, and reviewed the informed consent agreements with them, answering their questions along the way. Study patients have a much better understanding of what is being done to them, and for them, than most patients in hospitals or general medical practice.

This reflects poorly on the general state of medical care, I know. But from the blasé surgeon who says, "Trust me. You'll be back on your feet in no time!" to the harried staff who are short-handed and simply unable to spend the time to explain care adequately, few explain treatment better than Principal Investigators or their coordinators. Their thorough and carefully documented explanations are the best defense against lawsuits.

Clinical trial protocols often require frequent and extensive patient assessments. The investigators, because they are often less comfortable with a new medication or treatment than with familiar ones, are also often more attentive. The result is that study volunteers may well be watched more attentively than are "regular" patients.

Finally, many lawsuits arise out of misunderstandings and lack of documentation. Nothing is better documented about patients than discussions and assessments made during a clinical trial.

Jargon

First, for the uninitiated, let's briefly introduce the subject of clinical research jargon, or acronym soup. Regulatory and protocol terms are presented in the text; many more complete definitions may be found in the "Glossary and Acronym Guide" at the end of the book. *Clinical research* itself has been described as "a component of medical and health research intended to produce knowledge valuable for understanding human disease, preventing and treating illness, and promoting health."[2]

Two former leaders at the National Institutes of Health (NIH), Dr. Lawrence E. Shulman and Dr. Harold Varmus, defined clinical research more personally as "research performed by a scientist and a human subject working together, both being warm and alive."*[3]

Who's Who

As well as knowing the terms, you also need to be familiar with the major players required to conduct a research trial. The major roles and responsibilities for each member of the team are outlined below.

The *Principal Investigator* (PI), aka "top dog," is dryly defined as the person responsible for the conduct of the clinical trial at the study site, as outlined in the *Code of Federal Regulations* (21 CFR 312.60).[4] The PI's role is to

- Assume overall responsibility for the management of the study.
- Assign responsibilities for other members of the team.

---

* Dr. Shulman is the founding director of the NIH's National Institute of Arthritis and Musculoskeletal and Skin Diseases. Dr. Varmus is the former director of the NIH and corecipient of the Nobel Prize for his studies on cancer.

- Ensure that informed consent is properly obtained from the study volunteers.
- Be the liaison for major patient care issues with the sponsor and the institutional review board (IRB), an oversight committee, and ensure that the IRB is informed of all safety issues.
- Make the medical assessments, evaluating the efficacy of the study medication and whether adverse events are study related or not.
- Ensure the accuracy of the data that are submitted.

Subinvestigators receive second billing. They assume the responsibility for patient care assessments but are less likely to be saddled with the administrative responsibilities of the PI.

The *clinical research coordinator* (CRC) or *study coordinator* is the person in charge of managing the individual study site. The coordinator

- Helps assess study feasibility.
- Handles, prepares, and tracks document submission.
- Manages the day-to-day logistics of everything.

Subjects are the trial participants. I prefer the more respectful terms *patient* and *volunteer* to the clinical term *subject.* Subjects are occasionally disparagingly referred to as "guinea pigs" by the public and news media.

At the study site, the pharmacist is responsible for maintaining the drug inventory and the accountability for and accurate dispensing of the investigational medicine. The pharmacist also educates the study staff regarding administration of the investigational med.

The *sponsor* is the pharmaceutical company (drug company), or the group that holds the purse strings. This is the overall developer of the drug, which oversees the drug's growth from initial identification of the chemical entity through manufacturing and testing of the product in people. The sponsor's role is to

- Finance the study of a new medicine or device and provide management of the trial. This includes designing the trial, providing materials, collecting data, monitoring the trial, and auditing all procedures and data submitted to support the application for approval from the government.

- Keep the investigators informed of new information about the drug, with particular attention to prompt reporting of information that might adversely affect patient health or willingness to continue participating in the study.

The sponsor's team may include the following members:

- The *clinical research associate* (CRA), often referred to as the *monitor*, acts as an agent of the drug company. The primary requirement for this position appears to be an obsessive-compulsive personality. CRAs monitor how the trial is being conducted at the study sites.
- The *medical research associate* (MRA) functions like a CRA, only in-house at the sponsor's facility.
- The *medical monitor* is the physician on call for protocol questions or safety issues. Ideally, the medical monitor knows something about the investigational area in question. If not, the monitor should be willing to learn on the job.

The sponsor may hire a *contract research organization* (CRO), or middleman, to serve as a broker and administrator for the drug company if it doesn't have its own staff to handle the administrative work for the trial. Similarly, it might instead work through a *site management organization* (SMO), a euphemism for a middleman who takes a larger cut or offers, for you, a special deal. An SMO is to research what an HMO is to healthcare. An SMO provides managerial services for a number of individual study sites that form its network.

An independent *Data Safety Monitoring Board* (DSMB) may also be included on important trials. The DSMB is generally composed of experts in the field, statisticians, and others who can analyze the particular treatment under study. The board follows a trial at prearranged intervals. The DSMB can recommend changes during the conduct of the trial or rarely may stop a trial prematurely due to safety concerns.

In terms of regulatory issues, the *institutional review board* is a committee designated to review the participation of subjects in research studies. The IRB's responsibility is to oversee the regulatory, ethical, and safety aspects of a trial at the individual study site and to decide what constitutes informed consent.

In contrast, the *Food and Drug Administration* (FDA) of the U.S. government is charged with providing regulatory oversight for the pharmaceutical industry and assurances to the public for the quality and safety of all the drugs dispensed in this country.

Complex relationships exist between the sponsor and each individual study site. Each site requires the development of an infrastructure and a network to support the studies. These relationships are illustrated in figures 1.1 and 1.2. The major relationships are indicated by the heavier lines.

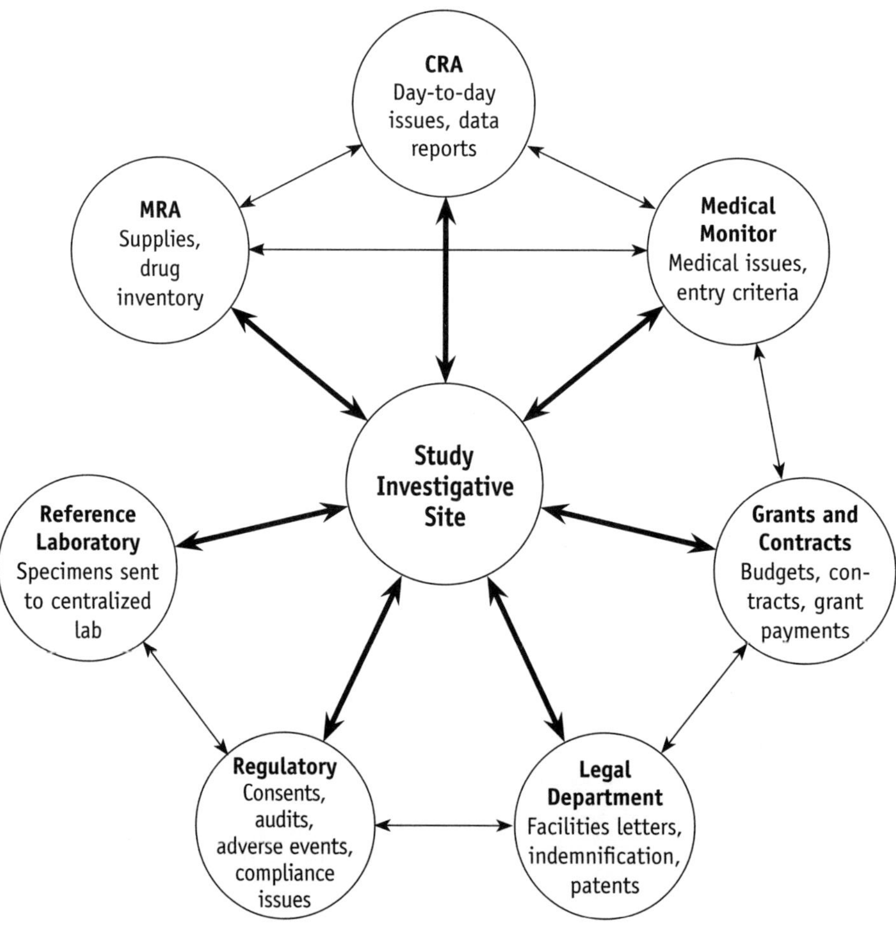

Figure 1.1 Sponsor-site relationships

Note that you will work with many departments of a sponsor company. At your own site, you will require the cooperation of a team from widely different departments to complete the study protocols successfully. This is illustrated in figure 1.2.

The Principal Investigator and study coordinator need to work well with a variety of departments to ensure a successful study.

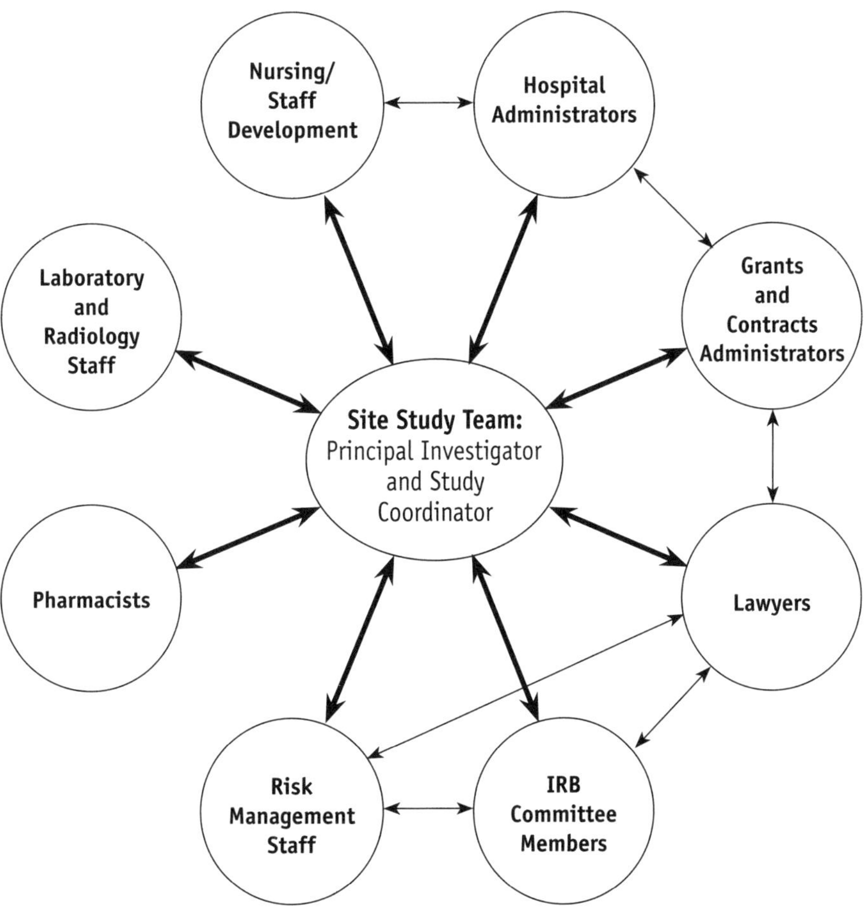

Figure 1.2 On-site relationships

Study Activities

On a clinical trial, each patient goes through different phases of participation. These periods of activity may be described as a life cycle:

1. Pretreatment (pre-Rx or prestudy drug) and screening
2. Study start-up or enrollment
3. On-treatment (on-Rx or on-study drug) procedures
4. End of therapy (EOT)
5. Long-term follow-up (LTFU)

Phases of Drug Development

To help you know what you are getting into, first it helps to know a little bit about the stages of drug (and device) development. Every drug goes through progressive testing phases. Each phase of clinical trials is under the supervision of the FDA and is conducted in accordance with international standards. Each phase is intended to capture data about the drug's efficacy and safety.[5]

The FDA is divided into several focused centers. The Center for Drug Evaluation and Research (CDER) is responsible for the safety of chemically synthesized drugs. The Center for Biologics Evaluation and Research (CBER) has corresponding responsibility for vaccines, blood and tissue products, and cellular or gene therapies. *Biologics* are biotechnology-manufactured mixtures derived from living sources (animals or microorganisms).

Similarly, the Center for Devices and Radiological Health (CDRH) oversees products such as intravenous (IV) catheters, pacemakers, implantable pumps for insulin or other medications, synthetic grafts, and breast implants. Devices are regulated a bit differently than drugs, depending on their use and the degree of safety and efficacy assurances required. For example, devices such as elastic bandages, which have little potential for harm, are understandably less regulated than pacemakers or life-support devices.

While this book refers to drug development, please note that similar development phases occur in testing biologic products, which are then subject to approval by the CBER of the FDA, and for devices, which are regulated by the CDRH.

Early Development

First is the preclinical development, the test tube or computer-based discovery phase. Then new agents are tested in animals, usually mice or rats. Next, the drugs are given to larger animals, such as dogs. These phases are intended to study a drug's action and metabolism and to evaluate the drug for obvious toxicities before it is given to people. Permission to give the drug to humans is requested from the FDA via the Investigational New Drug (IND) application. This application includes the outline for proposed clinical studies. When the IND application is filed, the drug is patented for 20 years; the clock is ticking. The drug development process is illustrated in figure 1.3 and table 1.1.

If the preclinical steps are successful, the drug company progresses to giving the new medicine to people under close observation. That's where we—clinical researchers—come in.

Phase 1

In phase 1, 20–100 healthy volunteers are given incrementally larger amounts of the study compound to test its safety, tolerability, pharmacokinetics, or PK (how long the drug lasts in the body; details about its absorption, distribution,

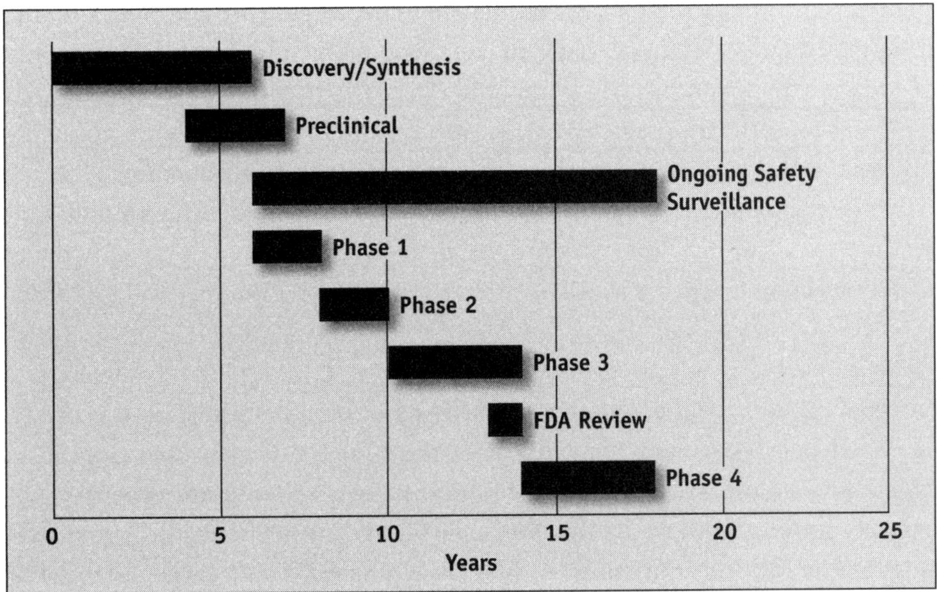

Figure 1.3 Time line of drug development

Table 1.1 Phases of drug development[6, 7]

Phase	Intent	Number of subjects studied	Duration of study	Average cost per patient
Preclinical	Test tube and animals		3–6 years	
Phase 1	Safety and pharmacokinetics	20–100	Months	$15,023
Phase 2	Efficacy and safety	Hundreds	Months to years	$21.009
Phase 3	Large scale efficacy and safety	Thousands	2–3 years	$25,494
Phase 4	After the NDA is approved by FDA	Varies	3–4 years	$13,011

metabolism, and excretion), and pharmacodynamics, or PD (details of the drug's activity).

For first-in-human trials, dosing is started at less than one-tenth of the human equivalent dose at the NOAEL (no observable adverse effect level) seen in the most sensitive species in two different animal studies.[8]

Early phase 1 and 2 studies also look at factors affecting absorption (product formulation, food, or antacid), metabolism, and excretion (for dosing for patients with liver or renal impairment). Volunteers are now required to undergo cardiac tests to look for possible life-threatening arrhythmias. Finally, drug interaction studies are done to look for possible problems, as commonly occur with the blood thinner Coumadin. Knowing how a drug is metabolized can help researchers predict whether serious interaction problems are likely and will be important in drug labeling and prescribing information.

A new early phase 1 trial is now sometimes substituted for this traditional testing. It is called a "microdosing" or phase 0 trial. (See "Costs of Clinical Trials" in chapter 7).

Phase 2

In phase 2, the drug company (sponsor) determines efficacy for the drug's intended use and tries to find the best dose for the target indication. This phase is also known as the "dose-finding" phase. Patients are generally not very ill, nor do they have many other illnesses or medications that could lead to confounding and confusing results. Early phase 2 trials can be somewhat spooky as this is the first time the untested medicine is given to sick folks. You just don't know exactly what might happen and should keep the responsibility that goes with this uncertainty firmly in mind. The investigator should watch the patient carefully and unhesitatingly drop a patient from the study if he or she is not responding to therapy as well as one would expect or if a safety issue arises.

Both phase 2 and phase 3 studies may include comparator drugs or a placebo; the latter is more likely in phase 2.

Phase 3

Phase 3 broadens the population that receives the new drug, including more real-world patients who do have other medical problems (underlying diseases). In phase 3, patients receive either the new study medication or one that is already on the market. Depending on the illness under study, one group may receive a placebo (a fake).

A common area of misunderstanding concerns the placebo arm or treatment group of a trial. Some studies may compare treatment X to a placebo (or no treatment), such as studies assessing the value of adding a vitamin or symptomatic treatment to a patient's regimen. It is important to emphasize that placebos are never given to patients who are seriously ill if an alternative therapy is available. To do so would not only be unethical; it is also illegal.

Phase 3, which focuses on gaining more safety and dosing experience, is the definitive phase before submitting a New Drug Application (NDA) to the FDA. The NDA claims the drug's effectiveness in treating a particular illness.[9]

The first effective drug for an ailment generally becomes the standard of care to which newer drugs are compared. This contributes to a marked competitiveness among companies to develop the first drug for an indication.

Phase 3 studies are often large (thousands of patients) and multicentered (conducted at multiple sites, usually covering a wide geographic area) and are considered primary efficacy studies, or pivotal trials in demonstrating a drug's efficacy. Generally, two successful phase 3 trials are required in order to obtain approval from the FDA (or similar international regulatory agency such as the European Union's EMEA). The rules are less stringent for oncology trials, where one successful efficacy trial is required.[10] Because phase 3 trials are so important to the drug's (and the company's) success, outcome and safety data are often monitored by an independent Data Safety Monitoring Board, especially if members of the sponsor's team are blinded. The DSMB may occasionally recommend changes during a trial. It can also halt the trial at any time because of safety concerns or because its analysis of outcomes shows that one treatment group is faring significantly better than the other, and therefore it would be unethical to continue the trial.

Phase 4

Marketing, rather than intellectual curiosity, drives many phase 4 trials. These trials compare the new drug, already approved by the FDA, to one that is viewed as the major competitor for the same indication. In phase 4 trials, further safety data are gathered, sometimes at the FDA's insistence or as a condition of approval of the NDA. For example, as a condition of approval for the blockbuster drug Xigris for treating early severe sepsis, Eli Lilly and Company was required to continue to study its drug, postapproval, in many thousands more patients who are less critically ill.

The drug maker tries to expand the approved uses to other indications at this time.[11] Phase 4, or postmarketing studies, can also lead to a change in a drug's status from prescription only to over the counter. And phase 4 studies may target new groups of different ages, sexes, or ethnicities.

The advantage of this type of required postmarketing study, or commitment study, is that the pharmaceutical (or biotech) company gains earlier approval than it would otherwise if the FDA delayed approval pending further safety studies. Unfortunately, not all companies follow through on their commitments and over the past several years, the FDA has been lax in follow-up and enforcement. An investigation by the Office of Inspector General explored the FDA's monitoring and noted that in 2004, a third of the required annual status reports were missing or lacked information on postmarketing study commitments. The next year, companies missed the deadline for submitting annual status reports almost half the time. Furthermore, almost two-thirds of open postmarketing studies had not even been started.[12]

This began to change with the FDA Amendments Act of 2007, which established financial penalties for companies that failed to meet the timetables for their commitments. The penalties start at $250,000 per violation and "double every 30 days up to $1,000,000/30-day period or $10 million for all violations adjudicated in a single proceeding."[13] An FDA draft guidance in 2009 proposes a "hierarchy of progressively more rigorous processes of postmarket data collection to identify and assess serious risks to health."[14] Stay tuned for further modifications.

Even after a drug is marketed, surveillance for safety continues. Occasionally, this postmarketing surveillance uncovers serious side effects that have not been previously recognized, resulting in the drug being removed from the market (as occurred with thalidomide, or, more recently with Ketek) or warnings being added.

Despite careful reviews at each level to assess efficacy and safety, trials involve relatively small numbers of volunteers in relatively controlled settings. For example, for medications for chronic conditions, the International Conference on Harmonisation guidelines the number of subjects required at approximately 1,500. Most adverse events occur within the first 6 months of exposure, so you need 300–600 patients treated for at least that length of time to detect events occurring at a frequency of 0.5-5 percent. To detect AEs with a cumulative 1-year incidence of 3 percent or less, more than 100 patients treated for more than a year are required.[15] Since most trials are shorter in duration or involve fewer patients, side effects and toxicities may go undetected and become apparent only after the drug is in wide use.[16]

In 1992, the Prescription Drug User Fee Act (PDUFA) was implemented, and the fees generated were used to hire more reviewers to speed the approval process. Despite criticism that PDUFA funding of the FDA is akin to having the fox guard the henhouse—the major concern is that safety might be sacrificed to expedite drug approval and result in more late withdrawals—PDUFA was reauthorized in late 2007. Between 1975 and 2001, 22 drugs were removed from the market after FDA approval.[17] Since then, no significant increase in drug withdrawals was noted between the pre-PDUFA and post-PDUFA reauthorization periods.[18, 19] However, the Institute of Medicine criticized PDUFA, noting that the user fees "are excessively oriented toward supporting speed of approval and insufficiently attentive to safety." The IOM recommended that specific safety-related performance goals be added to PDUFA, which was done.[20]

Safety withdrawals occur for approximately 3 percent of drugs and are not lower in the United States than in Europe, where the approvals are speedier.

Some of these withdrawn drugs, such as Redux, Seldane, Hismanal, Propulsid, Rezulin, bromfenac, and fenfluramine, were prescribed *millions* of times. According to Dr. Alastair J. J. Wood, assistant vice chancellor for research at the Vanderbilt University Medical Center, "First, a staggering 19.8

million patients (almost 10% of the United States population) were estimated to have been exposed to just 5 of the 10 drugs withdrawn in the past 10 years. Second, none of the drugs was indicated for a life-threatening condition nor, in many cases, were they the only drugs available for that indication."[21]

The FDA is in the position of being damned, on the one hand, for not subjecting drug candidates to closer scrutiny for safety and, on the other, for deaths and morbidities from delays in approval. Daniel B. Klein and Alexander Tabarrok give a fascinating review of this dilemma, concluding that far more lives are lost by the delays in new product releases than are saved by the added safety observations.[22]

More recently, several high-profile drug safety withdrawals have occurred in the past few years, including those for Baycol (cerivastatin), Vioxx (rofecoxib), and Ketek (telithromycin), the latter of which prompted a congressional investigation about the FDA's approval process. Concerns about drug safety also led to another safety study by the Institute of Medicine. Its recommendations included

- Labeling requirements and advertising limits for new medications
- Clarified authority and additional enforcement tools for the agency
- Clarification of FDA's role in gathering and communicating additional information on marketed products' risks and benefits
- Mandatory registration of clinical trial results to facilitate public access to drug safety information
- An increased role for FDA's drug safety staff
- A large boost in funding and staffing for the agency[23]

Protocol Design Part 1: Parts of a Protocol

When working on a trial, the sponsor provides every site with an identical protocol, which cannot be modified by the individual sites. (Occasionally, sponsors may reserve some funds for small, investigator-initiated studies, especially if they want to create goodwill at a particular site. More often, investigator-driven protocols are designed and conducted at academic medical centers, with funding obtained through grants. In these limited cases, the investigator must write the protocol and a grant proposal.)

For those whose appetite for detail is insatiable, I offer the following "recipe," which describes the ingredients required to prepare a protocol whether sponsored by a pharmaceutical company or a government grant.[24]

- Introduction: What is the illness you are targeting? Why do we need this drug?
- Objectives: Why bother conducting this trial? The intent of a trial may be to answer serious questions about disease processes and mechanisms of action or about the effect of interventions. As outlined earlier in "Phases of Drug Development," basic clinical research elements are most likely to be addressed in phase 1 (safety and pharmacokinetics) and phase 2 (safety and efficacy) trials. Phase 3 trials are intended to be the definitive efficacy trials. By phase 4, the objective is more likely to show that "My drug is better than your drug."
- Trial plan: How large is this trial? What type of population is targeted (e.g., diabetics, patients with a specific kind of cancer)? How many arms, or treatment groups, will the study include?
- Inclusion and exclusion criteria: What is your definition for the group of people who have the disease you want to study? This definition should clearly eliminate those groups that may confuse the outcome and hurt your chance of a successful trial. Careful diagnostic criteria are critical to successful study design.
- Study design and methodology: What exactly are you going to do with the volunteer patients, and when?

The Power of Numbers

On May 31, 2002, the Women's Health Initiative, a federal hormone replacement trial with 16,000 participants, was unexpectedly stopped when the Data Safety Monitoring Board analyzing the response of the participants found a small but significant—8 more women per 10,000 participants per year—increase in the risk of breast cancer. This was seen among the women who had received estrogen and progesterone hormone replacement therapy for more than 5 years. There were also small increases in the incidences of heart attacks, strokes, and blood clots. However, the DSMB found a similarly reduced number of colorectal cancers and hip fractures during this period.[25]

An estimated 6 million women take estrogen-progesterone either for menopausal symptoms or to prevent osteoporosis. Although they have taken these hormones for decades, this was the first study to examine the outcome of that therapy in a careful, controlled, scientific manner. The findings would not have been possible without this being a huge multicenter trial with oversight by a Data Safety Monitoring Board.[26]

- Treatment termination criteria: What end points, or outcome, will you establish for ending the study, based on both safety and efficacy? A statistician often determines the end points.
- Adverse events: How will you define and report adverse events?
- Laboratory procedures.
- Administrative section: How will you delineate the responsibilities of the site, the sponsor, the CRO, the regulatory agencies, and so on?
- Statistical plan: What is the trial's rationale in terms of mathematical justification or validation? The statistical plan also helps determine how many patients are needed (how large the trial itself must be) to show any differences in outcomes between treatment groups. (See Darryl Huff's *How to Lie with Statistics* for a good introduction to this topic.[27])
- Study personnel.
- Appendices.
- Informed consent template.

Protocol Design Part 2: Patient Mix

Having the right mix of patients is essential to the success of any protocol.

In the inclusion criteria, you need to define the illness being studied carefully to make sure that you are selecting a population that can provide the answer to the central question asked by the study.

The exclusion criteria, in addition to excluding patients who do not have the illness in question, further refine the patient pool. Exclusion criteria generally include protection for patients

- Who are allergic to the study drug.
- Who are at risk for serious adverse events due to the study drug interacting with their other medications.

Exclusion criteria also serve to protect the protocol integrity by excluding patients

- Who are too ill to demonstrate a benefit from the study drug.

- Who have other underlying diseases or need treatments that would seriously interfere with evaluation of the study drug's efficacy or safety.
- Who have received medication for the same condition without an adequate washout period, which is a period of time that a patient does not take a drug for the condition being studied. This is to ensure that all of the first drug's effects are eliminated before the patient begins the new treatment, so any changes from the newly introduced study medication can be clearly attributable to it.

Product Quality: Seals of Approval

As the elements of a protocol are being finalized by the sponsor, before implementing a study, the sponsor may turn to the FDA for assurances that its plan is sound and to improve the likelihood that a study's results will later be accepted by the agency and that the study will not have to be repeated due to a design flaw. Then the protocols are sent to each site that will be conducting the trial, as each protocol requires approval at the local level from the Principal Investigator and from a number of different departments at the sites. For example, contracts will need to be reviewed by the grants office and legal departments, particularly if the site is a large hospital or university. The nursing department and pharmacy will want to be sure that the protocol requirements won't strain their staff excessively. The departments likely to be involved are illustrated in figure 1.2.

Additionally, an approval is required for each site conducting the study by an institutional review board. The IRB is a committee that must review and approve each protocol for safety and ethical considerations and each volunteer informed consent form for clarity, accuracy, and completeness. The IRB must include at least five members of diverse backgrounds, including a layperson and someone not associated with the institution (organization). Details of IRB structure and requirements are given in the regulatory section in chapter 4.

The IRB is unlikely to be allowed to modify a pharmaceutical company's protocol as this would affect every other study site; instead, the IRB may reject a protocol's application for its own site. This is more likely to happen on investigator-initiated studies, especially if the IRB has any concern about the scientific validity of the proposal. The IRB can, however, insist on wording changes to the sponsor's volunteer informed consent agreement, as the IRB's primary responsibility is to ensure patient safety.

Protocol Design Part 3: Mixing the Ingredients

Study patients are randomly assigned, or randomized, to treatment groups in one of several ways.

In a *parallel study*, illustrated in figure 1.4, each participant is assigned to a specific treatment arm but all other study activities are the same for all participants.

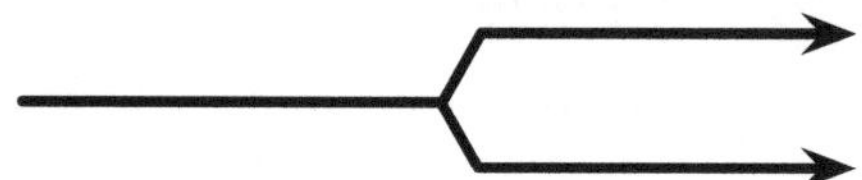

Figure 1.4 Parallel study design

A volunteer begins a study and then is assigned to one of two or more treatment options. For example, one group might receive drug A and the other drug B, and the two outcomes are compared.

The first known prospective controlled trial such as this occurred in 1747. After reviewing available evidence, James Lind randomized sailors to receive different dietary supplements. He thus established the treatment of scurvy with citrus fruit. (This was also the first trial to be criticized on a number of ethical grounds, including lack of consent.)[28]

In contrast, in a *crossover study*, shown in figure 1.5, patients receive one medication for part of the trial and then a second one for the remainder. In other words, some subjects begin on drug A and then switch to drug B; others do the opposite. In this way, each patient serves as his or her own control, or reference. Any changes seen in a given volunteer can be attributed to the study intervention rather than person-to-person variability.

"Double-dummy" protocols are also common. (This does not mean that the researchers don't know what they are doing!) The term means that in order to reduce bias, the study medications are disguised so that the subjects don't know if they are receiving drug A or drug B. In this type of study, some patients receive study drug A, with an active medication, and also a look-alike placebo for drug B. Others receive a placebo for drug A and the

Figure 1.5 Crossover study design

active medication in drug B. In each case, the volunteers receive an active drug—they just can't tell which one by its appearance.

Furthermore, studies may be blinded or not. If a study is unblinded, or *open label*, all participants know which treatment the volunteers are receiving. This is most likely to occur if there is no good comparative agent, such as in a cancer trial or *orphan drug* treatment. (An orphan drug is one that is targeted toward rare diseases and therefore has a very limited pool of potential study patients.)

In a single-blind study, the participants do not know the treatment assignment but the investigator and sponsor do. If the trial is double-blinded, then neither the investigator nor the subjects know the treatment assignments until well after the trial's completion. A code is available for emergencies, however.

A phase 3 trial usually is a double-blinded study, in which neither the volunteers nor the study personnel making the assessments are aware of which people are receiving the study drug. Blinding is illustrated in table 1.2. The pharmacist often knows who is getting which medicine but may also be blinded if the medicines are blinded, or made to look alike. Don't worry! An emergency code, explaining which treatment a particular subject received, is always available, no matter who is blinded to the study. The reason for blinding a study is to prevent the introduction of bias due to the expectations of the patient or the investigator—be it wishful thinking or an unconscious bias against some element of the study. Sometimes others involved in the trial, even those at the pharmaceutical company who are analyzing the data, are blinded, too. Only the study statistician knows the drug assignments for sure. (Though again, a code is available at all times, if needed for the patient's safety. In almost 20 years of conducting clinical trials, I have never had to break a patient's code.)

Some other types of trial designs are used on occasion, such as compassionate use trials, which provide investigational therapies to patients

Table 1.2 Protocol design: blinding

Study type	Participant	Knows treatment assigned	Doesn't know which treatment
Open label	Volunteer	x	
	Investigator	x	
Single-blind	Volunteer		x
	Investigator	x	
Double-blind	Volunteer		x
	Investigator		x
	Sponsor	x	
Triple-blind	Volunteer		x
	Investigator		x
	Sponsor analyst		x
	Data Safety Monitoring Board	x	

before FDA approval if the patients have no other options. However, the major trial types are noted above.

It is imperative that the investigator carefully review a protocol's dry sections that describe the population the drug is intended to treat as well as the clinical eligibility and evaluability criteria, as these definitions determine the success of the trial as a whole and at the investigator's site.

Medical Device Trials

The medical device industry is a major contributor to the world economy and accounts for billions of dollars in U.S. trade surplus and venture capital investing. Like drugs, medical devices have to go through a series of safety and efficacy trials prior to approval, though with some important differences. The most obvious difference is that the classification of devices is based on their intended use and risk, and this dictates which types of regulations apply.

But first, a device is defined as "an instrument, apparatus, implement, machine, contrivance, implant, in vitro reagent, or other similar or related article" that is "recognized in the official National Formulary, or the United States Pharmacopeia, or any supplement to them; intended for use in the diagnosis of disease or other conditions, or in the cure, mitigation, treatment, or prevention of disease, in man or other animals; or intended to affect the structure or any function of the body . . . and which does not achieve any of its primary intended purposes through chemical action . . . and which is not dependent upon being metabolized for the achievement of any of its primary intended purposes."[29]

What are the classes and their implications? In 1976, the Medical Device Amendments Act defined the classes according to their intended use and indication:

- Class 1 devices have minimal risk and are usually exempt from marketing applications and regulatory controls. Most of these were manufactured before 1976 and have been grandfathered in. They include items such as elastic bandages and exam gloves. Good manufacturing practice and labeling regulations apply as "general controls." Many (47 percent) medical devices fall under this category. If a new device is substantially equivalent to one that is already marketed, it can be considered exempt from a premarket notification application.[30]
- Class 2 devices (43 percent of medical devices) pose a moderate risk to the patients or users. If a new product is substantially equivalent to a device already marketed, the FDA requires a letter of premarket notification, or 510(k). Class 2 devices include EKG machines, contact lenses, conventional intravenous catheters, Foley catheters, endoscopes, and laparoscopes. Additional labeling requirements or performance standards may apply for this class.
- Class 3, or significant-risk, devices are implanted or intrusive into the body and pose a high risk of injury, or they are required to sustain life. They consequently require a premarket approval application (PMA), including, as is the case for drugs, studies and review of their safety and manufacturing processes as well as the effectiveness of the devices. Prosthetic heart valves, artificial joints, invasive monitoring devices, angioplasty catheters, and ventilators are examples of these more highly regulated devices.[31] Surprisingly, sponsors make the initial decision as to what represents "significant risk," although their decision can be challenged by the IRB or FDA.[32]

Similar to orphan drugs, a device can have a humanitarian device exemption (HDE) classification if the device will be used in fewer than 4,000 patients per year.

Many of the regulations relating to device trials—largely those pertaining to human subject protection and recordkeeping—are the same as for drugs. Regulatory requirements are outlined in the Investigational Device Exemption (IDE), 21 CFR part 812, the device equivalent of the IND application. Almost two-thirds of devices are approved on the first attempt for an IDE. Most disapprovals arise because of inadequate bench or animal safety studies.[33]

One other major difference between drug and device trials is that the latter may depend on the technical skills of the investigator, causing considerable variation between sites or requiring additional training.

Both INDs and IDEs permit the use of an investigational product to study safety and efficacy. Trials of devices that pose significant risk require clinical trials with IDE and FDA approval; those that pose a nonsignificant risk require IRB approval but not FDA approval. Just as there are requirements for serious adverse event reporting for drugs, there are requirements for devices (unanticipated adverse device effect, or UADE) with some differences in reporting times.[34]

Adverse events can lead to product recalls. A recall is problematic if the device is a critical implant, such as a defibrillator with faulty leads. Such a recall is understandably traumatic for patients as well as the manufacturer. This happened with the Sprint Fidelis defibrillator leads, which were plagued by fractures and more failures than other leads, resulting in unnecessary shocks or deaths.[35]

Unfortunately, patients have no protection against faulty devices, as the probusiness Supreme Court ruled in *Riegel v. Medtronic* that a manufacturer cannot be sued under state law if its device received marketing approval from the FDA. As a result, thousands of claims have been dismissed. In contrast, in *Wyeth v. Levine*, the Supreme Court justices did not uphold the argument of preemption, which says that federal regulations trump the states'. The court also did not dismiss Diana Levine's suit for "failure to warn" about the faulty administration of the drug Phenergan. (Levine, a musician, developed gangrene after the administration, which required amputation of her forearm.)

So, as it currently stands, device manufacturers have no incentive to be cautiously focused on safety because they are shielded from consequences. Fortunately, the Medical Device Safety Act of 2009, which would level the playing field and hold device manufacturers accountable for product defects, has been introduced in both houses of Congress. Being opposed by industry, it is languishing in committees as of May 2010.[36] Table 1.3 highlights the many differences between drug development and device development. The regulations controlling the two, on the other hand, are very similar.

As part of the Critical Path Initiative, the Medical Device Innovation Initiative was announced in May 2006 by the CDRH to expedite device development. Device trials are much shorter than drug trials, with a total development time that may be less than 18 months.[37] Similarly, the life cycle of the final product may well be less than 2 years, as new technologies lead to modifications and rapid obsolescence. This is very different than with drugs, many of which continue to be used for decades.

Table 1.3 Major differences between drug and device development[38]

Investigational drugs (CDER)	Investigational devices (CDRH)
One regulatory path (NDA)	Two regulatory paths, depending on the risk classification (510(k) vs. PMA)
FDA and IRB approval	Only IRB approval if the device has a nonsignificant risk
More than one trial demonstrating safety and efficacy	Single confirmatory trial
Placebo control	Sham control (not usual)
Randomization typical	Randomization not usual
Blinded trials typical	Blinding not usual
Form FDA 1572 agreement with investigator	Investigator agreement with sponsor
Limited influence of physician on outcome; little specific expertise required	Technical expertise required—more limited pool of investigators
Outcome dependent on interaction between drug and patient, not physician	Outcome also heavily dependent on experience of the user
Quick withdrawal possible	Withdrawal difficult, as device is often surgically implanted
	Larger influence of marketing on site selection (PI as "customer")
Slow changes in technology	Rapid development of new technologies and obsolescence of old ones
Extensive clinical trials required	Design through incremental innovation; bench testing or animal testing may be sufficient to allow approval without further clinical trials
Orphan = 200,000 patients	Orphan = 4,000 patients

The development process has been analyzed in detail by John Lindhan and Jan Pietzshe. Possible clinical needs are identified by observation, interview, or review of the FDA's MAUDE (Manufacturer and User Facility Device Experience) complaint database. The likelihood of a viable commercial product balanced by the associated risk is then assessed. The feasibility phase looks at both technical requirements and feedback from customers in an iterative loop of refinements. The FDA requires a formal design plan (21 CFR 820.30) and a risk analysis and mitigation plan (ISO [International Organization of Standardization] 14971). Refining the design and manufacturing processes occurs next, along with clinical trials for verification and validation of the device. With regulatory approval in sight, manufacturing is scaled up and plans are made for a sales launch. A major thread throughout device design is planning for obtaining reimbursement from Medicare and private insurers. After launch, continued physician training to broaden adoption, as well as postmarket surveillance to identify problems, may be needed.[39, 40]

The regulatory process for device development in Europe appears to be a bit less stringent than in the United States. Class 1 and 2 devices may not require clinical trials if safety and efficacy can be demonstrated by bench and animal testing and by data from an equivalent device. More variation in the regulatory approval process exists, as approvals are performed by any one of a number of nongovernmental "notified bodies," and a sponsor can shop for which NB to use. European device trials tend to be nonrandomized feasibility studies with less than 100 patients and are designed to demonstrate safety. In the United States, trials need to demonstrate efficacy; they are generally prospective, randomized controlled trials involving hundreds of patients.[41] As a result, new devices, for better or for worse, are often available much more quickly outside of the United States.

One other twist in device development is combination products, such as prefilled syringes, metered dose inhalers, and transdermal patches. These are a combination of a drug prepackaged in an administration device. They are more difficult to develop and pose some additional regulatory challenges, but they have promising potential to reduce the toxicity of many drugs by allowing targeted delivery, particularly important in cardiology and oncology trials. One notable success has been with Johnson & Johnson's CYPHER Sirolimus-Eluting Coronary Stent, which combined two previously approved products to reduce restenosis following coronary stenting by the localized addition of the immunosuppressant sirolimus.

Whether or not a combination product is reviewed by CDRH or CDER can have major implications, particularly as to the number and types of trials that are required. Assignment is determined by the product's "primary mode of action." For example, the drug-eluting cardiac stents had been regulated as devices, but drug-eluting disks for targeted chemotherapy are regulated as drugs.[42]

Device trials have some logistical problems that are seen less often in drug trials. For example, indemnification is a huge issue with devices, as they are often surgically implanted. The trials often require investigator training or proctoring; typically, the time for these activities is not compensated. Grants for device trials are also lower; a major institutional incentive may be the promise of appearing "state of the art." Similarly, postmarket surveillance may be required for up to 5 years; tracking patients can be quite time-consuming and costly.

Payment for the device is another stumbling block. Medicare will not pay for investigational drugs but may pay for some devices if they are considered reasonable and necessary and if all other applicable Medicare coverage requirements are met. The coverage applies to class 2 devices.[43] Just as with drug trials, private payers may not follow suit. Payment is under closer scrutiny in the current economy as devices cost $76 billion annually in the United States alone, and the profit margin for devices like defibrillators and prosthetic hips is over 20 percent. To add insult, device manufacturers have had gag clauses in their contracts with hospitals that preclude discussion of a device's price.[44]

In most developed countries, medical device registries track the failure or complication rates of products, making comparisons readily accessible. Appropriately, an increasing emphasis is being placed on comparative effectiveness trials and demonstrations of cost effectiveness in the United States, which lags far behind other countries in this arena.

Device trials may have more financial conflict-of-interest issues than drug trials because clinicians or inventors may have significant equity interests in the device and, because of their technical skills, be vital members of the initial device development team.

Informed consent may also be more problematic than on later stage drug trials because people's experience with devices is limited; far fewer patients are required for device trials. Recruitment and consent may be uniquely problematic for novel-device trials, where patients might face being randomized to be treated with an open surgical approach, conventional medical therapy, or a new minimally invasive technique. This occurred with the trials of RESPECT (percutaneous closure of patent foramen ovale in patients with a cryptogenic stroke versus anticoagulant therapy) and EVEREST II (Endovascular Valve Edge-to-Edge Repair Study done via a clip placed on the mitral valve via cardiac catheterization versus open heart surgery).[45]

In summary, devices with minimal risks require relatively little regulatory oversight and rapidly reach market. Significant-risk devices go down the PMA regulatory path, which has requirements similar to the IND hurdles for drugs, with a considerably shortened time frame and need for only one pivotal safety and efficacy trial. Because of the focus on and advances in engineering, devices are constantly being refined and have a very short life cycle.

Vaccines and Other Biologics

Another major FDA branch is CBER, or the Center for Biologics Evaluation and Research. Biologics are different from drugs in that they are derived from live tissues or organisms and therefore have an inherent risk of contamination. More complicated and more numerous steps are involved in development and production as well. With drugs, studies look at the maximal tolerated dose, and a linear dose response exists; with biologics, an optimal physiologically active dose is sought, and dosing is less predictable. Drugs may have significant cytochrome p450 enzyme interactions that affect their metabolism; biologics do not. Another notable difference is that biologics are often immunogenic (they boost an immune response), but drugs generally are not.[46] Finally, biologic products can be much more sensitive to impurities, even from seemingly minor changes in packaging.

In terms of risk, the most concerning problems to date have been due to contamination of the source tissue with a virus or a rare, unexpected, severe immune response, as in the TeGenero trial (see chapter 3).

A variety of investigational new therapies involving gene therapy, monoclonal antibodies, and stem cell therapies all come under CBER's purview. Each of these has unique development requirements.

We'll look at vaccine development to illustrate some of the differences in developing biologic therapies.

Developing a new vaccine from scratch is considerably trickier than many other types of drug development for several reasons. For one, unlike most drugs, vaccines are not inert chemicals but require growth of an organism for production. Vaccine development also requires considerable knowledge about a specific target pathogen and a good understanding of immunology, as vaccines work by stimulating the immune response to make a healthy defense. Vaccines can target either bacterial or viral pathogens or noninfectious diseases such as cancer. Public attention has been focused for years on attempts, thus far unsuccessful, on developing a vaccine to prevent AIDS. More recently, much news has shifted the public's attention to influenza vaccines, particularly against the threat of pandemic influenza. We'll focus on the HIV and influenza viruses and look at some of the differences between biologic development and drug development.

Table 1.4 shows how much slower vaccine development is than drug development.

Coincidentally, and for perspective, my own fellowship research involved attempts to produce a successful oral influenza vaccine that would work by stimulating secretory immunity. That was in 1981–1983; the initial attempt at oral immunization was conducted in the mid-1970s by J. R. McGhee and J. Mestechy.[47] We were able to stimulate secretory immunity in response to our vaccine, but almost 30 years later, no product has yet come to fruition.[48]

The same sort of time line can be seen with HIV. Just as there are much longer time lines for development of biologic agents than for development of chemical drugs, there are also some different developmental hurdles. In the preclinical phase, attention may be focused on identifying particular antigens, or proteins on the virus's surface, that might be the best target. For example, first developing clinical trials materials require prolonged efforts.

Table 1.4 Time line of H2N2 flu vaccine development[49]

1958	Flu pandemic (H2N2) results in more than 69,000 deaths.
1967	Dr. Hunein Maassab develops a live flu virus for use in a vaccine.
1976–91	NIAID sponsors clinical trials of the safety and efficacy of a live attenuated flu vaccine.
2000	The initial application is submitted to the FDA for licensure.
2003	FluMist is available for ages 5–49.
2007	FluMist is approved for ages 2–49.

You have many different choices in what part of the virus to use, what to include in the final vaccine, and how to manufacture the vaccine.[50] Do you use a live whole virus vaccine? A live attenuated (made weak, so as not to cause infection) virus (LAV) vaccine? An inactive attenuated virus (IATV) vaccine? A subunit vaccine, using an isolated bit of protein to stimulate antibody response? A recombinant DNA vaccine that doesn't require tissue culture but is grown in bacteria?[51] Such DNA vaccines are derived from plasmids, or rings of double-stranded units of DNA that replicate within a cell independently of the chromosomal DNA. They are faster and less costly to produce on a large scale. While they work for stimulating immune responses to proteins, they cannot be used for polysaccharide-based subunit vaccines.[52]

KEY POINT
Live vaccines can't be given to people with weakened immune systems, but they provide lifelong immunity.

Do you use an adjuvant (another drug that helps boost the immune response)? This has been done for years with tetanus, using alum. A bit more publicly controversial is whether preservatives such as thimerosal, which contains mercury, should be used. Because of vocal public concern as to whether the thimerosal causes autism (no, it doesn't), it is no longer used in the United States for childhood vaccinations except for influenza.[53]

How will your vaccine be administered? Vaccines can be given by injection, by oral (typhoid and cholera vaccines) pills or dissolvable wafers, nasally (FluMist), sublingually, and transdermally. Newer technologies also include improvements in packaging and reconstitution and time-temperature stability indicators. A dizzying array of delivery innovations is available for injectables, including intradermal devices and safety syringes.[54]

The development of vaccines is similar to that of drugs, but with some additional requirements, as shown below.[55]

- Phase 1 looks at safety and immunogenicity.
- Phases 2 and 3 look at safety, immunogenicity, and dose finding.
- The Biologics License Application (BLA) has two parts:
  - Product license application
  - Manufacturing plant (establishment) license
- Phase 4 continues inspections of each lot of vaccine and the plant, with more ongoing surveillance than with drugs.

Initial preclinical development is followed by preclinical animal safety studies. Then you have to demonstrate "proof of concept" (POC), the phase I was working on, and demonstrate that your vaccine is both safe and immunogenic. The next step is to validate chemistry and manufacturing controls (CMC) and good manufacturing practice (GMP) on a larger scale, including safety and consistency between lots.

Safety is a big concern, both because of the vaccine itself and because often the vaccine has been grown in live tissues, raising concerns of cross-contamination. You will have to demonstrate your product's purity and likely have to develop new laboratory assays to assess your product's efficacy. Unlike with drugs, samples of every lot of vaccine are examined prior to being released. Only three lots have been recalled in the past 10 years: "one was mislabeled, another was contaminated during production, and the third was recalled after the FDA discovered potential manufacturing problems at a production plant."[56]

Although a new flu vaccine must be developed every year due to mutations in the virus, the approach and process have been pretty well standardized. The new strain of virus is isolated, and this "seed stock" is used to grow the virus in millions of eggs. Sometimes, however, viruses grow more slowly than expected, delaying production of that season's influenza vaccine. This has been one of the problems plaguing the response to the Influenza H1N1 ("swine flu") virus.

Early efforts were troubled by contamination with other viruses carried in the cells used for culture. For example, contamination of early (pre-1963) polio vaccines led to inadvertent exposure of 10 to 30 million Americans to potentially cancer-inducing Simian virus 40. No clear link has been found yet, but the IOM and National Cancer Institute (NCI) are still looking.

Now specific and more refined cells are used, and there is better control over the process. In addition, extensive requirements have been put in place for the production facilities, including unidirectional flow of the product and segregated manufacturing areas to prevent contamination, as well as specialized air handling and biowaste systems. Still, accidents do happen, such as with Chiron, which lost 48 million doses of influenza vaccine due to bacterial contamination at one of its plants in England.[57] This was about half of the expected U.S. flu vaccine supply for that year, and the case highlighted the problems of the FDA's politicization, lack of oversight of the plant, and reliance on limited supply sources, some overseas.[58]

After the POC and quality hurdles are passed, you progress to phase 2 dose-finding and phase 3 efficacy studies, as with drugs. Efficacy studies are more problematic than regular trials because to prove efficacy, you may have to "challenge," or expose the volunteers to an infectious agent they have not yet encountered. Since this is not always ethical, you can sometimes demonstrate efficacy by clinical effectiveness (prevention of disease) or use of a surrogate end point for immune response, as was done with the Hib (Hemophilus influenza b) and hepatitis B vaccines. Animal studies of protection may be allowed under some circumstances, as for studies of more deadly infectious agents such as smallpox, anthrax, plague, botulism, tularemia, and Ebola.

Special problems are encountered in attempting to develop drugs for bioterrorism agents, where, once again, it would be unethical to do traditional phase 3 challenge studies to demonstrate efficacy. Phase 1 (safety) and phase 2 (dose-finding) trials are conducted along with measuring surrogate markers for efficacy, such as antibody responses. Challenge studies are done, however, in primates.[59]

Some vaccine trials are preventive and observational, such as the HIV vaccine trials that look at whether the vaccine candidate actually prevents infection in high-risk individuals or the Northern California Kaiser Permanente efficacy trial of the heptavalent pneumococcal conjugate vaccine, which followed 38,000 infants to see if invasive pneumococcal disease was prevented, since no accepted surrogate markers existed.

If a trial is successful, you go on to the FDA's BLA, which examines both the product and the manufacturing process. Unlike with drug trials, one good multicenter efficacy trial is generally adequate, rather than two.[60] One other obstacle in vaccine trials is that one vaccine is often administered at the same time as others, so additional studies need to be done to assess possible interactions.

In addition to FDA review, vaccines face other hurdles. The data have to go to the Advisory Committee on Immunization Practices (ACIP), which gives its recommendations to the Centers for Disease Control and Prevention (CDC). Further specialty groups also weigh in as to whom should receive the vaccine.

After licensure and the beginning of marketing, additional safety monitoring is done. As with drugs, the incidence of some side effects is too small to be detected, so a continued Vaccine Adverse Events Reporting

System (VAERS) is in place. There is also a valuable Vaccine Safety Datalink (VSD), which includes about 6 million people in six large HMOs. These large databases are critical in detecting unexpected adverse events early.[61] The most conspicuous example of these systems' effectiveness is the rapid detection of intussusception, a rare bowel blockage in infants, related to the administration of a rotavirus vaccine. With this first rotavirus vaccine, 11,000 children were tested, but the subsequent analysis showed that the incidence of vaccine-related intussusception was 1 per 10,000, so this side effect went undetected preapproval. That vaccine was promptly removed from the market. Its successor had to be tested in 60,000 children prior to approval.[62]

Vaccine development has had both successes and more publicized problems. The first success was in 1796 when Edward Jenner showed that a cowpox vaccination prevented smallpox. In 1813, the Vaccine Act was passed, regulating vaccines. In 1901, diphtheria antitoxin was made from a horse named Jim. The serum was made with no uniform controls or standards for purity and potency and it became contaminated with tetanus, resulting in the death of 13 children. This led to the 1902 Biologics Control Act (CBER's predecessor), which granted government authority to license related products and facilities. In the 1930s, administration of an early (inadequately) inactivated polio vaccine (IPV) resulted in 20,000 vaccinees' developing polio. Similarly, in the 1955 "Cutter" incident, an inadequately inactivated Salk IPV resulted in polio in 60 vaccinees and 89 family members. Occasionally other efforts went awry: the 1960s formalin inactivated measles vaccine led to atypically worse disease upon exposure to wild measles. Most publicized were the cases of Guillain-Barré Syndrome (GBS) and paralysis occurring at a rate of about 1 in 100,000 vaccinees following swine influenza vaccinations in 1976. The most recent big disappointment was in 2007, when Merck was forced to abandon its promising HIV vaccine trial due to lack of efficacy.[63]

Many vaccines have been in use for decades, are quite safe, and are very effective (see table 1.5). These include vaccines targeting childhood diseases, such as those caused by measles, mumps, and rubella viruses and some bacterial infections—tetanus, diphtheria (previously one of the most common causes of death in school-age children), pertussis (whooping cough), and bacterial meningitis.

They are so effective that in the United States, physicians rarely encounter these infections and often have to learn about them from textbooks.[64] (Having cared for two critically ill patients with tetanus and teens who died from

Table 1.5 Vaccine success[65]

Viral disease	Year of peak	Peak number of cases per year	Annual number of cases after introduction of vaccine
Hepatitis A	1971	59,606	5,683
Hepatitis B	1985	26,654	6,212
Measles	1958–1962	503,282	37
Mumps	1967	185,691	258
Polio	1951–1954	16,316	0
Rubella	1966–1968	47,745	1
Congenital rubella	1966–1968	823	1
Smallpox	1900–1904	48,164	0

preventable meningococcal infections, I can assure you that the vaccines are preferable.)

Similarly, because of the success of vaccines, most of the public has no experience with serious or life-threatening infections, particularly in previously healthy children. Understandably, many people therefore mistrust vaccines and blame autism, seizures, or similar childhood problems on vaccinations. Because of this and large vaccine injury liability claims, some manufacturers stopped production, resulting in predictable shortages. As a result, Congress passed the National Childhood Vaccine Injury Act (NCVIA) in 1986. This bill requires providers to give an information sheet to each vaccine recipient (or parent/guardian) with risk and benefit information. Providers are also required to report adverse events following vaccination to the VAERS. In addition, the National Vaccine Injury Compensation Program (NVICP) was created to compensate those injured by vaccines on a "no fault" basis.[66]

More challenges face vaccine manufacturers than those who produce drugs or devices. Some of the challenges relate to introducing new technologies.[67] Others pertain to deciding what the acceptable risk ratios are in settings where disease burdens are high (e.g., rotavirus or polio). Additional very controversial areas relate to mandatory vaccinations for school entrance (the balance of individual versus public health needs by providing herd immunity) and for military personnel (the anthrax vaccine). Many people lack the education, experience, or perspective to understand the need for

Swine Flu Vaccine Time Line

Despite a sense of urgency and a desire to vaccinate as many people as possible before students returned to school—a major mixing bowl for germs and a cesspool for transmission—in fall 2009, production of the Influenza H1N1 (aka "swine flu") vaccine was delayed. The problems of vaccine development are well-illustrated by this case.

Initial decision points:

Whom will you want to vaccinate?

What is your goal for a target date?

Do you have the infrastructure to meet this goal?

What are the public perception and political issues?

Let's look at the time line of swine flu vaccine development.

May 26, 2009: The World Health Organization recommends use of the A/California/7/2009(H1N1)v virus seed strain for developing the H1N1 vaccine and begins to distribute the seed strain to manufacturers. Annual flu vaccine production takes at least 5 to 6 months from this point.

June 4: The CDC provides the seed strain to U.S. manufacturers.

June 11: WHO declares a pandemic of Influenza H1N1.

July: Early vaccine production is occurring. A major problem is found: this year's H1N1 seed strain is growing unexpectedly poorly and slowly in eggs.

July 9: Flu Summit: Health and Human Services Secretary Kathleen Sebelius pledges $7.5 billion in preparedness funds and $350 million in direct grants to states and territories to help expedite the proposed massive vaccination campaign.

July 13: WHO provides recommendations as to prioritization for vaccination.

July 29: CDC's vaccine advisory committee meets to prioritize who should receive the vaccine.

Further decision points:

How fast can you produce enough vaccine?

How large a dose is needed (how much protein antigen is needed to stimulate immunity)?

Do you use an adjuvant, which boosts the response, enabling you to use a lower dose of flu antigen, thereby spreading out your supply? Canada elects to use vaccine without adjuvant for pregnant women; it contracts with GlaxoSmithKline for vaccine both with and without adjuvant.

Will you need one dose of vaccine or two to boost immunity adequately? Children or those not previously exposed to a particular vaccine often need two doses. Influenza H1N1 is a new virus and therefore might require two vaccine doses. But it is related to a previous H1N1 variant that circulated in 1957, so another question to ask is, can you get by with one dose in people born before 1957?[68]

Remember: you have to make all these decisions without clinical trial data or refined predictive data about the anticipated epidemic. And no matter what you decide, you will be criticized for the outcome:

- If an epidemic doesn't materialize, you are condemned for unnecessarily fear mongering and duping the public.
- If you expedite the vaccine release before extensive clinical testing, you risk more adverse reactions slipping through, as happened in 1976 with the Guillain-Barré association with immunization.
- If you wait for large-scale clinical testing (and you need large numbers to detect infrequent adverse events) and an epidemic materializes before then, you are damned for having failed to protect the public.

You also encounter conspiracy theories, for example, that the vaccine is being developed for Anglo-American genocide.[69, 70, 71]

All along, you have to juggle scientific, logistical, and political concerns, along with careful risk communication. And whatever the ultimate decision, any bad outcome will erode public trust for years to come.

August 7: Testing by the National Institute of Allergy and Infectious Diseases begins at eight university Vaccine and Treatment Evaluation Units.

August 14: Industry-sponsored clinical trials begin in Germany.

August 18: Pediatric trials begin in the United States, after no safety problems were reported in trials with adults.

September 14: Glaxo releases its initial results, which show slightly better antibody response with adjuvant.

September 15: The FDA approves the H1N1 flu vaccine. In his assessment, Eye on FDA's attorney Mark Senak said, "The FDA has done its job with H1N1 development. But Health and Human Services still has a job in front of them. That is to research the public on their intention to take the vaccine, their reasons for doing so and their reasons for not doing so, and launch a communications initiative that applies those lessons strategically."[72]

October 16: Glaxo's second trial shows that one dose yields an adequate immune response, thus enabling the supply to be stretched to be available to more people.

October 19: The first vaccine doses are shipped in Canada.

October 29: Canadian provinces have to ration the vaccine. Sole provider Glaxo has only one production line and has to stop it to produce non-adjuvant-containing vaccine, then resume regular production.[73]

October 30: WHO's Strategic Advisory Group of Experts (SAGE) on Immunization reports no unusual or increased side effects detected to date.

childhood immunizations. Interventions for healthy children is a hot-button issue anywhere and requires enormous trust. This situation is all the more difficult when there are political overtones and resistance to research or public health interventions (e.g., opposition to the polio vaccine in Nigeria). Risk communication is much more difficult and urgent with vaccines than with drugs because of both the scale of the exposure and the emotional overlay, particularly with children.

In summary, vaccine development has a long history and has been enormously successful in terms of reducing morbidity and mortality for a wide spectrum of illnesses. Vaccines can target either bacterial or viral pathogens or noninfectious diseases such as cancer. Vaccine development and testing, while analogous in many ways to the development and testing of other drugs, has its own set of rules, as vaccines are not inert chemicals but instead require growth of an organism for production. Vaccine development also requires considerable knowledge about a specific target pathogen and a good understanding of immunology, as vaccines work by stimulating the immune response to make a healthy defense.

The Evolution of U.S. Drug Law

In order to better understand how trials are conducted and why they are done in certain ways, it is helpful to place U.S. drug laws in a historical and social context. The Vaccine Act of 1813 was the first federal law addressing consumer protection and therapeutic substances.[74] Smallpox epidemics were regular occurrences in the 1700s and 1800s. Efforts were made to develop a vaccine from cowpox scabs imported from England. As the cowpox virus could not live very long in dried scabs, the virus was propagated by arm-to-arm transmission in successive person-to-person inoculations: an infected vaccination lesion on one person was scraped and used as the source of material with which to inoculate the next person. (This is no longer done because of the risk of transmitting other unwanted infections.) Often other infectious diseases were transmitted as well as the cowpox vaccine, dampening the enthusiasm for vaccination efforts. Uncontaminated vaccine was needed. Congress mandated that an adequate supply of purer cowpox be maintained and that the vaccine be supplied to any citizen. Under the Vaccine Act, Dr. James Smith, a Baltimore physician, was appointed the first vaccine agent. He propagated cowpox for 20 years via arm-to-arm transmission every 8 days.[75] Unfortunately, in 1821 Dr. Smith mistakenly sent smallpox crusts instead of cowpox vaccine to North Carolina. The inoculation of locals with live smallpox precipitated a smallpox epidemic as well as the subsequent repeal of the Vaccine Act of 1813.

The Import Drugs Act of 1848, which established customs laboratories, responded to counterfeit, contaminated, or adulterated drugs being foisted on the United States. In particular, American troops in Mexico had received counterfeit and ineffective medications for malaria.[76]

In 1905, Upton Sinclair's *The Jungle* exposed the unsanitary conditions of Chicago's meat-packing industry and precipitated legislation requiring processing inspections and forbidding interstate and foreign commerce in both impure and mislabeled food and drugs.[77] The Food and Drugs Act of 1906, which followed this exposé, was the first comprehensive U.S. drug law. While it did not require drugs to be efficacious, the law did require "that drugs meet standards of strength and purity. The burden of proof was on FDA to show that a drug's labeling was false and fraudulent before it could be taken off the market."[78]

Before 1907, drugs were bought and sold like any other goods, with no requirement to disclose the ingredients. The contents were considered a trade secret, and thus drugs became known as patent medicine.[79*]

It wasn't until 1938, after 107 deaths from "Elixir Sulfanilamide" had occurred, that the FDA was able to require "a manufacturer to prove the safety of a drug before it could be marketed."[80]

In 1947, the first international ethical guidelines for clinical research, the Nuremberg Code, were formed in response to Nazi abuses inflicted during World War II. The Nuremberg Code required that volunteers provide informed consent prior to participating in experiments and that the benefits of the research be weighed against the risks and discomforts of the subjects.[81]

Another milestone of particular interest is the Kefauver-Harris Amendment of 1962, sponsored by Senator Estes Kefauver, the Populist activist chairman of the U.S. Senate's Antitrust and Monopoly Subcommittee. The initial Kefauver bill proposed requirements for showing the safety and efficacy of drugs as well as provisions for patent sharing among companies to reduce unfair marketing practices. The initial bill was, not surprisingly, defeated. In response to the thalidomide disaster, in which thousands of babies were born with absent or flipperlike limbs after their mothers took a new sleeping pill during pregnancy, the bill was later passed, after the patent-sharing and pricing provisions were deleted. The public shock at the images of babies with such severely deformed or absent limbs led to requirements for studies of the teratogenicity and reproductive effects of drugs before they could be marketed.[82] Informed consent for patients receiving nonapproved drugs was also mandated.

About the same time as the thalidomide disaster, the Bay of Pigs invasion occurred. In that 1961 fiasco, 1,200 men were captured during a U.S.-backed invasion of Cuba. A ransom deal was worked out with Cuban president Fidel Castro whereby Cuba received $50 million worth of drugs and supplies donated by U.S. pharmaceutical companies. The companies realized significant benefits as the donations were valued as tax deductible at the wholesale price, and they also received significant political returns. Their reward for helping

---

* We may soon regress to this same process being applied to our foods, as manufacturers are opposing disclosure and labeling requirements regarding growth hormones, genetically engineered products, growing conditions (organic or not), and sterilization processes (including irradiation).

the government save face was reportedly the Drug Abuse Control Amendments of 1965, or the counterfeit drug ban bill. (Estes Kefauver had died in the interim.) The counterfeit drug ban bill made drug copyright infringement, or misbranding, a federal crime with penalties including fines and imprisonment and seizure of assets.[83]

One other particularly interesting episode in the U.S. drug law story is that of the Tylenol tampering case in 1982. Seven people in Chicago died as a result of Tylenol capsules having been adulterated with cyanide. Johnson & Johnson, the drug's manufacturer, handled the incident extraordinarily well and survived as a more-respected company due to quick actions that put public safety first. The company alerted the public not to consume any more of its product until the source of the tampering was identified and eliminated. In addition to stopping production, Johnson & Johnson recalled 31 million bottles of Tylenol capsules, valued at more than $100 million. The company was widely praised for its ethical and forthright response to this crisis. Subsequently, it led in the designing of tamperproof bottles.[84] A new law, called the "Anti-Tampering Act," passed in 1983, required tamper-resistant packaging and made tampering a crime.

The focus of the FDA has also undergone a gradual evolution. During the 1970s to 1980s, the emphasis was on efficacy and the development of processes for studies, such as randomization and blinding. As a result of high-profile drug withdrawals, safety and human subject research protection received more attention later in this period. In the 1990s, drug metabolism and special problems related to organ dysfunction gained more attention.

Safety reemerged in the early 2000s, again because of very high-profile problems: suicides with certain antidepressants, muscle and kidney damage from some statin drugs for lipid abnormalities, and excess deaths due to Aprotinin's use to reduce surgical blood loss and COX-2 inhibitors' use to treat arthritis. In 2007, the FDA Amendments Act put an emphasis on risk mitigation and pharmacovigilance—ongoing efforts for surveillance and reduction of side effects.

The current swing is toward comparative effectiveness research. Who knows what the next fad will be? I hope that it will be to focus on solving important medical problems rather than allowing more look-alike lifestyle drugs.[85]

An expanded time line of milestones is found in the "Time Line of Drug Development and Drug Law Milestones" in appendix A.[86]

Problems with Antibiotics

One of the most pressing problems in drug development is the huge void in the development of new antibiotics. The 1930s and 1940s saw the development of the first classes of antibiotics—penicillins (beta-lactams), sulfas, aminoglycosides, and chloramphenicol. In the next two decades, six more classes of antibiotics were developed, including tetracyclines, macrolides (erythromycin) and quinolones. Yet from the 1970s to the 1990s, no new classes of antibiotics were licensed—all new antibiotics were derivatives or look-alike, "me too" drugs.[87] Since 1998, the FDA has approved only 8 new antibiotics. In 2002, of the 89 new drugs approved, none were antibiotics.[88] As of 2002, while there were about 25 antibiotics in the early phases of clinical development, none of these were new classes of antibiotics, and none were broad spectrum. Out of more than 400 drugs now in development, only 5 are antibiotics.[89] It was noted at a recent workshop, "In fact, there has been only one new class of antibiotic developed in the past two decades, and resistance to it emerged before it came to market. This is alarming given the increasing accessibility of the tools and knowledge needed to develop antibiotic-resistant strains of bioterrorist agents."[90] This has been, and still is, the topic of considerable and heated discussion in infectious disease literature and at national meetings.

In an oft-cited letter, Robert Moellering and David Shlaes, two prominent infectious disease researchers,* blamed "the end of antibiotics" on changes in the FDA's statistical analysis requirements, which drastically increased the number of patients required for a trial. This new standard would be impractical and prohibitively expensive to implement.[91] Subsequently, the FDA met with members of the Pharmaceutical Research and Manufacturers of America (PhRMA) and the Infectious Diseases Society of America (IDSA). The FDA agreed not to use a rigid, specific statistical limit as a blanket requirement, and alternatives are being considered.[92]

In a most thoughtful recent paper, the Infectious Diseases Society outlines other reasons why almost all of the major pharmaceutical companies have withdrawn, either fully or substantially, from antibiotic research and

* Dr. Shlaes works in the pharmaceutical industry. Dr. Moellering is professor of medicine at Harvard Medical School and physician-in-chief and chairman of the Department of Medicine at the Beth Israel Deaconess Medical Center, Boston.

development. These companies include Aventis Pharmaceuticals, Bristol-Myers Squibb, Eli Lilly and Company, GlaxoSmithKline, Procter & Gamble, Roche, and Wyeth. The problems outlined revolve around the lack of financial incentive for the industry:

- Clinical trials for antibiotics are more expensive to conduct than are those for other drugs because efficacy has to be shown both against specific bacteria and for different sites of infection. (Antibiotics penetrate different types of tissue with differing ease, so urinary tract infections are generally easier to treat than pneumonia, for example.)
- As previously noted, drug companies are interested in developing drugs for common chronic diseases, for which use will be long term, rather than drugs that will be in use only for a short period.
- As resistance emerges, the antibacterial agent becomes less effective and therefore less profitable. Also, when there are few effective antibiotics, infectious disease experts urge restrictions on their use and hospital formularies also limit access to specific drugs. This cuts into a drug's profitability. The attempt to maximize the duration of a drug's usefulness conflicts with the pharmaceutical company's desire (and duty to its investors) to profit from the drug.[93]

Still too little effort is being made even regarding the critically urgent need for antibiotics for resistant organisms (the ESKAPE pathogens *Enterococcus faecium, Staphylococcus aureus, Klebsiella pneumoniae, Acinetobacter baumanii, Pseudomonas aeruginosa*, and *Enterobacter species*), the increasingly important cause of hospital-acquired infections. Yet the one study found that only three potentially useful antibiotics are now in phase 2 and 3 studies, with none effective against the growing number of panresistant organisms.[94]

An exciting creative solution to improve patient care was recently announced. Two companies—Bristol-Myers Squibb and Gilead Sciences—have joined together to produce a once-a-day pill for treating AIDS. When the antiretroviral cocktails were first developed in the 1990s, patients had to take a complicated and cumbersome regimen of up to 50–60 pills per day. More recently, as better drugs have been developed, the regimens have been streamlined and often begin with just 3 pills per day—but this is still difficult and discouraging for patients, many of whom also need medications for other problems. The two companies collaborated to combine their products into a single pill. They had to overcome psychological obstacles surrounding the business culture of competition, legal/antitrust issues, and the technical obstacles of formulating a stable compound.

Another striking example of the benefit of collaboration was described by Dan Weiner and Mark Hovde: "With HIV research, the introduction of CD4 and viral load as biomarkers for efficacy led to the approval of an entire class of lifesaving drugs in three years or so . . . Merck published the X-ray crystallography showing the structure of protease, allowing other companies to cut time and money from their protease-inhibitor development efforts."[95]

Such innovative cooperation between competitors has wide-ranging implications for patients, public health, and the sponsor companies. Patients win by having the convenience of fewer pills to take and lower copayments. Public health wins by reducing the likelihood that resistance to the anti-AIDS drugs will emerge by increasing the probability of patients' compliance. And the pharmaceutical companies win by producing a better product that will guarantee them increased market share and profits.[96] Similar efforts would be enormously valuable in treating other illnesses, particularly multidrug resistant (MDR) tuberculosis. Imagine if this type of collaboration were the norm. Further examples are given in chapter 9.

I raise these considerations to help you understand the arguments from both sides and learn how these issues lead to pressures on the drug industry, which then affect investigators.

Conclusion

So far, we have reviewed the stages of drug development from test tube discovery to therapy and the complexities of the multiple jobs and people that need to come together to successfully bring a drug to market.

We've looked at basic differences between development of drugs and that of vaccines and devices. Now let's continue by looking at the activities involved in carrying out a study, from landing your first study and negotiating with the drug company through recruiting and treating the volunteers to navigating the regulatory details. We'll conclude with an overview of ethical issues that may come into play.

CHAPTER 2

Scrounging Your First Study

You cannot acquire experience by making experiments.
You cannot create experience. You must undergo it.
—ALBERT CAMUS

Landing your first study is somewhat akin to finding your first job. Remember the want ads, all of which said, "inexperienced need not apply"? Yet you can't get experience because you don't have experience. Just another Catch-22.

What Do You Need to Get Started?

Before you can apply to conduct studies, here's what you will need—at a minimum:

- An MD (or similar terminal degree) who will be the responsible party, or Principal Investigator (PI): The *Code of Federal Regulations* (21 CFR 312.60) makes it clear that "an investigator is responsible for ensuring that an investigation is conducted according to the signed investigator statement, the investigational plan, and applicable regulations; for protecting the rights, safety, and welfare of subjects under the investigator's care; and for the control of drugs under investigation."[1]
- A study coordinator: This may either be an RN or your secretary, if this person is of the type formerly known as a jack-of-all-trades. In hiring such a person, remember the old adage, "Hire brains." In this case, it also helps if the person is pleasant, flexible, charming, compulsive, detail oriented, and extraordinarily well organized. Good study coordinators are rare jewels. Medical knowledge is a nice plus, but it is not at all essential as it

is more readily acquired than the rest of the desired qualities. Bank tellers or others who are detail oriented can become excellent coordinators.

- An institutional review board: This may be either local (at the individual study site) or centralized (a commercial IRB that provides services for multiple sites).
- A telephone.
- Internet access and e-mail capability.
- A fax machine (preferably with a time warp feature, as everything will have to be sent yesterday).
- Storage facilities for supplies: You might want to look for a former aircraft hangar, warehouse, or decommissioned nuclear power plant, given the volume of supplies and the need to store case report forms (CRFs) and other study records for eons. Extra locked facilities are mandatory if the investigational medications are being stored on site and for maintaining the confidentiality of patient records. If you are doing more than one study with electronic data capture (EDC), be aware that each sponsor will require the use of its own dedicated computer.
- A pharmacist, a phlebotomist, and lab, radiology, or other technical support personnel, depending on the protocol specifics.
- Money, money, money.

Your study site needs to be equipped with all of these before you can even try to conduct studies.

Starting in the research business is no different from starting any other business. You are likely to have significant start-up expenses and experience a cash flow crunch. Be aware that it will likely be months into a study before you see any useful amounts of money arrive from the sponsor or CRO.

Consider where you might borrow money. Options include credit unions, a local bank, microfinancing sources, and a winning lottery ticket. The Small Business Association (http://www.sba.gov) has a wealth of information on business plans and loans. In addition, business assistance programs are available for minority, woman, rural, and other special needs business owners.

View from the Trenches

This is how I got my first break.

After my fellowship in Morgantown, West Virginia, I moved to the middle of nowhere, the former Gateway to the West: Cumberland, Maryland. I had first encountered the town driving home from college some considerable number of years earlier, driving alone cross-country in a cheap "drive away" auto transport deal, when I had a tire blowout outside of town. It was an omen, a portentous sign to stop and settle here. After I struck out into solo practice, a mentor, the dean of the medical school where I had completed my fellowship, recommended me to his CRA, Ron Montgomery. The dean had been offered a study that he was too busy to do. Ron had to drive through Cumberland anyway to get to Morgantown, so he stopped, and over a period of months, checked out our site and me. Since we were on the route to points west, it was convenient for Ron to place the study here. It was also extremely low risk. It added no travel time for him, for example. From that initial break, the rest evolved.

With that first study, I established my reputation as a hard worker, generating good, solid data. The CRA and sponsor wanted to do repeat business, since developing our site was in their interest, and we were offered a wider range of trials.

I learned, on that study, that CRAs and medical monitors as a whole are an incredibly fickle and mobile group. They often move from company to company on a regular basis and are regularly reassigned within a company. You hope they will all take their little black books and their PDAs with them so that you can expand your horizons along with them.

What I hadn't counted on was that the first pharmaceutical company's monitors wanted to keep our site a secret from the competition. (They later described it as a veritable gold mine.) Unfortunately, they did too good a job. (Congress, or the White House, could learn a lot about avoiding leaks from these guys!)

Be sure to analyze your expenses, including employees' wages, taxes, and benefits; unemployment, workers' compensation, and liability insurance; and facility costs—rent and utilities, equipment, supplies, and shipping. Also, try to minimize your overhead. Start small and initially work with part-time or contract employees if you can so you are not locked into a crushing overhead.

Most importantly, perhaps, you need to have some insight into your strengths and weaknesses. Be willing to start out by focusing on your "specialty" and strengths; then broaden your business as you gain experience.

Navigating Site Selection: Landing Your First Study

You might consider several approaches for acquiring your first study.

Ask a Friend or Mentor

Word of mouth is your best friend, next to nepotism. Networking is extremely effective in coming by studies.

Rise Up the Food Chain: Overcoming the Catch-22

Being on the bottom of the medical staff food chain holds great risk: you might be taken advantage of either financially or in terms of receiving adequate credit for your contribution—in a sense, being devoured by the more senior staff. Traditionally, you could climb higher on the food chain in several ways. The most time-honored tradition of gaining the necessary experience is that of "medical training," a euphemism for indentured servitude. You work for slave wages under inhumane conditions to gain experience and, if you are lucky, to make some contacts.

The next link up is that of apprenticeship. I have trained colleagues in doing trials, largely out of friendship and collegiality, so they could see what they were getting into without having to make a large commitment. The hope was also that we would then help one another on future multisite trials and be able to provide backup coverage for each other. This arrangement has produced mixed results. A new investigator should consider proposing this kind of pact to a more senior physician in order to gain experience and access. The offer may well be accepted as extra help and, perhaps, regarded as an investment in the future, especially if the new person does not pose a significant financial threat (that is, if the new person is working in a different subspecialty or if the alpha male is nearing retirement). The downside of such an arrangement for the senior investigator is described by the old adage, "Give me a medical student who only triples my work, and I'll kiss his feet!"[2]

With luck and hard work, you can attain the status of subinvestigator. While these achievements may be small and incremental, they are useful for listing on your curriculum vitae and are a passport to greater opportunities.

One unfortunate change in the industry is that CRAs have lost much of their clout in placing studies. This change in strategy is not one of the smarter decisions made by the sponsors. CRAs know their territories well, have the leisure (relatively speaking) to check out potential new sites, and know their investigators' abilities. They are excellent judges of where to place a trial. Now decisions are largely made in-house, by a centralized team distanced from the action and therefore unaware of site nuances or the unique personalities of sites and investigators. This is an unfortunate development for all.

Network

Informal networks are also quite an effective way to get studies. Ask colleagues at medical and investigator's meetings, for example, to ask their CRAs if any additional sites are needed for a current study. When you are later offered a different study, you can return the favor. Or you might be able to suggest far distant sites, with friends or colleagues that you have known for years. Reputation, networking, and the personal touch have, over the years, continued to prove the most constant and reliable source of studies.

Try CROs or SMOs

Some drug manufacturers not only design their studies but conduct them as well, having their own in-house management team and CRAs. Others farm the work out, subcontracting with other businesses to identify study sites, recruit patients, and perhaps manage the lab work or advertising while remaining as the general contractor on their (drug) building project. For example, the major subcontractors on clinical research trials are contract research organizations. These companies are agents for the sponsor, hired to find appropriate sites and to conduct the studies for the sponsor. CROs work for many different drug companies. (Site management organizations are similar but much less common. They work by marketing groups of sites to a drug company and by providing the management services to oversee a study for the sponsor.) The advantage of working with a CRO is that you are then entered into the organization's database, which is used for offering services to multiple drug companies. In the future, when the CRO needs a site for a specific type of study, it is likely to approach you again.

Newer Methods for Landing a Study

The techniques described above for attracting studies all evolved in simpler days. Other options for selling your site are now available and expedient, but they are neither as personal nor as gratifying. The primary route in vogue is registering with an on-line broker, as discussed below.

Medical sales representatives, or "drug reps," will be detailing you as a physician to sell their wares. Tell them that you have just completed a trial in a particular indication or that you are interested in a specific research area, and ask if they will suggest your site to their company's clinical development department. It's worth a try, but this is not a particularly effective route. (This method perhaps works better if the drug you recently tested was from one of their major corporate competitors.) In addition, investigators can occasionally attract studies by advertising, either in journals or by "hustling" at medical conference booths, but this approach also appears to be a less-effective route.

You should also do your own research, reading and studying industry forecasts for your area of interest. You can learn about ongoing and upcoming studies by exploring ClinicalTrials.gov and then contacting the pharmaceutical sponsor of interest. Conferences that are specialty or disease specific and abstracts of early research findings can provide important leads. Company Web sites and some commercial sites, such as those of CenterWatch, the Association of Clinical Research Professionals (ACRP), and the Drug Information Association (DIA) can give you important leads.

My favorite pharma news sources are Pharmalot's Ed Silverman (http://www.pharmalot.com), who can now also be found posting on the In Vivo

View from the Trenches

Life in the Wilderness

Although living in the relative wilds of western Maryland has its charms—such as the bear visiting me in my garden paradise while I was writing this book—it can feel rather isolated at times. Fortunately, with the Internet, you can research most topics from anywhere. My favorite pharma news sources on my Google Reader feed are Pharmalot's Ed Silverman (http://www.pharmalot.com), Mark Senak's Eye on FDA (http://www.eyeonfda.com), and Wired's Med-Tech (http://feeds.wired.com/wired/medtech). It's also really easy to set up Google News Alerts for almost any topic you might imagine—including investigational trials for whatever condition might interest you.

Other handy sites include Clinpage (http://www.clinpage.com), FDA News (http://www.fdanews.com), DIA Daily (http://www.dia.custombriefings.com), FiercePharma (http://www.fiercepharma.com), Contract Pharma (http://www.contractpharma.com), and Outsourcing Pharma (http://www.outsourcing-pharma.com).

Blog (http://invivoblog.blogspot.com), Mark Senak's Eye on FDA (http://www.eyeonfda.com/), and Wired's Med-Tech (http://feeds.wired.com/wired/medtech). It's also really easy to set up Google News Alerts for almost any topic you might imagine—including investigational trials for whatever condition might interest you.

Register with an On-Line Site-Listing Service

Increasingly, investigators with study sites to offer have successfully turned to on-line site-listing services, such as CenterWatch, Research Investigator's Source, Inclinix, or Site Management Solutions, where they can list their experience and areas of research interest. This information becomes part of a database, which can then be searched by the drug company sponsoring an upcoming trial. The use of a database is somewhat limiting, however, as the format does not allow for any description of unique attributes or qualifications of the site. But this format may still be useful for attracting initial attention to a well-trained investigator with little experience. (I particularly liked the now-defunct Clinmark, because I could readily see who had accessed my listing.) The downside of registering with a commercial database is that the listers are often required to pay several hundred dollars. While this cost can be recouped, it is expensive for the beginning investigator and seems akin to a dowry offering.

Register with an On-Line Broker

You might also consider listing your research site with a study broker, especially if you are new to trials. A study broker is a middleman who connects sites and sponsors—for a fee. Unfortunately—and to my mind, unfairly—the fee comes from the investigator rather than the more well-to-do sponsor or CRO. Part of the broker's business is keeping up with the constant personnel changes in the industry; part is monitoring drug development and becoming aware of new opportunities. Investigators can do this themselves, at less expense, through their own industry research or through subscription services such as TrialWatch, but it is considerably more time-consuming than relying on a broker.

So the broker plays matchmaker, introducing the sponsor and investigator. If those two parties agree, the investigative site pays the broker a fee, typically 10 to 20 percent of the grant. If all parties are happy, they will repeat the process in the future.

Unlike a site management organization, a broker is generally not involved with the logistics of the pretrial activities—the budget and contract negotiations and the regulatory hoops. The site and sponsor handle these details directly. But the broker might, on occasion, serve as a sort of marriage counselor, helping the two sides work out differences in expectations.

A significant advantage of using a broker is having the opportunity to learn about more studies so you can fill unexpected gaps in your workflow. In theory, if all goes well with the arranged trial, you may have future opportunities to contract directly with the sponsor, without the middleman. However, lapses in institutional memory mean that the sponsor may not remember your good work and, in the worst case, you would have to work through a broker again. But, as Joe Bollert, president of Investigator Location Services, notes, "90% of something is better than 100% of nothing."[3]

Be a Coauthor

Being listed on a publication is an elusive but useful goal and something worth negotiating for in a contract. For example, if you are listed in the fine print on a publication about a pneumonia trial, another sponsor might follow this lead and call you, looking to place a different pneumonia trial. Most sponsors will not agree to list you on a publication as coauthor, but some will, stipulating that coauthorship will be based on enrollment. Only the top two to three PIs will win this valuable prize; this is another incentive for the PI to work hard on the study. Get it in writing! Don't rely on an oral commitment. In one case, although one investigator was far and away the leading enroller, that investigator was not part of the sponsor's long-term strategy or marketing plan, which relied on name recognition of investigators on publications and presentations. Therefore, the sponsor did not want the investigator to be the coauthor and did not list that person on the study. This disillusioning experience was one of the investigator's more embittering lessons. Remember—get everything in writing.

When a New Drug Application receives approval, the list of investigators working on the protocol becomes public information that is then occasionally mined by other drug companies. But it takes years after a trial has begun before the NDA is approved—if it ever is approved—so you shouldn't count on this route to recognition.

Why It's So Difficult to Get Studies

Several factors contribute to the difficulty some investigators may have attracting studies even when they have been previously successful. Twenty years ago, site-sponsor relationships seemed more friendly and cooperative. Since then, as pharmaceutical companies have swallowed each other up, many internal processes have become centralized in an organizational attempt to become more lean and mean. As the companies became more enamored of the bottom line, they further consolidated. This centralization results in the sponsors becoming increasingly distanced from the study sites, and the personal touch has become less important. As Ron Montgomery, an experienced former CRA and consultant, aptly observes, "Developing long-term relationships has become secondary to getting the job done for the least amount of money and grief. They talk about developing relationships but in fact do the hard line, confrontational, 'business-like' thing more often. Time is money, and 'what have you done for me today?' applies."[4]

Also, there is now a more rapid turnover of company personnel and less loyalty to and from a company. This turnover of staff contributes to the lack of "institutional memory" that may plague the attempts of an investigator to attract further studies. This holds true even when an investigator has performed well, if the product has not. In that case, the product may be abandoned and the sponsor's team scattered to work on other drugs in development. The sponsor's team may not associate your site with the ability to study other indications successfully. Surprisingly, many pharmaceutical companies reportedly do not maintain their own databases regarding their investigative sites.[5]

KEY POINT
Having a large patient pool and rapid turnaround time for IRB and administrative details will win you studies.

Unfortunately, sponsors and CROs are also increasingly using databases to weed out sites, not just to identify potential fertile new ground. Sponsors are increasingly removing the human element and instead relying on healthcare data to determine site selection and help with patient recruitment.

Data Mining

Using electronic healthcare claims data, one company claims to have "de-identified medical and prescription claims records for over 220 million U.S. patients. This longitudinal data, dating back to 1991, is comprehensive, precise, and updated in real time as healthcare claims are submitted nationwide from 355,000 physicians, 1,500 hospitals, and over 25,000 pharmacies." So 220 million patients are linked "to their individual diseases and drug histories over the past 10 years" and these data are available to sponsors and CROs to identify potential sites and patients for specific studies.[6] For example, in oncology consortiums using electronic medical records, patients with a specific stage of a specific tumor can be readily identified, along with details about their geographic location, attending physician, and prior healthcare utilization.[7]

The level of commercially available detail about potential patients is astonishing to me. Most surprisingly, the company mentioned above claims that "methodologies and data sources are fully compliant with the federal regulations of the Health Insurance Portability and Accountability Act."[8] Yet ironically, individual sites and small centers are unable to successfully identify potential subjects because of the stranglehold HIPAA has at the local level.

Opportunities Do Exist

Rather than using experienced CRAs in the field, site selection is increasingly conducted by a rigid set of yes/no criteria with little allowance for uniqueness. Also, experience and enthusiasm are not the high priorities they once were. Rapid turnaround time and a large population base seem paramount. Name recognition also ranks higher than many other attributes. Switching from a personal assessment to rigid binary computer-based screening seems shortsighted, but it correlates with the increasingly frenetic pace at which sponsors want everything to be done.

Despite this shift in how companies place studies, an interested physician can attract studies successfully. As noted in chapter 7, there is an increasing need for Principal Investigators. In 1995, almost 12,000 doctors were listed as PIs for the first time on Form FDA 1572, the "Statement of Investigator," by which they agree to abide by the federal regulations for use of investigational drugs.[9] This number rose to 26,000 investigators globally in 2007, but only about 14,000 of them were in the United States.[10] While the absolute number of investigators has not decreased, the number of new investigators is not keeping up with the pace of new trials (1.7 trials per investigator in 1985 versus 3.3 in 2005).[11] More and more of these physicians are office-based rather than academic. Furthermore, 52 percent of investigators conduct only one clinical trial; only 14 percent conducted more than four trials between

1988 and 1997, suggesting that success begets further success.[12] Some investigators have nearly given up their regular patient practice and are focusing almost entirely on conducting clinical trials. This business-oriented approach has shifted the norm of conducting 2 to 4 trials at a site at a given time to conducting 13 to 14 at a relatively new type of site: a "study mill."[13] The turnover among investigators is rather high, so good opportunities are available for entering the field of clinical trials. Being experienced in the indication and having performed well for a sponsor are likely to get you further studies.

Site Selection: Be Careful What You Wish for—You Might Get It

In a recent article, Hassan Movahhed, then senior clinical director at Amgen, noted that "one-third of the doctors who sign up for its trials each year never return, a huge loss in institutional knowledge and money."[14] This is quite intriguing. Others note that 54 percent of new investigators are never used again.[15] Given this finding, it's even more surprising that the drug companies haven't been more creative and innovative in identifying study sites. One would think that sponsors would turn to doctors and sites that not only enjoy doing studies but also do them responsibly and competently. The drug companies should cultivate that type of site to run a variety of

View from the Trenches

In a sense, my specialty becomes almost irrelevant to my ability to conduct many types of trials. I like being the Principal Investigator on trials, especially working on new types of therapy. *I know how to conduct trials well at my site.* I have the capability of networking with other doctors in other specialties and gaining access to their patients and their knowledge of their specialty. Much of the specific pathophysiology, or medicine, I can learn (and demonstrate competence in, if need be), just as I have to learn new things every day as part of my regular patient care practice. The ability to conduct clinical studies should be regarded as a specialty of sorts, in and of itself.

I saw an interesting model of this some years ago at a study site I visited to better learn the ropes. In this particular case, an RN study coordinator ran the site within a large multispecialty practice. She conducted all aspects of the trials except for the medical assessments that required a physician, whom she hired as a subcontractor and trained.

studies. This would be far more efficient for both the sponsor and the site personnel. Learning each other's quirks and idiosyncrasies eliminates a lot of inefficiency and waste. However, the FDA would also have to be willing to try this model, since one of the current triggers for an FDA audit is, in fact, a PI conducting a trial outside of his or her area of expertise.

The extraordinarily wasteful and rapid turnover of sites appears to be caused by several factors at work. Some site teams may not be able to complete a project as readily as they envision. A rule of thumb is that one-third of centers (sites) will recruit no patients, one-third will recruit 20 percent of all patients enrolled in a study, and one-third will account for 80 percent of the enrollment.[16] A more recent Harvard Business School study confirmed this adage, noting that 30 percent of sites failed to make a significant contribution to subject recruitment, and 70 percent of PIs perform only one trial with a sponsor.[17] Often, the key opinion leaders (famous doctors in a field who can mold opinion) do not contribute any significant portion of the enrollment—they provide the experience and prestige instead of the patients.

Another factor is money. The opening and closing of nonproductive sites now costs more than $30,000. This amount includes personnel costs and travel to the site for qualification, training, and initiation visits. Delays in enrollment or completion of a study result in an additional $40,000 per day in direct sponsor costs.[18] Sponsors are thus not likely to reinvest in a poorly performing site. On the other hand, even if you have worked with the sponsors or CROs before, they are likely to duplicate site visits because little communication exists between the different teams of monitors. (We recently had two qualification visits from the same CRO during one week, despite my suggestion that they combine forces!)

Some investigators probably have misjudged the amount of work and aggravation involved, the initial capital needed, the amount of lag time before they receive payment, and the cost of conducting trials. Dr. Harold Glass, founder of DataEdge and professor of pharmaceutical business at the University of the Sciences in Philadelphia, has analyzed this problem further. He concludes that a site must have about four or five studies running to be profitable, both in financial terms and in terms of the effort required to build a solid infrastructure.[19] Experience has shown that a small practice can do well with only two to three studies running at one time, depending on the type of protocol.

Site Selection: Why a Site Is Chosen, or a Marriage of Convenience

Once a sponsor has shown a nibble of interest, other attributes are factored into the question of placing a study at a particular site. One is the geographic convenience of the site for the sponsor or CRA. It is expensive for the sponsor to place a study in an obscure place. A convenient location is a good selling point and would undoubtedly help in your initial success. (Being charming, as well as exuding competence when a sponsor's CRA visits your site, can then clinch the deal.)

Being able to make a convenient driving loop of small sites made placing studies at my site attractive to several CRAs and sponsors, as it met their needs for efficiency and reduced wear and tear on the monitor (CRA).

Being available for the site qualification visit is crucial in landing a study as well as in establishing your image and reputation. Be prepared. Read the protocol and make notes on things you don't understand. Ask about inclusion and exclusion criteria that appear to be problems based either on your previous experience with studies or on your knowledge of your patient population. Have the protocol and your list of questions ready. Do your homework. Show your interest, and ask questions! A surprising number of CRAs and medical monitors express amazement that an investigator has

View from the Trenches

I have always regarded CRAs as my guests and tried, from the initial phone contact, to make them comfortable and meet their needs with a personal touch. I know they are tired of traveling and of being in cookie-cutter motel rooms in towns that may appear interchangeable. Make your site a pleasant interlude for them. I advise them about the best route from wherever they are coming from and direct them to scenic locations, pit stops, and good places to rest and eat en route. I try to match their interests and budgets with distinctive places to stay here in town. Occasionally, CRAs will mention hobbies or personal interests, which I will then try to follow up on as their host and tour guide. Our town is quiet, to put it mildly. A traffic jam is three cars ahead of you at the stoplight. But that slow pace and the beautiful scenery is a welcome break for many CRAs who are otherwise quite stressed from their frenzied, pressured job and urban travel adventures.

It never ceases to amaze me when CRAs express astonishment that a PI will meet with them at all, let alone try to be friendly and helpful. It just comes down to regarding them as people, with unique personalities and needs, and trying to be a hospitable host. I guess my mom instilled that in me.

actually read the protocol and paid attention to some of the finer details. How could it be otherwise? A deliberative approach is not only the rational way to approach protocols but shows a business suitor that although you may be inexperienced, you are thinking, credible, and compulsive.

If your mind is engaged, you can always learn. Curiosity is the first step; attentiveness is the second. If you have no interest in the protocol, you will transmit your attitude to the CRA, who will then not bother to place the study with you. An old adage, shared with me as I set out from training into the real world, advises that the keys to success as a consultant are "availability, affability, and ability," unfortunately, in that order. The same is true in relationships between a site and a sponsor.

Site Qualification Survey—Recording Your Experience

Before committing considerable time and resources to your site, the sponsor or CRO will do an initial assessment of your capabilities by sending you a site qualification survey. The sponsor doesn't always require previous research experience. It wants to know whether you have the types of patients the study requires and if you have a large enough patient pool.

After your first study, to make acquiring subsequent studies easier, it is extraordinarily useful to develop your own outcome data. Tracking your own experience helps demonstrate your credibility as a serious researcher. It also helps you assess study feasibility and budgeting for future protocols.

One reliable way to sell a study site is to develop a research experience summary or site profile. Make your profile look professional, and highlight the unique strengths of your site, be they special facilities, background, training, or certifications. Emphasize your experience, especially if you exceeded any goals. Some suggest developing a marketing package including a one-page cover letter with your logo, the name of the person you have in common with the recipient (or who is introducing you), references, standardized curriculum vitae for your site's personnel, and your outcome data.[20] Your research experience summary or site profile should include the following items:

- Indication (e.g., sepsis, community acquired pneumonia [CAP], or intra-abdominal infection) and type of drug (e.g., monoclonal antibody or antibiotic).

- Screening-to-enrollment ratio, or the number of patients screened for acceptance in the study compared to the number of patients who are then enrolled in the study.
- Number of patients agreed to in the study contract.
- Number of patients actually enrolled per unit time (e.g., one to two patients enrolled per month).
- Evaluability, or the percentage of patients who meet all the inclusion and exclusion criteria and complete all the protocol requirements. If the patients are nonevaluable, they won't be able to support the study drug's claims. If your site has a high percentage of evaluable patients, even if only a small number of patients, then it is a valuable and cost-effective site for the sponsor. If you enroll many patients who are not evaluable, the data are not useful and your site may be viewed as inefficient and unnecessarily costly.

This summary will also be quite helpful to you in answering the next sponsor's site qualification (also called site feasibility) survey. This survey doesn't always require previous research experience. The sponsor wants to know whether you have the types of patients the study requires and if you have a large enough patient pool. It is important that you try to answer the survey accurately. While this form can be a nuisance to complete, doing so will likely gain you entrée to the next stage, the first site visit. (For a sample "Research Experience Summary" and a sample "Site Qualification Survey," visit http://conductingclinicalresearch.com.)

Site Qualification Visit, or "Shall We Dance?"

The site qualification visit is somewhat akin to meeting a blind date. At the beginning, it is a ritual courtship. Monitors will be checking you out. They will review the protocol to assess your interest, level of understanding, and capability, as well as the overall experience of your team. Similarly, they will assess and review your understanding of regulatory requirements and good clinical practices (GCPs). The monitors will also view the general neatness and ambience of your office as a microcosm representing other aspects of your practice.

Monitors will check whether you have adequate staff to conduct the study and whether you are running competing studies. They will tour the site to evaluate your facilities, such as the lab, radiology, and pharmacy. In particular, they will focus on the security and storage conditions for the investigational med, as well as the pharmacy's capability for managing drug accountability. Often, they will want to meet other members of the study team, such as the lab manager, microbiologist, and study pharmacist, again to assess their level of commitment, enthusiasm, and experience.

The CRA will also be quite interested in seeing what, if any, space you have for him or her during a monitoring visit. It needn't be fancy, but comfortable surroundings are definitely a plus. Monitors, too, like creature comforts—a small but clearly designated workspace, such as a study or dictation carrel, and access to a photocopier, a fax machine, a telephone, coffee, and a bathroom. Many monitors claim to be oblivious to light, so a small niche in the dark recesses of the medical records department or a converted closet will do if need be. On the other hand, an attractive setting (such as our rural site with views of beautiful mountains and almost no traffic or crime) can be an added enticement that may serve to mitigate other inconveniences.

Monitors will assess what kind of patient population you have and whether patients are likely to be compliant. They will ask from where you draw your patient base, how many patients you have with the health problem of interest, and how you have derived your estimates. You might have gathered this information from a computer search of your own or the hospital's medical records, or from data showing your previous enrollment on a protocol for a similar indication. The monitor will review protocol requirements and assess recruitment strategies for your target population, again with an emphasis on compliance with GCP. Protocol requirements will be detailed.

The CRA will request a CV, the equivalent of a pedigree, and licenses for all involved. He or she will also review required regulatory documentation, such as Form FDA 1572. (For a sample "Site Qualification Visit Agenda," visit http://conductingclinicalresearch.com.)

Try to get to know the visitor to sense whether you are an appropriate match so that there will be less chance of "morning-after" regrets for either party. You might guide the CRA or suitor around your hospital personally, rather than delegating the tour to your staff. The time invested here presents a good opportunity for assessing the CRA and the sponsor company's projected persona, as well as serving as an opportunity for bonding and for selling your site.

What the CRA or Sponsor Will Be Looking for at Your Site

To help you prepare for your initial site visit, here is a list of the types of information the CRA or sponsor will be looking for:

- Evidence that the right patient population exists.
- Pedigree of the investigator and staff (aka credentials).
- IRB turnaround time or the ability to use a central IRB.
- Turnaround time for grants and contract negotiation.
- From where (and how) patients are likely to come: sources may include the investigator's practice, other referrals, advertising, or other sources.
- Ongoing conflicting or competing studies.
- Experience level of the PI and the coordinator.
- Attitude: You need to convince the CRA that you really are enthusiastic and committed to doing the study. Otherwise, why should the sponsor bother with your site, since you are unlikely to meet your commitment toward the enrollment goal? Remember, it costs the pharmaceutical company a great deal of money to set up and monitor a site.
- Willingness to follow GCP guidelines and the sponsor's SOPs (standard operating procedures).
- Contracts and facility letter requirements: who must approve this study?
- Office organization.
- Facilities (e.g., lab and x-ray facilities).
- Ability to use a central reference lab and handle "send-outs," or specimens that need to be shipped to a central reference laboratory, and whether your facility will allow this. Occasionally, hospitals might insist that specimens also be run in duplicate (i.e., one run at the hospital as well as a second sample sent to the reference lab).
- General atmosphere.

- Creature comforts for the CRA: Is there a workspace available? Access to medical records? Necessary equipment and accommodations?

The adage that the keys to success as a physician are availability, affability, and, lastly, ability has been modified for investigators as follows:

Recipe for Site Qualification Visit Success

2 cups availability

2 cups affability

1 cup ability

3 cups enthusiasm

2 cups obsessive-compulsiveness and attentiveness to detail

Flavor with appropriate amounts of essence of organization, ambience, and other auras, as desired. Top with a large dose of being genuinely nice and a personal touch.

We've focused a lot on how you can prepare for qualification visits and try to attract studies to your site. You should also ask yourself how comfortable you will be working with the sponsor and the CRO or sponsor staff that you have met. Consider what information you might still need to decide whether you want to work with them. Are they a good fit stylistically, or have warning signs been raised by their attitude or manners? Do they appear to be responsible and ethical in their approach to the study question and design? And, most importantly, do you want to work on this problem, and with these people, for the next year or more?

Do Size and Setting Matter?

A decade ago, most clinical trials were conducted at universities. By 2000, the academic centers' share had declined from 75 percent to less than 40 percent.[21] From 1994 to 2009, the market share of independent, community-based research sites increased from 37 percent to 76 percent.[22] While many would decry the shift from academic to clinical practice settings, this concern is largely unwarranted. The shift reflects the reality of patient care and presents a more real-world view of future experience with the drug under study.[23] Many university patients are indigent, with multiple medical problems that have often been neglected for years. This population tends to have more problems with compliance and loss to follow-up, that is, patients fail to return and cannot be reached by telephone or mail. Some of this is related to lower levels of education among these patients and some to inadequate social support. Certainly, huge cultural barriers have reduced trust and compliance in many settings, particularly in cities. Patients drawn from your practice or referred by colleagues are more likely to be compliant and to complete a study than are patients with whom you have no underlying stable relationship. I strongly believe that the type of patient seen in many community practices provides a more accurate portrayal of future drug use and experience than do inner city populations.

Community clinicians are often disparaged by academicians as "LMDs" (local medical doctors). But the quality of trial data is in large part determined by the quality of the protocol and is independent of the site where the patients are accrued. Prominent academicians are often too far removed from actual patient care. Keep in mind, too, that for most phase 3 protocols, a typical rate of expected patient accrual might be one or two patients per month. It makes sense for the sponsors to maintain wide networks of sites, similar to the way idle computer power is harnessed through decentralized Internet webs. So the two types of settings—academic centers and community-based practices—may well serve to complement each other.

KEY POINT
The main ingredients for scrounging a study are the leading characters at the site, the PI and the coordinator. Remember—a good coordinator is a rare find. Treasure him or her.

Enthusiastically promoting your site, especially if you are new or rural, is critical to landing a study. When selling a small site in competition with a name brand university, you can outline the advantages of being small and rural as follows:

- Community and private practice advantages:
  - Probably greater accessibility and convenience for patients, factors that encourage treatment compliance, study retention, and follow-up.
  - Small-town, down-home, personal atmosphere.
  - Personal treatment, attention, and even pampering for both the study participants and the visiting CRAs.
  - Consistency of evaluations due to fewer people making assessments.
  - Compliant patients, known to the individual investigator and rarely lost to follow-up. This is a significant advantage and should be emphasized.

VIEW FROM THE TRENCHES

I offer an unparalleled consistency because, with rare exceptions, I do all the study visits myself. (These are visits required by the protocol, where specific protocol-related examinations and testing are done.) The house staff does not change from day to day; one individual can more readily notice and assess subtle changes in patients.

If investigators draw patients from their own practices, they can be good judges of the patients' likely compliance and retention in the study. Also, investigators are trusted and respected by their patients and can thus further influence patients' compliance.

- Think of your own site's advantages or unique attributes and add them to this list.

- Major university's advantages:
  - Name recognition.
  - Aura of academia.
  - Larger pool of available subjects.
  - Generally more convenient and readily accessible for monitoring.
- Community and private practice site disadvantages:
  - Lack of panache.
  - Smaller pool of available volunteers.
  - Possibly greater inconvenience and expense for the sponsor to conduct site visits.
- Major university's disadvantages:
  - Cumbersome bureaucratic administration.
  - Poor maneuverability and responsiveness. The university may have a slower response to change due to its larger size and numerous layers of people to deal with (e.g., a large, lumbering elephant versus a speedy, agile mouse).
  - Slow IRB and legal reviews.
  - High fixed costs.
  - Attitude of entitlement.
  - Disdain for clinical research as opposed to pure bench work in "real," or basic, science.

- Cost of conducting a clinical trial approximately 10 percent higher than at unaffiliated sites.[24]

Private study sites have greater flexibility and maneuverability because fewer people and fewer administrative levels are involved. Interest and enthusiasm about the study is higher: "We're doing the study because we want to, not in obedience to a decree from above." Overhead is lower, a major advantage. Start-up time is shorter because fewer people and fewer levels of bureaucracy generally mean more rapid approval of contracts, protocols, and similar details.

So a persuasive argument can be made to the CROs or sponsors for placing studies in smaller, more rural settings. While this decision might add some initial inconvenience, the sponsors may well get a better return on their investment in rural sites than they would in sites in the bigger cities.[25] Trial organizers can draw from a larger and potentially more diverse group of patients if they are placed over a broader network of communities.

Conclusion

In summary, word of mouth and networking are the most reliable, successful, and pleasant routes for landing your first study. When you have acquired your first study, establish your reputation for providing quality work. The old-fashioned, simple ways of hard work and excellence are still the best.

CHAPTER 3

Reality Testing: Feasibility, Budgets, and Contracts

Every discovery of what is false
leads us to seek earnestly after what is true,
and every fresh experience points out some form of error
which we shall afterwards carefully avoid.
—JOHN KEATS

At this point, you have made initial contact with a drug company. Perhaps you even have a tentative nibble on your hook. What happens next (aka "What have I gotten myself into?")? In this chapter, we'll discuss study feasibility and planning for the study start-up.

Just as sponsors will be checking you out before deciding to place a study at your site, you should assess the sponsors and their protocols before committing yourself to a study. There are a number of factors to consider—but you will need to sign a confidentiality letter before you can get the most useful information or are even shown the protocol. (For a sample "Confidentiality Letter or Nondisclosure Agreement," visit http://conductingclinicalresearch.com.) The sponsor provides the confidentiality letter so that you make a binding agreement not to reveal the company's trade secrets. All you have to do here is sign on the dotted line.

Feasibility Overview

A protocol can be examined from different perspectives. While this chapter focuses on the practicalities and feasibility of protocol implementation for your site, it is important to consider other aspects as well. These aspects are scientific, regulatory, and ethical considerations.

Scientific considerations are likely to be the most difficult to understand, at least if you're working with novel compounds. It's important to try to be more than a technician and try to understand the background and rationale of the study. Does the study make sense, given what you know about the condition under study and the existing science? Are the objectives clear? And are the objectives in line with the study's design? Is the appropriate data being collected to meet the objectives? The NIH provides excellent resources on this topic.[1] Regulatory considerations are not likely to be an issue if you work with commercial sponsors, as most independent sites will do.[2, 3] Pay particular attention to the description of the study design, the inclusion-exclusion criteria, and the assessments.

Ethical considerations weave their way through everything else and are of paramount importance to me when assessing a study. These issues are discussed in more detail in chapters 8 and 9. In doing your initial review of a potential study, be mindful of the ethical tenets. Is access to the study and its potential benefits equitable? Are specific groups unnecessarily excluded? (Geriatric populations are often excluded, for example, as are women of child-bearing potential.) What are the safety and efficacy end points? Do they seem reasonable? How are they measured? Does the risk-benefit ratio for the participants seem reasonable? What plans are in place to minimize risks to the participants? What is the comparator? If it's a placebo or if, as is often the case, it's a lower-than-usual dose of an already marketed drug or a drug with significant known toxicities, then you should be more careful. How does the design fit with what is the standard of care in your community or country? Similarly, is there a washout period prior to participation that could be difficult or hazardous to participants? What happens to participants after the trial ends? Will they have continued access to a drug that they could not otherwise afford?

Protocol Feasibility

First, assess the practicality of the proposed protocol. Is the sponsor looking for a readily identifiable and available population, such as patients with diabetes or high blood pressure? Or is the sponsor looking for patients with rare illnesses? How many of these patients have you seen in your practice or hospital? (Can you run a quick search on medical records? Can you retrieve relevant data from your coding and billing software? Can you work cooperatively with other physicians and access their patient records?) All of these questions and more can be answered by a thorough feasibility review, which is akin to a business plan. Typical questions are outlined below.

After you and your staff receive and initially review a protocol, farm out relevant sections of it to other departments for their feasibility review. Then plan a meeting (or a telephone call) to discuss potential problems and brainstorm solutions.

Make a study feasibility checklist, broken down to include the following elements (see the sample "Study Feasibility Checklist" at http://conductingclinicalresearch.com):

- Administrative support: In addition to your own practice manager's perspective of how much support will be required, you should also assess the level of support you might expect from your hospital administration. If you don't have enthusiastic support from your staff and buy-in from your institution, you will be fighting an uphill battle.
- Subject recruitment and retention: Is an adequate number of volunteers available? How will you recruit volunteers? Do the inclusion-exclusion criteria seem reasonable? Or are enrollment criteria too restrictive? (Keep in mind that even for studies of common diseases with reasonable criteria, a typical enrollment rate is only one patient per month.) Does the sponsor provide any support for recruitment? How ill are the patients you will be working with? If they have significant underlying illnesses, they are more likely to have a number of adverse events (AEs) and serious adverse events (SAEs), which are likely to be quite stressful and time-consuming for all parties. Are there known significant risks with the study agents or similar classes of drugs? Once you have volunteers, will you be able to keep them? How interesting or difficult does the study seem to your volunteers? Is compensation given? If so, is it fair and noncoercive? What happens to the volunteers after the trial ends, in terms of access to care and medication?
- Study activities: Will compliance for the volunteers be too difficult because of the study requirements? Do some procedures seem too uncomfortable or too risky? Are certain procedures or scheduled activities likely to cause

a high dropout rate? Are volunteers likely to have to miss school or work? Must certain study activities be done at inconvenient times (such as nights, weekends, holidays, or changes of shift)? If so, how will this affect your having staff or institutional support? How will that affect costs or compliance? Is the drug dosing inconvenient, unpleasant, or difficult? (For example, one influenza drug we worked with had a very difficult-to-use dispenser that required skill and training just for the administration of the inhaled drug. Very good drug, poor design.) How large is the time window for conducting the study procedures? Rigid requirements can be very, very problematic.

- Personnel: Do you have an adequate number of personnel and do they have the necessary skills? How does your staff feel about this protocol? Have them review it, ask for feedback, and make them partners in the decision as to whether to undertake the study.
- Staff orientation: How will you train staff to carry out the study activities? Who will provide the training? How much time will that require—and take away from other commitments? Do you have backup trained personnel in case of coordinator illness or turnover?
- Regulatory requirements: Can you meet your IRB submission and consent requirements?
- Budget: Have you done thorough feasibility and reality testing? Are you able to conduct the trial with some breathing room in the budget for unforeseen problems?
- Contract issues: Does the contract appear fair? Are there any potential problems, such as with indemnification clauses or facilities letters? Do the payment terms appear reasonable? Will payment be received for screen failures? This is particularly important to consider if the enrollment requirements are quite restrictive. Will the sponsor pay for prestudy activities (e.g., IRB submission, meetings, chart reviews), even if no patients are enrolled, if there has been a good-faith effort (as evidenced by screening logs, for example)? Some factors are more difficult to anticipate and budget for, such as a higher-than-expected number of SAEs. These are potentially tremendous sinkholes. The same applies to audits. Will the sponsor consider add-on charges for such events?

- Pharmacy: Is a pharmacist required 24-7? Will you be able to enroll volunteers during certain hours only? How difficult will the drug preparation and administration be? Are these activities likely to interfere with other patient care activities for a harried pharmacist?
- Laboratory: Are the lab tests done locally or centrally? If centrally, how will you be alerted as to safety concerns and abnormal results? Are there any unusual lab requirements that your site can't meet, such as specific and rapid turnaround times for critical (to enrollment or safety) tests? Will shipping to a reference lab pose any problems? Is staffing likely to be a problem (e.g., night/weekend requirements)?
- Space and equipment issues: What, if any, special facilities or equipment are required? Are space or storage requirements prohibitive? If special equipment is required, will you need to buy it or will the sponsor provide it?
- Data submission: What are the data submission requirements? Are the documents electronic or paper? Ask to see a sample of the case report form to check for unexpected requirements or to see how difficult it might be.
- Monitoring: How often will monitoring occur? Will there be a monitoring visit after the first or second patient is enrolled to make sure that your site is doing everything correctly? Will a DSMB review the data? If so, at what intervals do they meet?

Organized by such "areas of attack," responsibilities can then be apportioned between the PI and the coordinator or other staff.

Some of the factors you should consider are objective and concrete, as above. Others reflect your impressions of the sponsor company and the team with whom you will be working. How do they handle your questions? What kind of affect do the monitors show? How pressured and hurried do they appear? Are they always late getting things to you and then wanting everything done "yesterday"?

You have to decide how interested you are in participating in this particular protocol and whether it is worth the aggravation and the risk that it will bring. It is better to opt out of a study that looks too difficult or for which you feel you might not be able to "deliver" the agreed-upon number of patients than to make a commitment you are unable to complete. If you think the requirements are not feasible or if you don't have the appropriate population for this specific protocol, gently let the sponsors know. Simply thank them as you decline the offer and ask them to keep you in mind in the future. They will probably appreciate the forthrightness.

An overview of the primary areas to consider in evaluating a potential protocol follows. For further details, see "Project Management Techniques" in chapter 6 or visit http://conductingclinicalresearch.com.

Patient Pool

KEY POINT
Estimate the number of volunteers by dividing your expected population in half—and then half again.

A primary question to answer is, how many patients will need to be screened to find one that is enrollable? This is in large part dependent on the answer to the questions, how realistic are the inclusion and exclusion criteria and can they be met by the population of patients I see? A quick estimate can be derived from your clinical experience as a practitioner, or your "gestalt." Ron Montgomery, my first study monitor and mentor, suggests the following recipe for evaluating your patient pool:

Ron's Reliable Recipe for Estimating Patient Numbers

Take the gross number of potential patients.

Divide that number in half.

Cut this number in half again to exclude women of childbearing potential.

Cut that number in half for patients who will not (or cannot) consent.

Cut that number in half for patients who will be eliminated by each of the top three inclusion and exclusion criteria.

Bake until done and you may have a realistic estimate.[4]

This formula boils down to your enrolling about 1 out of every 16 patients you thought you had in hand. One in the hand is worth 16 in the population. If you are lucky, you may have to screen only 10 patients to find one who can be enrolled.

One of the important tricks of the trade is to keep track of recruitment information for each study that you conduct. Your research experience summary might include your ratio of volunteers screened to those enrolled, how many completed study activities and were evaluable, how your recruitment compared to the contracted enrollment goal, and other such records. If you have a high rate of evaluable volunteers, this information will help you sell your site to future potential suitors. You are especially likely to land a study if you can demonstrate that you met or exceeded the number of subjects you contracted for on a similar protocol. (See "Site Selection: Why a Site Is Chosen" in chapter 2.) Knowing your screen-to-enrollment ratio and your dropout rates from various causes (e.g., adverse events or treatment failures) will also help you to refine budget estimates more precisely. Keep in mind that the selection criteria for many studies are so restrictive that you can expect to find only one or two patients per month for your site.

KEY POINT
Keep track of all your recruitment figures—they will be enormously helpful to you for later planning.

Despite experience, you may show initial interest in a study that turns out to be impractical or nearly impossible to do. Before bailing out altogether (if the contract has not yet been signed), discuss your misgivings with the sponsor's medical monitor. Oftentimes, sponsors will ease the inclusion or exclusion criteria that you feel are overly restrictive. Ideally, they will ease the criteria before the study begins if they get similar feedback from several experienced investigators. But restrictions are often eased later on, when the sponsors see that they are not getting their expected enrollment.

Occasionally, an investigator has not recognized the impossibility of a protocol until going to the investigator's meeting. (This is a meeting the sponsor holds for investigators and coordinators prior to beginning recruitment in the study. The protocol is reviewed and investigators have a chance to express their concerns and offer suggestions, as well as to learn about the disease process being studied.) It would still be better to bail out at that point than to proceed to the initiation of the study and then fail at the study. Contracting for more patients than you are able to deliver is likely to be a fatal error, virtually guaranteeing that you will not work again with that sponsor.

Staffing

Questions that you have to answer very early in the courtship process include the following:

- Do you have the time, energy, and training required to undertake the specific trial? (The sample "Schedule of Activities Worksheet" available at http://conductingclinicalresearch.com will be helpful in assessing the time and staffing required for each patient. The sponsor will provide you with this type of schedule for each protocol.)

KEY POINT
Hire for brains and common sense—not necessarily in that order.

- Will the sponsor provide training in specific procedures?
- Are you involved in other conflicting studies or obligations?
- Can you hire out some of the work? You might consider this for study activities such as home visits, meetings with a dietician, specific test procedures, or specimen processing. Transcribing data into case report forms is also something that can be done on a piecework basis. See the sidebar on page 76 for an amusing example of the advantages of hiring the right person for the job.

Roles and Responsibilities of Team Members

The Principal Investigator role is as follows:

- Assumes overall responsibility for the management of the study
- Agrees to follow good clinical practices guidelines
- Is responsible for ensuring that proper informed consent is obtained
- Agrees to promptly report adverse events that may be causally related to the study medication and to report serious adverse events within 24 hours
- Is the liaison for major patient care issues with the sponsor and the IRB
- Makes medical assessments of efficacy of the study medication and of whether adverse events are study related; similarly assesses the significance of changes in lab test results and whether they are related to the investigational medicine
- Networks and acts as a broker between different members of the research team

The study coordinator role is as follows:

- Helps to assess study feasibility and whether the site can or should undertake the specific study
- Handles, prepares, submits, and tracks documents:
  - Form FDA 1572 (see sample at http://conductingclinicalresearch.com), which lists the name of the protocol and outlines who the responsible parties are
  - CVs for all those listed on Form FDA 1572
  - IRB submission packet, including protocol, consent, and the Investigator's Brochure
  - Licenses, which must be annually updated for all, including for each lab that may be involved as well as for the study team

Continued on next page

Orientation of Staff

As you do your feasibility assessment, you will need to be sure that you either hire staff with the requisite skills necessary for the specific protocol that you are undertaking or that your current staff members are bright enough and flexible enough to be trained to perform the new tasks.

Research studies are now more regulated than in the "good old days." If you hire anyone to work regularly or to do anything substantive with patients or specimens, it is wise to provide him or her with some documented orientation, including competence in both specific skills and the more general following topics (see the "Orientation for New Employees Worksheet" at http://conductingclinicalresearch.com):

- Roles and responsibilities of each study team member
- Ethics

Continued from previous page

  - Regulatory binder
  - IRB and sponsor correspondence, including IND and site reports
  - Study guides and worksheets
- Manages the logistics of everything:
  - Scheduling monitor visits and patient visits
  - Tracking patient visits and the study activities required at each visit
  - Maintaining study supplies
  - Preparing advertising if need be
  - Screening patients by the strict inclusion and exclusion criteria, leaving the more nebulous or "flexible" criteria to the PI
  - Obtaining informed consent and, if an RN or PA, performing medical exams
- Coordinates monitor visits:
  - Preparing the case report forms
  - Making sure all source documents are available
  - Arranging for the care and feeding of the monitor (e.g., finding a reasonable workspace, preferably near a watering hole)
  - Handling queries and edit requests promptly and courteously, despite the natural inclination to do otherwise
  - Working as the liaison between the lab, pharmacy, radiology, administration, IRB, staff development, and whatever other departments are relevant to a particular study (dietary, housekeeping, etc.)

The Cat in the Hat, juggling many activities at once, is a suitable image of a good coordinator.

- Informed consent
- Confidentiality
- HIPAA regulations
- FAA (Federal Aviation Administration) shipping regulations
- OSHA (Occupational Safety and Health Administration) regulations

Don't forget to provide each employee with hepatitis vaccinations and appropriate personal protective gear, such as lab coats, goggles, and latex gloves for handling specimens.

Regulatory Considerations: IRBs

As with other aspects of clinical research, obtaining regulatory approval for your study isn't getting any easier. And now you must also evaluate what type of IRB you should choose for your site: an in-house IRB or an outside, commercial IRB.

IRB committees used to be more informal and have fewer layers of bureaucracy, and they were often locally based. However, the IRB function is being outsourced to professional IRBs with increasing frequency. Outsourcing can be done in two ways. Some institutions contract with a commercial IRB to review all of the studies from their sites. Or, because it is less expensive,

View from the Trenches

I have found it helpful to hire part-time people to supplement my regular staff or to do particular aspects of a trial. This practice "hedges one's bets," and it reduces overhead to a manageable level as the staffing can expand or contract with the amount of work necessary at any given time. Hiring temporary staff also enables me to hire the right people for specific jobs.

For example, the saving grace on the impotence study I did was that I hired a wonderful staff nurse to moonlight and do many of the study evaluations under my supervision. As it turned out, she had been an army nurse. She was used to handling men, and nothing fazed her. She was perfect for that particular trial. We made a great team.

In other words, supplement your staff with individuals specifically suited to a given need.

local institutions may defer to a central IRB chosen by the sponsor for each study. Which type of IRB might be best for your site?

Both types of IRBs have pluses and minuses. Having a local IRB may include advantages such as a pretty rapid turnaround time for review and a familiarity with the IRB members that fosters better communication, especially when discussing potentially thorny issues. In addition, the local IRB is likely to be more attuned to community concerns that might not be apparent to a national IRB but might relate to your investigation—regarding volunteer selection, for example. Historically, rapid IRB turnaround has been a major advantage for small sites in attracting clinical trials and in competing for them with universities. (For an example of an "IRB Submission Checklist," see http://conductingclinicalresearch.com.)

The downsides include the obverse. The personal familiarity can lead some people to engage in power plays or to make decisions based on personal conflict rather than rational, objective factors. Often significant rivalries arise, as do everyday conflicts of interest.

Also, given that IRB members are generally volunteers, getting a quorum for meetings at community study sites can be a struggle. Delays in meetings and approvals are extraordinarily costly, for both the sponsor and the site. Having a rapid turnaround time (generally 1 month) was critical to my site's success and gave it a significant advantage over academic centers, where approvals could be bogged down for months.

The availability of experience can be another limiting factor at smaller institutions. Smaller IRBs are less likely to have the academic breadth of experience on which to base their decisions. The committees are required to have only five members with diverse backgrounds, and understanding the science behind the protocols and evaluating safety data may be unreasonable burdens on such small committees.

Farming out the IRB work is increasingly appealing for sites such as small community hospitals, as it frees the staff from a tremendous amount of work and responsibility. They can, in theory, be assured that the commercial IRB will be handling regulatory issues professionally and competently. Centralized IRBs generally have up-to-date training regarding the changing regulatory playing field. Their staffs meet regularly, often at weekly or biweekly intervals, rather than quarterly, as often happens at smaller sites.

A growing consideration is the cost of running an IRB. Jane Green, a research consultant, addressed this question, projecting that for a moderately active IRB that reviews three protocols per month, the administrative cost per study is over $8,000.[5] Given that sponsors reimburse roughly $2,000 for IRB costs, the local institution is likely to be significantly in the hole for providing this service. Using a central IRB also greatly reduces the costs for the local investigator, as well as for his or her institution, as the sponsor generally submits all of the paperwork to the IRB, saving considerable work.

In reviewing all of the factors—including the availability of personnel, the other commitments of the personnel, the true monetary costs, the ethical considerations, and the simple hassle factor—I think that using a central IRB makes growing sense now, especially for smaller, private institutions.

Now that the decision has been made regarding the type of IRB, how do you proceed?

Managing the IRB Submission Process

It's easy to feel overwhelmed by all the information that needs to be submitted for IRB approval prior to your being able to actually start a study. Here are some suggestions to help you keep your submission tasks straight and save you time and stress.

Submittal for IRB Approval of the Study

The IRB submission packet must include the protocol and any amendments, the informed consent, and the Investigator's Brochure. If you're using a central IRB, this will be taken care of by the sponsor. Form FDA 1572 shows the IRB who your subinvestigators are; CVs are required to help verify their qualifications. All advertising materials also require approval. Payments to subjects require approval and may be a source of contention between the investigator and IRB.

To expedite your submission to the IRB and make sure that nothing that is required for approval is missing, you might want to use a checklist (see a sample at http://conductingclinicalresearch.com). Listing the contents makes it easy for all involved to double-check that the submission is complete. Compose a letter that outlines the contents of the IRB submission packet and that requests approval.

Be sure you know how far in advance of the IRB meetings you must submit all the documentation. You don't want to get bumped off the IRB schedule because of something like a missed deadline! Also, find out whether the PI is invited to the IRB meeting to explain the protocol or to answer any questions.

Pitfall Alert

Ideally, you should negotiate a budget and the contract details with the sponsor prior to IRB submission. This avoids a lot of wasted effort if last-minute negotiations fail. Some sponsors are very reluctant to finalize an investigator contract prior to approval, however.

Some sponsors will not allow any changes to their informed consent forms. Some IRBs are equally intractable. If you can, familiarize yourself with your IRB's quirks so you can try to hammer out likely points of contention with the sponsor before the formal IRB submission is made.

Keep in mind that not only will you be dependent on your IRB's approval, but you might also be required to get approval from your institution's contracts department, financial office, nursing service, and lab. Negotiating with these groups concurrently may work the best.

Review of the IRB Approval Package and Miscellaneous Correspondence

Be sure the letter of approval you receive from your IRB contains the following information:

- Name and address of the IRB and its chair
- Name of the contact person and other details pertaining to your IRB
- Name of the protocol (e.g., Study of X in Treatment of Y)
- Protocol identification numbers (e.g., SuperPharma SPX054)
- Principal Investigator's name and contact information
- Date of the IRB approval
- List of the documents reviewed (e.g., protocol and version number, amendments)
- IRB decision (approval or not, any modifications required)
- IRB certification and list of members
- Signature of the IRB chair
- Expiration date of the approval
- Location where the study may be conducted

If the PI is a member of the IRB, it is critical to note that he or she was recused from the vote.

Ongoing IRB Review

Don't think your work with the IRB is done simply because you've received your approval letter. You still have your ongoing regulatory requirements to meet, as noted in chapter 6, "Study Activities."

But with a good routine, an organized binder of IRB correspondence, and a checklist of tasks to be completed, tracking of your IRB submissions will be routine rather than unnecessarily burdensome.

Specific regulatory requirements that surround the informed consent form are addressed elsewhere.

Regulatory Considerations: Billing for Clinical Trials

Who would have suspected that billing could get you in major trouble with federal regulators? Major booby traps you might inadvertently step into relate to subject injury and to Medicare.

Here's a relatively new wrinkle related to subject injury you must be aware of. The 2004 Medicare Secondary Payer (MSP) Rule and the 2007 Medicare Extension Act added reporting requirements for the sponsor and institution as well as significant financial penalties for delays or improper claims. The MSP Rule says that when a trial sponsor promises to pay for research-related injuries, it becomes the "primary" insurer, and therefore Medicare will no longer be responsible for any payments. This can also create a billing and reporting nightmare for the sites.

KEY POINT
Before you invest a lot of time, energy, and expense, obtain a copy of the contract and look for any deal-breaker clauses. Unfortunately, they are occurring more frequently than in the past.

(A related warning for those of you who might think you are just trying to be nice to your patients: You can't waive or pay the copayment for a Medicare patient because such payment is considered an inducement to utilize a government service under the Federal False Claims Act.)[6]

In an effort to ensure access to clinical trials for Medicare beneficiaries, the Medicare National Coverage Decision was enacted in 2000, allowing coverage for some "routine costs." Because of confusion, the rules were revised in 2007 as follows:

> *Medicare covers the routine costs of qualifying clinical trials, as such costs are defined below, as well as reasonable and necessary items*

and services used to diagnose and treat complications arising from participation in all clinical trials. All other Medicare rules apply.

Routine costs of a clinical trial include all items and services that are otherwise generally available to Medicare beneficiaries (i.e., there exists a benefit category, it is not statutorily excluded, and there is not a national non-coverage decision) that are provided in either the experimental or the control arms of a clinical trial except:

- *The investigational item or service, itself unless otherwise covered outside of the clinical trial;*
- *Items and services provided solely to satisfy data collection and analysis needs and that are not used in the direct clinical management of the patient (e.g., monthly CT scans for a condition usually requiring only a single scan); and*
- *Items and services customarily provided by the research sponsors free of charge for any enrollee in the trial.*

Routine costs in clinical trials include:

- *Items or services that are typically provided absent a clinical trial (e.g., conventional care);*
- *Items or services required solely for the provision of the investigational item or service (e.g., administration of a non-covered chemotherapeutic agent), the clinically appropriate monitoring of the effects of the item or service, or the prevention of complications; and*
- *Items or services needed for reasonable and necessary care arising from the provision of an investigational item or service—in particular, for the diagnosis or treatment of complications.*[7]

Rush University became an illustrative lesson in the consequences of Medicare billing errors in a widely publicized settlement. In 2003, Rush undertook an internal review and discovered that some services had been inadvertently billed to Medicare when they should not have been. To its credit, Rush promptly put a hold on further clinical trial billing and reported its error to the government. The subsequent settlement included a 50 percent penalty and added reporting obligations under a compliance program. Now a new department at Rush coordinates the research and billing arms of its operations. This Research and Clinical Trials Administration Office also reviews informed consents with an eye as to which procedures are billable and which are not, in addition to performing traditional budget reviews.[8]

Other sites have added dedicated clinical trial billing personnel to their study staff in an effort to remain compliant with the ever-evolving and confusing Medicare rules and to avoid "double-dipping," or billing an insurer for a service provided by the sponsor.

One helpful tip is to itemize all lab procedures required by the study protocol's activity requirements and be sure that these are all covered in your grant. Do not bill Medicare for these services. If a procedure is required solely for research, rather than for a patient's care, do not bill Medicare or other insurers.[9] Keeping track of lab billing was actually easier for us before computerized order entry. We made color-coded lab requisitions for each study, alerting the lab that any order on a colored sheet was to be billed to us and not to the patient's insurer or Medicare. Life was so much easier then.

Antikickback, False Claims, and Stark Laws

The last recent boogeyman that deserves mention regarding clinical trial agreements is that of antikickback statutes, or Stark laws and Sarbanes-Oxley laws. These laws are not very likely to become an issue for investigators participating in phase 2 or phase 3 trials, which receive closer FDA and IRB review. The issue of paying physicians excessive fees may, however, arise in phase 4 trials.[10]

These regulations require some attention when drafting clinical trial agreements.[11] For example, to avoid question, the specific and detailed purposes of initial start-up payments should be given in the agreements in order to document compliance. For example, you might want to specify that the start-up payments are reimbursement for time spent in submitting regulatory documents and attending the investigator's meeting, to compensate for lost time from patient care.

LEGAL LAND MINE
Specify what items start-up payments cover.

For light reading, try the laws, rules, and regulations regarding the federal antikickback statute (42 USC 1320a-7b(b)); the Limitation on Certain Physician Referrals, also referred to as the "Stark law" (42 USC 1395nn); and the Sarbanes-Oxley laws. Only don't do so before bedtime, or you are likely to risk night terrors.

Budget Feasibility

Next, before investing vast amounts of time, try to see if the sponsor is offering a plausible budget. Budgeting accurately is a difficult task and comes only with hard experience because nothing in a protocol is ever "as advertised."

Increasingly, sponsors seem to be reluctant to discuss budgets until after you have made a major time investment—such as after the site qualification visit, a preliminary planning meeting with your study team, and even the investigator's meeting. Similarly, sponsors often seem to have no clue as to the amount of work and time that are involved in executing their protocols. While this attitude is perhaps understandable because the sponsors are isolated from the realities of actually trying to implement the protocols, it may be a major obstacle to reaching an agreement. It's important to get at least a rough idea of the range early on.

Sponsors either ask you to develop and submit a budget or, more often of late, make you an offer that is nonnegotiable or has little wiggle room. You would find it useful to have a fairly complete idea about the protocol details and what you are getting into before you finalize a budget; however, in reality, that rarely happens. Although the budgets that sponsors will present you with may appear straightforward, listing the procedures specified in the protocol and the total cost per procedure or study visit, they are sorely lacking. Unfortunately, these templates ignore the numerous hidden costs of conducting a trial—costs that Norm Goldfarb estimates may make up 80 percent of a study's expense for a site.[12]

Fortunately, investigative sites have several resources available to help calculate a more realistic budget. In addition to the traditional Current Procedural Terminology (CPT) codes, Goldfarb describes Clinical Research Terminology (CRT) codes that specifically describe study-related activities. He notes the most time-consuming activities are completing the CRF, reading and processing correspondence, writing and sending correspondence, and reviewing charts for potential subjects. Note that most of the time is administrative rather than involving direct contact with the volunteers. Study visits account for only 20 percent of the time provided for in site budgets.[13]

Even more information about hidden costs in trials is detailed by Guy Johnson, formerly of the George Washington University Clinical Research Administration Program. Johnson stresses the need to include all employee benefits in your calculation—and these can easily amount to an additional

30 percent of the employees' base pay. His analysis and accompanying Coordinator Cost Calculator are very valuable tools.[14, 15]

It is very important to have a fairly complete idea of the protocol details and what you are getting into before you finalize a budget. Unfortunately, that information isn't always available at this stage in the process.

Begin your estimation by including all your known fixed costs (e.g., for medical procedures) and time estimates based on your usual practice patterns. At least double your normal time estimate for seeing each patient, as study patients are much more time-consuming to evaluate. The hardest part of budgeting is estimating the number of screen failures you are likely to have—patients whom you will spend time screening but who then aren't eligible for enrollment. Don't forget to also estimate time for preparing for and meeting with the IRB, for meeting with other involved departments, and for inservicing (training) hospital staff. If you are having difficulties in budget negotiations, remember that you can exert some leverage by not starting any administrative or clinical processes before the budget is final or by putting a hold on them if you have already started (which we often do, in an expression of good faith). Delays cost the sponsor a lot of money.

Spreadsheets are your best friend, enabling you to try several "what if" scenarios relatively easily. Improv (by Lotus) has been my favorite, allowing me to use a standard template and then modify it for particular protocol requirements. It, however, has gone the way of other user friendly and intuitive formats and has been replaced by "improved" spreadsheets. Sample budget worksheets are provided at http://conductingclinicalresearch.com and are available on the Web.[16, 17]

Sponsors often use a database from Medidata (formerly DataEdge) called Pharmaceutical Information Cost Assessment Service (PICAS) to generate the budgets they proffer to sites. PICAS provides extensive cost-related data from

View from the Trenches

On my very first protocol, I submitted my proposed budget to the CRA with fear and trepidation that it would be rejected as too high. Instead, he made a little choking sound, paused, and said he would increase it slightly. My estimate, I later learned, was still a ludicrously low reimbursement for the amount of work involved. Some time later, he told me he couldn't in good conscience pay me as little as I had asked. Ask for budgeting advice from someone with more experience than the person I had asked!

U.S. and European sites and can be used by sponsors to insert figures for each study procedure into a template while developing budgets for specific indications. PICAS also helps the sponsor anticipate its costs at different locales. PICAS data not only include procedure costs but also personnel and institutional overhead costs for widely varying settings. Pharmaceutical companies can obtain cost data for specific disease indications and even for different phases of drug development trials. The PICAS data are proprietary and not specifically available to individual investigators. When a sponsor offers you a detailed budget template, you should keep track of the amount offered as reimbursement for specific procedures; this will serve as a surrogate for the PICAS data. It will also give you a good starting point when submitting your own budget proposal on this or future trials. (Similarly, sponsors may also use the CRO Capability Assessment Service [CROCAS] to obtain detailed information about a CRO's experience with different types of trials.)[18]

Medidata reports that its surveyed sites' charges are higher than those from PICAS, perhaps a case of wishful thinking. But Kenneth Getz and his colleagues document the depressing news that investigator compensation per procedure has declined 3 percent annually since 1999 while the sites' work burden increased 10.5 percent annually.[19] My experience certainly confirms this, so I am not terribly sympathetic to an overreliance on PICAS data.

The spreadsheets I have developed for our site—as you should similarly do—include standard charges for lab tests as well as estimates of time involved. Keep in mind that phase 2 studies are invariably more complicated than phase 3 (which are harder than phase 4), and will be more stressful and time-consuming than the later trials. You need to try to account for this when you negotiate for a study—as well as for any unique attributes of your site that affect your time and costs. For example, I stress that I don't have "hot and cold running house staff" to see the patients and that I conduct all patient assessments myself. Given the unusual consistency in evaluations and my atypically high level of involvement as a Principal Investigator, I can occasionally negotiate a grant at the higher end of the range.

Money, as they say, is not everything. You must consider nonmonetary factors as well. Dr. Harold Glass has developed models to assess "price elasticity" and the factors leading to participation of investigators in a trial. He notes that an investigator is likely to sacrifice 25 percent of a typical grant to work with a novel, innovative compound. That's consistent with my own experience. Other important factors include the sponsor's reputation, the potential for obtaining more desirable studies from the sponsor in the future, and coauthorship.[20]

More idealistically, you may just want to be able to provide a particularly promising opportunity to your patients, as I did in working with drugs targeted at life-threatening sepsis or superbugs. Keep these intangible factors in mind as you develop your budget proposal. It is one thing to knowingly accept an unprofitable study, or SUMP (subsidized unprofitable medical project), because of anticipated nonmonetary gains, but don't allow yourself to be taken advantage of.

Study grants, or budgets, reflect payments for each patient who completes a study, start-up costs, overhead, and administrative time. Additional, less obvious factors that you should consider when making your feasibility assessment include the complexity of the study, patient acuity (how sick the patient is), preparation requirements, and the reasonableness of the inclusion and exclusion criteria. You might draft a budget by one of the methods discussed below. Several Web sites, listed in appendix B, present excellent alternative approaches you may also wish to explore.[21] One particularly valuable site is the Clinical Trials Networks Best Practices site.[22] With all these aids, you are in a much better position to predict your time and expenses and negotiate a budget that is fair to your site.

Budgeting Advice for Neophytes

Not surprisingly, estimating and drafting a budget can be quite difficult, especially for an inexperienced investigator. That might help explain why only

View from the Trenches

An intriguing study by Dr. Harold Glass suggests exploring "price elasticity," or trade-offs, that a site will be willing to make to land a study. His data parallel my experience with one exception. Based on his model, Glass states that site personnel do not have a preference between working directly with a sponsor and working with an intermediary contract research organization; I strongly disagree. I suspect Dr. Glass's opinion stems from the fact that investigators often are insulated from the day-to-day dealings with the monitors and administrative personnel of the sponsor, so they may not be as aware of the differences between the two situations as their coordinators are likely to be. An experienced site team might well prefer to work directly with a sponsor, although it is not likely to make a financial sacrifice to do so.

10 percent of investigators stay in the business for 5 years or more.[23] You might benefit from others having learned the hard way if you consider the following suggestions as a basis for estimating your costs. Costs will vary depending on your locale and circumstances. Just as "Ron's Reliable Recipe for Estimating Patient Numbers" above halved the initial estimate and then halved it again, you might now do well to double the following recipe, especially if you are new to this challenge.

KEY POINT When budgeting, be realistic—don't shortchange yourself.

The Laboratory

Ask the lab manager for the listed charges for the specific tests needed (e.g., CBC, chemistry panel). Also ask for the listed fees for shipping and handling "send-out" specimens (typically $25–$50) as well as the cost of dry ice. You will also need to know specimen collection fees ($10) and lab bookkeeping fees. Ask what the Medicare reimbursement rate is for each test, and perhaps the rate negotiated by managed care players. Then ask the manager whether you might negotiate a discount based on volume, the fact that your study is considered an "outside account," or the fact that helping you (or science) is just the right thing to do. When you submit a budget, use the list price. The spread, or difference between the list price and your negotiated price, may be your only profit margin on some (not most) studies. You might similarly negotiate with your institution regarding discounts for use of other resources (radiology, clinic space, etc.) and for special payment terms. For example, we were able to help our cash flow by negotiating a delay in our payment to the hospital until we had received final payment from the sponsor. Watch for hidden costs, such as complex processing or shipping requirements, lab paperwork, and telephone calls to reference labs. At the risk of discouraging you, an extensive list of these costs and proposed research codes has been compiled.[24] These are largely behind-the-scenes costs that sponsors write off as the cost of doing business. I agree with Goldfarb that these are very real costs that should be included in the budget as legitimate study-related activities for sites. Other readily overlooked costs are equipment maintenance or replacement, error and omission liability insurance, and legal review of contracts.

The Pharmacy

For some inpatient protocols, the pharmacy costs may be lower for study patients than for nonstudy patients. The drug company either provides the medications or reimburses the site's acquisition costs for the study drug. The study might require fewer daily drug administrations than other regimens require, reducing preparation time. Significant time is spent for drug accountability and some time for training pharmacy staff. So a pharmacy fee can be negotiated based on the difficulty and labor intensiveness of the protocol.

Equipment and Supplies

Call vendors for prices of equipment and supplies you will need. Evaluate what, if any, special facilities are required. For example, in 1991, new OSHA requirements came into effect (the Bloodborne Pathogens Standard, 29 CFR 1910.1030).[25] These require extensive new training and separate facilities for handling and processing lab specimens from patients. Because of these requirements and more recent FAA (yes, the Federal Aviation Administration, not the FDA) requirements for special training for shipping specimens, you might consider maintaining a contractual relationship with a hospital or independent laboratory to handle these aspects of your studies. OSHA regulations make it prohibitively cumbersome and expensive for a small-practice investigator to become more independent, running outpatient studies without involving a hospital at all. (See the "Specimen Collection and Preparation Worksheet" at http://conductingclinicalresearch.com for an example of the type of lab specimen processing involved just for blood tests before deciding to process lab samples in your office.)

The IRB

Increasingly, institutions are requesting reimbursement by trial sponsors to cover their administrative time running the IRB that oversees the studies. Currently, reimbursement from the sponsor for IRB administration is likely to be in the $1,500–$2,500 range. Your own IRB preparation time is not reimbursed unless you have included it as overhead. You should estimate at least 1 hour preparation time for the initial IRB meeting, 1 hour for attending the actual IRB meeting, and 1–2 hours to review safety update submissions to the IRB. Be sure that your contract specifies terms not only for initial IRB fees but for annual renewal fees and protocol amendments as well. Rather than specify exact figures, it is generally better to say that the site will invoice the sponsor for any IRB fees as they occur, and the sponsor will reimburse these promptly (within 30 days). If you use a central IRB, the sponsor pays the IRB fees directly and submits all the required reports. This is a big help for individual sites.

Administration

You'll need to budget for the following administrative costs:

- Contract negotiation: approximately 2 hours
- Legal review: 1 hour
- Meeting with pharmacy, lab, nursing, and information systems: approximately 2 hours
- Administrative changes due to protocol revisions: 1–5 hours, depending on the complexity of the protocol
- Study monitoring visits (see "Case Report Forms" below)

Radiology and Special Studies

Although radiology and special studies costs tend to be less negotiable, you can use the same procedure you used to figure the lab costs. A recent cost example is that of a hospital charge of $1,000 for an echocardiogram. Medicare reimbursement for this procedure is $200 plus $100 for the physician's interpretation.

Medical Evaluations

For most protocols, a good estimate is approximately 1 hour for the initial history and physical exam and 1 hour for answering the volunteer's (and family's) questions, obtaining consent, and initiating study orders. For each subsequent medical visit, figure 1 hour for coordinator activities plus 1 hour for data entry by the coordinator. Follow-up visits tend to run approximately half an hour per visit, including the exam and the required documentation.

Add half an hour extra for each adverse event, if mild. These adverse events might include nausea, mild rash, or headache, for example, and are often three or four per subject. For serious adverse events (SAEs), plan at least 2–3 hours to treat the patient and report the event to the sponsor. This will take much longer if the event has not been previously reported as a side effect of the medication or device. SAEs are more likely to occur in phase 2 trials or in trials with a more ill or elderly patient population. It is hard to budget for these. Try to budget for the worst-case scenario, which might anticipate that perhaps one in five patients will develop a serious and unexpected condition; usually the occurrence is far less, given a healthier patient population. It's also worth trying to have SAEs as an add-on to the budget, at a given hourly rate, as their frequency and the amount of time they will consume are so unpredictable.

Case Report Forms

Plan 8–10 hours per patient for paperwork, on average. For a complicated phase 2 study, double that estimate. Paperwork time depends partly on how well designed the CRF is. You would do well to ask for a sample before finalizing the budget agreement, especially on early phase trials.

You might also add several hours to your budget for query resolutions, particularly for an early phase study, and 1 hour per patient for record archiving. (Queries are requests for clarification regarding data submitted via the case report form. They may relate to obviously incorrect data or to inconsistencies in the data. A careful, compulsive person completing the CRF is essential to minimizing queries and the attendant expense for both the site and the sponsor. Queries sometimes result from turnover in monitors, with different monitors requesting that CRFs be completed differently. Should this occur, you might try to work out an additional payment to cover your site's added time. Queries are further discussed in chapter 6 and are illustrated at http://conductingclinicalresearch.com.)

Site-Sponsor Meetings

A new Principal Investigator should probably plan, as a rough estimate, approximately 1–2 hours for the first site visit, or site qualification meeting. Other meetings to budget for include

- Investigator's meeting: plan on losing 2–3 full days of work, including travel.
- Initiation meeting: plan 1–2 hours—longer for the coordinator.
- Monitoring visits: plan 1 hour for the PI, 2–3 hours for the coordinator.
- Closeout visit: plan 1 hour for the PI, 2–3 hours for the coordinator.

View from the Trenches

Our experience is that remote data entry (RDE), or electronic case report forms, are more time-consuming and cumbersome for our site than paper forms. Except for the storage and environmental impact, paper is still preferable. The industry trend is strongly moving toward electronic data entry, however, as this greatly reduces the time and expense for the sponsor's staff.

- Audits: for an in-house audit (see "Audits" in chapter 4), plan at least half a day for the PI and 1–2 days for the coordinator. For an FDA audit, the time required is anybody's guess.

Start-Up Fees

While start-up fees are addressed in other sections, the importance of trying to negotiate a fee to cover the following expenses can't be overemphasized:

- Your time for protocol feasibility and reality testing and for budget reviews
- IRB preparation time
- Time for developing a patient recruitment plan
- Screen failures

Ideally, these payments should be nonrefundable as you incur tangible costs whether or not your enrollment efforts are successful or whether the study is cancelled by the sponsor.

KEY POINT
Negotiate aggressively for a start-up fee covering major administrative costs and meeting time.

Miscellaneous Costs

Additional costs not mentioned above can add up. You'll need to budget for

- Patient time and travel: A typical allowance is $25 per visit for outpatient studies to reimburse for travel and for the inconvenience and discomfort of the blood draws. Invasive studies tend to pay more—be careful not to be coercive and to obtain IRB approval for all payments to subjects.
- Finder's fees: Many investigators, including me, don't view finder's fees as ethical and don't use them. They are commonly used, however—especially, it appears, for incentives for house staff or nurses to recruit patients—and tend to run in the $25–$100 range, depending on the difficulty of identifying and recruiting subjects. Be careful to check with your institution and IRB so you don't run afoul of their policies.
- Food for inservices (training site personnel to conduct a specific trial): serving food can readily run $50–$100 per week if you choose to serve food to make attendance at your programs more palatable.

- Advertising: Generally, advertising is a separate item, not included in per-patient reimbursement. Costs vary from $50 to several hundred dollars per study, per site.
- Storage: Especially with the industry's merger mania in the past several years, it can be difficult and time-consuming to track down whom to contact at the sponsor regarding the need for continued record storage. Sites generally have no reliable way to determine when the legal period for record retention ends, so you may want to budget for long-term storage.[26] A possible alternative for a site is to return the study records to the sponsor or the sponsor's third-party designee after a specified amount of time. Be aware that it will take hours to prepare the files for archiving, as the sponsor will likely want a detailed list of what subject records are in each box.
- Overhead: Typically, the sponsor factors in 20–25 percent of the budget totals for overhead in its grant proposal. For an internist, a representative practice overhead is approximately 50 percent. Look at what additional costs you will be incurring beyond your regular practice requirements to conduct the study. Some of the factors to consider are whether you need to rent additional space; buy or lease special equipment; add telephone, fax, or dedicated computer lines; hire additional personnel; or purchase additional insurance. One major advantage of a small, independent site over an academic institution is that a university may tack on an overhead of 50–100 percent, making it more expensive.
- Unanticipated costs: You need to add language in the contract noting that unanticipated costs are likely and that they will be compensated for, without including specific figures in the contract, if possible. Items to consider include the inevitable protocol amendments, a higher-than-anticipated screen failure rate, and changes in charges from your suppliers (e.g., radiology).[27]

Budgeting by Activity

One approach for estimating budgets is to determine costs for each specific study activity. All activity budget worksheets should include the following elements, which are further detailed in the sample "Budgeting by Activity Worksheet" at http://conductingclinicalresearch.com.

Medical Evaluations

Medical evaluations include the initial history and physical examination, follow-up assessments, administration of medications under observation, and any special tests or procedures that require your presence as the physician.

KEY POINT
Administrative costs are largely fixed. Front-load them in your budget.

Administrative and Overhead Costs

Your administrative time and practice overhead costs are roughly the same whether you enroll 1 patient or 30. If you are not able to successfully negotiate for "one time," or start-up and administrative, costs, try to adjust the per-patient costs to reflect the anticipated amount of time and effort required. It is preferable to negotiate a start-up fee (see "One-Time Fees" below) that will cover initial administrative fees and fixed costs. Ideally, this fee should be independent of enrollment numbers and nonrefundable; these terms, however, are very difficult to get.

When drafting a budget, remember to "front-load" your administrative costs so that these costs will be covered if a patient fails to complete the study. Some patients, inevitably, will not complete the trial. Similarly, be aware that sponsors will try to "back-load" the grant to encourage you to have every patient be fully evaluable as well as to lower their overall costs, again because some patients, unavoidably, will not complete the trial.

Procedural Costs of Study Activities

The procedures required by the study will incur costs such as laboratory charges, radiology charges, equipment and supply costs, special procedure expenses, and patient payment.

One-Time Fees

Administrative start-up fees include costs for assessing the feasibility of the protocol and budget, developing a patient recruitment plan, submitting the study proposal to the IRB, negotiating with the lab and pharmacy, preparing source documents, and so on. You should include time for attending the investigator's meeting here. Also, add time and reimbursement for changes due to protocol revisions. This fee is difficult to estimate—consider planning for 1-2 hours for straightforward-appearing protocols and at least 5 hours for complex trials.

Many sponsors will provide a start-up fee to cover your initial administrative time, and this should be nonrefundable. Insist that this fee be included in the contract.

It's important to differentiate this administrative start-up fee from an advance payment, which is usually refundable if the study is cancelled for any reason and is otherwise credited against future earnings. The advance payment is generally equal to the fee for one study patient, and its purpose is to help your cash flow pending patient completions. Be sure to insist on this payment if you expect enrollment to be very slow.[28]

Special circumstances will add other costs, such as those due to serious adverse events and other unexpected occurrences that are not the fault of the investigator, audits, protocol amendments that require new assessments, and screen failures.

You should also include the time required for the investigator's meeting, which will cost you 2–3 days of missed work and occasional teleconference time as the study progresses.

Grants from Sponsors or CROs

I have been told that a sponsor's budget for investigative sites comes from a separate "pot" than that for CROs. This has apparently not always been the case. Budgets for protocols administered by CROs appear to have been generally smaller than budgets handled directly by the pharmaceutical companies; this observation has also been made by others, who have noted that the budgets were 15 percent smaller.[29] Some CROs appear to have paid per completed procedure and kept the "spread," the difference between the total per-patient grant from the sponsor and the activities or lab tests actually performed. (Some procedures may not have been done because a patient did not complete all of the visits; some may simply have been missed due to human error.) Payment per procedure or study activity is a logistical nightmare and enormously expensive in terms of wasted time and administrative cost.

Budgeting by Evaluability

Another approach for estimating budgets is by subject evaluability. It is far easier to track payments that are made based on a simple algorithm for evaluability, as described below. Overall, this appears to be simpler and actually fairer than budgeting by activity. I generally propose this kind of arrangement, but sponsors are often reluctant to adopt this approach. You also need to remember that you are still negotiating the study at this point and therefore using your experience as your only guide as to what the subject outcomes are likely to be, how many of your patients are likely to be compliant and complete all the study visits, and so on. Predicting the future is a dicey endeavor.

Budgeting by evaluability is also generally less cumbersome and time-consuming (translation: less expensive) for a site. However, you need to look carefully at what is defined as an evaluable patient in the protocol and contract, or you are likely to receive unwelcome surprises. The following definitions are commonly used to categorize the evaluability of study patients, and therefore to assess the level of reimbursement that might be expected.

- Evaluable patient: A patient who completes the entire study and all evaluations. Try to add the phrase "or who drops out due to an adverse event (AE)" to the clause defining "evaluability" in your contract with the sponsor. Inserting this caveat into the contract is recommended because if the adverse reaction is significant enough that the patient must be dropped from the study, considerable additional work will be involved in following up and reporting the event to the IRB and the sponsor. This is especially important to get for early phase 2 studies, in which you are dealing with an unknown drug and have less of an idea as to how frequent adverse events will be and how serious they may be.
- Supportive patient: A patient for whom you have significantly incomplete data, usually due to early termination, but whose case is still useful for

Bait-and-Switch Clauses

Be especially careful about criteria that adversely affect a patient who has already enrolled in a trial and would be forced to drop out. From my perspective, these are the worst contract clauses. An example is a clause that makes the patient's continued participation dependent on a specific lab result, such as a positive culture. This condition is upsetting because it carries the connotation of a "bait-and-switch" tactic to patients. They don't understand why they are being dropped, losing the benefits of the study. It is similarly upsetting to the referring doctor and does not positively reinforce referring patients for protocols in the future. Some sponsors insist that such patients be dropped from a trial, as that will cost them less for that patient, without appreciating the broader implications and the cost of trial delays that may result from this practice.

KEY POINT
Watch out for bait-and-switch clauses or requirements to drop patients based on results that don't affect safety.

safety data. On infectious disease studies, sponsors often include patients with negative cultures (cultures that do not grow a pathogen) in this category, for example.

- Unevaluable patient: A patient who is not useful to the study. Unevaluable patients are still included in the "intent to treat" analysis (which examines all randomized patients, whether or not they ultimately received the drug or the experimental treatment), even though the data will not support the application.

You still have to go through an itemized budget worksheet to help ensure that you have included all the factors (see the sample "Budgeting by Activity Worksheet" at http://conductingclinicalresearch.com). However, in terms of grants and for ease of bookkeeping, you can then simplify your definitions. So, working from the sample budget example, the study contract might say

Evaluable patient: $4,100

Supportive patient: $2,500–$3,000

Unevaluable patient: $1,000–$1,200 (This covers your up-front expenses.)

Contract clauses that are dependent on factors over which the investigator has no control are particularly bothersome. For example, for infectious disease trials, some grants are structured so that evaluability is dependent on whether the patient's culture grows organisms or even a specific organism.* (This provokes the response, "Do I look like I have a crystal ball?" or, "Do you think I'd be doing this if I could predict the future?")

Investigators should be responsible only for things over which they have control.

Budgeting by Position

For specific individuals and positions, you can, if need be, further break down budget estimates; for example, by salary if salaries are to be applied to different department cost centers. Otherwise, if there is no specific need to do so, don't bother. Factors to include are listed in the sample "Budgeting by Position Worksheet" at http://conductingclinicalresearch.com.

---

* Predicting culture results is very chancy. Predicting the likelihood of a patient's being compliant with the drug or returning for follow-up, and therefore being clinically evaluable, is a bit safer bet.

Multiply the estimated time required for each activity by the number of occurrences in subject visits and then by the expected number of patients. Multiply this subtotal by each person's salary (don't forget benefits!) to get an estimate of personnel costs. It's amazing how quickly they add up.

CROs and SMOs: Dealing with the Middleman

Any choice involves pros and cons. One of the early decisions you might face is whether to work with, or through, a contract research organization or a site management organization. CROs act as brokers who contract with the pharmaceutical companies to conduct and monitor a particular study. If you can work well with a CRO, the upside is that you will then have access to more trials in the future than you might have "going it alone" as the organization is likely to turn to you for other trials. The downside includes the organization's taking a cut of the profits. According to Mark Hovde of DataEdge, investigators receive about 15 percent less on a grant through a CRO than on one directly from the sponsor.[30] CROs also tend to have a higher turnover of monitors, many of whom are extraordinarily inexperienced. This inexperience and rapid turnover can be quite costly and aggravating for the study site. You wind up providing on-the-job training to young monitors for the CRO.

A more global problem is that "most project managers at CROs seem to believe that a study simply will conduct itself if people and resources are thrown into the mix," notes Cullen Vogelson, an experienced study coordinator, monitor, and manager and former assistant editor of *Modern Drug Discovery*.[31] Similarly, another overall problem with the CRO model is that, as with government contracts, the project often appears to be awarded to the lowest bidder. Reassuring, isn't it? The CRO may try to bid low and then experience considerable cost overruns due to poor planning or delays in enrollment, which can drag a study out for months beyond what was

View from the Trenches

We have occasionally had a series of monitors on a (usually CRO-placed) study, each wanting CRFs redone in a different fashion by my coordinator—even though the company should have employed one uniform standard and direction. Our record is 13 CRAs (monitors) in a 12-month trial—well more CRAs than patients! This turnover was enormously costly and annoying for our site.

initially anticipated. In their defense, CROs often are saddled with the more difficult or hurried studies, in which everything has to be done "yesterday." The sponsor pressures the CRO, who, in turn, puts heat on the site.

Why do sponsors use CROs? you might wonder. One major advantage for the drug company is that subcontracting some element of the work allows greater flexibility for the sponsor. On any project, or in any business, the amount of staffing personnel and work are likely to vary dramatically over time. Maintaining a large cadre of well-trained, experienced staff is likely to be extraordinarily costly and wasteful of a sponsor's resources. Using CROs (akin to adding holiday help in the mall) as temporary help to fill gaps in staffing reduces fixed overhead costs considerably.

Site management organizations may be even more problematic. They try to offer a group of sites to a sponsor, suggesting that by providing the administrative functions, the SMO will ensure more uniform procedures among the sites, as well as in data collection. But investigators have observed that SMOs are even more difficult to negotiate with than are CROs. SMOs are also extremely rigid about what contact site personnel may have with a sponsor and tend to prohibit site staff from discussing any budget issue directly with the sponsor. Furthermore, they levy sites an additional 10 percent of the grant total as their brokerage fee.[32] SMOs may also retain restrictive covenants precluding the site's participation in further trials for some time. It seems that the sponsors generally don't realize either the severity of the restrictions that the SMO has placed on their sites or the impact those restrictions may have on their trial.

Why should you consider working through a CRO? For a new investigator, a CRO has distinct advantages because it offers access to trials and the potential of being favorably placed in the CRO database, thereby being more likely to attract additional studies. On the other hand, overall, working directly with the pharmaceutical companies has proven to be preferable. Their monitors are better trained and more experienced, and the medical monitor at the pharmaceutical company tends to be the monitor for all indications for the new compound and thus has more experience with it. In contrast, a CRO's medical monitor is generally less familiar with the drug, dealing with it only on one protocol, and may be juggling more than one protocol. Perhaps this opinion reflects my obsessive-compulsiveness about the protocols and my sense of responsibility to my patients.

As an experienced investigator, I prefer dealing directly with the sponsor. Once you are established, I would recommend this approach. However, more and more drug companies are turning to CROs to administer their protocols, and working with a CRO is a particularly good entrée for a beginning investigator.

The annual number of New Drug Applications has almost doubled since the 1980s, and the number of patients required for each NDA has also doubled. The number of active investigators has increased almost fourfold to 30,000.[33] Because of this rapid increase in workload, sponsors have increasingly turned to CROs to fill their need for workers. Over 600 CROs are now operating. A handful are full-service providers, generally multinational, and represent 40 percent of the market. These include Covance, Quintiles, Paraxel, IBAH, and Inveresk (formerly ClinTrials). Because they provide a full array of services, they are increasingly large companies that mirror their sponsors. This size leads to increased fixed costs and thus to their being less competitive in terms of cost—they charge about 20 percent more than the smaller CROs do. They make up for this premium by their wider experience.

Niche providers are much smaller and specialize in one particular aspect of a trial, such as regulatory affairs or patient recruitment. Numerous small, privately run CROs act as consultancies. An interesting study from DataEdge looked at how various CRO attributes are weighed by sponsors making their selection. As might be expected, sponsors weighed their previous experience with the CRO as the most important factor. The CRO's experience with the indication being pursued ranked second. Surprisingly, the CRO's bid was actually sixth of seven parameters assessed, according to DataEdge.[34]

CROs are often the training ground for folks who want to become monitors, or clinical research associates. They are willing to hire inexperienced new graduates; the pharmaceutical companies almost invariably want experienced staff. Because of this and their desire to keep costs down and be competitive, CROs tend to pay their monitors less than sponsors do and to work them harder.[35] Other interesting differences in how sponsors and CROs manage their clinical research associates include, for example, the fact that monitors of CROs have less experience to begin with but are deployed in the field much more extensively than those who are in-house with the sponsor. They rapidly gain experience, particularly in initiating and closing study sites.

To conclude, SMOs may provide a useful introduction for clinicians interested in learning to conduct trials for pharmaceutical companies, as much of the administrative detail is taken care of by the SMO. Working well with a CRO is likely to help you become better known most quickly and gain you more rapid access to future trials. Working directly with the sponsor is the best option for the more experienced investigators: you can generally negotiate a better contract and you are likely to work with more experienced players.

Contract Basics

KEY POINT
I strongly recommend that you seek experienced legal advice before you agree to a contract.

Please note that the following contract information is provided to reflect issues that might be helpful as an overview for readers. It is intended neither to be all-inclusive nor to provide legal advice or assurances, but is rather a description of factors to consider before undertaking clinical research. Regulations change rapidly. While references are given for further details, the reader must assume responsibility for checking the most current requirements and other legal and contractual issues.

Clauses to Watch Out For

Negotiating a contract can be even more difficult and time-consuming than dealing with the regulatory submission process. Contracts used to be written in English and were relatively straightforward. They now are often written in legalese and can be an expensive stumbling block if the sponsor is inflexible. Ask to see a sample contract before you invest major amounts of time or resources that could turn out to be for naught.

Several particularly problematic areas for investigators are discussed below:

Grant Payment Schedules

Even if you believe that you have come to an agreement with the sponsor on a budget, the contract will generally be "stacked" to benefit the sponsor. This is becoming increasingly true as the drug companies are facing increased competition and are tightening their belts, too. For example, the schedule of payments is likely to provide for the bulk of the payments to be made at the end of the study, while the investigator's expenses are front-loaded. Try to address this issue early on in the negotiations. If the payments are made at the end of the study, you will be operating in the red for a long time.[36]

The best payment schedules provide for payment as work is completed—but define that carefully. Next best are regularly scheduled payments. Milestones can be used reasonably for payment schedules. The major clauses to avoid call for withholding a percentage of the grant or otherwise delaying payments.[37] Similarly, ask for a start-up payment to be made when the contract is finalized, rather than at enrollment of the first patient. This helps with cash flow and covering your start-up costs for patient recruitment and early screening efforts. To make your life easier, specify in the contract that the grant payments will be broken down by patient, either according to evaluability or per visit milestone or by some other readily identifiable point. Insist that payments include a remittance advice, or detailed breakdown of what the funds are for. Otherwise, tracking payments can become a bookkeeping nightmare, especially if your site has multiple investigators, sponsors, and studies.

KEY POINT
Read the fine print—more than once! Contract terms may well be negotiable.

Beware of certain innocent-sounding clauses regarding payments. The sponsor will often propose payment for the entire study in several "easy" payments, to make bookkeeping less cumbersome—say, for example, start-up, after an enrollment target is reached, after the last patient is enrolled, and after the CRF queries are all resolved. An example of a target might be an agreement that the sponsor will make grant payments after every fifth patient is enrolled. On some studies, that may work. On others, enrollment may be unexpectedly low or delayed, which will result in the investigator essentially "floating a loan" to a sponsor—a large corporation—and can cause a major cash flow problem for the investigator. It may be over a year before the first target enrollment is reached. In the meantime, the site investigator will have received next to no payment yet have to pay all the study employees and creditors. Even after milestones for payment are reached, it may be some time before the sponsor pays the site. Cash flow problems also occur because the collection periods from sponsors average more than 100 days longer than the site's payment period to its employees and vendors.[38] Similarly, start-up payments, intended to cover up-front salary and administrative costs, are often not made until after enrollment has begun.

The most desirable grant payment schedules call for an advance start-up sum, usually the equivalent of one evaluable patient, followed by payments

View from the Trenches

I have long wanted to level the playing field a bit by including a clause that charges the sponsor interest for late payments. After all, we have to pay our employees, rent, and other bills, and creditors charge us interest. Surprisingly, the wealthier sponsors don't see it this way. Late payments, or reinterpreting the criteria for payment, appear to be occurring more frequently and may lead to a divorce between a site and a sponsor based on irreconcilable differences, complete with the rancor normally reserved for abusive relationships.

made for work completed. Be careful to check whose definition of "completed" is used—the sponsor's or the site's. Does it mean when the monitor retrieves the CRF, or not until all queries are resolved at all sites? Payments upon receipt of invoice are also generally good, as are regular (monthly) payments.

A less desirable but adequate schedule provides for payments at predetermined milestones. The worst agreements lack such milestones and call for a significant withholding until all queries are resolved.[39] A very useful contract clause, especially on complicated studies, is one that requires the monitor to visit the site within 2 weeks of your having enrolled your first patient. It's helpful to have the initial patients closely monitored to make sure that you are enrolling patients appropriately and performing all the study evaluations correctly. Catching errors early on will help avoid unevaluable patients that are painfully costly for both the site and the sponsor.

Again, be careful when budgeting by evaluability and, with newer drugs in the pipeline, of getting adequate (if any) reimbursement for patients who experience serious adverse events (SAEs), which are an administrative sinkhole.

Special Terms for Start-Ups

I recently became aware of a previously unheard-of problem: sponsors defaulting on payments to investigators! Because of the current recession, some smaller companies have declared bankruptcy, leaving their hardworking sites in the lurch. As a result, Larry Brownstein and Kate Leonard recommend completing a financial review of the sponsor or CRO if you have not worked with that party previously, including working capital (current assets minus current liabilities), cash balance, and history. They also suggest adding the following protective terms to your contract:

- Recovery of all attorney fees and related costs, in case of nonpayment.
- The ability to withhold data from the sponsor for nonpayment until payment is received.
- Retrieval of CRFs at frequent regular intervals (specify them). Milestone payments should note that if the CRFs are not retrieved regularly, the sponsor will provide the site with an interim payment for patient visits completed.
- Insurance for the sponsor: "throughout the term of this Agreement and for a period of two (2) years thereafter a policy of insurance covering any and all liabilities hereunder. Such insurance policy must include coverage for products liability and any liability arising out of clinical trials, including contractual liability, for no less than $5,000,000."[40]

As if we needed something else to worry about. But I do appreciate the alert and advice.

Publications Clauses

Clauses often prohibit investigators from publishing data collected at their site, under the ruse that the study results are proprietary information whose publication would jeopardize the sponsor. Confidentiality and patent protection are legitimate concerns, but they must be balanced with the right of investigators to publish negative results and to maintain their identity as ethical, responsible, unbiased researchers. (See "The Betty Dong Affair" sidebar.)

You might like to enhance your career by publishing your own case experience and find yourself thwarted in doing so as it would be inconsistent with long-term strategic marketing goals of the pharmaceutical company.[41] Understandably—from their perspective—companies are going to try to protect their investment. Unfortunately, this goal is often at odds with the best interests of the public. More favorable publications clauses can sometimes be negotiated. Sample wording is available in the "Contract or Clinical Trial Agreement" example at http://conductingclinicalresearch.com and from several other Web sites.[42]

Patent and Inventions Clauses

Contracts stipulate who "owns" discoveries that may lead to new indications and, therefore, more profits. Patent and inventions clauses (sometimes referred to as rights and patents clauses) are not often recognized as important by

The Betty Dong Affair

The Betty Dong affair is one of the most egregious examples of the abuse by pharmaceutical companies of the publications clause in investigator contracts.

In this case, Dr. Dong conducted a clinical trial for Boots Pharmaceutical to study the bioequivalence of Synthroid to its generic competitors. When her study concluded that the drugs were, in fact, equivalent and that use of generic versions might save U.S. healthcare costs $356 million annually, Boots aggressively attempted to suppress the data from the $250,000 trial it had funded. The company aggressively criticized Dr. Dong's work, and attempted to discredit her and prevent publication of her work in *JAMA* (*Journal of the American Medical Association*). When that attempt failed, Boots threatened Dr. Dong with a suit for breach of contract related to its publications clause. Faced with a backbreaking suit after 8 years of research, Dr. Dong was forced to withdraw her findings from publication in *JAMA*. After adverse publicity and pressure from the FDA, Knoll Pharmaceutical (which had since acquired Boots) relented, and Dr. Dong's findings were ultimately reported in 1997—10 years after the saga began—alongside a thoughtful commentary on the entire affair.[43]

Most publications clauses are less restrictive now, but they still require presubmission of the article to the drug company. A period of time is defined during which the sponsor can review and challenge the findings. Complete obstruction and squelching of unfavorable results appears to be less likely.

less experienced investigators. An example of their relevance is the case of the medication Minoxidil. This medication was initially developed for severe hypertension. Subsequently, two dermatologists claimed that they had discovered Minoxidil's benefit in combating baldness, an unexpected side effect of the drug. They had to sue the Upjohn Company for their rights. As of 1996, when the drug, marketed as Rogaine, went off patent, the two dermatologists had received $26 million in royalties.[44]

Patents and inventions clauses are notoriously one-sided. (The sponsors apparently didn't learn the value of sharing in kindergarten.) In the company's defense, it will already have spent millions of dollars just to get a compound to the large clinical trials phase. However, patents and inventions clauses that grant exclusive benefits to the sponsor are not in either party's best interest.

In terms of patents, investigators are considered employees of the sponsor company. They have not made any financial investment toward developing the new agent or device and thus they are not considered to have any entitlement. However, sponsors do not appear to have a good understanding of human nature. Investigators who discover a potential new use for an agent believe they should share in the credit for discovery. As people—including the PI—generally need an incentive to pursue a goal or discovery, more balanced wording is increasingly appearing in contracts. Similarly, contract language may also include rights of institutions to new uses discovered during trials. Recommended wording that benefits both parties is outlined in the sample "Contract or Clinical Trial Agreement" at http://conductingclinicalresearch.com.

Indemnification Clauses, or Investigator, Beware!

Having a good indemnification clause in your study contract is imperative in protecting you in case of a liability suit. This is perhaps the most important clause to have vetted by an attorney. Sample phrasing from actual contracts includes "unless there is willful negligence" on the part of the investigator, or protection if "substantive specifications" of the protocol are adhered to (as opposed to the blanket "all" specifications of the protocol). A new area of concern relates to the ownership of tissue and what should be put in clinical trial agreements (CTAs) and informed consent clauses about that. (See "Whose Body Is It?" in chapter 8.) An inexperienced investigator is likely to overlook many other problematic clauses. A discussion of these is available at the MAGI Web site along with a sample contract.[45, 46]

One of the nastiest covert clauses, now appearing more frequently, relates to "cross-indemnification." Previously, companies would, if asked, provide a "letter of indemnification" to the study site, saying that if the investigator followed the protocol and a patient experienced a significant adverse event, the company would indemnify, or cover, the site and the investigator in the event of a liability suit. Now the companies are asking that the investigator's site indemnify them! This is akin to David providing protection for Goliath and is patently absurd. Can you imagine an investigator, like me, in solo practice, or you (even worse!), providing liability coverage for a multibillion dollar corporation?

Ask to see a contract template early in the dating relationship with a sponsor and simply refuse a study (especially in an early phase trial) that requires you to indemnify Goliath Drug Co. These clauses are offensive and absurd. Most doctors seem to be naïve and inexperienced in business matters. *Learn to protect yourself. No one else will.*

What would be fair and reasonable would be a clause that says, in essence, "If we, the site investigator or institution, foul up in a grossly negligent way, we will take responsibility for our error. If the problem is with the drug or sponsor's product, they will provide liability coverage and take responsibility for their product." Review contracts very carefully for this frightening new stealth clause. Again, insist on receiving a draft contract prior to investing a lot of time in the protocol. For further discussion, see the provocative commentary "Should Clinical Trial Sites Unionize?" by John Ervin[47] and the Society of Principal Investigators Web site at http://www.sopi.org.

Insurance for Clinical Trials

It used to be commonly believed that indemnification from the sponsor adequately covered the investigator and the site's potential liability. This situation began to change with the suit over volunteer Jesse Gelsinger's death in 1999. Since that time, the Gelsinger family attorney, Alan C. Milstein, has alone successfully filed and settled 20 suits. Milstein explained his success: "Signed consent forms are no longer worth the paper they are written on."[48]

Subsequently, a Joint Commission report supported Milstein's assertions, noting that 44 percent of patients who signed consents for surgery didn't know the exact nature of the operations; 60–70 percent either did not read or did not understand the consents.[49]

Another factor raising concern about the adequacy of informed consent is the issue of coercion. While this is most often heard about in relation to exploitation of subjects overseas, it is increasingly a problem in the United States, as more and more people are uninsured, can't afford medical care, and seek "treatment" through access to clinical trials.

Suits aren't restricted to subject injuries. They may seek coverage for denied insurance claims or relate to issues such as breach of contract, intellectual property rights, financial/SEC breaches, and more.

Some suits have occurred due to denial of access to a trial or an investigational drug. For example, Amgen was sued (*Abney* and *Suthers* cases) by participants in a phase 2 trial for Parkinson's disease for having terminated the study because Amgen felt the investigational agent was neither safe nor efficacious. The patients sued Amgen for continued access—and lost.[50] Perhaps the most recent are suits from participants claiming a property interest in inventions and discoveries derived from their blood or genes.

With the proliferation of social media sites, blogging, and Twitter, word about trials gone awry spreads like wildfire, fueling further suits and a new industry.

Because the indemnification clauses in CTAs do not cover alleged physician error and most malpractice insurance policies exclude coverage for clinical trials, you might want to consider purchasing an insurance policy specific to clinical trials. Costs vary depending on factors such as the type of research, the phase of the trial, and your past experience with conducting clinical trials. Coverage is now available through at least two avenues: Clinical Trials Reciprocal Insurance Company and Clinical Research Liability Insurance (CRLI).[51, 52]

You can't be as trusting as in the old days, when I began to conduct trials. Remember lawyer Milstein's words: "Signed consent forms are no longer worth the paper they are written on." Protect yourself, and look into this insurance option.

Subject Injury

One of the more contentious and complicated issues that has received increased attention over the past several years is that of subject injury and compensation for same. This issue was brought to light following the Gelsinger lawsuit. Two other prominent and more recent cases are that of Suzanne Davenport, who became seriously disabled following participation in a Parkinson's disease trial, and the more widely publicized TeGenero, or "elephant man," trial, in which six healthy young men almost died from their participation in a phase 1, or first-in-human trial of an immune modulator drug, TGN1412.[53, 54, 55] Each of these examples of trials gone awry has resulted in huge and protracted lawsuits from the injured volunteers and has changed the clinical trial climate both by further impeding investigator-sponsor-university contractual negotiations and by further scaring potential volunteers.

The main contractual issues revolve around the blame game and whether the injuries are related to

- Subject negligence or noncompliance in following instructions
- Investigator or site (e.g., hospital) negligence or misconduct
- Sponsor negligence or misconduct

One additional problem brought to light by the TeGenero case was that the sponsor's insurance coverage, $3.7 million, was inadequate to cover catastrophic outcomes. The National Bioethics Advisory Commission stated in 2001, "Participants who are harmed as a direct result of research should be cared for and compensated" as a matter of justice.[56] On the other hand, no U.S. law requires such compensation, nor is there a requirement for compensation in the GCP (5.8), the Declaration of Helsinki, or the World Health Organization/Council for International Organizations of Medical Sciences *International Ethical Guidelines*.[57]

The most rational response to this issue is the report from the prestigious Institute of Medicine, which recommended in 2002 the creation of a no-fault compensation system for injured subjects.[58] Such a system already exists in many European countries, which "mandate the provision of clinical-trials insurance, through which subjects are often covered regardless of fault."[59]

Because of these cases, investigators must now be much more careful about the subject injury clause in clinical trial agreements, and this clause, as well as indemnification, can readily be a deal breaker.

Part of the debate is that while the informed consent form may say that the sponsor will reimburse the subject, the sponsor does not sign that agreement and may not be legally bound by the consent. Similarly, while the contract between the site and sponsor may state that there is identical subject reimbursement, the volunteer is not a party to that contract. One conclusion: "Because the investigator—the site's representative—signed the ICF, it is generally easier for the subject to enforce a monetary claim against the site than against the sponsor."[60]

KEY POINT
Be sure that the wording is consistent between the protocol, informed consent, and CTA.

Who wins in all of this? Only the legal industry.

You can now find warnings about potential damaging phrasing and a variety of recommendations for suggested wording.[61–64] Be sure to investigate these.

Confidentiality Clauses

Contracts should include a statement that if the site investigators need to provide any information to the sponsor in which a patient is identifiable, the sponsor agrees to maintain confidentiality. This is important in light of the recently enacted federal privacy regulations known as HIPAA.

Facilities Letters

To provide indemnification for hospitals, facilities letters acknowledge that the hospital agrees to allow an independent investigator to perform a study at the facility. Negotiating these letters has suddenly become problematic because of the recent adverse publicity surrounding clinical trials and the hospitals' perception that liability for them has now increased.[65] (See the sample "Facilities Letter" at http://conductingclinicalresearch.com.)

These clauses are illustrated in more detail in the corresponding samples at http://conductingclinicalresearch.com.

The Dark Side of Contracts, or Things Your Mother Never Told You

In recent years, clinical research has undergone a marked shift in the relationships between investigators and drug companies. The general tenor has shifted from being collegial and cooperative, with at least the illusion of working as a team, to being sometimes adversarial. Sponsors show less loyalty to investigators, and study sites are now often treated as expendable, interchangeable parts on a factory line. This change can be attributed in part to corporate downsizing, the "lean-and-mean" paradigm as the model for industry. It also reflects the change in healthcare delivery overall, exemplified by HMOs, with the emphasis on business and the bottom-line cost rather than on patient care and quality. Hospitals have replaced "patient" with "customer" or "consumer."

This shift has significantly affected both the budgeting and the contracting processes. For example, where simple letters of agreement used to suffice, now contracts have extensive clauses that contain many undesirable terms. Previously, the contract was a straightforward agreement: the investigator promised to do X amount of work for X payment per patient. Now, unfortunately, the contract is more difficult to negotiate and may well be more time-consuming and stressful than the IRB and regulatory aspects of a study. This makes it frustratingly common for the investigator to have invested enormous amounts of time and energy before the sponsor is even willing to share the details of the contract, thereby "hooking" the site, which may be reluctant to pull out of the study and cut its losses.

Contracting represents an increasingly difficult balancing act for any investigator. On the one hand, due to the increased competition and the rising cost of research and development, drug companies are in need of more investigators who can rapidly conduct a trial and provide quality data. On the other hand, there are many more investigators than a decade ago and the pool is growing. As noted, investigators are increasingly regarded as commodities that can be readily replaced. So if you are too insistent in advocating for a more equitable partnership, you are likely to be replaced. Individual investigators must weigh the risk-to-benefit ratio of a particular protocol or relationship, considering many personal factors.

Win-Win Relationships

Most often, the pharmaceutical companies with which investigators seem to have had difficulty negotiating a contract or budget have been smaller, relative newcomers to the industry. Many of the more experienced players recognize that it is in their interest to sign a contract that is fair to both parties and that will encourage repeat business and long-term relationships with their investigative sites. For example, you can often anticipate areas where disagreements tend to occur during contracting negotiations and be prepared with alternative language options. We tend to do this with contraceptive, indemnification, and patent clauses, in particular, with a menu of sample wording that has been acceptable to prior sponsors and that we know will be acceptable by our institution's lawyers and administrators. Another solution is to develop master agreements with a sponsor if you are likely to work with the company repeatedly and then tailor the generic master to study-specific issues. One company surveyed reported that it was able to develop master agreements with 50 to 60 percent of its investigator sites.[66]

View from the Trenches:

The Things They Never Taught You in Medical School

To run a successful research study, you need to consider and attend to a morass of details, none of which you would ever have imagined needing. It may be helpful to assign the various tasks to be juggled to different people and track these responsibilities on one of the ubiquitous checklists. Many PIs may choose to delegate most of these activities to the study coordinator, leaving the physician with just the patient care activities. I tried that in my earlier days. Since I am a perfectionist, however, and want to keep track of the make-or-break global issues or those that may come back to haunt me and my staff, our responsibilities are currently outlined as noted in the "Prestudy Activities Worksheet" available at http://conductingclinicalresearch.com.

Developing a relationship with a new site is quite expensive for the sponsors, too, and it is in the sponsor's interest to maintain those relationships. In fact, Hassan Movahhed, formerly of Amgen (now vice president at Geron), worked hard at changing his company's structure to better cultivate relationships with its investigative sites. For example, monitors (CRAs) are traditionally assigned by protocol or by area of research and will cover a wide geographic territory of all sites studying that indication. In contrast, Amgen is shifting its model to having the CRA cover specific sites rather than indications for use, thereby having the CRA become extremely familiar with a site and its capabilities. The company can help develop a site's capabilities and, in turn, can expect lower costs from a site knowledgeable and experienced in meeting its particular requirements. Movahhed noted that Amgen had successful experience with this model for assigning CRAs to sites, with improved relationships and resultant increase yield in patients per site.[67]

Movahhed was already astutely implementing a strategy popularized by the auto industry called "knowledge-based sourcing," which emphasizes a collaborative relationship designed to grow over time, rather than a one-time, less balanced deal. Jackson and Pfitzmann describe this approach used so successfully by Honda: "Manufacturers and suppliers share a long-term commitment to improving each other's capabilities, starting by working together to eliminate wasted effort and inefficiencies. The two sides, instead of being at odds, collaborate openly on lowering costs and raising overall performance, with the expectation that this mutuality will continue over many years, benefiting both companies."[68]

Imagine if this attitude were the norm in the pharmaceutical industry. Undoubtedly the rapid turnover in investigators and CRAs would not exist, and productive, long-term, and mutually beneficial relationships would likely evolve. Advantages of this type of sponsor-site relationship and strategies to implement it are discussed in a thoughtful review by Tracy Blumenfeld and Darren Zinner.[69] Pharmaceutical sponsors are slowly becoming more attuned to this seemingly novel concept of treating investigators as partners.

Winning Contracts

Part of having a successful long-term relationship between a site and a sponsor is having a contract that is equitable to both parties. In summary, fair terms might include the following elements:

- Regular grant payment schedules: for example, within a month of each CRA monitoring visit, or quarterly payments for work completed to date
- Publications clauses that allow investigators to publish any of their findings with several months' notice to the sponsor
- Patent and inventions clauses that provide incentives for discoveries
- Indemnification clauses that protect the investigator and study site

An example of an equitable contract appears in the "Contract or Clinical Trial Agreement" available at http://conductingclinicalresearch.com. A more detailed one, particularly important to review because of the commentary and optional clauses, is that of the MAGI Model Clinical Trial agreement, available on-line.[70]

Conclusion

If you remain undaunted, after signing the contract and obtaining IRB approval and while awaiting start-up supplies and your study initiation visit, you can design and implement protocol-specific study aides, as well as put together generic study folders. Are you ready to start?

The devil is in the details. Visit chapter 4 if you dare meet him.

CHAPTER 4

Regulatory Issues

Hell, there are no rules here—
we're trying to accomplish something.
—THOMAS A. EDISON

The regulatory landscape of clinical trial conduct is evolving, changing due to public pressure, economics, and globalization. Different standards for good clinical practices and regulatory requirements presently exist in different parts of the world. For example, the United States follows the FDA good clinical practices (GCP) regulations. The European Union follows the EU Directives, and the European Union, United States, and Japan all agree to follow the International Conference on Harmonisation (ICH) guidelines. Each set of standards is a little different. The ICH guidelines cover studies in 17 industrialized countries and 15 percent of the global population.[1] They are often used as a reference in other countries. For all practical intents, there are few differences between the FDA and the ICH standards. If a protocol meets ICH guidelines, it will meet FDA requirements, but the ICH addresses some issues, such as nontherapeutic trials, in greater detail.[2] The ICH also requires more elements in an informed consent than the FDA does. Both sets of standards provide a guide to the design, conduct, performance, monitoring, analysis, and reporting of clinical trials. Both also attempt to ensure the truthfulness of the data and to provide protections to study participants.

Currently, 20–30 percent of clinical trials are being conducted in developing, or "ascending," countries, primarily in eastern Europe, Asia, and Latin America. In a CenterWatch survey, eastern European study sites were rated "excellent" in the categories of investigator experience, investigator disease knowledge, and GCP experience. Asia is more problematic as many countries there don't have IRBs, though they do have other drug development regulations. Some of these local regulations are said to provide a climate that is not particularly conducive to pharmaceutical development. India ranks quite high among the developing countries in the areas of investigator experience, coordinator quality, and site operations efficiency, but its GCP experience lags. The Indian government is said to be promoting a "clinical research culture," making the regulatory climate more favorable and promoting GCP training. Latin America has lagged in the race for clinical trials due to its regulatory climate, areas of political instability, and the economics of developing drugs there.[3]

One recent change in good clinical practice guidelines is the addition of a requirement that new studies be listed in a clinical trial registry. These registries will require that all results—positive or negative—from a clinical trial be made available. Currently, only half of clinical trial study results are published. Sometimes this lack of publication may seem to be a deliberate attempt to stifle information, as in the Betty Dong case featured in chapter 3. In a recent survey, when Dr. Kay Dickersin, director of the Center for Clinical Trials at Johns Hopkins Bloomberg School of Public Health, "asked a group of investigators why they didn't publish some of their findings, 22 percent said they had never finished the work; 11 percent said publicity had not been their aim; and a full 30 percent said the results were 'uninteresting' (meaning, in most cases, 'negative')."[4] Certainly another unmentioned explanation is simply that it takes a tremendous amount of work to write and publish an article in a peer reviewed journal. Recent proposals have resulted in new trials being registered at inception or as a condition of funding or publication. Hopefully, the new transparency of having all results available in a timely fashion will increase the public's willingness to participate in clinical trials.

All the rules and regulations won't feel quite so burdensome if you keep their intent in mind: the overriding concern behind them is assuring the safety of the volunteer. Let's look at some of the activities in this context.

The *protocol*'s focus should be on minimizing risk and having risk commensurate with the stage of research and study objectives. For example, studies with healthy volunteers should have minimal risk; those targeting urgent, life-threatening conditions might have a higher threshold. A well-designed protocol should give a clear and sound rationale for the study based on a careful review of the literature and basic science. Safety nets should be in place, beginning with the entry criteria and including appropriate lab tests and monitoring. Stopping rules should be in place should a study not go as hoped for.

Similarly, the levels of safety review must be greater in riskier studies and include DSMB meetings at frequent intervals. Safety evaluations, both clinical and lab, should be similarly proportional. Plans should be made for proactively managing toxicities, with contingency plans to provide more expert backup if necessary. Real-time data collection and accountability are critical.

For perspective, consider the several tragic high-profile cases that illustrate trials gone awry and the need for strict safety measures. (See the table in appendix A.) The main issues in these cases can be categorized as related to protocol, IRB review, recruitment and informed consent, and trial implementation, both in study conduct and in data reporting. While some of the lapses were due to inexperience, others reflected a lack of ethics and a culture that emphasized discovery and profits (financial and academic) rather than patient safety.

One of the recurrent themes is that more safeguards are appropriate, trials involving healthy volunteers who have no expectation of benefit (other than financial) should have more safeguards regarding their amount of risk exposure. Often, the focus appears to have been on the ability to consent rather than the potential harm to the volunteer. The need to balance paternalism and experience with naïveté, youthful enthusiasm, and financial need will be occurring more frequently. Let's try to learn from these tragedies.

In this chapter, we'll look at some of the regulatory details you are likely to encounter as you undertake your clinical trials.

New Regulations

The past few years have seen an increase in the number and scope of new regulations. Some people are calling for much greater scrutiny of the FDA itself as well. Here are the highlights of changes in the regulatory environment. Note: These rules change at a dizzying speed. Be sure to check the latest FDA guidances before embarking on any trial.

KEY POINT
Subscribe to an FDA list server to receive alerts about new guidances.

Food and Drug Administration Amendments Act (2007)

The Food and Drug Administration Amendments Act (FDAAA), also called Public Law 110-85, amends the Pediatric Research Equity Act, among others, and requires a plan for pediatric testing of a drug unless the drug is to treat a condition occurring only in adults, such as Alzheimer's. Sponsors can no longer wait for studies in adults to be complete to begin planning their pediatric trials; pediatric drug development should start early in the process. For some indications, such as meningitis and otitis, which occur much more frequently in children than in adults, studies in adults and approval are not required prior to studying the drug in children.

The FDAAA also includes the Sentinel Initiative, Clinical Trials Registry, and Clinical Trials Transformation Initiative (CTTI).

Sentinel Initiative

The Sentinel Initiative markedly expands the scope of postmarketing surveillance studies and requires "active surveillance" for risks. A goal is access to data from 100 million patients by 2012, with active real-time surveillance for adverse events, rather than the passive reporting system now in place. The intent is to have live monitoring of large group health systems' electronic medical records (EMRs) and insurance claims databases to detect adverse events. This should greatly enhance the identification of major safety issues.

While not the stated intent, this legislation will also allow the FDA to readily identify the off-label use of drugs. One of the limitations of the Sentinel Initiative is that, at present, it has access to only Medicare data. In order to have information regarding a broader population, a partnership with the private sector will need to be developed. This will mean overcoming issues of information technology infrastructure, privacy, and security.[5]

Clinical Trials Registry

The Clinical Trials Registry requires registration of drug and device trials with the FDA.[6]

> *The law includes a section on clinical trial databases (Title VIII) that expands the types of clinical trials that must be registered in ClinicalTrials.gov, increases the number of data elements that must be submitted, and also requires submission of certain results data . . . Under the statute, the "applicable clinical trials" trials generally include:*

- *Trials of Drugs and Biologics: Controlled, clinical investigations, other than Phase 1 investigations, of a product subject to FDA regulation; and*
- *Trials of Devices: Controlled trials with health outcomes, other than small feasibility studies, and pediatric postmarket surveillance.*[7]

This registry is an excellent addition, as it will prevent negative outcomes in trials from being buried.[8] A similar IRB registry is now required if the research is conducted or supported by DHHS.[9] It is not yet required for industry-sponsored research.

Clinical Trials Transformation Initiative

CTTI is a public-private task force, including members of industry, government (FDA and NIH), universities, investigators, and others. CTTI's projects include

- Reporting and interpreting serious adverse events
- Improving monitoring practices

Genetic Information Nondiscrimination Act (2008)

The good news: the Genetic Information Nondiscrimination Act says that genetic information cannot be used to make decisions regarding health insurance underwriting or the hiring, firing, and promotion of employees. Research volunteers are informed more clearly about privacy risks regarding their genetic data. The bad news: a huge gap in GINA doesn't address availability of life or disability insurance after disclosures.

FDA's Acceptance of Foreign Clinical Trial Data (2008)

Prior to October 2008, the FDA's position regarding the acceptance of foreign clinical trial data in support of a U.S. marketing application (for both drugs and devices) was to require that all studies be conducted in compliance with the Declaration of Helsinki standards. Now the rules have been relaxed, and studies must be in compliance with ICH-GCP guidelines and older Helsinki standards (1989 standards per 21 CFR 312.120(c)(1) for drugs or 1983 standards per 21 CFR 814.15(a) and (b) for devices).[10] Other recommendations for the use of foreign data reflect concerns regarding the oversight of trials by review boards, the level of experience of researchers, and the difficulty the FDA has providing oversight itself, given its limited resources.[11]

For drug trials, a concern has been that the participants' demographics reflect those of the local populations, as ethnic differences—as well as illnesses, compliance, cultural differences, or regional variations in standards of care—may confound responses to medications. Thus, the ICH issued guidelines in 1998 regarding accepting data generated in one region for use in another. These guidelines were modified in 2006.[12, 13] The intent was to expedite research by avoiding duplication of studies in different regions and to identify and describe any differences due to ethnic factors. (See "Shifting Studies to Developing Countries" in chapter 9).

The FDA issued further guidance in 2008 for non-IND studies, largely suggesting that studies follow ICH-GCP regulations regarding human subject protection and the availability and completeness of data.[14] This was optimistically called a "Final Rule." Noncompliant data may still be reviewed or used if they contain data relevant to safety considerations.

The use of data from multiregional clinical trials is not of concern just to the FDA. Similar concerns have been raised by the EMEA regarding the applicability of studies conducted outside Europe to the EU population.[15] An excellent overview of the issues regarding multiregional trials is given by Bruce Binkowitz.[16]

For device trials, an additional concern was that the FDA should consider studies that reflect U.S. medical practices prior to a device's acceptance in the United States.[17]

Non-U.S. study sites may be audited by the FDA, particularly if the application relies substantially on non-U.S. data, if major discrepancies between the United States and non-U.S. data exist or if fraud or abuse is suspected. This is not very likely to happen, however, given the funding constraints of the FDA. For example, between 2000 and 2005, the FDA audited less than 1 percent of the 350,000 trial sites estimated to be active worldwide.[18]

To overcome concerns about the use of data from different regions of the world, *ICH Topic E5: Ethnic Factors in the Acceptability of Foreign Clinical Data* was issued. These guidelines allow use of a bridging study, defined as "a study performed in the new region to provide pharmacodynamic or clinical data on efficacy, safety, dosage and dose regimen in the new region that will allow extrapolation of the foreign clinical data to the population in the new region. A bridging study for efficacy could provide additional pharmacokinetic information in the population of the new region."[19]

Bridging studies avoid duplicating large, complicated trials by using small studies in specific ethnic populations to extrapolate expected results. These are specifically required by Japanese regulatory agencies, for example because significant differences in metabolism, dosing, and adverse reactions have been shown with a variety of drugs (cancer, arthritis, antibiotics).[20]

American Recovery and Reinvestment Act (2009)

The American Recovery and Reinvestment Act (ARRA, also known as the "stimulus package") provides $10 billion for "scientific research and facilities" through September 2010. NIH is the major beneficiary. Special attention is also given to information technology with the Health Information Technology for Economic and Clinical Health Act (HITECH Act), also part of ARRA.

One of the specified intents of the HITECH Act is to facilitate health outcomes and clinical research. Under HITECH is a Health Information Technology Standards Panel (HITSP) subgroup focusing on improving the infrastructure needs of research. Areas of interest include requirements, design and standards selection, networks, and registries. It is anticipated that this subgroup will also provide for more information about trials being communicated to participants and healthcare providers.

Healthcare providers are being pushed into using electronic medical records. Medicare reimbursements to providers will increase significantly if there is "meaningful use" of the EMRs, defined as data used for health purposes (e.g., public health, quality reporting, or research), and decrease if there is not "meaningful use."[21]

Medicare has one significant and related problem—"pay for performance"—that has already impacted my site. By linking payment to adopting evidence-based pathways, Medicare is discouraging institutional as well as individual participation in clinical trials. Deviations from a "clinical pathway" for research are allowed without penalty if they meet certain documentation requirements, but therein lies the rub. The requirement is that "There is documentation that the patient was involved in a clinical trial during this hospital stay relevant to the measure set for this admission."[22] For example, the only acceptable documentation of trial participation is the informed consent or protocol physically on the medical record. A research chart, however, is not considered an official medical record.

Pay for performance has other holes that we needn't go into here. The upshot is that this strongly promotes algorithm-driven healthcare. In my institution's case, there was a very strong push to have uniform order sets for pneumonia, for example, that included standards that were to be met for the timing of cultures and beginning of treatment after a patient's arrival in the emergency room and specified which antibiotics were considered appropriate, such as option A, ceftriaxone, or option B, levofloxacin. There was no politically acceptable option C: enrollment in a pneumonia trial. (Another, unintended consequence included the decerebrate, indiscriminate prescribing of an antibiotic with significant central nervous system side effects, one I would not customarily prescribe to our elderly patients otherwise seen in consultation because of this side effect profile.)

Research will also be integrated with EHRs, with electronic case report forms having some data entered automatically. Other fields will have prompts to help ensure correct completion. If the system actually works, wouldn't that be a dream! I suspect it will be a mere pipe dream for the foreseeable future. One major advantage of such a system would be the real-time reporting of data to DSMBs, which would be able to more quickly evaluate and respond to safety reports.

Standardization in formats would also greatly reduce time and data entry errors, as noted in "Breaking the Scientific Bottleneck" in chapter 7.

ARRA also creates a new Federal Coordinating Council for Comparative Effectiveness Research, with $1.1 billion allocated, including $1.5 million to the IOM to prioritize the most effective areas for study.

And, while it's not technically part of ARRA, another important recent project, the Clinical Research Information Exchange (CRIX), represents a "collaborative effort among government, the bio-pharmaceutical industry and academia to implement a common, secure standards-based electronic infrastructure to support the sharing of clinical research data for faster, more efficient development of new drugs." We certainly could use standardization and a reduction in paperwork.[23]

Executive Order 13505: "Removing Barriers to Responsible Scientific Research Involving Human Stem Cells" (June 2009)

Executive Order 13505 rescinded the restrictions on federal funding for human embryonic stem cell research, allowing "conduct (of) responsible, scientifically worthy human stem cell research including human embryonic stem cells to the extent permitted by law." The NIH Guidelines for Human

Stem Cell Research became effective on July 7, 2009. They include a registry and centralization of procedures for review. Many states have responded to the executive order with their own, more restrictive laws.[24]

Form FDA 1572—What Are You Really Signing?

The famed Form FDA 1572 may seem like just another routine piece of paper that you need to sign. Often, the form is even already conveniently filled out for you, ready for you to make your mark. Nothing to it, right?

Stop! The 1572 is a binding contract between the investigator and the FDA, whereby the investigator makes certain commitments. You must read and understand these obligations or the FDA can take legal action against you. You wouldn't sign a contract to buy a used car without examining the document and the car, would you? Let's look under the hood of the 1572.

KEY POINT
Sponsors can delegate their responsibilities to CROs. PIs cannot delegate to anyone.

You'll be asked to sign a Form FDA 1572 for any phase 1 through phase 3 studies that are under the supervision of the FDA. The 1572 is essentially a marriage contract between the investigator and the FDA whereby the investigator vows to fulfill the following obligations:

- Conduct the trial in accordance with the protocol. You can change the protocol if a patient's safety, rights, or welfare is at stake but not otherwise. If you make a change, you must notify the sponsor.
- Personally conduct or supervise the investigation. You cannot be an uninvolved figurehead. If you delegate responsibilities or assessments, you are still responsible—and you must list your subinvestigators on the 1572. It's important to remember that you have to revise the 1572 if your subinvestigators change, and this change must be reported to your institutional review board (IRB). Some sponsors specifically note that they will indemnify anyone listed on the 1572, another reason to make sure the list is complete.
- Inform patients that the drugs are being used for investigational purposes. I prefer obtaining informed consent from volunteers myself because it is such a significant responsibility. After all, informed consent is a process, not a signature obtained like a trophy.

- Report adverse events to the sponsor. If they are serious AEs, you are obligated to report them within 24 hours.
- Read and understand the Investigator's Brochure. It's not just a reference manual to gather dust on the shelf. You are supposed to understand everything that is already known about the drug.
- Ensure that other staff members who are assisting in the trial understand their obligations. You may not be able to make them comply with every guideline, but you must have informed them of everything.
- Maintain accurate records.
- Report all unanticipated problems promptly to the IRB.
- Ensure that the IRB "that complies with the requirements of 21 CFR part 56" will provide continuing review for the clinical investigation. No one has yet successfully explained this one to me. How is each lone investigator supposed to do this? I keep my fingers crossed and take a giant leap of faith.

Updates to these requirements are generally issued in April and October and can be found at the FDA's Web site (http://www.fda.gov), as can 21 CFR part 312.[25]

If you really want to understand the two-page Form FDA 1572 in astonishing detail, a 134-page book, *The Form FDA 1572: A Reference Guide for Clinical Researchers, Sponsors, and Monitors*, is now available to answer even the most oddball questions.[26]

Your commitments to the FDA are listed in tiny print on the back of Form FDA 1572 (although you might expect the important stuff to be on the first page). Make sure you read them all because the obligations are real. Errors can result in your receiving warning letters from the FDA. Serious violations can result in your being prohibited from participating in further clinical trials. The final warning on the form is that "a willfully false statement is a criminal offense." So, when the sponsor conveniently presents you with a 1572 that is already filled out and ready for your signature, be sure to stop and read it.

IRBs

An institutional review board is a committee designated to review the participation of subjects in research studies. The IRB's responsibility is to oversee the ethical and safety aspects of the study and to decide what constitutes informed consent. Its members assess whether the foreseeable risks are reasonable compared to any potential benefit for the volunteer. The IRB must approve the protocol, the companion informed consent form, and all advertisements prior to their use. The IRB must also review each protocol annually, at a minimum. Furthermore, the IRB reviews all IND safety reports as well as trial outcomes at the study site and decides if any intervention is necessary.

The criteria for IRB structure include a minimum of five members with diverse backgrounds. There must be at least one layperson without a scientific background and one not affiliated with the investigator's institution. The members must not be all of one sex. Investigators may sit on an IRB, but they must then recuse themselves from participating in decisions on their own protocol. IRB members at hospitals may be appointed by the medical staff, as are other committees, or serve at the pleasure of the president of the medical staff or be appointed by the governing board of the hospital. The Principal Investigator does not make decisions regarding appointing members to the IRB.

IRBs may be commercial, centralized, and for-profit enterprises or nonprofit boards maintained by local hospitals or academic institutions. Commercial boards often are used for large trials that are conducted at multiple sites and might involve outpatient studies. They are convenient for both the individual sites and the sponsor, which can make one submission (of study-related materials requiring IRB approval) to cover all the participating sites. Sponsors are also guaranteed rapid turnaround for their submissions to a commercial IRB, and these IRBs have the advantage of being more experienced and often have access to a greater depth of expertise than local IRBs. A major advantage of using a central IRB is that the individual study sites are relieved of many of the administrative headaches and responsibilities as the sponsor will make submissions to the IRB for them.

The FDA, in the *Code of Federal Regulations* (21 CFR part 50), outlines specific parameters IRBs should consider when reviewing a protocol.[27] These considerations include the following:

- Is the use of humans in this trial relevant and appropriate?
- Does the design or conduct of the protocol raise any ethical concerns?

- Are the risks to volunteers minimized? These include emotional, financial, and legal concerns as well as the more obvious physical risks.
- Are the risks reasonable and proportional to any expected benefit?
- How are the subjects selected? Is this method equitable in regard to gender and race? Are vulnerable populations included (e.g., pregnant women, prisoners, children, those with decreased mental capacity, or those who are disadvantaged)? What safeguards are in place for their participation?
- Are provisions for monitoring safety adequate? Are side effects or risks described in the Investigator's Brochure noted in the informed consent agreement? If a washout period from previous medication is planned, what safeguards are in place for monitoring the subject during that time? How will worsening medical conditions be handled?
- What provisions are in place for confidentiality?

Further considerations, particularly for studies involving vulnerable populations, are noted on the University of Iowa's excellent Web site.[28]

IRBs came under considerable scrutiny and unfavorable publicity in 1998. Several oversight bodies—the President's National Bioethics Advisory Commission, the General Accounting Office (GAO), and the Department of Health and Human Services Office of Inspector General—all questioned the ability of IRBs to ensure volunteer safety. The National Institutes of Health (NIH) Office for Protection from Research Risks (OPRR) even went so far as to totally close down clinical research at several prominent hospitals, including Johns Hopkins University, Rush-Presbyterian-St. Luke's Medical Center, and Duke University—over this issue and the lack of adequate oversight.[29]

IRBs have enormous responsibility and often limited resources with which to make their decisions. Another problem facing them is that the committees are made up of members with diverse backgrounds. Understanding the science behind the protocols and evaluating safety data often appear to be unreasonable burdens on them. On the other hand, if an informed consent is written clearly, any reasonably educated person should be able to evaluate whether the protocol appears to be reasonable and ethical. As a result of the recent criticisms, IRB programs are being improved by ensuring more resources for the committees and more education for individual members. Public Responsibility in Medicine and Research (PRIM&R) and its affiliated organization, the Applied Research Ethics National Association (ARENA), are the major sponsors of education for IRB professionals. ARENA offers certification programs for IRB members and administrators.[30]

HIPAA

One of the most confusing areas for researchers and IRBs is that relating to the HIPAA rules. In 1996, Congress enacted the Health Insurance Portability and Accountability Act (HIPAA).[31] While the intent—allowing for the protection of individual personal health information—is noble, its implementation has been a bureaucratic nightmare. HIPAA enforcement is under the direction of the Department of Health and Human Services. Full details are available in the *Code of Federal Regulations* Title 45—Public Welfare—and are beyond the scope of this book.[32] Some aspects of the act affect the ability of investigators to do research and are detailed below. However, the government attempted to make a carve-out for researchers, having understood that clinical science would otherwise come to an abrupt halt.

The HIPAA privacy rules impose onerous new requirements on researchers. These requirements include petitioning the IRB for waivers to gather information preparatory to research (to ascertain if a proposed study can identify enough patients, for example), restrictions on subject recruitment, and limitations on data use.

The most important point is that requests to review records, to use "protected health information" (PHI), and to identify subjects (other than through self-disclosure) must all be approved by an IRB. Some hospital IRBs will waive some privacy requirements in order to help identify patients who might benefit from a new treatment. However, the customary practice at a number of institutions is that only a patient's personal physician can initiate contact with the patient about research; if the patient gives permission, then the coordinator or investigator can contact the patient, but not otherwise.* Other institutions have the patient sign a release on admission to that facility or

* According to the Privacy/Data Protection Project of the University of Miami Web page, "It is still permissible under HIPAA to discuss recruitment into research with patients for whom such involvement might be appropriate. This common practice is considered to fall within the definition of treatment. Typically such a conversation would be undertaken by one of the patient's regular health care providers . . . By contrast, a patient's information cannot be disclosed to a third party (even another care provider) for purposes of recruitment into a research study without an authorization from the individual or an approved waiver/ exception of authorization."

for use of its services as part of the release already in place allowing insurance companies access to information. Specific HIPAA consents are now required as part of the volunteer's informed consent for investigational studies. For a "HIPAA Consent Template," see http://conductingclinicalresearch.com.

Because of the considerable confusion that followed the new regulations, I prepared a simplified explanation of HIPAA for our hospital's staff: see the "Understanding HIPAA and Research Handout" at http://conductingclinicalresearch.com.

The most relevant points for researchers are excerpted here from the HIPAA regulations. The same sections are presented with more detail at http://conductingclinicalresearch.com: see "HIPAA Highlights for Researchers."

The Unexpected Toll of HIPAA

HIPAA has had several unintended consequences (beyond the nuisance factor), the most serious of which is its negative impact on research. While those of us in the trenches immediately and directly felt the burden, a new report from the Association of Academic Health Centers (AAHC), *The HIPAA Privacy Rule: Lacks Patient Benefit, Impedes Research Growth*, affirms our suspicions about its chilling effect on research.[33]

It was painfully apparent that HIPAA really hurt the number of volunteer referrals from my local hospital. For example, even when the IRB provided a carve-out allowing us to be alerted about potential patients for a sepsis study, many hospital staff members had knee-jerk "we can't tell you anything" reactions, fearing for their jobs and concerned about heavy financial penalties. Some resentful staff fomented misunderstandings about HIPAA seemingly deliberately as one way of derailing the study. Mostly, HIPAA caused rampant confusion that cost us a number of potential patients, which is especially painful given that qualified candidates were as rare as hen's teeth—as they often were for the studies I generally got asked to do.

The AAHC study confirms these subjective findings, giving further explanation. The HIPAA rules are unclear and are subject to misinterpretation. Many researchers don't understand that a waiver of authorization can be provided by the IRB. As the AAHC notes, "The fear of regulatory punishment is driving IRB, Privacy Officer and Organizational decision-making in clinical research."[34]

The fear of liability dissuades many other parties from supporting research and distracts everyone from the goal of helping to develop new treatments. In addition, valuable personnel time and money are wasted on the unnecessary and excessive new administrative burdens.

Other studies have also demonstrated the dramatic reduction in recruitment rates for research since HIPAA was introduced. One University of Pittsburgh study cited by the AAHC showed recruitment was slashed by more than 50 percent after HIPAA. Similarly, a University of Michigan study showed consents dropped from 96 percent to 34 percent after HIPAA.

The AAHC notes that besides limiting overall recruitment, HIPAA has had a particularly negative impact on minorities and less-educated volunteers, who may be intimidated or overwhelmed by the complexity of the regulations. "This negative impact on participant recruitment and the diversity of research participants has fundamentally changed the conduct of research. With a less diverse participant pool, the scientific credibility of research is at risk for the future," the report states.[35]

Sometimes it seems as if the only beneficiaries of HIPAA are insurers, from whom we ironically have no privacy. The AAHC report concludes, "Finally, the patient whom HIPAA is designed to protect does not appear to recognize, understand, or care about this complex law as it applies to research."[36]

In one of his provocative articles, Norman Goldfarb did an interesting review of the HIPAA complaints that were related to clinical research between 2003 and 2007. Of the 32,487 privacy complaints received by the Department of Health and Human Services during this period, guess how many were related to clinical research? A whopping 17! Goldfarb does some interesting math, concluding that "there is a 100- to 1,000-fold lower frequency of HIPAA complaints" for research than for regular patient care. He attributes this, probably rightly so, to the good subject-coordinator relationships that generally exist. Intriguingly, he also extrapolates that if obtaining a HIPAA consent takes 5 minutes and a research site's time is postulated as $60 per hour, this translates to at least $10 million per year spent just to obtain this cumbersome, and often misunderstood, authorization.[37]

A new report from the prestigious Institute of Medicine further expands on HIPAA's unintended interference with research and gives several recommendations. It suggests that a distinction needs to be made between "the unique needs of information-based research, which uses medical records or stored biological samples, and interventional clinical research, which involves people who participate in experimental treatment. Applying the same protections in these two fundamentally different scenarios is neither appropriate nor justifiable." The report further recommends that the Common Rule's human research protections be applied to interventional clinical research and that there be new federal oversight of information-based research.[38]

With the growing consensus gathered from clinical researchers, reviews of patient complaints, surveys of academicians, and the imprimatur of the nation's leading scientists that HIPAA is not only failing to provide any protection for clinical research subjects but is increasing research costs and probably reducing participation, we can only hope that reason will prevail and the HIPAA rules will be eliminated for clinical research.

"Minimum Necessary"

[45 CFR §§ 164.506, 164.502(b), 164.514(d)]

> ***General Requirement***
>
> *The Privacy Rule generally requires covered entities to take reasonable steps to limit the use or disclosure of, and requests for protected health information (PHI) to the minimum necessary to accomplish the intended purpose. The minimum necessary provisions do not apply to the following:*
>
> > *. . . Disclosures to or requests by a healthcare provider for treatment purposes.*[39]

Research (Guidance)

> *A covered entity may use or disclose PHI for research purposes pursuant to a waiver of authorization by an IRB or Privacy Board provided it has obtained documentation of all of the following:*

- *A statement that the alteration or waiver of authorization was approved by an IRB or Privacy Board . . .*
- *A statement that the IRB or Privacy Board has determined that the alteration or waiver of authorization, in whole or in part, satisfies the following major criteria:*
- *The use or disclosure of PHI involves no more than minimal risk to the individuals:*
  - *There is an adequate plan to protect the identifiers from disclosure.*
  - *There is an adequate plan to destroy the identifiers as immediately as is practicable, given the nature of the research.*
  - *There are written assurances that the PHI will not be disclosed to others*

- *The alteration or waiver will not adversely affect the privacy rights and the welfare of the individuals;*
- *The research could not practicably be conducted without the alteration or waiver;*
- *The research could not practicably be conducted without access to and use of the PHI;*
- *The privacy risks to individuals whose PHI is to be used or disclosed are reasonable in relation to the anticipated benefits, if any, to the individuals, and the importance of the knowledge that may reasonably be expected to result from the research.*[40]

Tutorials and documents regarding HIPAA are available from several excellent Web sites, such as those of the NIH; the University of California, San Francisco; and the University of Iowa.[41] See appendix B for further resources.

Drug Accountability

Recordkeeping for study drugs is akin to keeping track of narcotics; every dose must be accounted for. This is potentially a problem in that you, the investigator, are held accountable for the inventory even though you may never see or handle the drug if this is an inpatient study. If you are dispensing the drug from your office, you must make sure that you have secured storage facilities. Be sure, too, that you have considered any special storage requirements.

Be specific in verifying shipping. For example, note how many blister packs or vials of a drug are received and how many pills are in each vial. When volunteers return for follow-up visits, have the study coordinator review the pill count with them—this helps verify and encourage compliance as well as makes it easier to account for discrepancies. Have the patients return all unused supplies, even "empties," to check them against the dispensing logs.

View from the Trenches

During my fellowship, when we did a homemade, blinded, placebo-controlled study, we solved the drug tracking problem by working as a team, making little "seal-a-meal" packs and labeling each as they were completed, while one person watched to help provide verification.

It is particularly difficult to track medications in a blinded, double-dummy "look-alike" trial unless the sponsor provides the medications in blister packs for each patient. If you are dispensing medication yourself, prepare small packs ahead of time, each containing the active drug and the corresponding placebo—and never return a pill to the bulk supply, even if you think you know which group it came from.

On most studies, tracking supplies by a "balance on hand" log tends to be the easiest and most accurate method. (See the "Drug Accountability or Dispensing Log" at http://conductingclinicalresearch.com.) If you've tracked medications concurrently and accurately, your upcoming audit should be relatively pain free.

Financial Disclosure, or Whose Business Is It Anyway?

Since 1999, nongovernmental investigators have been required to disclose potential financial conflicts of interest both at the onset and at the conclusion of studies for either drugs and biologics or devices. The requirements are detailed in the 21 CFR 54 Financial Disclosure by Clinical Investigators.[42]

Before you commit to undertaking a clinical trial, understand that this financial information will be required. If you are offended by the intrusive questions, stop now. Also, be aware that the financial disclosure requirements might be the deal breaker in an agreement between you and a colleague you might have been planning to work with as a coinvestigator. My experience has been that physicians' perceived invasion of their privacy by this regulation has caused many to stop agreeing to be coinvestigators or even the emergency backup for drug studies. Even your coordinator, if listed on Form FDA 1572, is required to complete a financial disclosure. It's best to explore this issue upfront when you are making sure that you have adequate staffing for your studies. The financial disclosure also applies to the spouse and dependent children of the investigators, and disclosures continue for a year after the completion of a study.

By signing the financial disclosure form (Form FDA 3454), the investigator certifies that the following statements are true:

- The investigator and all subinvestigators named in item 6 of the 1572 have no significant financial arrangement with the sponsor where the study outcome could affect compensation.

- The investigator does not have a significant (more than $50,000) equity interest in the sponsor.
- The investigator does not have a proprietary interest in a related patent, trademark, copyright, or licensing agreement.
- The investigator (or the investigator's site) has not received more than $25,000 for consulting work, speaking engagements, equipment, new construction, or other compensation from the sponsor.[43]

Any potential conflict must be disclosed. If financial benefits in excess of the limits on the Form FDA 3454 are in play, a different form, Form FDA 3455, will need to be filed, detailing the financial arrangements between the investigator and sponsor.[44] (These forms are available from the FDA Web site, and they will be supplied to the investigator's site by the sponsor's regulatory department.)

Historically, some question of impropriety might have been triggered when a site received a piece of expensive equipment or capital improvements in lieu of payment. Thus Form FDA 3455 applies if the PI or other staff or the institution itself has any financial interest in the sponsor's company.

Financial disclosure is required for all studies filed under a U.S. IND application, even if the studies are carried out outside of the United States. In fact, foreign investigators must file financial disclosures, too.

In 2008, Norman Goldfarb filed a Freedom of Information Act (FOIA) request seeking information to analyze these sponsor-site financial relationships. Here are some of the findings from his report:

- Less than 2 percent of investigators disclosed financial conflicts of interest.
- A total of 26 (53 percent) of the New Drug Applications (NDAs) disclosed financial conflicts.
- Most of the conflicts of interest came from only a few sites: "Five (10%) of the NDAs accounted for 151 (67%) of the disclosed conflicts. One NDA accounted for 50 (22%) of the 226 disclosed conflicts."[45]

And yet failure to declare financial interests may result in an FDA audit and the exclusion of that investigator's data from the analysis and support for the NDA. So, the FDA wants to know about your business, not just to be snoopy, but also to help ensure that the data being analyzed in support of a new drug's evaluation are objective and not biased by potential financial gains for the investigator.

Audits

One of the things I've learned over the years is that there is a significant downside to performing research well and accruing stellar enrollment. One of the unadvertised special prizes is being awarded with audits.

A clinical study can undergo two kinds of audits, the in-house ones and the out-house ones. The former are conducted or contracted for by the sponsor. Sometimes they are used as in-house checks on the sponsor's own procedures and personnel, to confirm that everything is operating in a standard fashion. (For example, on one such audit, the auditors were somewhat surprised and concerned that the various CRAs did not have a uniform way of having the CRFs completed and there had therefore been many revisions and corrections because of the lack of internal consistency.) Audits can also be called for if a sponsor thinks the PI is not conducting the study properly.

KEY POINT
Careful drug accountability will save you from needing sedatives.

These internal audits are also, in a sense, a dress rehearsal for the "big time" external audits and are awarded to study sites with high enrollment, particularly on pivotal or primary efficacy studies—those whose results the company will use as part of its NDA application to the FDA.

Internal audits are not generally intended to be punitive. Rather, they are conducted by ever higher levels of obsessive-compulsive people, each double-checking that people in the lower echelons have done their bookkeeping jobs at least passably well.

FDA Audits

The FDA may conduct audits to ensure that patients' rights and safety are being adequately protected, that the study is being conducted in compliance with applicable regulations, or that the study data are valid. These external audits may involve a specific investigator or site, an IRB, a specific study, or a trial sponsor.

Your chance of being audited is higher now than it was a few years ago, under the Bush administration. From 2004 to 2008 the number of FDA inspections declined steadily from approximately 22,000 to 15,000 annually. At the same time, warning letters decreased from 725 to 445 and injunctions declined to just 5 in 2008.[46]

LEGAL LAND MINE
Audits target adherence to protocol and delegation.

During this period, the FDA became highly politicized, and more of its decisions came under attack than previously. Newly appointed FDA Commissioner Margaret Hamburg has vowed to increase effective FDA enforcement, including more regular and vigilant inspections, a greater focus on the most significant risks and violations accompanied by stronger penalties, a more rapid response, and a more visible response, to send a strong message confirming her intent.

It's easier to show attempts at being compliant with the regulations than to take corrective action in response to a negative audit. One way to show good faith is to seek accreditation from the Association for the Accreditation of Human Research Protection Programs (AAHRPP) because investigators who are accredited have a better record in FDA audits than those who have not taken this step. Another is to be proactive in setting up your own staff training, procedures, recordkeeping, SOPs, and quality assurance systems and to periodically assess ways you might improve your processes. Ongoing education is critical, as this field's requirements are rapidly changing. Be sure to document your efforts because if they are not written, they didn't happen. You might consider performing a mock audit on your own to validate your practice's procedures.

LEGAL LAND MINE
Make ongoing quality assurance a priority.

In 2007, another *Guidance for Industry* was issued by the FDA, with specific attention to the supervisory responsibilities of investigators. It contains two critical points. The first is "When tasks are delegated by the investigator, the investigator is responsible for providing adequate supervision of those to whom tasks are delegated and the investigator is accountable for regulatory violations resulting from failure to adequately supervise the conduct of the clinical study."[47]

LEGAL LAND MINE
The Principle Investigator is all-responsible.

Note that inappropriate delegation includes "Screening evaluations, including obtaining medical histories and assessment of inclusion/exclusion criteria, conducted by individuals with inadequate

Your compliance plan should address the following key questions:[48]

- Who is the responsible party? (Be sure to designate and provide detailed information on delegations of responsibility and authority.)
- Is there a consistent review mechanism and group to do reviews?
- What is your training for PIs? CRCs? IRBs? Other staff?
- How often do you perform risk assessments, looking at gaps in your procedures?
- How will you monitor for problems and implementation of correction plans?
- How will you ensure compliance (e.g., peer review or mock audit)?
- How is reporting—or the ever important paper trail—handled?

LEGAL LAND MINE
Document consent carefully.

medical training (e.g., a medical assistant)." It also includes "Informed consent obtained by individuals who lack the medical training, knowledge of the clinical protocol, or familiarity of the investigational product needed to be able to discuss the risks and benefits of a clinical trial with prospective subjects." I found this interesting because some of my colleagues had suggested that someone impartial and not involved with the investigation obtain consent from patients to avoid any possible appearance of conflict of interest. I responded that it would be absurd to have someone not deeply knowledgeable about the protocol try to obtain consent, which is more complex than reading a form to a patient. Our compromise: I had a nurse witness the consent process (not just the signing ceremony). I wanted to do this anyway, as the sepsis trials, in particular, enrolled only patients with a 40–50 percent predicted mortality. I wanted it very clear to patients and families that the patients might not do well, no matter what their decision.

If you don't have OCD and you're doing the assessments yourself, as I did, you must read this recent FDA guidance.[49]

If you are audited, it is now more important to respond to the findings promptly (within 2 weeks) because that is one of the FDA's increased areas of attention. When responding to allegations, focus not only on the specific complaint but also on the implications of the problem and the regulatory requirement that was not met. You should consider a root-cause analysis examining the systemwide problems that led to the adverse finding. FDA audit closeout reports will be posted on the agency's Web site, so it's critical to promptly respond with an action plan outlining corrective measures and the time frames for doing so.[50] Basically, the FDA conducts two kinds of audits: those that are routine and those that are "for cause."

Routine FDA Audits

Generally, the FDA gives 3–10 days advance notice for routine FDA audits. Routine site audits focus on a specific study rather than all protocols being conducted at a given site. These audits target the same sites the internal company audits do—those that have high enrollment or that are running pivotal primary efficacy phase 3 studies—the "make it or break it" trials.

The FDA generally conducts 225–250 of these audits of U.S. clinical investigators annually, 140 audits of IRBs, and fewer (28 in 2001) of sponsors or CROs.[51]

What will the FDA examine? FDA auditors will want to see the paper trail of the study, beginning with Form FDA 1572 and investigator clinical trial agreements. They will also want to verify oversight and review documents such as the protocol and any amendments, the informed consent forms, and CRFs. They will validate drug accountability records. IRB correspondence and approvals are likely to be examined, and the timely reporting of adverse events will be verified.

For case report forms, data will be compared with source documents (e.g., hospital or office charts) to make sure the data are accurate, legible, and contemporaneous. The auditor will look at the quality of supporting documentation and how corrections are made in CRFs.

When examining informed consent forms, auditors are likely to ask, Are all required elements included in the consent form? Did the IRB approve the consent? Did each participant sign and date the consent form himself or herself? Was the appropriate version of the consent form used for the subjects?

View from the Trenches

On my second internal audit, the inspector looked around my office at the rows of fat CRFs and directed his first question to me: How did you get all these patients?

I, ever tactful, sarcastically retorted, "What do you think? I made them up!"

Do not try this sort of mouthy response! These guys, too, appear to be humorless—an apparent occupational requirement. After he stopped gasping, the auditor did acknowledge the truth—that it would have been far more difficult to create these patients and the attendant source documents than to just do the work in actuality, as I had done.

Inspectors will also want to examine your SOPs manual. It is important to note how your practice will handle various procedures and demonstrate consistency, but your SOPs should not be so detailed as to readily get you hung for not following them. It's a rather delicate balance. Key SOPs include steps for obtaining and documenting informed consent, interacting with the IRB and handling protocol amendments and IND reports, handling adverse events, site monitoring, and handling the investigational drug and supplies.[52]

Auditors may also inspect facilities and staff at the study site. Study personnel may be interviewed. The drug storage area will be checked for appropriate temperature and security.

The auditors will also compare data and drug records from the sponsor and the study site. In addition to verifying the number of participants and the outcomes, the auditors will ask questions, such as, Was there bias in subject selection? Were all eligible participants entered on the study? Did subjects meet the inclusion criteria? Auditors will also verify drug administration and accountability, asking, Was the investigational medicine properly disposed of? Was the blind kept properly? Were the patients properly randomized?[53]

The most common FDA audit findings are errors in drug accountability logs, concomitant medication lists, failure to update Form FDA 1572, and transcription mistakes—innocent human errors that are inevitable in dealing with large amounts of data.

The most frequent serious problems cited in FDA audits of study sites include the following:

- Adverse events not reported or followed up on. (In the investigator's defense, adverse events are considerably easier to recognize in hindsight. They may appear to be insignificant at the time, especially if either the patient is terribly ill and on multiple other therapies, as is common with sepsis study patients, or if a concurrent outbreak of infection, such as influenza, occurs in the community.) Be sure you report adverse events, especially if serious, immediately. (See table 4.1.)
- Failure to promptly and properly inform the IRB of the updated data.
- Failure to account for all doses of the study drug.
- Absence of equipment necessary to conduct the study properly.

Table 4.1 Reporting of adverse events[54]

Event	Regulation	Who reports event?	To whom?	How fast?
AE related or probably related to drug	21 CFR 312.64	PI	Sponsor	Immediately if "alarming"
Serious AE, related, unexpected	21 CFR 312.32(c)	Sponsor	FDA and all PIs via IND safety report	
Unreasonable significant risk	21 CFR 312.56	Sponsor	IRB, PI, and other investigators	5 working days
Unanticipated problem or "adverse events that should be considered unanticipated problems."	21 CFR 56.108(b) (1), 21 CFR 312.53(c)(1) (vii), 21 CFR 312.66	PI	IRB	"Promptly" (undefined by FDA, 1 week recommended by Office for Human Research Protections (OHRP) if serious, 2 weeks if not)

- Failure to provide adequate supervision to staff. You are responsible for your staff members' training and actions. You cannot delegate some tasks to them, a big one being attribution of adverse event causality. They can be responsible for completing related sections of the CRF but not for making the assessments.[55]
- Arrogance and gross ignorance of regulations. An example is an investigator modifying the protocol without sponsor or IRB approval.
- Irregularities in the informed consent process or documentation of the consent. This is a huge focus of the FDA. If you are not using the most recent version of the informed consent, the FDA will nail you for not adequately informing the volunteers of risks. This mistake can easily happen when you are drowning in papers. Be sure you have a plan in place to address version control of consent forms and to update any study enrollment packets that you have previously prepared. If you find you used the wrong consent form, you must go back and get consent again from the patient, using the corrected and current version, and document when the patient consented again. If the consent changes for an ongoing study that patients are still on (perhaps a long-term study), also go back and get consent again from them, so you can be

LEGAL LAND MINE
Version control is critical on informed consent.

sure they have been apprised of all known risks and wish to continue their participation.[56]

- Fraud. According to Cullen Vogelson, 0.1–0.4 percent of all clinical research is conducted fraudulently, with either finances or academic advancements being the primary motivation.[57]

Error or Fraud?

Everybody makes errors, and though most times we don't intend to make them, the consequences can be serious. One example is that of signature errors, as well as the related but more complex issue of the signature as a reflection of informed consent.

While signature concerns usually center on informed consent, they can apply to other study documentation, such as medication administration or notes in source documents. Everything in medical trials is subject to audit and verification—that is why it is important to maintain a signature log for all study participants.

A terrific overview of some types of errors is provided by Stan Woollen. I love his hierarchy of the attribution of sins as due to

- Innocent ignorance
- Surprising sloppiness
- Malicious malfeasance

In terms of innocent ignorance relating to signatures, Woollen gives an example of an investigator misguidedly "backdating the subject's signature on a consent form because the subject forgot to date the form originally and the monitor is coming tomorrow!"[58]

Sometimes problems arise because volunteers are too ill to initial and date every page of a consent form. Commonly, patients ask site personnel to date the consent form for them. However, I explain that the FDA would be most disapproving if we "helped" and ask them to muster the strength to note the date. They have always obliged, although not happily.

Errors from innocence or sloppiness can occur when you have a volunteer sign the wrong version of a consent form, for example. In such cases, you can only document your explanation and any corrective action you take, such as having the volunteer reconsent. One ameliorating action is to be sure you write a progress note in the patient's chart documenting when consent was obtained. I usually also note the presence of any witnesses and ask hospital nurses to document their witnessing of the consent discussion, not just the signing ceremony itself.

The most dramatic errors are euphemistically called "malicious malfeasance" by Woollen but are more prominently reported in headlines as "investigator fraud." Sanofi-Aventis earned this unfortunate headline with its Ketek studies. Reading the notes from the Office of Criminal Investigations gives one a sort of perverse pleasure—and insight on the importance of accurate signatures.[59, 60]

While errors in the innocent ignorance and surprising sloppiness categories are understandable and perhaps forgivable, those in the malicious malfeasance category are neither understandable nor forgivable. All of us involved in clinical research can only hope that instances of such malfeasance are rare and are quickly uncovered and suitably corrected. Hopefully this will happen more readily with the commitment of the current FDA chief, Margaret Hamburg, to enforcement and restoring of the agency's credibility.

The Ketek scandal: malicious malfeasance

Anne Kirkman-Campbell, a Ketek study PI, enrolled 400 patients, forged consent forms, and faked the data. She ultimately pleaded guilty to mail fraud and received a sentence of 57 months in prison.

One of the pieces of evidence recounted by journalist Ed Silverman was that "patient consent forms had been signed every few minutes and, at times, when the office was closed."[61]

Each of these actions is shockingly egregious—and the false nature of the work was reportedly known to the sponsor, Sanofi-Aventis, which neither reported the fraud nor retracted the data. And then the fraudulent data were knowingly presented to the FDA, which approved the drug. Conscientious medical reviewers, such as Dr. David Ross, were allegedly threatened by then-FDA Commissioner Andrew von Eschenbach and were told not to express their opposition to Ketek's approval or they would be "traded from the team."[62]

Unfortunately, while it took years for this scandal to unravel, a number of patients died, and some fine and ethical FDA reviewers were forced from their jobs. This was a tremendous loss for patient safety—all for want of a valid signature. Monitoring of source documents, which detected the falsification of signatures, was one of the first clues in this sorry tale. Such a seemingly small and trivial detail, a signature, turned out to be the proverbial smoking gun.

For-Cause FDA Audits

On the other hand are the "for-cause" audits, such as that headlined in the 2001 news about a study at Johns Hopkins Hospital. In this case, a 24-year-old healthy volunteer, Ellen Roche, died as a result of participation in an asthma experiment in which she was exposed to an inhaled chemical irritant, hexamethonium. Numerous questions were raised, particularly about the adequacy of the oversight process. The Office for Human Research Protections (OHRP) temporarily shut down all studies at Hopkins.[63] For-cause audits may be precipitated by findings from an earlier routine inspection or from adverse publicity and media pressure. Similarly, eyebrows may be raised by surprisingly favorable data or unexpectedly high enrollment at a given site or by an investigator who conducts a large number of studies outside his or her area of expertise. These audits are not study specific and may encompass a broad review of many trials running at one site. For-cause audits are generally conducted without notice.

The FDA audit may result in the issuing of the dreaded Form FDA 483 to the investigator, a citation for sins committed or alleged. Findings cited on this form require an urgent response. The investigator will perhaps do best, in this case, to get advice from the more experienced CRO or sponsor as well as his or her attorney, as the stakes here are high.

Form FDA 483 is subclassified as follows:

- NAI—No Action Indicated
- VAI—Voluntary Action Indicated
- OAI—Official Action Indicated

NAI and VAI findings constitute about 91 percent of Form FDA 483 citations, and OAI constitutes about 9 percent (44 percent NAI, 52 percent VAI, and 3 percent OAI in 1999).[64] Although the numbers below are based on a relatively small sample, it is interesting to note that clinical investigators who are accredited by AAHRPP fare better in FDA audits than those who are not:

	NAI	VAI	OAI
Accredited	73%	27%	0%
Nonaccredited	53%	46%	<1%[65]

Consequences of adverse audits cover a spectrum from further investigation to warning letters to criminal prosecution, along with all the negative adverse publicity, humiliation, and unanticipated social or marital effects. One of the most serious consequences is that the investigator can be restricted in conducting further trials or debarred from participation at all and may never, ever, conduct a trial again. Blacklists of restricted and disqualified investigators are available from the FDA or on the Internet.[66] Rarely, an investigator might be fined or jailed.

Sponsor Audits

Sponsors may undergo similar inspections to those described above, and these are also likely to include comparisons of the sponsor's copy of the CRF to the sites' copies.

Sponsors are responsible for ensuring that they select investigators who are qualified by training or experience to investigate the drug. They are also responsible for ensuring that adequate monitoring is taking place.

A recently publicized case vividly illustrating this issue is the August 2009 warning letter issued by the FDA's Bioresearch Monitoring Program to Johnson & Johnson. The letter noted egregious breaches by the coordinator, astonishingly not detected by the monitor, including the following:

- Documentation showed administration of the study drug to multiple subjects at the exact same time.
- Subjects who did not meet eligibility requirements were enrolled in the study and given the drug.
- Documentation was poor, including the use of correction fluid to cover data.
- Significant discrepancies were found between the CRF and source documents.
- The unblinded site pharmacist did not receive baseline creatinine clearance in time to ensure appropriate study drug dosing calculations.[67]

The most serious implications for a sponsor are that a particular investigator's data are discarded, that the company's NDA review and approval processes are delayed, or that an NDA is not approved at all. Each of these outcomes is extraordinarily costly to the pharmaceutical company. Each day's delay is estimated to cost the company $1 million.

IRB Audits

Specific regulatory requirements are in place for IRB composition and function, outlined in 21 CFR part 56. Historically, the most common audit citations for IRB irregularities have been for

- Lack of a quorum
- Inadequate meeting minutes
- Lack of ongoing review and oversight of a study
- Lack of written SOPs and failure to follow SOPs[68]

In 2008, 52 percent of IRB audits resulted in No Action Indicated and 44 in Voluntary Action Indicated. In addition to the FDA audits of IRBs, civil suits have been brought against IRBs, as well as individuals, for negligence. The most recently well-publicized cases were *Gelsinger v. Trustees of University of Pennsylvania* and *Grimes v. Kennedy Krieger Institute.*[69, 70]

Because of the high rate of IRB errors found by FDA auditors and the increasing risk of civil suits, it might be prudent to have ongoing education for IRB members, including a formal orientation and instruction on GCP and human subjects protections (readily available at the NIH Web site).

International Audits

With the globalization of clinical trials and the increasing shift of many trials overseas, interest has developed as to how well different countries perform clinical trials. One study reviewed 3,178 FDA audits conducted between 1994 and 2004; 2,765 were conducted in the United States. The classification of No Action Indicated was made in 38 percent of the U.S. trials, a bit better than in other areas except central and eastern Europe (CEE). Official Action Indicated (OAI) notations ranged from none in CEE, Australia, and Canada to 2 percent of the U.S. inspections and up to 7 percent in western Europe and Latin America. These more serious offenses cited failure to obtain informed consent from patients or inadequate consent forms (16 percent); inadequate drug accountability (12 percent); failure to adhere to protocol, known as protocol violations (20 percent); and inadequate and incorrect records (21 percent). Interestingly, these patterns of deficiencies were generally similar regardless of the region. An exception was that in Asia, failure to report adverse drug reactions was more common (29 percent) compared to the other regions. The rate of problems with informed consent was also higher (21 percent) in Asia.[71]

How to Prepare for an Audit

First, remember to breathe in and out slowly. Then notify the sponsor and/or the CRO of the impending onslaught. A routine FDA audit is only for the specific study under inspection and some material, such as contracts and grant payments, are not included in the audit.

Perhaps the most important response that will lead to a good outcome is demonstrating your commitment to quality, reflected in your day-to-day operations and systems to monitor quality. It's tough to be retrospectively compliant (unless you employ the time warp feature you used in completing queries). So your staff should be prepared with materials, including the SOPs manual and regulatory binder, and consents. All staff members should be able to describe their job responsibilities and training and how problems are corrected.[72]

You should review your procedures at least annually and can even do your own mock audit. A handy masochist's FDA *Compliance Program Guidance Manual* is available at the FDA's Inspections, Compliance, Enforcement, and Criminal Investigations Web page. It includes rule books so anyone can play—sponsors, CROs, and monitors, too.[73] (If you want to have nightmares or see what may happen if you don't play by the rules, visit the Inspections, Compliance, Enforcement, and Criminal Investigations Warning Letters page at the FDA's site.)[74]

You can't wait until the last minute to produce all this documentation—you need to show that "quality improvement" reviews and training are an integral part of your practice. Dr. Janet Woodcock, of the FDA, summarizes it as "Say what you do, do what you say, prove it and improve it."[75]

Recipe for Preparation for an Audit

Ingredients to gather in preparation for an audit:

- *1 complete regulatory binder, including the current signed protocol, amendments, and current informed consent version*
- *SOPs manual*
- *All IND safety reports from the sponsor company and adverse event reports from the study site to the company*
- *All IRB correspondence and communications, including the original approval for the protocol and consent and subsequent renewals or changes*

- *Other regulatory documents, such as the signed Form FDA 1572*
- *Current CVs and licenses of all those listed on the 1572*
- *Monitoring logs*
- *Drug shipping and accountability records for the investigational medication*
- *Telephone logs and other correspondence*

  Do not add contracts or grant information. Do not forget to add large pinches of humor and patience, seasoning generously.

  Add liberal doses of help from CRO, sponsor, and friends, as the oven temperature may vary from day to day.

Before the audit, organize all study materials and documents:

- Make sure the regulatory binder is complete, with the current protocol, amendments, consent agreements, and safety information.
- List all study personnel and check the Delegation of Responsibility Log for completeness. (See the sample "Delegation of Responsibility Log" at http://conductingclinicalresearch.com.)
- Prepare a list of all the study subjects, and make sure that their informed consent agreements are available.

LEGAL LAND MINE
The threats of FDA inspections (including audits), debarment, financial sanctions, and possible criminal charges against the investigator all hold true for the IRB, site, and sponsor, with similarly huge stakes.

During the audit, be nice: not overly nice, but professional, polite, and cooperative. Provide the auditor or inspector with a place to work. Have medical records and source documents available. Do not volunteer information; just answer questions honestly and accurately. Confirm with the inspector what his or her expectations are for the meeting, and later, when responding, verify that your answers are satisfactory. If unsure of what is being requested, ask for clarification. If providing any documents, keep copies. Arrange to have a closing meeting to receive the inspector's feedback and clarify any outstanding issues. Limit your hospitality. Do not offer to buy meals or even so much as a cup of coffee; any offer might be misconstrued as currying favor. (See the "Preparing for an FDA Audit Checklist" at http://conductingclinicalresearch.com.)

When you receive the findings from the inspection, formulate your response carefully, simply listing each finding and your objective response, accompanied by the all-important Corrective and Preventive Action Plan (CAPA Plan).

Don't admit wrongdoing! Rather, focus on the regulatory requirement associated with the allegation and provide information as to how you have specifically modified your procedures. Be sure to keep the plan limited, focused, and realistic. Describe when the corrections will occur and how you will monitor for their effectiveness. An easy mnemonic to guide your response is "the FDA wants to hear your DRUMM"—that your response will be "direct, related, universal, management, and monitoring."[76] Then be sure you actually implement the plan, as the inspector will likely be back to confirm whether you have corrected your deficiencies.

Conclusion

Now you've seen the scariest parts of what you'll likely encounter if you undertake clinical trials. You have learned how to approach the regulatory maze and to anticipate and resolve potential problems, either with the drug company sponsor or with the regulatory agents. Let's move on to the details of implementing the study.

CHAPTER 5

Study Start-Up

> If you wish success in life, make perseverance your bosom friend, experience your wise counselor, caution your elder brother and hope your guardian genius.
>
> —JOSEPH ADDISON

When you start a study, a whirlwind of activities vies for your attention. Planning or theoretical considerations, an analysis of the logistics of implementing the protocol, and then the realities of the study in actual practice all demand your focus. As you gear up, there are just a few things remaining before you can finally enroll your first patient. You must prepare for the sponsor's initiation, or "launch," visit and draft, obtain approval of, and assemble the informed consent form and a plan for identifying and recruiting volunteers. You will then receive your supplies and complete your initiation visit. This chapter discusses how to perform each of these tasks.

Informed Consent—Safe, Sane, and Consensual

The informed consent is similar to a contract made between the study volunteer, the Principal Investigator, and the sponsor. It documents the volunteer's agreement to participate in the trial, undergo procedures, and receive treatments. All of the study procedures are explained in detail on the informed consent form. Each of the required elements on the form is intended to ensure the subjects' rights and to verify their understanding and agreement. The most important difference between a consent form and a contract is that the volunteer may opt out of participation in a study at any time, without any adverse consequences or penalties.

Informed consent is truly one of the most critical elements in conducting a study, and one that carries the gravest responsibility. Because of this importance, the PI should usually obtain the consent personally, although, on occasion, the PI can carefully review with a coinvestigator how to present the consent form to the volunteers. Most often, the drug company will provide a sample informed consent form. Many investigators prefer to write their own. Writing your own form is particularly useful if you are conducting several trials, as you can ensure that the consent forms are consistent in their format, which helps ensure that all points are covered. Writing your own informed consent agreement also enables you to tailor the language to the educational level and specific needs of your local volunteer population. The consent form must be written in simple, clear, understandable language.

KEY POINT
The informed consent form must be approved by both the sponsor and the IRB before being presented to the volunteers.

Avoid euphemisms. Doctors often use cheery euphemisms ("procedure" instead of "surgery," for example) to try to minimize anxiety for their patients, but if you're a clinical investigator it's critical to write consent forms that are clear and detailed.[1] In writing a good consent form, tell the volunteer the who, what, why, when, where, and how of participation, though not necessarily in that order. Regulatory agencies describe the elements more formally.[2]

The following elements of the informed consent agreement are required by the FDA and the International Conference on Harmonisation and are further detailed in the "Informed Consent Form Requirements Checklist" at http://conductingclinicalresearch.com:

- A statement that the study involves research
- The purpose of the research
- A description of the study procedures
- The time frame in which participation will occur

View from the Trenches

It's frustrating when a patient declines to participate in a trial because of fear, but then asks nothing and prefers to know nothing about his or her approved regular medicines that, in fact, may be more toxic than the investigational medicine. On the other hand, I remind myself that you can only explain things to a point. Because of education level, previous experiences, or fear, some patients will not have the perspective or the ability to make what appears to be the best choice about their care.

- A description of the procedures or treatments that are experimental
- A description of anticipated risks and discomforts, and a caveat that there may be significant unknown risks
- A description of what, if any, benefits might be reasonably expected
- Alternatives to participation that are available
- A confidentiality statement, explaining who will have access to the records and for what purpose
- An explanation of compensation (and limits) for treatment or injury
- Direction as to whom to contact for further information, including both the Principal Investigator and the IRB
- A declaration by the volunteer acknowledging that his or her participation is voluntary, that he or she is aware that no benefits will be lost should he or she choose not to participate, and that there is no penalty for early withdrawal from the study

Other elements are strongly suggested. The following elements are optional under the FDA regulations but are required by the ICH.

- An explanation that the volunteer may be dropped from the study without his or her consent, by the investigator or by the sponsor, should that appear to be in the volunteer's medical interest or should the study be terminated early
- A description of any costs that might be incurred by the volunteer

A humorous description of the informed consent, but with inappropriate enticements and promises that would never be allowed in a real consent, follows (to the melody of "The Music of the Night"):

Research sharpens, heightens each sensation
Placebos stir and wake imagination
Silently the senses abandon their defenses

Slowly, wryly the drug unfurls within you
Feel it, sense it, know that it will heal you

Turn yourself away from the treatment of the day
Turn your thoughts from old well-meaning friends
And listen to the promises I bend

Take your health on a journey through a brave new world
Leave all the fear you knew before
Let our drug take you where you long to be
Only then can you belong to me

Floating, falling, sweet intoxication
Touch it, taste it, savor this sensation
Let the trip begin, let your pain and fear give in
To the truth of the promises I give
The promise of a longer life to live.[3]

- An assurance that the volunteer will be informed of significant new findings during the study that might affect his or her decision to continue participation
- A statement that the volunteer has received a copy of the informed consent document

Table 5.1 presents a summary of the important differences between FDA and ICH-GCP guidelines about informed consent.

Several universities, such as the University of Michigan and the University of Southern California, and other organizations offer sample informed consent forms on their Web sites.[4] You'll find a more complete list of resources in appendix B and informed consent form elements in the "Informed Consent Form Requirements Checklist" at http://conductingclinicalresearch.com.

In writing your consent form, use short words, short sentences, and bulleted lists. Avoid multisyllabic (like this) words, conceptual terms ("normal range," "incidence," "condition has stabilized"), category terms ("ACE inhibitor," "H2 blocker"), and value words ("excessive," "regularly"). Longer entences should be broken down into small sections, using commonly understood terms—such as *throw up* instead of *vomit*, *pee* instead of *urine*, *draw blood* instead of *venipuncture*. Sample phrases and lists of synonyms are available on the Internet to help you write your consent form.[5] Federal guidelines say that patient material must be written at no higher than a fifth-grade level, so test the readability of your consent. Besides the Flesch-Kincaid test used in Microsoft's grammar checker, the SMOG (Simplified Measure of Gobbledygoop) test is easy to use and is recommended.[6]

The "Informed Consent Form Template" available at http://conductingclinicalresearch.com includes all the elements required by the ICH and the FDA.

You must obtain informed consent before performing any study procedures, including screening laboratory studies or procedures.* You must also now

* Some sponsors and state laws allow you to obtain informed consent before a potential volunteer actually meets all of the strict inclusion or exclusion criteria for a trial; others do not. This permission is useful in cases where the enrollment might depend on an intraoperative finding, for example, and the patient would not be able to consent at that time because of sedation or ventilatory support. It is also especially useful in sepsis trials, where a patient's condition might be expected to worsen, and anticipatory consent would make sense—again because the patient might not be able to consent at the time enrollment criteria are met. If you receive anticipatory consent, you should document it (assent) and reaffirm consent when the patient regains the ability to make such decisions.

Table 5.1 Battle of the regs[7]

Issue	FDA	ICH-GCP guidelines
Who can obtain informed consent?	No clear regulation	PI can delegate
Copy to patient?	Yes, but need not be signed	Yes, signed and dated by person obtaining consent
Impartial witness	Not required except for short form (oral presentation)	Always required
Consent elements		
Risks and benefits of alternative treatment	No	Yes
Probability of random assignment	No	Yes
Subject responsibility	No	Yes
Who can access medical records?	FDA	Many—foreign regulatory agencies
Second-party consent information level?	Not specified	Unknown
Compensation for injury	Studies involving greater than minimal risk	All studies
Informing of PCP?	No	Yes
Protocol		
Identification of what data are to be recorded directly on CRF as source document	No	Yes
Sponsor		
Notification to PI as to when records can be destroyed?	No	Yes
Indemnification of investigator or provision of insurance?	No	Yes
Disclose financial COI	Yes	No
IRB		
PI statement that IRB is ICH compliant?	No	Yes

document in the medical records (e.g., in the progress notes) the fact that consent was obtained before study procedures were performed.[8] If your IRB has granted a Waiver of Authorization, you are allowed to screen medical records to identify subjects and determine their eligibility for a trial and then approach the patients to obtain their consent for participation. Otherwise, the informed consent is supposed to be obtained after it is determined that a patient meets all inclusion and exclusion criteria and will be enrolled. The footnote on page 150 explains the exception to this rule.

KEY POINT
Be certain to obtain informed consent before doing any study procedures!

Other tips for documenting that consent was obtained properly are listed here:

- Patients must sign and date the informed consent form themselves. This is a cumbersome but important detail.
- The patient must receive a copy of his or her informed consent form.
- Though not required by the FDA or the ICH, for your own protection you should have an objective witness who is not your employee present when the patient signs the consent form (e.g., a hospital's RN). You should document all of the consent process in the patient's medical record.
- Since documenting consent is so critical, you should keep a second copy of the patient's informed consent form at a different location.

Informed consent has always been a favorite target or focus point for FDA audits, with errors found in more than 50 percent of audited clinical trials.[9] In light of recent well-publicized deaths on clinical trials (e.g., healthy volunteer Ellen Roche at Johns Hopkins Hospital and Jesse Gelsinger in the University of Pennsylvania's gene therapy study, discussed further in chapter 8), consent procedures will likely receive even closer scrutiny.

We have seen some new trends in obtaining informed consent, and new guidance is reportedly on its way. Consent forms have become more complex—no surprise given our litigious climate—often now reaching 10 pages or more. Some are suggesting the use of a more focused form, the ABC model. Part A contains the essential elements, including risks and benefits and alternatives, and should be no more than two pages. B gives the details. C verifies consent. This model enables volunteers to focus on the most important elements first, before they lose attention or become overwhelmed.

Withdrawal of consent is becoming a hot issue and is receiving increased attention because of the implications for privacy and for profit. As part of the HIPAA regulations, volunteers can withdraw authorization to use data *that have not already been submitted to the sponsor.* That's the key element and reportedly a major driving force behind the shift to electronic data capture.

Plan for stages or levels of withdrawal of consent. Otherwise, you won't be able to use any of a patient's data. If patients don't want to continue therapy and test procedures, ask if they will still allow use of their data and contact for limited telephone follow-up.[10]

Subjects can also withdraw permission to use samples of their blood or tissue. This has become an issue because some sponsors are deriving large profits from patients' tissue specific cell lines, for example. (See chapter 8 for more about ethical issues.)

HIPAA confidentiality language actually works in patients' interests in one way: it specifies that test results obtained only for research will not be part of a patient's record. This is useful so that patients won't lose insurance because of an abnormal lab result, but it is a logistical nightmare because research lab reports need to be kept separate and may be overlooked. This also means that research labs should be kept as a separate or outside account to reduce billing errors and the chance that a result might end up on the patient's hospital chart.

Remember, both the sponsor and the IRB must approve the informed consent form. Here is a creative example of an IRB rejection:

"Unapprovable" (to the tune of "Unforgettable")

Unnn-approvable
That's what they say
It's un-doable
In short, no way.
My consent form was too technical
The benefits were theoretical
They sent me to see
Some guy, (insert your choice) . . .

Expeditable
That's what I thought
I'm indictable
If I get caught
I say goodbye to my relations
If I don't follow the regulations
Then my pardon
Will be unapprovable, too.[11]

Health Literacy and Informed Consent

The preceding several years have seen both increasing globalization of clinical trials and an increase in outreach to minority groups in the United States. Mandates require that minorities be specifically recruited as subjects for research, yet at the same time obtaining consent has become increasingly difficult. In the United States, a new emphasis has been placed on health literacy in a broad range of medical encounters. Why the change? More mandates, of course.

On August 11, 2000, President Clinton signed Executive Order 13166, "Improving Access to Services for Persons with Limited English Proficiency."[12] And with this comes another Guidance, the Guidance Document of the U.S.

Department of Justice, "Enforcement of Title VI of the Civil Rights Act of 1964—National Origin Discrimination against Persons with Limited English Proficiency" (LEP Guidance). Under federal antidiscrimination laws, any agency that receives federal funding must implement a system to serve the needs of LEP individuals.

A common misconception is that most illiteracy is found in groups of immigrants, minorities, and the poor. In fact, the majority of low-literacy patients are Caucasian and native born, although the percentage of illiteracy is higher in other ethnic groups. The IOM estimates that 90 million people in the United States have limited health literacy, which includes not just the ability to read and write but also the ability to obtain, process, understand, and appropriately act on the information provided.[13]

In a 2002 survey, 21 percent of adult Americans were functionally illiterate (read at a fifth-grade level or lower), with 60 percent being over 60 years old. An additional 25 percent were marginally literate. The illiteracy rates are probably worse now.[14]

Health literacy, or lack thereof, is pertinent to a wide range of clinical trial activities. In an often-cited white paper, the Joint Commission reported that 44 percent of patients who signed an informed consent form did not know the exact nature of the operation to be performed, and 60 to 70 percent did not read or understand the information on the form.[15] Health literacy is also shaped by beliefs that derive from cultural, social, and family influences and evolve over time. An in-depth, highly recommended review is the IOM's report *Health Literacy: A Prescription to End Confusion.*[16]

KEY POINT
Cultural competency (or sensitivity) applies when dealing with immigrants or any special population.

An excellent tutorial from the University of Virginia's Claudette Dalton provides a variety of examples of where illiteracy causes medical encounters to go awry. For instance, she notes that while 50 percent of all patients make medication errors, such errors happen five times more often with illiterate patients. She reports that "*literacy is the single best predictor of health status—better than educational level or other demographics.*" Lack of compliance may thus be due to an inability to read the instructions rather than a behavioral or attitudinal problem. Patients may be unable to make or keep appointments or navigate from one department to another for scheduled procedures. Dalton emphasizes that diabetics (who are a large proportion of our patients) may have particular problems with literacy—because of retinopathy, because of the complexity of their disease, and because the ability to remember information varies with an individual's current blood glucose level. Furthermore, there is an association between literacy problems and health outcomes: literate patients had an average HgbA1c (an indicator of blood sugar control over time) of 7.2 percent; the illiterate patients had an average of 9.5 percent.[17]

Dalton relays other generalizable suggestions. Some are techniques for assessing literacy that help avoid embarrassment, pertinent for all our healthcare encounters. For example, rather than asking directly, "Can you read?" you might screen all patients by asking "How do you get your information?" or "What things do you like to read?" or "How satisfied are you with how you read?" Similarly, staff might be encouraged to offer help in completing registration forms.

Using models or sketches ("cued" literacy) can help considerably in explaining procedures. Clip art is widely available and easily recognized. In written materials, use simple phrases and start with the most important information first. Some advise putting the risks and benefits on the first page of consent forms, in simple bullet points, followed by the cumbersome details. In addition, color coding medications can help improve compliance, as can linking taking medications with some other part of the patient's routine.

If you are working with many non-English-speaking or LEP patients, it is imperative that you have a trained interpreter available. Don't rely on the patient's family for translation. You also need to have a consent form in the patient's native language. Ideally, the consent should be from a certified translator.

In terms of instructions, rather than asking "Do you understand?" (which will almost inevitably be answered yes) or other yes/no questions, have the patient repeat back the instructions. Multiple studies show the efficacy of this "teach back" technique in improving understanding and compliance, as well as reducing cost. And surprisingly, little additional time is involved. Have patients repeat each major point in their own words. Be sure you do this for the risks, benefits, alternatives, and procedure, and then be equally certain that you document this. The National Quality Forum has emphasized this as a critical safety step for any informed consent, not just for research. Its Safe Practice Standard 10 is "Ask each patient or their legal surrogate to recount what he or she has been told during the informed consent discussion."[18]

One exciting development is a multimedia patient education and informed consent program. Such an interactive program has been shown to improve comprehension, understanding of risks, and patient satisfaction. This type of program is invaluable in risk management because the audit trail of patient responses captured provides good evidence of consent.[19, 20]

One such solution (which I've not yet seen in action to directly verify) reportedly has the following elements:[21]

- The electronic informed consent has audio and visual components, all IRB approved. Video graphics can be embedded to explain various procedures. Multimedia consents have been shown to improve comprehension compared to paper-based forms.[22]
- Security for volunteers is achieved by having them create their own passwords using a color-coded keyboard. Crayons and paper enable them to record their password for themselves.
- The system's auditing functions show how long a subject stayed on each section of the consent, which is useful for refining the site's procedures and better understanding enrollment barriers.
- Thumbprints are used for volunteer e-signatures.
- Versioning controls provide alerts regarding the need to get consent again from subjects.
- Importantly, the interactive voice response system (IVRS) system will not allow a patient to be randomized to a study drug if the consent is not completed.

We've seen how challenges in obtaining informed consent are evolving as demographics change and clinical trials enroll a wider range of participants. Fortunately, we also seem to be seeing some very innovative and elegant approaches to meeting these challenges.

Cross-Cultural Issues in Informed Consent

A variety of cross-cultural issues affect informed consent. Obstacles include the need to build a collaborative relationship between people with different cultural backgrounds and interpretations and to develop an infrastructure, including an IRB, specialized informed consent procedures (translation, multimedia formats), data collection and management systems, and research protocols that are feasible in local, often much less technologically advanced, settings. Anthropologists note that even the words "research" and "consent" have widely different interpretations.

A particularly illustrative example of cultural issues is given by Vincanne Adams and her colleagues, who looked at a trial comparing misoprostol to a traditional Tibetan treatment for postpartum hemorrhage. First, the clinical researchers' work required fluency and literacy in English, Tibetan, and Mandarin—and there was a limited pool of such highly trained people to work on this project. Also, Tibetan medicine practitioners' decisions regarding therapy include evaluating a patient's cultural and even spiritual factors, reflecting profound and basic differences from the Western practices.[23]

Other difficulties were encountered as well, including establishing an IRB, and developing an informed consent form. Conceptual problems occurred with regard to randomization, blinding, description of the risks involved, use of a placebo, standardization of the comparator drug, and creation of a "no medicine" group. The Western interpretation of these elements was often viewed as unethical by Tibetans and had to be modified.

In other cultures, practices such as phlebotomy may pose a hurdle. Protocols may have to limit certain procedures because people of some cultures, such as Maori, believe that drawing blood is "taking away the life force." Consents may have to specify that tissue and body fluids will be accorded special ritual handling.[24]

Maori culture also includes the belief in a collective accountability. Participation in and details of protocols must have approval from a subject's extended family, subtribe and tribe, or advisory team members.[25] This issue also raises questions about the voluntariness of an individual's participation. Similar practices are common in many African cultures.

KEY POINT
You may need to provide considerable education in research ethics, be flexible in negotiations, and provide ongoing education for local investigators, IRBs, and communities.

Documentation of consent was an issue in Adams's study, as it is in many other settings where researchers are working with an illiterate population.

For further discussion of related topics, please see chapter 9.

Start-Up in Theory

The enrollment phase is akin to a racetrack with competitors lined up at the starting line. Often there is a scramble (and perhaps a stampede) to enroll patients rapidly. Several reasons contribute to this urgency, mostly related to cost; a slow start is costly for both the site and the sponsor.

The Sponsor

The sponsor experiences considerable pressure to beat the competition, especially for drugs that are the first in their class and will therefore have an edge on publicity, name recognition, and prescription writing habits and will become the standard drug for any further comparator entries. All of these factors will obviously boost sales enormously as well as maximize the time before the drug patent expires.

Drug companies are almost always behind on their time lines. They also want you, the study site, to commit only to them. On the other hand, sponsors have little or no loyalty to your site and might "end the marriage" at any point, leaving your site in the lurch with neither options nor "alimony." This is most likely to occur if your enrollment is significantly lower than that for which you have contracted. Your involvement may also be ended if the patients you enroll are not helpful for their application—if too many patients are not evaluable (e.g., if no bugs are isolated on an infectious disease trial, which means that the subject is therefore not microbiologically evaluable), if follow-up is poor, and so on.

The Investigator

From the investigator's perspective, delays are also quite costly. Enrollment is generally quite competitive and limited. Rather than contracting for a specific number of patients from a given site, sponsors close enrollment when they reach the target number of patients for a trial. Your administrative investment is roughly the same whether you recruit one or many patients. In addition, you need to recoup up-front staffing and supply costs, as they are not yet specifically reimbursed from the pharmaceutical company (and most likely never will be). Sponsors may also offer incentives to meet enrollment goals by a specific target date. I recommend avoiding this kind of arrangement unless the target population is extremely limited and well defined, as it may be too tempting for most investigators, and it encourages abuses.

While you should not intentionally contract for competing studies, the lead time is such that you need to plan for your future productions, trying to forecast at least 6–12 months in the future so that as one study ends, another will be ready to fill the gap. When the sponsor of the new study then delays start-up, often by 6–12 months, studies may overlap. When a company asks you to commit to a start-up by date X, it is safe to assume that, in fact, the study will not be ready to start for a minimum of 4 months after that time.

This is like safe sex. Learn to protect yourself. Plan for your future; no one else will. Perhaps that is why this phase is known as "initiation."

Start-Up in Practice: The Paper Trail—Implementing Regulatory Details

By the close of the initiation visit, the CRA will want to ensure that the regulatory (or study) binder, the primary organization system for regulatory documents, is set up correctly and that the coordinator knows how—and why—to maintain it. Study binders are generally provided by the pharmaceutical company and are intended to hold all of the regulatory documents in one repository. They generally contain sections for the following documents:

- Signed study protocol and amendments
- Investigator's (investigational drug) Brochure
- Form FDA 1572
- CVs for all personnel listed on Form FDA 1572
- Approval letter from the institutional review board and all IRB correspondence
- All IND safety reports and acknowledgment of their receipt by the IRB
- Site safety reports to the IRB
- Informed consent form approved by the IRB
- Copies of advertisements and their approval by the IRB
- IRB membership list
- Investigational drug inventories and shipping logs
- Telephone logs
- Copies of lab certification and lab normals or reference ranges
- Study closeout letter

- Visit logs for the CRAs to sign and date to document their visits

A more complete "Regulatory Binder Contents Checklist" and sample forms are available at http://conductingclinicalresearch.com.

The CRA (monitor) will often check the regulatory binder's completeness at each visit, and he or she will carefully note any deficiencies at the closeout visit, which you will need to correct. While keeping the binder current is tedious, it really is helpful to have all the documents together as a ready reference. Note, too, that during an audit, comparisons are likely to be made between the study site's records and those of the sponsor.

The CRA will also introduce the case report form (CRF) at the initiation visit. The CRF is a notebook that attempts to capture all of the relevant data for an individual study subject—including the patient's history and course on a trial—in a format that can then be entered into a database for analysis. The study coordinator (or other designee) transcribes the data from hospital medical records, office records, lab and x-ray results, and worksheets, onto two-part or three-part carbonless forms that are coded. No personally identifiable information may appear on these forms. You can find an example of a "Case Report Form" at http://conductingclinicalresearch.com.

The CRF should be used to collect the data necessary to meet the objectives and end points of the protocol and, in sequence and essence, it should mimic the actual protocol. At subsequent monitoring visits, the monitor will collect one copy of each CRF, after comparison and verification against the source document, or original medical records. Someone then transcribes the data again and enters them into the CRO's or sponsor's computer program. Increasingly, sponsors are turning to electronic data capture to eliminate this cumbersome transcription step.

Initiation Visit

As you prepare to launch your trial, the sponsor will again visit your site. This occurs after the study site receives supplies and before enrollment begins. In many ways, this visit is a recap of the site qualification visit, which probably occurred months earlier and whose details have been long forgotten. The protocol inclusion and exclusion criteria, study activities, and procedures are reviewed at the site by the sponsor's monitors. The sponsor highlights any changes that have been made because of concerns raised at the investigator's meeting, because of your reality testing, or because somebody has cold feet about specific aspects of the trial. Volunteer recruitment strategies may be reviewed. The CRA may help identify pools of potential patients as well as suggest strategies to avoid bias in patient selection, which would make the study results data worthless. The monitor will again review good clinical practice guidelines. Also, this is a good time to make a contingency list of whom to call when the inevitable problems arise (see "Contact Worksheet for Sponsor and Vendors" at http://conductingclinicalresearch.com).

Electronic Medical Records

In chapter 4, we saw the major push from government and insurers to have all providers use electronic medical records (EMRs). Some of the new initiatives are laudable, like the Health Information Technology for Economic and Clinical Health Act (HITECH Act) and Clinical Research Information Exchange (CRIX), especially with their focus on improving the infrastructure needs of research.[26] EMRs have advantages for research, particularly for timely recognition of adverse events that might otherwise remain undetected in postmarketing surveillance. For example, the International Serious Adverse Events Consortium (SAEC) has announced a valuable project with the HMO Research Network to identify patients with genetic mutations that are associated with specific serious adverse events.[27] Similarly, data mining of extensive primary care medical records in England analyzed with a new technique to reduce confounding (prior event rate ratio) was said to be as useful as randomized controlled trials in assessing drug efficacy. A similar study from the University of Pennsylvania also raises the possibility of using such extensive data analysis to supplant the need for some clinical trials.[28]

EMRs have the particularly promising potential to help identify and recruit study participants. Inclusion and exclusion criteria are becoming increasingly restrictive, resulting in expected accrual rates of less than one patient per month on many trials for even common illnesses. However, lab data can be successfully and efficiently used to screen large numbers of prospective patients.

For example, University of South Carolina researchers screened 7,296,708 lab results from 69,288 patients, identifying 70 potential candidates who met automated criteria, 3 of whom ultimately participated in the trial. Since current research regulations preclude a third party from alerting an investigator about a potential study volunteer without that patient's advance consent, however, the researchers developed a compliant but convoluted work-around with the IRB. If the lab identified a potential subject, the ordering physician was notified of the patient's potential eligibility. Then the ordering physician had to decide whether to make the effort to contact the patient to obtain permission to contact the clinical trial staff and then to follow through.[29]

Similar electronic screening has been done with alerts by diagnosis or by pharmacy orders. This type of procedure for contacting patients is a cumbersome and time-consuming one. In my setting, it would be unworkable for a variety of reasons, including the uncompensated time of the primary physician, the hassle factor, and the narrow time window for enrollment on trials for acute infections. In addition, many physicians are not familiar with either the needs of research or the benefits to their patients.

Screening health information is also particularly promising at sites that conduct multiple trials because it can alert investigators to multiple opportunities and guide patients to the most appropriate study. When health information technology is used to screen for potential patients, the personal touch is critical in obtaining consent and enrollment. One solution to the various obstacles is to incorporate alerts about possible clinical trials into the EMR used at the time of a patient's encounter with a physician. This method has the advantage of reminding physicians about trials while minimizing the additional work for them. It also overcomes HIPAA concerns because the physicians communicate directly with their patients, and it increases the likelihood of enrollment because having their doctors' recommendation has been shown to be a key factor in volunteers' decision to participate. Furthermore, screen prompts help guide physicians through verifying that the eligibility criteria have been met. If a patient is agreeable, a referral order is generated in the electronic order entry, sending a message to the study coordinator with permission to do further chart review and contact the patient.[30]

However, EMRs also pose unique problems for research. Privacy issues have received the greatest attention. These affect researchers' ability to review records, recruit patients, and monitor study participants. Confusion also results from the different consent requirements of different groups and because the standard consent clause that allows the sponsor's representatives to review the records does not meet the HIPAA rule's requirements.

The FDA has issued regulations and recommendations regarding electronic records: first, 21 CFR part 11, Electronic Records; Electronic Signatures; Final Rule (1997); then the clarification in the Guidance for Industry, 21 CFR part 11, Electronic Records; Electronic Signatures—Scope and Application (2003); and, most recently, the Guidance for Industry, Computerized Systems Used in Clinical Investigations (2007).[31, 32] (Remember that guidances are FDA recommendations, not regulations.) Electronic source data still have to meet the ALCOA elements (attributable, legible, contemporaneous, original, and accurate) expected of paper source documents so the FDA can verify all data submissions.[33] Security safeguards are also required with limited, password-protected access and audit trails of the access and any data changes.[34]

The OHRP recently extended privacy rules to "research" done as part of infection control and quality improvement activities. In an irrational and counterproductive move, it closed down research at Johns Hopkins University and a network of hospitals throughout Michigan regarding the use and efficacy of a checklist in reducing life-threatening hospital-acquired infections. The data from each hospital were deidentified before being sent to Hopkins for analysis, yet the OHRP ruled that individual consents were required. An excellent and scathing review by Dr. Atul Gawande noted, "The government's decision was bizarre and dangerous. But there was a certain blinkered logic to it, which went like this: A checklist is an alteration in medical care no less than an experimental drug is. Studying an experimental drug in people without federal monitoring and explicit written permission from each patient is unethical and illegal. Therefore it is no less unethical and illegal to do the same with a checklist. Indeed, a checklist may require even more stringent oversight, the administration ruled, because the data gathered in testing it could put not only the patients but also the doctors at risk—by exposing how poorly some of them follow basic infection-prevention procedures."[35] The OHRP ultimately overturned its ruling on February 14, 2008, but not before having wreaked havoc and further muddying the question of when IRBs can waive consent requirements.

EMRs also pose problems for monitors, both because the monitors have limited access to data stored electronically and because of problems verifying that the data have not been altered. The electronic date and time stamped audit trails are important here. While log-on names and passwords are not supposed to be shared, this is probably commonly done during monitoring visits since there is no other practical way of getting timely access to read-only records for the monitor. Sometimes, EMRs are printed out and "certified" as being accurate source documents.

So on the one hand, we have the push from the government and insurers to have electronic medical records and health outcomes research (HITECH Act), the Sentinel Initiative for postmarketing surveillance of electronic medical records for adverse events, and Medicare reimbursements linked to "meaningful use" (i.e., providing data) of the EMR. On the other hand, we have the specter of HIPAA and more draconian penalties for breaches of personal privacy. Ironically, health insurers are the most likely to abuse personal health information by asking intrusive questions and denying claims or care. Hopefully, the benefit of allowing access to medical records for research, given appropriate safeguards regarding privacy and permissions for reuse, will gain broader acceptance and boost the current dismal participation rate of less than 5 percent.

KEY POINT
Be sure your IRB approves any review of medical records for study recruitment.

The focus now shifts to scrounging patients, an issue that everyone wants to have done yesterday or, better yet, the day before yesterday.

Volunteer Recruitment Strategies

Often, the most difficult—and expensive—part of a trial for the investigator is that of recruiting your patients. For the sponsor, this phase accounts for 27 percent of the clinical costs of drug development, which translates to almost $2 billion per year.[36] Part of the problem is that the FDA is requiring more specific patient selection criteria to meet statistical end points and prove drug efficacy. At the same time, multiple companies are looking to recruit patients from the smaller pools. For the study site, this is also quite expensive, as you may need to screen 10–20 patients to find 1 who matches the enrollment criteria. Sponsors generally do not adequately reimburse the sites for screening. Once you identify potential participants, you still need to obtain their agreement to participate via the informed consent.

Identifying Potential Volunteers

The first goal in recruiting volunteers is to identify and define your target population. Are they inpatients or outpatients? Acutely ill or not ill at all?

Once you have defined your target population, you are ready to recruit. Some general recruitment strategies are to

KEY POINT
Build a broad network of helpers throughout the institution to identify potential volunteers.

- Recruit from your own practice.
- Ask for referrals from colleagues.
- Review computerized databases (e.g., hospital records) or lab results pertinent to your study, admission diagnoses logs, surgical schedules, and so forth. You now need IRB approval to do this.
- Investigate community support groups.
- Advertise.

The approaches you use for identifying potential volunteers depend on your setting and the type of protocol you are recruiting for. As you design your strategy, you will find it useful to remember the "Social Marketing Approach" described by Linda Lillington: "Identify and understand 'target populations,' including: insight into what they value, where to reach them, how to speak a language they understand for the purpose of making them an 'offer' that they may consider important." Ms. Lillington aptly notes that "any given clinical trial is . . . an 'offer' that has both perceived 'costs' and perceived 'benefits' which are identified through target population research for the purpose of developing and positioning the 'offer' effectively."[37]

Incentives to Patient Recruitment, or Why Would Someone Want to Participate in a Research Study?

People choose to participate in a clinical trial for a variety of reasons. You should consider several factors when you are deciding how to approach recruiting someone, including the following:

- Personal implications of the disease (i.e., will this trial help the person or his or her children or not be personally useful?)
- How to "pitch" the protocol in terms the person will understand and relate to

During the enrollment process, the investigator should strive to understand a particular patient's reasons for volunteering. Why should this person want to participate and help you? This is important in assessing whether the patient can truly understand and give informed consent as well as whether participation is really voluntary or is due to inapparent coercion. What are the perceived costs and benefits to the volunteer? Some reasons for being on studies might include

- Access to novel therapies where no therapies currently exist (e.g., therapies for septic shock or inborn errors of metabolism). Such access was noted to be the major incentive for patients surveyed recently.[38]
- Access to expertise that would not otherwise be available (but be certain that you are not being coercive; see "Ethical Principles" in chapter 8).
- Closer medical monitoring: While in many cases it is true that patients participating in studies receive better care than they would otherwise, some would argue that you should not imply to prospective patients that they will receive better care by being on this particular study—even if you believe it to be true. Access to better medical care was cited by 47 percent of CenterWatch survey participants in 2009.*
- Extra TLC, attention, and emotional support.
- A desire to please the family physician or family members. (Watch out for coercion here!)
- Expanding knowledge: Volunteers might learn more about their own medical conditions or helping others understand a disease process better.
- Income: Being a regular study participant can be an interesting job or way to supplement one's income, especially for young people. The pay, conditions, and hours are generally better than at minimum wage jobs, and it is an opportunity to learn a great deal. This was cited by 34 percent of CenterWatch survey participants (2006–2009).[39] Occasionally, this can lead to problems, as with the recent death of a college student

Patient Care or Profit

Better care during clinical trial participation is an unfortunate reality. Hospitals have turned to a for-profit business model of healthcare, resulting in downsizing and short staffing, away from the patient-care service orientation they previously strived to maintain. Often, there is in fact more adequate staffing and better attentiveness to patients participating in a trial.

* This survey was Web based, with 86 percent of respondents being white and only 1 percent having less than a high school education.[40]

participating in a clinical trial—one question was whether the benefits were too coercive.[41]

- Free medication and medical care: This was a major factor influencing study participation for 32 percent of trial volunteers.[42] It will be interesting to see how these numbers change, given the stark rise in both unemployment and the uninsured in 2009.
- Altruism: A recent survey found that 76 percent of respondents expressed a willingness to participate in research even if the research would not be personally beneficial.[43] A Canadian investigator recently confirmed this attitude when asked how he recruits volunteers in a country with universal healthcare coverage, saying that in his setting, patients rarely decline participation although they lack the financial incentives inherent in the United States.

So how are patients learning about trials? While awareness of trials and participation are generally low, a significant shift has occurred in the past few years. Learning from drug marketing, sponsors are increasingly turning to direct-to-consumer ads and announcements about clinical trials. Many patients—by far the majority in the highly educated CenterWatch survey pool—find trials through Internet searches. What is disconcerting—and telling—is that 58 percent of respondents did not learn about trials from their physicians. Friends and family were also more likely to influence patients' decision to participate than their physicians.[44]

Barriers to Patient Recruitment

A variety of factors can be barriers that make it difficult to recruit patients for trials:

- Unrealistically restrictive inclusion and/or exclusion criteria.
- Unrealistic protocol requirements ("You want me to do what?").
- Politics, as manifested by rivalry between groups of physicians or between the hospital and a given researcher, which may interfere with patient referrals.
- Bad publicity about clinical trials, which can frighten off potential volunteers.

- Physician or hospital concerns about potential liability. For example, for a phase 2 study of complicated skin and soft tissue infections, the surgeon of a patient with an unexpected postoperative wound infection may have misgivings about the patient participating in the trial of a novel agent, fearing further complications and unwarranted blame.
- Insurance or HMO policies that may preclude reimbursement for any care if a patient is participating on a protocol. This resistance can very occasionally be overcome by a call to the holder of the purse strings. For example, in nonstudy situations, Medicare won't pay for home IV antibiotics, and the patients' secondary carriers generally follow suit. Sometimes you can call and say something like this: "You mean you won't pay $200 for the patient to be at home, but you are willing to pay $1,000 per day to keep this patient in the hospital and put him or her at risk of additional infections or complications? I don't understand . . . Can you explain this to me?" This technique may work for late phase 3 or phase 4 studies, but rarely earlier.

A few states, such as Maryland, have laws that mandate insurance coverage for participation in trials for life-threatening illnesses or cancer but not for other illnesses. Certain restrictions apply.[45] Unfortunately, there appears to be no ready definition of what constitutes a "life-threatening" illness. In many cases, such as when patients present with acute illnesses or infections, necessary treatment allows no time for pursuing this issue with the insurance carrier.

Why Would Someone Refer a Patient for a Study?

Accruing patients for a trial through referrals is preferable to advertising, as you are more likely to have a compliant volunteer who will complete the study visits and you generally have a better idea about the patient's overall health from information provided by the referring physician.

Motives for patient referrals run the gamut from avarice to altruism. On the more cynical end are finder's fees, not recommended because of the perception of impropriety. On the other hand, screening fees are appropriate when the referring doctor (or nurse) has to do a fair amount of work. In this case, the referring individuals must actually conduct the screening for major inclusion and exclusion criteria (like drug allergies, concomitant medications, or illnesses, etc.) and fill out a form to document their work. Small contributions to a department, rather than to an individual, are perhaps preferable—for example, to buy educational materials or for a continuing education travel fund for the emergency room or nursing staff to use at their discretion.

Next on the scale toward altruism is an investigator's desire to provide funding for his or her department or for research in other areas. Participation can also create learning opportunities for patients or staff. Involvement in clinical trials sometimes leads to a higher rung on the education and career development ladder.

Most referrals come about because the referring doctor believes that the study will provide good care and is in the patient's best interest. Occasionally, a referral to a trial is made out of desperation, offering patients access to a novel drug or procedure when few or no alternatives are available. (It is important that patients understand that the intervention is investigational to avoid the problem of "therapeutic misconception," whereby they construe an experimental procedure as accepted therapy.) My biggest compliment is having a study patient who asks to participate on another trial or who refers a family member. Investigational medications usually provide state-of-the-art care, an important issue both in reality and in perception, especially in a small or rural community.

Many volunteers and physicians are eager to participate in trials simply to advance medical knowledge and to help others, even though they will not personally benefit.

Recruiting Patients: The Personal Touch

One key to recruiting patients is identifying key people throughout the institution (for inpatient studies) or the community (for outpatient studies) and developing a rapport with them. By key people, I do not mean the CEO of the institution. Rather, concentrate your energies on the admitting office clerk, unit secretaries, radiology transcriptionist, and so on. These folks, generally unappreciated, can provide your earliest alert to potential patients. Give them readily available and visible pocket cards, with the major inclusion/exclusion criteria and contact information for the coordinator and PI, that can serve as handy reminders to them.

View from the Trenches

I make it a point to go in and out of the hospital by way of the emergency room (ER) and the admitting office. The few minutes I spend with Jeannie, the admitting clerk, serves several purposes—it establishes a rapport with her, shows her that I value her contribution to the project and her talent as a scout, and serves to remind her about the study. Above all, our visit is a brief but pleasant interlude in an otherwise stressful day for both of us.

When I tour the hospital with pharmaceutical reps during site visits, I introduce Jeannie as my "secret weapon." Jeannie, in turn, views identifying potential study patients as her contribution to this important project as well as a personal favor to me. She sometimes even makes it into an informal competition with the other clerks, seeing who can identify and contribute the most patients for a protocol.

One other strategy that has been effective for me in the past is to hire ER nurses to moonlight as part-time coordinators. Not only did they help check that study-related activities were done and complete CRFs, but because they were so attuned to the studies, rarely did potential study patients get through the ER without my knowing about them and having an opportunity to screen them. It's a wonderful system, all in all.

Advertising

Remember that the IRB must preapprove any advertising for trial recruitment and that the ads must meet specific FDA requirements. This includes posters, patient information, notices in doctors' offices, and Internet ads—anything that prospective volunteers see. Advertising can be a useful tool for recruiting patients for some types of studies. For example, for outpatient studies, brief ads on radio or local television may be productive. Depending on where you live, these are not generally too expensive. If you place ads in a newspaper, work with the paper to give your ad the most appropriate exposure for the target population. As an example, for an impotence study, we had the ads placed on the sports page. Other prime spaces in our small community are the pages opposite the letters to the editor or those opposite the obituaries.

Before you place ads, study your market and determine what types of material have local appeal.

While advertising and the Internet are growing in importance as avenues of recruitment, according to Cutting Edge's survey of clinical development executives, "physician referral remains the most effective for securing patients

View from the Trenches

On my first study, with her permission, we excitedly took a picture of my first patient, while she was in the ICU, to prepare for a story announcing clinical trials in the newspaper. We asked that the story run in the local section, opposite the obituaries, as that space draws major readership. The patient, an elderly woman, did well on the study, recovered, and went home. By ill luck, she died on the day her long-term follow-up visit was due (which meant that her death was our first SAE). Fortunately, we thought to call the newspaper and ask to have her picture pulled from the story, as we felt including it would be disrespectful and in poor taste. We were just in time! The story announcing our hospital's debut with these studies was on one page, and our first patient's obituary was facing it on the opposite page.

to take part in studies, as it was in 2006." Many sponsors now provide investigators with recruitment kits and tools for local marketing.[46]

Advertising Requirements and Regulations

KEY POINT
All advertising for clinical trials must meet FDA regulations and be approved by the IRB before being displayed.

Numerous regulations govern recruiting and advertising for study volunteers, as with every other aspect of a protocol. Advertisements to recruit volunteers should be limited to the information subjects might require to determine their eligibility and interest. The capsule summary of advertising criteria from the FDA includes the following elements:

- The procedure for recruitment must not be coercive.
- There must be no implication of favorable outcome or benefits beyond those described in the informed consent agreement.
- No claims of efficacy or safety can be made in the ads.
- Ads must explicitly state that the test material is "investigational" or "experimental" rather than use the phrase "new treatment," which implies proven worth.
- Ads may mention but not emphasize the amount paid to subjects.
- Ads must not promise free medical care.
- The fonts used and the general appearance of ads must not unduly influence the decision to participate.[47]

This is a good example of an appropriate trial ad.

Do You Have Diabetes?

A new investigational medicine is being evaluated in a medical research study.

Benefits include, at no cost:

- Study-related doctor visits, lab tests, and study medication
- Travel expenses

For info, call Dr. Investigator at 1-800-2Enroll

The medicine is clearly labeled as investigational or experimental.

Benefits are limited and free care is not promised.

This type of reimbursement is not generally considered coercive.

This ad is a good template. It is general and makes no promises. The fonts and appearance are not very enticing.

Remember that these rules for advertisements apply to all advertising to recruit patients in any form of media—television, radio, the Internet, posters in the hospital or doctor's office—not just print media. An important exception is that doctor-to-doctor letters, even when soliciting study volunteers, are not considered advertising. For example, alerting hospital personnel to the availability of drug studies is helpful. (See the "Drug Study Announcement Memo" at http://conductingclinicalresearch.com.) In a larger loophole, advertising requirements exclude news and "Dear Doctor letters," which are letters from drug companies to physicians and other health professionals to inform them of important new product issues, such as new safety information or warnings or important changes to prescribing information.[48]

Centralized Advertising Venues

For large trials, a new trend is for sponsors to use centralized patient recruitment, largely because of the economies of scale. The centralization also helps the sponsor or CRO measure and assess the response to various strategies. "Metrics" is the mantra at the moment.[49]

For some large multicenter protocols, the sponsors may hire and use an advertising agency. For example, they may run an ad on television or in major newspapers and ask prospective patients to call a central number. They can cover large geographic areas that way and readily collect data indicating what advertising and targeting strategies are most effective. This approach, too, has pluses and minuses for the individual study sites. It can be devastating if your

This ad (by Jeff Cooper) didn't make it.
Can you identify the improper elements?

Wondercillin Ad

"Wondercillin! From STDs to TMJ, it helps your heart, takes warts away.

Just a pill from our pink tin, makes healthy hair and glowing skin! Yes, friends, this pill can do almost everything. I know you're asking yourselves 'What is this going to cost me?' Well friends, I have good news. Wondercillin isn't going to cost you the MSRP of $350, it's not going to cost you $175.

Friends, we're going to pay YOU $1500 to take Wondercillin. Yes, we will pay you to take this fantastic new medication and just sit around all day.

Call 1-800-GET-CASH! Call 1-800-GET-CASH! Positions are limited and going fast. Operators are standing by now for your call. So call 1-800-GET-CASH now!

Not available in stores . . . May cause sterility, deafness, and sudden death in susceptible individuals. In case of research related injury, the sponsor might pay for some reasonable medical expenses provided that you have followed the directions of the sponsor without error, can recite the consent document backwards from memory, notify us within 5 minutes of the injury and have a very competent attorney threaten us with a law suit.

Sponsor otherwise absolutely will not pay for disability, pain, discomfort, acne, halitosis, lost wages, or reduced intelligence. Nothing in this disclaimer is meant to waive your legal rights as if you have any idea what they are anyway."[50]

See http://conductingclinicalresearch.com for a critique of this ad ("Critique of an Inappropriate Ad") and an "FDA Warning Letter" for an ad that the FDA found "false or misleading, in violation of the Federal Food, Drug, and Cosmetic Act."

region is not in the target area of the campaign. For example, our population watches local Hagerstown WHAG and not the DC/Baltimore stations where ad time was purchased for one large multicenter study in which we participated.

If the call-in center favors one site over another, that, too, can torpedo your site. If you are one of the beneficiaries, however, these ads are likely to reach a broader audience and have the benefit of production by an experienced and professional PR firm. Furthermore, the central screening site saves you considerable time and expense by prescreening the volunteers. The agency will only refer patients to you who appear compliant, are able to return for follow-up visits, and meet the basic enrollment criteria.

Finally, patients, investigators, and sponsors are all increasingly turning to the Internet.

View from the Trenches

Dressing for Success—a Different View

There are wide cultural differences regarding what is considered "appropriate" or "professional" attire. As anyone who knows me can attest, I have a somewhat unorthodox style, but one that has served me well. Both as a patient on the receiving end of care and as a physician on the better end, I have always detested the image of the "white coats"—from their use for projecting authority and superiority to their intimidation factor and their starkness. I much prefer a more humanistic, friendly image. I tend to see my patients while wearing colorful, cheery, floral T-shirts, nice slacks, and running shoes. This casual style has served me in good stead. Many patients comment to me that they find my clothing puts them at ease and is less threatening to them than a white coat; some say that they appreciate the human touch. Occasionally, patients look askance. I tell them that I prefer to concentrate completely on caring for them and not on my appearance, or that I can't think if my feet hurt. It breaks the ice. (I tell my male colleagues that I'll wear heels on hospital rounds when they do!) I think my "dressing down" also helps communicate to my patients that they can trust me, that I'm not some "city slicker."

On one occasion, I remember sitting down with a family to review a consent form for a trial in which I hoped to enroll their ill relative. They were somewhat conservative, older women, with their minister by their side. I figured I didn't have a snowball's chance in hell of their agreeing to the trial. After reviewing the consent form, they turned to their pastor and asked, "What do you think?" He paused for what seemed an eternity, looked down at my sneakers, and said, "It's okay. Go ahead. She's real working folk."

I save dressier, "professional" attire for business or state occasions, sometimes with surprising results. On one occasion, my willingness to be adventurous in trying new attire even landed me an entire study.

The Story of the "Black Dress"

After my initial success on infectious disease trials, I hoped to expand my practice to other types of studies by networking with colleagues, who would provide the patient base and be subinvestigators, while I would provide the logistical experience and support.

So Ron Montgomery and another monitor-turned-manager we'll call Tall Man placed a diabetes trial with me and came to discuss the possibilities of further expansion and to meet the other doctors for dinner later that day. Tall Man, my husband/business advisor, and I were meeting at our house during the afternoon. I was

Continued on next page

Web Advertising and Social Networking

Some Web sites provide general information to educate the public about clinical trials. A very good example of this is the video *Entering a Clinical Trial: Is It Right for You?*—a public service announcement produced by Harvard's Dana-Farber Cancer Institute, in collaboration with Brigham and Women's Hospital, Massachusetts General Hospital, and Beth Israel Deaconess Medical Center.[51] The Center for Information and Study on Clinical Research Participation (CISCRP) has produced an educational audiovisual program, *Participating in*

Continued from previous page

dressed in my usual casual attire. As a joke, I held up two outfits—one a simple dress, the other a rarely worn black cocktail dress—and asked Tall Man which he thought would be more appropriate for dinner. Ever chivalrous, he suggested the black dress. He then returned to the hospital, agreeing to meet us all at dinner.

Now, you must understand that nobody in Cumberland had ever seen me dressed to the hilt. I playfully donned this strapless black velvet cocktail dress and fumbled with make-up and hair, thereby arriving a bit late for dinner. As I walked in, eyes bugged out and jaws dropped in astonishment. Maria, the owner of this fine restaurant, L'Ostoria, insisted on my going downstairs to show me off to the hospital administrators, who happened to be having a party there. Tall Man, a strikingly attractive black man wearing a prominent diamond ring, escorted me to the hospital folk. Maria had to introduce me to the (then) CEO, who couldn't figure out who I was (and probably hasn't to this day). My, tongues did wag in this small town. It was great fun.

Over the course of dinner, we were discussing possible areas into which we might be able to expand. Tall Man, half jokingly, and in response to my uncharacteristically flattering attire, asked if I would do an impotence study. While normally I would have said, "Are you kidding?" I was feeling uncharacteristically adventurous that night and said, "Sure, why not?" I guess he never thought I would take him up on it. I figured if I could do the monster diabetes study and the impotence study, they would see that I could do anything, and we'd reach for the stars. So they yanked the impotence study from a university site that wasn't enrolling many patients, placed it with me, and we rapidly completed it.

Your CV isn't always the only thing that lands you a study—sometimes, it's just being in the right place at the right time, or demonstrating a willingness to be creative and try new things. So, consider your audience and the impact you hope to make, and choose your own style, however unconventional that may be, with that in mind.

a Clinical Trial. It also has DVDs available for purchase targeted specifically toward African-American and Hispanic populations, as well as a variety of brochures and posters.[52] Other groups produce similar materials.

Many research sites have their own Web pages describing available trials. Disease-specific advocacy sites often list available trials for those illnesses. Sites like Craigslist and Google ads also serve as advertising and recruiting venues. In addition, sites such as CenterWatch, ClinicalTrials.gov, and the International Federation of Pharmaceutical Manufacturers & Associations (IFPMA) Clinical Trials Portal are proliferating and becoming major brokers, the "Yentas" of the clinical trial world.[53]

Most recently, social networking sites are serving as both valuable information clearinghouses and social communities for prospective volunteers. These include Inspire, Click It Forward, MediciGlobal, Inclinix (a CRO specializing in enrollment), and PatientsLikeMe.[54, 55] Social networking sites—particularly ones with very actively involved and motivated memberships, such as PatientsLikeMe, are ripe prospects for targeted ads to prospective volunteers.

The PatientsLikeMe site is novel in that it collects a wealth of data freely offered by patients suffering from a variety of illnesses. Patients post details of their symptoms, treatments, and, in some cases, emotional responses, all of which are compiled and displayed graphically. Sponsors gain insight into patients' day-to-day experiences with their illnesses or treatments. They can also target recruitment ads or information to specific members registered in different communities on the site.

Internet communications, whether from a research center's Web site or through social networking groups, raise ethical questions. The Office of Inspector General (OIG) has weighed in on this issue, noting that while the sites generally do a good job of educating the public about clinical trials, they do less well at supporting informed consent. Of 110 trial listings OIG reviewed, it found shortcomings in the following areas:

- *Trial benefits and risks. Not one has any information about risks to human subjects, while 29 describe the benefits.*
- *Sponsor name. 77 fail to identify the sponsor for the clinical trial.*
- *Phase of trial. 69 do not indicate the phase of the clinical trial.*
- *Description of trial. 56 lack a general description of the protocol.*[56]

OIG also found privacy policies to be significantly lacking. It is also unclear what information on the Internet is subject to IRB review and approval. The OIG report made recommendations regarding clarifying the role of the IRB, suggesting establishment of voluntary standards and periodic review of the sites by independent agencies.[57]

If the recruitment process can be structured in an ethical and more standardized way, Web sites and the Internet hold great promise for more successfully educating and recruiting volunteers.

If the public is given better education about clinical trials, participation rates could possibly increase from their current 2–3 percent. Harris Interactive polls have found that "81 percent of the general population says that they have never had the opportunity to participate in a clinical study. Of those given the opportunity, 58 percent enrolled."[58] The value of public education is higher for cancer patients, where "out of the 85 percent of cancer patients unaware of clinical trials, 76 percent of them indicated that they would be willing to consider a clinical trial had they known about them as an option."[59]

Analyzing Your Approach

Evaluate the responses to various advertising approaches that you try. One useful tool is the screening and enrollment log. As part of the screening process, ask potential patients how they heard about your study. Did they hear about the study from a referral, an ad in the paper, a television announcement, or by word of mouth? These logs are beneficial for the site and the sponsor and not just another bookkeeping burden. They can also help in reality testing the current protocol with the sponsor (see "Protocol Feasibility" in chapter 3). For example, sponsors may vastly underestimate how many patients will need to be screened—or how low a percentage of patients will be microbiologically evaluable (i.e., a culture from the patient grows a bacterial pathogen). The pharmaceutical company will hopefully use the screening log data to design more realistic entry criteria in the future as well as for advertising studies.

If used properly, these logs can also help your site in future negotiations. Generating your own outcome data reflects that you are viewing the studies seriously and professionally and analyzing your experience. Screening and enrollment logs, as well as your research experience summary (as described in chapter 2), thus help establish your credibility as an experienced site and investigator. See the sample "Screening and Enrollment Log" and a sample "Research Experience Summary" at http://conductingclinicalresearch.com.

Approaching the Patient, or "You Want Me to Do What?"

Preliminary screening of prior lab tests or medical records can and should be done before making direct contact with the patient, but only if this prescreening has been approved by your IRB. Note that no study procedures or lab tests may be obtained prior to obtaining informed consent. If a patient comes to the office for a routine visit and the Principal Investigator discovers something that might qualify the patient for a study (e.g., a lab test result), the PI does not have to obtain consent before further discussing the study option with the patient. On the other hand, if the PI wants to search the practice's medical records to identify and contact a patient, this will first require IRB approval. If the patient is contacted specifically for consideration in a study, the PI must get consent prior to doing anything with the patient.

After a focused chart review to see if the patient has obvious exclusions from the protocol, one can approach the patient, hopefully presenting the informed consent agreement palatably.

Discussing Risks and Benefits

First, it is important to establish a rapport with a patient and to assess whether she or he may be an appropriate candidate for a particular study given underlying illnesses, concomitant medications, allergies, or social factors. I take a brief, focused history and physical. By that time, the patient and I have some "feel" for each other. After making the preliminary assessment, I explain that the patient's primary physician would like me to inform him or her about a study that we are conducting. I emphasize that it is a study, working with new medications that are not yet on the market. (The words "research" and "study" are preferable initially. The word "experiment" carries too many negative connotations.) I also explain, if needed by way of background, that every medicine on the market (and every medicine that the patient is already taking) has gone through the same research phases that the study medicine will go through. First, the medicine is tested in animals. Second, it is given to healthy volunteers, such as hungry college students.

Third, it is given to patients who do not have many other medical problems, to study its effectiveness and to determine the best dose. Fourth, it is given to patients with more complicated underlying illnesses. Finally, the drug is marketed and further experience is gathered.

If necessary, I also explain why it is important to develop new medicines. I ask if they've seen in magazines or heard on the news about "superbugs," which are resistant to multiple antibiotics, and explain that we are running out of antibiotics because the bacteria are "smarter" than the drug companies and doctors, developing resistance more rapidly than their pursuers can develop novel compounds.

In actually obtaining consent, I review the informed consent form with the patient. I summarize each section and paraphrase it in words that may be more familiar to him or her. It is imperative to review carefully the risks and alternatives and to explain that the patient may receive no benefit from the study medicine. However, I also put the risks in perspective.

For example, if the drug is a new quinolone, I might say that the study medicine is similar to or is the "son of" Cipro, which the patient may have heard about extensively from the publicity surrounding anthrax exposures. Or I ask what antibiotics the patient has previously taken to see if he or she has had experience with a similar type of drug.

To put the risks in context, I may tell the patient that the new medication is expected to be similar to the one that he or she may have previously received and that it carries a risk for certain side effects. Penicillins may cause rashes and quinolones may cause headaches or insomnia, for example. Always emphasize that these are expected, known risks of that class of drugs and that the new medicine may carry additional, unknown risks.

In terms of benefits, some patients seek the free care or medicines offered on a trial. With indigent patients, it is particularly important to determine whether the drug is an appropriate option for them and not just a means to receive the financial benefit. My threshold is whether I would take the medicine under similar circumstances or if I would have a family member take it. I have never accepted a protocol in which I would not take the medicine myself. In fact, I was a patient on my first protocol and my husband was a patient on two of my protocols. I would suggest the same standard for other investigators.

Occasionally, a patient may qualify for two ongoing studies that overlap temporally. Patients can be in only one trial, so you need to have a mechanism for deciding in which protocol the patient should participate. One can either offer the patient a choice or decide, based on his or her other medical problems, which study might be more appropriate. You can also have a mechanism for randomly assigning the patient to one of the two trials. This type of randomization plan is the most common solution. If you have no plan, you are likely to introduce bias into the study and risk invalidating the results.

Many patients are quite altruistic and appreciate the opportunity to participate in a trial to help develop medicines for others, even when there is likely to be little or no benefit to them. I have also found this outlook to be of some comfort to families of patients who are critically ill and unlikely to recover—they may derive consolation by volunteering and bequeathing their experience to others.

Conclusion

In past chapters we've covered how to land your first study and how to negotiate a budget and a contract, and we have alerted you to the regulatory obligations you will need to be familiar with. Let's move on to provide you with the skills that will help you deal with the details of implementing the study.

CHAPTER 6

Study Activities: Strategies and Tools

The difference between a great design and a lousy one
is in the meshing of the thousand details that either fit or don't,
and the spirit of the passionate intellect
that has tied them together, or tried.

—TED NELSON

As I'm sure you've noticed, a myriad of details must be tracked when conducting a clinical research study. In this chapter, we will look at some useful tools and review documents that must be maintained while a patient is "on treatment." Corresponding sample forms are available at http://conductingclinicalresearch.com.

SOPs—Why Bother?

Standard operating procedures (SOPs) provide a way of standardizing care at and between investigative sites. Many sponsors use the same format in preparing protocols, only they call it a MOP or a MOO (manual of procedures or manual of operations). Don't you love the images these acronyms create? But these manuals are quite useful in ensuring that procedures are conducted in a standardized, reproducible, and analyzable manner—as anyone who has done laboratory research can attest to. While it may seem like overkill at the site level, having SOPs in place—and using them—can serve as a useful safety net, to make sure you don't overlook details in conducting your trials, and as a valuable training resource for new staff. SOPs are perhaps best regarded as an insurance policy for your site, rather than a nuisance.

SOPs should be informative but not too specific because an FDA auditor could later penalize you for not following them exactly. Review your site's SOPs annually and keep a signature log to document that each topic was reviewed by your staff.

You can buy books and disks with ready-made SOPs and templates for prices that range from $84 to $1,200. An April 2005 review by Norman Goldfarb in the *Journal of Clinical Research Best Practices* covers these products, with an amusing warning that their value should not be based solely on the price per pound.[1] If you want to develop SOPs on your own, go first to the Clinical Trials Networks (CTN) Best Practices site for a good, detailed outline of elements to be included in each SOP. (In his review, Goldfarb also provides a handy table of suggested topics to include.) Suggested elements for each SOP are administrative trivia, such as author, approval dates, revision date, review date, and so on. Other elements you should include are the purpose, scope, responsibility, procedure, review, contingencies, definitions, and references.[2]

That covers what goes into each SOP, but what SOP topics should be documented? After years of experience, both in my practice and in perusing various articles on the subject, I would suggest you include these topics:

- Archiving: Procedures for archiving case report forms, other study records, training records, and communications.
- Data collection: Procedures that cover source document requirements, case report form completion, e-signatures, data collection, and study file maintenance. Give special care to procedures for controlling access to patient records and for obtaining and reviewing electronic medical records for research staff such as monitors and sponsors.
- Equipment and instruments: Procedures for maintaining temperature logs and for documenting the maintenance history for research equipment.
- Ethics: Standards that relate to misconduct and fraud.
- FDA inspections: Procedural information for training for this eventuality, whom to alert at the sponsor, how to host inspectors, the closing meeting, and follow-up procedures. Hopefully you will never need the policy for

responding to items listed on a Form FDA 483, the citation of audit findings.

- Informed consent: Procedures for carrying out the consent process, content development, and approvals, including any specific policies or procedures your IRB might mandate, and documenting the policies for subjects unable to personally consent.
- Insurance/billing issues: Procedures related to Medicare and commercial insurance and billing.
- Investigational product (IP): Procedures for documenting drug accountability, the IP shipment contact, and the receipt, handling, storage (e.g., temperature logs), dispensing, and return or disposal/destruction of investigational agents.
- IRB: Procedures that relate to IRB applications and their continuing review as well as completing and submitting study applications and renewals and the required documentation and tracking communications.
- Laboratory and OSHA regulations: Procedures for specimen collection, handling, and shipping, as well as documenting training.
- Monitoring and audit visits: Procedures for preparing for and coordinating the initiation, monitoring, closing out, and handling of the study audit visits.
- Noncompliant subjects and/or nonresponsive monitors/sponsors: Procedures for handling situations beyond your control.
- Protocol review and approval, and amendments: Procedures for reviewing potential protocols, navigating the approval process and making amendments (this overlaps with IRB procedures), and handling the Investigator's Brochure.
- Screening and enrollment of subjects: Procedures for screening, recruiting, and enrolling subjects as well as advertising. (This category overlaps with IRB procedures.)
- Personnel/staff roles and responsibilities: Issues related to your research team directory; the qualifications, roles, and responsibilities of participating research staff; delegation of authority; and study contact information for the site and contractors.

- Privacy issues and HIPAA: Procedures for ensuring patients' privacy regarding use of photographs. (This category overlaps with archiving and informed consent procedures.)
- Regulatory binder and files: Explanation of what to include in the binder and how to maintain it.
- SAE reporting: Explanations of how and when to document and report serious adverse events.
- SOP on SOPs: Information on the preparation, review, and maintenance of the SOPs themselves. (This reminds me of Dr. Seuss. Imagine the places he could go with this!)
- Training: Details on what type of training is required of staff for each study, as well as how to document the training and maintain records.
- Site-sponsor study documents: Procedures for study documents such as the confidentiality agreement and clinical trial agreement, the budget (and who is responsible for negotiation), financial disclosure, and indemnification for study personnel as well as instructions for documenting investigator meetings, site qualification visits, site initiation visits, site monitoring visits, sponsor audits, sponsor-CRO communications and visits, study start-up visits, and study closeout visits.
- Subject safety: Generally covered in SAE reporting procedures, but also includes information about after-hours coverage, IND safety report review and disposition, and protocol deviations.

Each SOP should designate the responsible person for SOP compliance. *What* is entailed in each procedure should be outlined, but do not specify exactly *how* so you don't get caught being in noncompliance with your own procedure. Similarly, avoid using "must" or "shall"; it is better just to describe what is done.

Another handy reference for developing your SOPs is Ruth Ann Nylen's *The Ultimate Step-by-Step Guide to Conducting Pharmaceutical Clinical Trials in the USA*. Her book is in a chart format, but it tells you what items to include and specifies the related regulations for each item.

Having SOPs in place and using them can serve a useful purpose: to make sure you don't overlook details in conducting your trials.

Study Tracking: What Day Is Today?

One bizarre and confusing question that everyone has trouble keeping straight, especially if they are juggling more than one study, is, "What is Day 1?" There is a surprising and bewildering array of answers to this question. And, while it sounds trivial, all study activities are based on the definition of Day 1. Some companies define Day 1 as the day of the patient's enrollment, up to midnight of that day. For others, it is the first 24-hour period after enrollment, regardless of the calendar day. Yet others call enrollment day "Day 0."

While many investigators generally track patient visits with a calendar or graph paper, and occasionally an Excel spreadsheet or a homemade Linux program, large sites might want to consider commercial study software packages. One such program, Study Manager, appears to be quite well designed and useful for protocols with regularly scheduled study activities.[3]

General Tracking Procedures

Several parameters, if tracked on a regular (routine) basis, will be helpful timesavers in the long run. These will also help you gather information for assessing future studies or marketing your site to potential sponsors.

Screening and Enrollment Log

First, remember the ever-important screening and enrollment log. The FDA requires you to keep this log to show that your enrollment wasn't biased toward a specific group of patients. Sponsors actually view having occasional patients decline to participate on your trial as a plus because it shows them (and the hierarchy of auditors leading up to the FDA) that no coercion was placed on the prospective patients. The sponsor may provide the screening log book. Otherwise, any log you develop should contain the elements shown in the "Screening and Enrollment Log" at http://conductingclinicalresearch.com.

If you have a patient who is close to meeting the study's entry criteria but doesn't quite fit, it is often worth calling the medical monitor to see if an exception might be granted. Company policies vary: some frequently allow exceptions for minor criteria; others never do. Such exceptions to protocol inclusion or exclusion criteria are often granted on protocols that are otherwise nearly impossible to do. Companies eventually are forced to do reality testing as protocols evolve, and they may realize that their entry criteria are too restrictive or that it will take until the next century to accrue enough patients. They will thus either modify the protocol via an amendment or allow exceptions, granted by the medical monitor.

Protocol exceptions *must* be well documented. Put a note in the source document and in the CRF, if possible. This note should include the date and time of the call to the medical monitor (or CRA), what the deviation from the inclusion or exclusion criteria was, and the fact that the exception was authorized by the medical monitor, giving the physician's name. Otherwise, when monitored, your assessments will be plastered with the reproachful "protocol violation" and the sponsor will not pay for an otherwise completely evaluable patient. This is a place where a newbie can easily get into trouble, especially with CROs, which tend to be less understanding than the sponsor drug company.

Patient Outcome Log

Next, keep a patient outcome log. This log will help both in tracking volunteers' outcomes and in making a final report either to the sponsor or to the IRB. Information is easily entered into a computer spreadsheet or a paper worksheet. Demographic items to be noted should include date, age, sex, and underlying disease. On infectious disease trials, it is also worth noting pertinent culture results, whether the patient was microbiologically and clinically evaluable, and whether the patient suffered any unexpected adverse events.

It's much easier to record these data as you receive them than to remember after the fact or to have to go back through all the CRFs at the end of the study to retrieve the information. When the study is completed, you can then readily generate a summary for submission to the IRB. If this outcome information is recorded in a database, then it is searchable or sortable by different criteria, which is helpful in planning for future protocols. See the "Patient Outcome Log" at http://conductingclinicalresearch.com.

Worksheets, Forms, and Study Folders: Getting in Touch with Your Inner OCD*

Worksheets are helpful in capturing information that you will later need to submit to the sponsor. Such information includes signs and symptoms of

* Obsessive-compulsive disorder.

each volunteer's illness, results of examinations, medications, and lab data. These worksheets should be included in your source documents and can be enormous timesavers.

I would suggest designing your own worksheets to save the PI (or coordinator) time and reduce the likelihood of missing evaluations or making errors. Alternatively, many template worksheets are now available, the best being at the CTN Best Practices site. You can adapt these to suit your own style. Your forms can either mimic the CRF (some companies don't allow duplicates of the CRF to be used as a source document) or be customized to suit the way your brain works, with someone else having to worry about transcribing the data to the actual CRF. For example, worksheets that record similar activities on the same sheet—observations of signs and symptoms—might help you evaluate whether your patients' conditions are slightly better or worse than the last time you saw them or compare the severity of their symptoms. (See the sample "Signs and Symptoms Worksheet" at http://conductingclinicalresearch.com.) The pharmaceutical industry seems to design and organize CRFs by visit now, rather than by activity. Perhaps this change is meant to subsidize the paper industry or, more likely, to make data entry easier for computer users (read less expensive); I suspect the latter.

One of the keys to coordinating research is organizing your project activities by study and keeping track of the separate studies. We designed a useful color-coded system for when multiple studies are running simultaneously. This helps "idiot proof" the study mechanics and is particularly useful as hospitals are increasingly short staffed or have higher turnover in personnel. The colors alert all the ancillary departments that a patient is on a drug study and readily differentiate between the protocols. A glance at the colors can serve as a mnemonic for what studies you are juggling, too. For example, a urinary tract infection (UTI) study is likely

View from the Trenches

On blinded studies in which mortality is predictably and depressingly high, such as sepsis protocols, the ICU nurses and I often make note of whether we expect the patients to live or not, and if they happen to make an unexpectedly good recovery. Years later, when we are "unblinded" and receive the code telling us each patient's treatment group, it's interesting to see whether the patient received the active study drug in addition to standard antibiotics and supportive care.

to be yellow, pneumonia to be green, a bloodstream infection to be red or pink, COPD blue, and so on.

So if a patient is on a UTI study, that patient's study order sheet (standing orders specific for a particular protocol) might be yellow. The pharmacy and the lab are alerted to the specific protocol by both the protocol name and the color. The micro lab techs place a yellow tape on the culture plates. This reminds them what discs to place on the plates for special antibiotic susceptibility testing, and it correlates to a list of how isolates are handled—for example, whether they are to be shipped out or frozen. Patient names are also jotted on a blackboard, sectioned by the colors, as an added safeguard and reminder so that study specimens are not inadvertently discarded.

KEY POINT
Aim to make your organization system mistake-proof. Try color-coding your studies.

A worthwhile practice is to make a folder for each study and keep it in a box in the ER, or wherever else you are likely to enroll patients, with all the material needed to enroll a patient on a particular protocol readily available and conveniently accessible. (We affectionately call ours my "hope chest.") While each study's materials are color-coded and specific to the study, the required folder contents are standardized and include

- Consent forms.
- Inclusion and exclusion criteria checklist.
- Study-specific order sheets for the patient chart.
- Lab reqs (requisition forms).
- Schedule of study activities. See the sample "Schedule of Activities Worksheet" at http://conductingclinicalresearch.com.
- Signs and symptoms checklist or other data that must be recorded at enrollment (e.g., the Apache, or severity of illness, worksheet). See the "Signs and Symptoms Worksheet" at http://conductingclinicalresearch.com.

The study folder then accompanies the ER patient to the hospital floor when he or she is admitted. Each packet is designed to be self-explanatory so that staff on different shifts can readily understand and pick up study-specific activities and tasks. Be sure to include all of the worksheets as part of your source documents.

It is also quite helpful to keep a pack of supplies specific for the study with your study folder. Having the necessary supplies at the patient point of care will save you considerable aggravation and helps ensure that no procedures are overlooked. (See the "Study Supply Checklist" at http://conductingclinicalresearch.com for an example of supplies needed for a diabetic foot infection study.)

Project Management Techniques

While you can plan and plan, some detail is always unanticipated and overlooked. The PERT–CPM model is great for helping avoid some unpleasant surprises by identifying rate limiting steps, or potential bottlenecks—be they the availability of an unusual piece of equipment or special training needed by a staff member. PERT (Program Evaluation and Review Technique), CPM (Critical Path Method), and Gantt charts are all useful tools to help you plan and conduct your clinical trial successfully. Each of these project management techniques helps you analyze and break down the project into individual tasks that are interconnected, and each helps you identify rate limiting steps.

PERT-Gantt techniques are further reviewed by Jack Byrd and by Martin Modell.[4] A Gantt chart is a simple graphical depiction of different tasks on one axis plotted against time. This can be initially sketched on graph paper or can be more formally represented by a graphical user interface model or time chart made on an Excel spreadsheet. The PERT-CPM model is more complex but shows which tasks are dependent on other ones.

Sometimes, however, only experience will teach you. There is something to be said for the old adage "See one. Do one. Teach one."

Software Programs

For larger sites, appealing computer programs are now available to help manage a variety of study logistics, including patient scheduling, drug inventories, and tracking of regulatory documents and study grant payments. These programs appear potentially quite useful for larger sites but are generally limited to protocols with a set, well-defined enrollment period. One well-designed program is Study Manager by Advanced Clinical Software.[5] A number of large study sites use this program. Many others are available, including TrialWorks and Oracle's

SiteMinder and open-source OpenClinica.*[6] Another highly recommended program is the Data Doctor Office Technology Systems' (DDOTS) Clinical Research Environmental Data Infomatics Tracking program, which also helps with patient communications, billing, and IRB-related activities. Make sure that any program you invest in will be able to meet the specific needs of your site. For example, the one glitch some programs have is being stymied by the rolling-window periods for enrollment common on some infectious disease trials (where enrollment is dependent on a patient with a specific test result returning or meeting the inclusion and exclusion criteria within a certain time period rather than one specific, inflexible time).

Coping with Minutiae

You will hopefully have addressed all the minutiae during your feasibility review and initial courtship visit, but you might want to review here some of the details that must be attended to. For example, if your study involves sending specimens to a centralized lab, be sure you have reviewed the details of the protocol carefully and that you have checked out some of the following concerns:

- Where can you get dry ice? Is it delivered once or twice a week or ordered as needed? How long in advance must the delivery be scheduled?
- Do you have adequate storage space for drug supplies, send-out kits (these are voluminous), and CRFs (which need to be kept in perpetuity)?
- How accessible are radiology services? Phlebotomy?
- Is your shipping contract with a particular vendor (e.g., FedEx or Airborne)? Does this carrier come to your town, let alone your facility? What is the schedule? For example, if the carrier picks up from your site at 9:00 a.m. only, then patients' specimens will sit around overnight and often arrive at the central lab "beyond stability." (See the "Specimen Shipping Log" at http://conductingclinicalresearch.com for a sample of the type of record you should maintain regarding shipments.) Whom do you contact regarding problems? What arrangements exist for getting and sending supplies on weekends and holidays?

KEY POINT
Make lists. Redundancy is good.

---

* See the *Applied Clinical Trials* Web site, http://www.actmagazine.com, for further discussion. OpenClinica is worthy of mention as it is a freely available, open-source Web-based software with modules that can be modified for specific sites or trials.

- Are you equipped and trained to ship biohazardous materials, aka blood and urine, or patients' microbiological isolates?
- Do all your office procedures meet OSHA regulations? HIPAA regulations?* Other regulations not yet invented but almost certain to be retroactive? What, if any, special facilities are required? Keep the OSHA requirements in mind. These regulations mandate extensive new training and separate facilities for handling and processing lab specimens from patients. Heavy fines are levied for violations.
- What is the turnaround time at the central lab? In other words, is the patient likely to die before you are aware of a critical test result? How will you be notified of test abnormalities? By fax? By phone? What happens on weekends and holidays? Are some lab tests run in duplicate—both on-site for rapid results and at a central or reference lab for standardization? Who pays for the duplicate testing?

Billing Compliance—Practicalities

How do you keep study charges separate from nonstudy charges for patients? As noted in chapter 3, the billing landscape is now interspersed with land mines such as subject injury and improper Medicare claims. In fact, billing has become so complex that many sites have to hire personnel specifically trained in coding and compliance.

LEGAL LAND MINE
Billing errors can result in charges of fraud.

For example, the CPT code and level of reimbursement vary significantly depending on whether a procedure is performed as an inpatient or outpatient procedure. Ambulatory procedures will include a facilities fee, not just the physician reimbursement that might be listed in the sponsor's budget. Many radiologic or outpatient procedures also require pretest labs (e.g., a creatinine before contrast) or medications that might have been overlooked in the proposed budget.[7, 8]

It is important to develop a billing system at your site before undertaking study activities. Meet with the institution's lab manager, pharmacy manager,

* OSHA (Occupational Safety and Health Administration) requirements can be found at http://www.osha.gov; information on HIPAA and clinical research can be found at http://privacyruleandresearch.nih.gov/clin_research.asp.

billing clerk, finance and registration offices, information technology guru, and your own staff early on, and involve them in designing a workable system. Have each department review the coverage to help ensure that the budget is adequate. Sometimes, when comparing the protocol, consent, and contract (CTA), you will find disturbingly conflicting information as to what will be covered by the sponsor and what is to be the patient's responsibility. Remember, the FDA regulations and Common Rule require the informed consent to include a statement of any additional costs to the subject that may result from research participation.

KEY POINT
Compare the protocol, consent, and CTA for consistency in regard to costs.

We kept it simple, using color-coded lab regulations as alerts so the lab staff knew to bill us for specific study lab tests rather than the patient or the insurance company. Anything that was required by the study was automatically billed to us and paid for by the study with these regulations. Unexpected study-related charges, such as for following up an adverse event, were communicated to the lab, so the lab knew to bill us rather than the patient's insurer, and we could then invoice the sponsor for add-ons.

KEY POINT
If a procedure is required solely for research, rather than for a patient's care, do not bill Medicare or other insurers.

You might consider a mock compliance audit on a sample of your patients to verify that your system is functional. With an adequate computer entry system (as opposed to our hospital's archaic one), special fields can be set up to flag these charges automatically, reducing some administrative time.

Drug Storage and Accountability

Tracking investigational medicine is akin to accounting for and tracking narcotics. The intent is that there be no way that an investigational medicine can be given to the wrong person. You must account for absolutely every dose of the study medicine. You must meticulously document transfers of medicine from the pharmaceutical company to the study site and then to the patient, and the final return of unused supplies to the sponsor. The investigational medicine must be kept in a very secure storage area with limited access. Temperature and humidity and, occasionally, light may also be storage issues. Inquire ahead of time.

View from the Trenches

Our hospital complex is a veritable maze as well as being somewhat sprawling. Most of my protocols involve inpatients, who return for one or two follow-up visits after hospital discharge. For the convenience of the patients, especially if they are elderly, immobile, or otherwise impaired, I arrange to rent a room in the ER area of the hospital for some of these follow-up visits. The phlebotomist or EKG tech will come to the patient, and x-rays are taken next door. The patients greatly appreciate the "one-stop shopping" and that I am sensitive to their needs and willing to come to them. For a small practice such as mine, this arrangement is also less expensive than hiring office staff or maintaining my own facilities. My office does have a small dedicated phlebotomy and "dirty" area, which is used for larger outpatient studies.

If your study medicine is kept in a pharmacy or other area with "regular," nonstudy medications, you must designate a distinctly defined area, clearly labeled, for the investigational medications.

Drug accountability is one of the FDA's favorite areas to check, ranking in the "top five" sources of errors that result in citations during audits and inspections of investigative sites.[9]

Maintaining Drug and Supply Inventories

While you can try to plan for maintaining inventory, perhaps using a PERT-CPM model or chart, unanticipated problems inevitably arise. A tickler file of some sort—whatever suits your style—can help you keep things simple. (*Organizing from the Inside Out* by Julie Morganstern offers helpful

View from the Trenches

On the diabetes study we committed to do, we were astonished to learn that for each patient, the study medicine was going to require two partitioned boxes, each measuring approximately 12 x 12 x 4 inches. With 40 patients on the study, and allowing that both boxes had to be accessible for each patient's visit, we were suddenly faced with a logistical nightmare, and we had to scramble for space. Fortunately, the hospital was able to arrange for us to use some unused storage space and generously fitted the space with a partition and locked door (within the locked room!), as well as floor-to-ceiling, warehouse-grade shelving. Fort Knox might have been more accessible!

View from the Trenches

We chose to keep our investigations medications next to the beer kept for patients, which occasionally caused raised eyebrows among monitors unaccustomed to the realities of patient care. (An occasional beer is far easier to administer to prevent withdrawal in alcoholics, and is safer than many other sedatives. It also enhances patient satisfaction.)

suggestions.[10]) Develop a system for identifying or marking send-out kits as they too become outdated. How will you check your inventory and maintain adequate supplies? Who will do this?

In general, if you enroll two or three patients on a given study, you should check with the hospital's pharmacy to verify its inventory of the study drug. If a holiday period is coming up, ask the pharmacy to stock up on the investigational drugs you'll need, and check your stock of other supplies.

Monitoring Visits

After the initiation, or start-up, visit by the sponsor's representative, monitoring will occur almost monthly. At each visit, the monitor (a CRA) will audit source documents to verify that inclusion and exclusion criteria have been met and to collect details about any adverse events, in particular. CRFs will be reviewed for accuracy and collected for submission. Recruitment efforts will be reviewed, and suggestions for different strategies might be offered.

What else will happen? The monitor will compare all entries on CRFs to the corresponding source documents and verify the accuracy of the entries. Any errors or discrepancies will be reviewed with the coordinator (CRC) and, if clinically significant (i.e., more than a minor transcription error), with the PI. On later site visits, the monitor may not always perform 100 percent verification of the case report form compared to the source documents but will always come very close to doing so.

To avoid complications and embarrassment during monitoring visits, remember the CRA's siren song:

(to the tune of "My Favorite Things" from *The Sound of Music*)

I'm really sorry to hear that you blew it
You should have listened to me and you knew it
Your tale is sad but excuse while I sing
Following rules is a *Very Good* Thing . . .[11]

VIEW FROM THE TRENCHES

For one of my more memorable studies, I agreed to participate in an influenza trial. It never occurred to me that supplies of the study drug were limited and would not be sent to a study site until influenza was actually documented in the community by lab assays. Our outbreak occurred at Christmastime. While I work 24-7 in solo practice, I learned that this multibillion dollar corporation had next to no one minding the shop over the holidays and was not prepared to ship the drug. When I was finally able to get the drug shipped, we then ran into problems with the limited holiday schedules of the shipping carriers. Then there was a blizzard, with many patients (even those I knew personally) saying they were too sick to visit the doctor during the bad weather. All in all, this was an unpleasant and costly experience that I hadn't anticipated.

Regulatory documents are reviewed by the monitor, as are informed consent agreements and screening and enrollment logs. Each dose of the investigational drug must be accounted for, along with, it seems, every scrap of paper. At all visits, the focus is on compliance with the protocol and good clinical practice guidelines. Emphasis is placed on enrollment criteria, informed consent, and adverse events reporting.

Any glitch in selecting volunteers, administering study procedures, obtaining specimens and lab test results, or documenting any aspect of the study in the CRF—and glitches are inevitable—is reviewed by the monitor with the site personnel and often generates a nasty form letter detailing the violations.

Volunteer Retention and Satisfaction

Simply identifying and enrolling your participants is not the end of your involvement with them. The next hurdle is keeping your volunteers compliant and making sure that they return for follow-up visits. Many skills are required for this, as well as some understanding of human nature. Especially on long-term studies, or if a study involves significant inconvenience or discomfort for the patients, it is important to remember that the patients are doing you a favor and a service as well as receiving benefits from participating in the study. I was surprised to learn that the industry standard for patient dropout and noncompliance is 25 percent.[12] We rarely had dropouts, perhaps because of the continuity of care and TLC we showered on our volunteers.

In an interesting survey, Elizabeth Moench found that study patients were almost universally dissatisfied with the amount of contact they had with the Principal Investigator—and that only 5 percent of physicians routinely saw their patients during study visits; the other physicians frequently left the visits to ancillary personnel. Hence, "PI" came to be translated as "practically invisible." While the visits did not require the presence of a physician, this practice did not mesh with the patients' expectations of the doctor's role, and it adversely affected patient retention.[13]

You will need to tailor your approach to the age and particular needs of your patients. For example, suburban women with young children are likely to have different psychosocial needs than senior citizens, gay men, or an inner city population. Strategies for improving patient satisfaction and retention include the following:

- Cluster the visits of study patients together. For example, on a diabetes study, patients were scheduled for major visits in groups of eight. This gave the investigators an opportunity to give nutritional counseling to a group, and the patients were able to share recipes and advice. The patients viewed this ongoing education as a significant benefit; it served as an important incentive to their continued participation. This education also demonstrated respect for the patients, and further made them partners in the process of caring for their illness.

- Provide support and TLC. After our diabetes study patients had their fasting blood drawn, they were given a nutritious breakfast snack to enjoy while they waited for other study activities. They very much appreciated the thoughtfulness and unexpected touch. As the study evolved, the visits also became a support group for the participants, who became quite close to each other.

- Consider providing or arranging transportation, if necessary. This might involve arranging for a community's van service or paying for a taxi. This is particularly important with mothers and the elderly.

- Provide convenient and flexible follow-up appointment times, including evenings and weekends, so as not to interfere with job obligations.

- Be prepared to make house calls for follow-up visits, particularly for elderly or debilitated patients. Patients greatly appreciate these visits, and home visits can provide you with a great deal of insight about a patient's support systems, or lack thereof; you might enjoy providing that kind of care.

- Provide a convenient and comfortable setting for the participants. If your office is not conveniently located, you might sometimes rent a room from the participating hospital and conduct the patient visits there, if that would be significantly easier for them.
- Provide a setting with childcare, if possible.
- Consider how much, if any, extra care you will provide patients beyond the protocol requirements. For example, will you take care of minor health problems that come up so patients do not need to make extra visits to their primary care physicians?
- Maintain good communication with the patients' primary care physicians. Treating the doctors as partners in the study process will help ensure their continued support. Try to emphasize to both the patient and the primary care doctor that participation is giving the patient access to state-of-the-art care, free medication, and lab tests.
- Call your patients at set intervals or event time points. This allows them to express any concerns they might have and the sponsor to gather valuable feedback. You might build these proactive retention initiatives into your budget. Similarly, some sponsors provide 24-hour support for volunteers through call centers.
- Consider setting up e-diaries, which can be remarkably effective in improving patient compliance. They provide reminders to patients to take their medications or record symptoms (or outcomes). If information is not promptly entered, call center staff can contact the patients, addressing any concerns they might have and heading off dropouts.[14]

If you are mindful of how you would like to be treated in similar situations and act accordingly, you will see satisfied patients who will complete their follow-up visits as requested. Be appreciative, be courteous, and minimize their waiting times—try to treat them as VIPs. After all, they are giving you—and all of us—an important gift, what Kenneth Getz, the founder of CISCRP, fittingly calls the "gift of participation."[15]

One caveat is to be aware, especially with long-term studies, that the patients may want to please you to the point of not wanting to confess to problems with compliance with the study regimen's medications or by minimizing their discomfort. This recently became an issue with a patient on a three-year rheumatoid arthritis study. Toward the end of that period, she developed progressive symptoms but did not want to drop out of the trial. I had to remind her that her health came first and that it was inappropriate for her to continue on this trial. This desire to please and to not disappoint the doctor is particularly a problem among patients drawn from your own private practice or with whom you have a longstanding relationship. Again, you need to be careful that the patient neither feels coercion to continue nor becomes worried about how dropping from a trial might affect future care.

Patient Instructions

It's quite useful and timesaving to develop a template for patient instructions on outpatient studies. On long-term studies in particular, you might like to provide patients with wallet cards for easy reference. Occasionally, misguided physicians stopped patients' study medications because they had never heard of the drugs, even when the patients told the doctors they were participating in trials. A card with your phone number can help avoid this type of costly glitch. (For sample "Patient Instructions" and a sample "Patient Wallet Card," visit http://conductingclinicalresearch.com.)

Patient instructions should include the following elements:

- Name of medication and indication
- Medication dosing and scheduling
- Any special storage instructions for the drug
- List of medications that must not be taken concurrently (e.g., MAO inhibitors or antacids)
- List of any foods that must not be eaten (e.g., foods containing tyramine)
- Reminders to return all medication vials or blister packs, even if used or empty (for drug accountability and compliance assessment)
- Reminders not to share the medication with anyone else and to keep the medicine in a secure place

A good PR idea, especially on long-term studies, is to provide the patients with cute little tote bags in which to store all of their supplies, diaries, and so on, to reduce the likelihood of their forgetting to bring a required item to a study visit.

"Con Meds"

Along with the reminders and detailed instructions regarding the investigational drug, be sure you address concomitant medications, or "con meds," with both your volunteers and their primary physicians. Otherwise, you will likely be surprised by what your patients forget to tell you. Generally volunteers aren't really trying to "con" you; they just don't deem some information to be important. This is particularly true regarding over-the-counter medications or herbal supplements they may be taking.

Why should you care? Because, of course, careful attention will provide better patient care and more useful data. But sloppiness can also result in FDA sanctions. Following are tips on how you can avoid major headaches for your site.

Con meds include drugs and biological products, such as vaccines or blood products. Often, nutritional supplements are considered food, rather than medication, but that is not the way they are categorized in most clinical trial reporting, and this distinction is important. For example, is glucosamine and chondroitin just a supplement? The concurrent use of this drug would certainly be relevant to note on an arthritis trial's study of an investigational agent.

A good way to overcome patient forgetfulness is by asking your volunteers to bring a bag containing all of their medications and supplements to each study visit. This will likely save time and help you avoid burdensome reconciliations later.

Thoroughly documenting all medications taken while a subject is on an investigational agent is critical for helping you attribute causality to symptoms or problems that might come up and to monitor for possible drug interactions. So sponsors will want you to track all such additional exposures in abundant detail.

Sponsors will likely have varying time periods for reporting exposure to these other agents, and, unfortunately, their formats for capturing this information will also vary. To avoid unnecessary aggravation and work, it's important to understand the ground rules before you enroll patients. For example, will sponsors want the individual dose size reported or the total daily dose? How do you document a dose that varies over a given time range? What if the dose changes? The following information must be recorded for each medication: name, dose, and indication. Beyond that, details vary for how to record it; Eric Ceh provides some good examples.[16]

Clearly, identifying the indication can be critical in capturing new symptoms or adverse events, as well as in determining the efficacy of the study medication. For example, it is common on influenza trials and long-term arthritis trials to provide "rescue meds" for pain. But analgesics and anti-inflammatory medications can mask the symptoms you want to monitor for efficacy. Note that for meds like nonsteroidal anti-inflammatory drugs, the indications may well vary, and each symptom or indication should be reported separately. For example, is the symptom of "pain" a headache, myalgia, arthritis, or other discomfort? (Emmanuel Maheu and others on the Osteoarthritis Research Society task force have written a good overview of symptom-modifying drugs versus structure-modifying drugs.)[17] Be sure to make careful note of the indication for each drug. Is it for symptom relief? Prophylaxis? A concurrent illness?

Diligently recording conmeds is a key factor in understanding and detecting adverse events, evaluating efficacy of symptom relief, and contributing important data for study analysis. While recording this information can feel like a nuisance, keeping its importance in perspective and having good formats for capturing this information concurrently can greatly reduce the difficulties of this task.

Lessons from Katrina—Have an Emergency Action Plan

Have you heard of IEPs, or individualized education plans, for kids? Well now you need a related plan, a unique EAP, or emergency action plan, for your site. Most of us were oblivious to that need until Hurricane Katrina hit.

At that time in 2005, 750 active clinical trials were taking place at the Ochsner Clinic in New Orleans and hundreds more elsewhere in the area.[18, 19] Studies included patients with serious illnesses such as cancer, diabetes, HIV, hemophilia, lung disease, and cardiac disease, as well as medical device trials.

Many of the lessons learned relate to the need for better communications plans and for backups. For example, almost all communication was seriously disrupted for some length of time after the hurricane, including cell phone service and Internet access. Digital text messaging reportedly worked the most consistently.[20] There was no immediate way to contact study participants, and many were lost to follow-up after they were evacuated to other communities scattered across the country.

In addition to the loss of contact with patients and loss of data and research specimens, the magnitude of the financial and personnel loss to universities was staggering. For example, Louisiana State University reported a loss from clinical trials of "more than $7,000,000 from fiscal year 2005 to fiscal year 2006. Seventeen NIH funded investigators have left the institution since the hurricane for a total loss of $5.7M per year."[21]

Some sponsors and sites had on-line survivor databases designed to unite patients and doctors. Tulane University's "Office of Human Subjects Protection required all investigators to report on the status of their studies and efforts being made to contact participants, to define potential harms to participants from the research interruption and to formulate plans to mitigate those harms."[22]

Take-home messages include the following:

- Obtain as much contact information as your volunteers will provide, including cell phone numbers, e-mail addresses, and emergency contacts (preferably outside the area). Note this information as part of your HIPAA consent. Store this information securely, and also back up the data off site.
- Require that sites provide subjects with contact information in the form of an identification card or wallet card, as previously described.
- Consider using radio communication with subjects after a disaster, as well as Web site postings. We used radio announcements very effectively when a large group of elementary school students took refuge in my house during a tornado warning years ago; the memory remains quite vivid. We called a local radio news station and asked that someone broadcast that the kids were safely at my home and would stay there until the authorities permitted otherwise. It would be a good idea to keep contact information for local radio and television news stations handy.
- Require a universal toll-free phone number on investigational product labels; patients would then likely have this with them wherever they might be evacuated to.[23]

- Partner with other sites in different geographic areas to plan for a backup location in case of emergency.
- Have remote data storage and backup electronic records off-site. Tulane had electronic medical records that were accessible from distant locations. The university also was able to set up a toll-free number for volunteers to call.

While all of this may sound excessive or unnecessary, there is much to be learned from Katrina; it would be wonderful to have something good come out of this debacle.

The Paper Trail Continues

Generally, the CRA will visit as soon as the first patient has completed the study visits at your site. Occasionally, an anxious CRA will visit shortly after the first patient is enrolled, sometimes even before the patient has completed the trial. This is more likely to occur with complicated studies or unfamiliar sites. The CRA will be eager to verify all aspects of the study's conduct and documentation and that is done by comparing the source documents to the case report forms.

What Is a Source Document?

In essence, source documents are the collection of a patient's medical record and any ancillary worksheets for the protocol. They also include memos, study diaries, and information recorded from EKGs or other electronic devices—any original data or records. Especially critical are verification that the patient has met the inclusion and exclusion criteria and verification that informed consent was properly obtained. Source documents also include documentation of drug dispensing and administration (the medicine administration record, or MAR) on the patient's chart, as well as records of all completed procedures, compliance issues, and any adverse events. Every step must be verifiable; auditors should be able to reconstruct a patient's course on a study by piecing together all of the data from the original source documents.

Some companies allow photocopies of blank CRFs to be used as study worksheets and source documents. Others don't. Be careful to check. Using a "mock-up" of the CRF is sometimes useful for making sure that you don't miss capturing any of the data that the sponsor wants and that may not be part of your routine. This format also makes it easier to transcribe the data onto the actual CRF. Often, however, the CRF design is not user friendly and may be cumbersome. I often prefer to design my own worksheets in a form that will expedite patient visits and safeguard capturing information critical to the study-required assessments. This may be more time-consuming for the coordinator to transcribe, but to me it is a "perk" I feel is both well earned and well deserved. It is critical to try to capture all required assessments and document them well. Remember, "If it isn't documented, it didn't happen."

Before going over what else will likely happen at the monitoring visit, let's review CRFs in detail.

What Is a Case Report Form?

A case report form is a report in which the site's research coordinator attempts to capture all of the relevant study data for an individual subject in a format easy to enter into a database. The data are then submitted to the sponsor.

Each CRF records the following data for a study volunteer:

- Visit schedule
- Inclusion and exclusion criteria
- Medical history
- Demographic information
- Lists of medications (see the sample "Concomitant Medications" list at http://conductingclinicalresearch.com)
- Lab data
- Special test results
- Clinical end points and outcomes
- Adverse events
- Study summary and the PI's evaluation of outcomes

It is imperative that all corrections on CRFs be made by drawing a single line to strike through the error and then placing the correction, initialed and dated, next to the offending item. This is *the* cardinal rule of CRFs and is to be inviolate. The reason for this is that *everything*—and that does mean everything—must be verifiable and available for a clear audit trail.

The monitor collects one copy of the forms after comparison and verification against the source documents or original medical record. Most of the data are relatively clear-cut and objective (e.g., past medical problems such as diabetes, hypertension, etc., or results of lab tests). These types of data are amenable to check boxes or "fill in the blanks" that can be coded. The coordinator transcribes the required data from office or hospital medical records, lab and x-ray results, and worksheets, onto forms (in duplicate or triplicate, with carbonless paper) that are coded, and on which there is no personally identifiable information.

Some of the data are not straightforward and are more difficult to capture, such as adverse events or symptoms, because patients often forget to mention symptoms at a particular visit but will recall them at a follow-up visit.

Symptom diaries are also quite problematic as intrinsic day-to-day variations and inconsistencies occur in evaluation and reporting. Following up on adverse events also tends to be more subjective, and is not as well documented, and can therefore be quite problematic. These problems will come back to harass you in the form of seemingly unending query forms or requests for clarification. If the sponsor's Grand Computer Data Cruncher is good, it will be programmed to identify problem areas, such as a new symptom or medication, and to look for inconsistencies between one section of the CRF and another, generating the dreaded query forms. Minimizing the hassle of queries is one good reason to keep a running list of adverse events readily available on each patient's chart and to use your own forms to log them (see the sample "Adverse Event/Intercurrent Illness Log" at http://conductingclinicalresearch.com). Keeping a patient problem list as additional confirmation is also helpful (see the sample "Patient Problem List" at http://conductingclinicalresearch.com). Be sure to include some amount in your budget to handle time for query resolution.

For consistency and to try to reduce day-to-day observer variation (even my own!), worksheets that place all subjective assessments on one form are preferable to those with separate packets for each visit. (Samples of a CRF, various worksheets, and a "Data Clarification or Query Form" are available at http://conductingclinicalresearch.com.) CRFs used to be designed this way but are now generally set up on a visit-by-visit basis. Having one form at hand will help you minimize queries. A similar worksheet is useful for tracking concomitant medications and noting AEs at the same time—as the patient reports a change in medication, questions about the need for the new medicine can be used to complete the AE report more accurately. One incentive for reducing CRF queries is that the sponsor will withhold the final grant payment until all the queries are resolved and the data are declared "clean."

For phase 3 trials in particular, 7,500–9,000 pieces of data may be entered for each patient. Multiply that by the 500–800 patients that may be on a trial (some I've participated in have had approximately 1,200), and you'll see that a trial is likely to generate well over 6—perhaps 9—million pieces of information to be interpreted.[24] These figures certainly give a sense of the amount of number crunching and sophistication needed to analyze trial data. They also bring us back to the importance of having a good study design to start with.[25] Finally, these numbers again help explain the enormous costs of clinical research trials. John Clay, director of e-technologies at Aventis Pharmaceuticals, reports that the costs of data collection, industry-wide, were approximately $4.8 billion in 2001 and that the cost per individual data query was $75–$100.[26]

View from the Trenches

CRFs—a Hazard to Your Health?

When I began doing studies, CRFs were simple documents, generally 12–15 pages long, with additional forms available to report AEs or SAEs if needed. They were essentially small folders, with data captured by subject area (e.g., symptom assessment or all vital signs) rather than by visit. Now, the CRFs are voluminous and heavy notebooks weighing up to 8 pounds per patient.

Let me warn you to be alert to repetitive use stress injuries from handling the CRFs themselves. I know. I've developed torn cartilages in both wrists from handling massive CRFs. This resulted in considerable pain and debility and required several operations. A triangular fibrocartilage complex (TFCC) injury produces an unusual syndrome, generally misdiagnosed, including at the "meccas." I learned that the hard way, too. Fortunately, I eventually found a terrific hand surgeon who immediately recognized the problem and, less immediately, fixed it—more or less. If you develop new problems, you just have to apply similar investigative skills to solving them as you do to your research and become a sleuth to discover the culprit.

Adverse Event Reporting: Tracking Regulatory Reports

Flattering child you shall know me, see why in towers I hide
Look round your lab and your binders, it is there inside.

—*Kathy Schulz*

Adverse events are any new, untoward signs or symptoms that develop while a patient is on a study, whether or not you believe they are related to the investigational medicine. They are considered one type of "unanticipated event."

"Unexpected" or "unanticipated" refers to any AE not listed in the Investigator's Brochure. If an AE is listed in the Investigator's Brochure, it is not unexpected—and no longer needs to be reported. Whether or not an AE requires any intervention, or whether it really represents an intercurrent (simultaneously occurring) illness, investigators have been required to report anything new or unanticipated. The OHRP notes that the phrase "unanticipated problems" is found in regulations but not defined and explains it as any incident that is "unexpected in nature, severity, or frequency . . . related or possibly related to participation in the research . . . and suggests that the research places subjects or others at a greater risk of harm than was previously known or recognized."[27]

And you must report any action taken and the presumed relationship of the symptom to the study medicine. Adverse events may be defined as serious or not serious, and they carry different reporting implications. To elicit adverse events, ask patients if they have experienced anything new since you last saw them. Try not to bias them by suggesting specific symptoms. Open-ended questions are preferable. You should also ask if they are taking any new medications or have sought other healthcare in the interim.

Serious adverse events are those that are fatal or immediately life threatening, are significantly or permanently disabling, require or prolong hospitalization, or are manifested as birth defects or a congenital anomaly. These definitions were developed by the International Conference on Harmonisation and are the definitions that the FDA also uses.[28] (The FDA now also emphasizes or "Requires Intervention to Prevent Permanent Impairment or Damage").[29]

By custom (and sponsor requirements), serious adverse events must be reported to the sponsor within 24 hours of discovery, and usually within 48 hours to the local IRB, which can establish its own requirements.

A sample "Serious Adverse Event Report" form is available at http://conductingclinicalresearch.com. The sponsor then has 7 calendar days to report the SAE to the FDA if the event was fatal, unexpected (meaning not in the Investigator's Brochure), and associated with the study drug. Nonfatal unexpected SAEs must be reported to the FDA within 15 days. These reports then become IND safety reports, which are promptly sent to all the investigators of the trial. However, in every year of a clinical trial, the sponsor has to submit new information supporting the IND. This includes updating the Investigator's Brochure—which then removes the finding from "unexpected" and reduces reporting requirements.[30]

These reporting requirements have been evolving and, frankly, are even more confusing now because the recommendations from the FDA, which changed in January 2009, are a bit at odds with those of the OHRP. Why does this matter? Largely, it is a matter of what will increase safety.

A corollary of this development is that the workload for the IRB and investigators has skyrocketed, raising the concern that all the reporting is actually creating an unsafe environment. A recent presentation subtitle from Western IRB is telling: "Improve safety by reporting less." The IDSA echoes this concern, noting in a complaint to the newly appointed FDA commissioner, Margaret Hamburg, that "local investigators and IRBs receive a flood of off-site adverse event reports. Importantly, neither the local investigator nor the local IRB has access to the information that would allow them to perform any meaningful analysis of individual adverse event reports (e.g., denominators that would allow calculation of rates of adverse events). As a result, the evaluation of off-site adverse event reports becomes a pointless exercise for local investigators and IRBs, and one that is estimated to consume 9% of the local IRBs' time and resources." The FDA wants to continue having the local IRBs assess a variety of unanticipated event reports from off site; the OHRP recommends that reporting to the IRB be limited to cases the sponsor or DSMB feels relate to patient safety.[32, 33]

KEY POINT
The only AEs that need to be reported to the IRB are those events that meet the definition of "unanticipated problems."[31]

Part of the confusion is that the "FDA regulations use different terms when referring to an *adverse event*. For example, *adverse effect* is used in 21 CFR 312.64; *adverse experience* is used in §312.32; and unanticipated problems is used in §312.66."[34] The FDA is currently just using "adverse event" to cover all.

Figure 6.1 provides perhaps the clearest explanation. If an adverse event is known (e.g., reported in the Investigator's Brochure), it need not be reported. Otherwise, consider it unanticipated and report it.

I had to plot out the information in table 6.1 to even try to understand the new guidance. (By the way, a guidance is considered a nonbinding recommendation, but who wants to take a chance during an audit?)

LEGAL LAND MINE
Err on the side of reporting, especially if event is "alarming" (unexpected, serious).

So what is a poor investigator to do? Most often, the confusion and difficulty stem from trying to assign causality—do you believe the investigational drug is responsible for the adverse event? Practically and ethically speaking, attributing causality of an AE is no easy matter. Particularly with critically ill patients who are on multiple medications, deciding if a change is due to an underlying illness, a medication interaction, or a new complication of the disease is extraordinarily difficult.

Carefully document every detail you can about each patient's symptoms or signs at the outset. Sometimes people don't remember details, but as an example, noting that someone has chronic headaches occurring one time per week can be very helpful later during the study. Be sure you mention the severity and frequency of each symptom.

A careful review of the patient's baseline medications—including over-the-counter and prn (as-needed) medications—will often yield clues to which of the underlying symptoms or conditions should be documented. Recording baseline physical examination findings carefully is equally important.

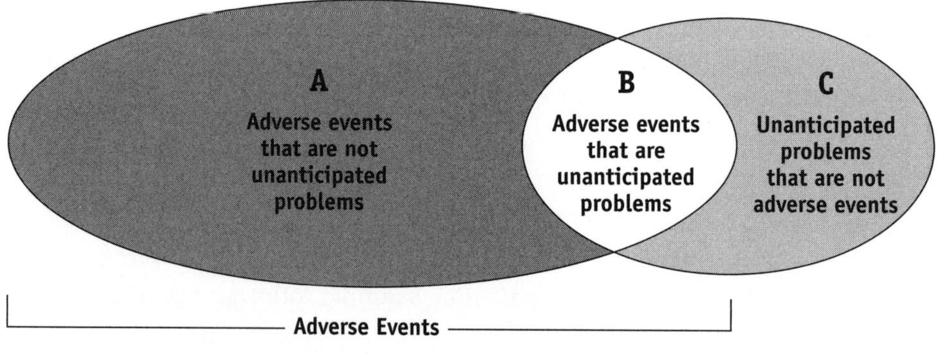

Figure 6.1 What problems do you report?[35]

Table 6.1 Reporting of adverse events[36]

Event	Regulation	Who reports event?	To whom?	How fast?
AE, related or probably related to drug	21 CFR 312.64	PI	Sponsor	Immediately if "alarming"
Serious AE, related, unexpected	21 CFR 312.32(c)	Sponsor	FDA and all PIs via IND safety report	
Unreasonable significant risk	21 CFR 312.56	Sponsor	IRB and PI	
Unanticipated problem or "adverse events that should be considered unanticipated problems"	21 CFR 56.108(b)(1), 21 CFR 312.53(c)(1)(vii), 21 CFR 312.66	PI	IRB	"Promptly" (undefined by FDA—1 week recommended by OHRP if serious, 2 weeks if not)

A separate issue gets back to the confusing and inconsistent recommendations regarding AE reporting. No deterrent exists for reporting an AE, but perhaps an inherent disincentive for the site is that each AE generates yet more work and another report. But if you try to ignore a symptom, it will likely be picked up by your CRA, especially if the patient received a new medication for symptom relief. Then you'll have to go back and ferret out all the details. This is more costly to your site, in both time and aggravation, than tracking this information as you go along and reporting it with the initial CRF.

I have a low threshold for reporting potential adverse events, especially if they are unexpected. If an event was mentioned in the Investigator's Brochure, then in theory, it is not unexpected. But if it is disconcerting to me or gives me indigestion, that exceeds my threshold and prompts me to file an AE report.

Clarify the ground rules with your sponsor's monitors and with your own IRB at the start. What are their definitions of events that are to be reported, especially regarding SAEs? Do they have a specific, standardized grading scale for classifying lab abnormalities, or is that left to your judgment? What is the time frame for reporting adverse events? Explicitly defining these details will save your site considerable time and stress—and help keep you from feeling like you might go insane completing AE reports. Most importantly, clear and rational AE reporting requirements might help detect important side effects of drugs that are in development.

To help guide you, see the following algorithm and some common examples.

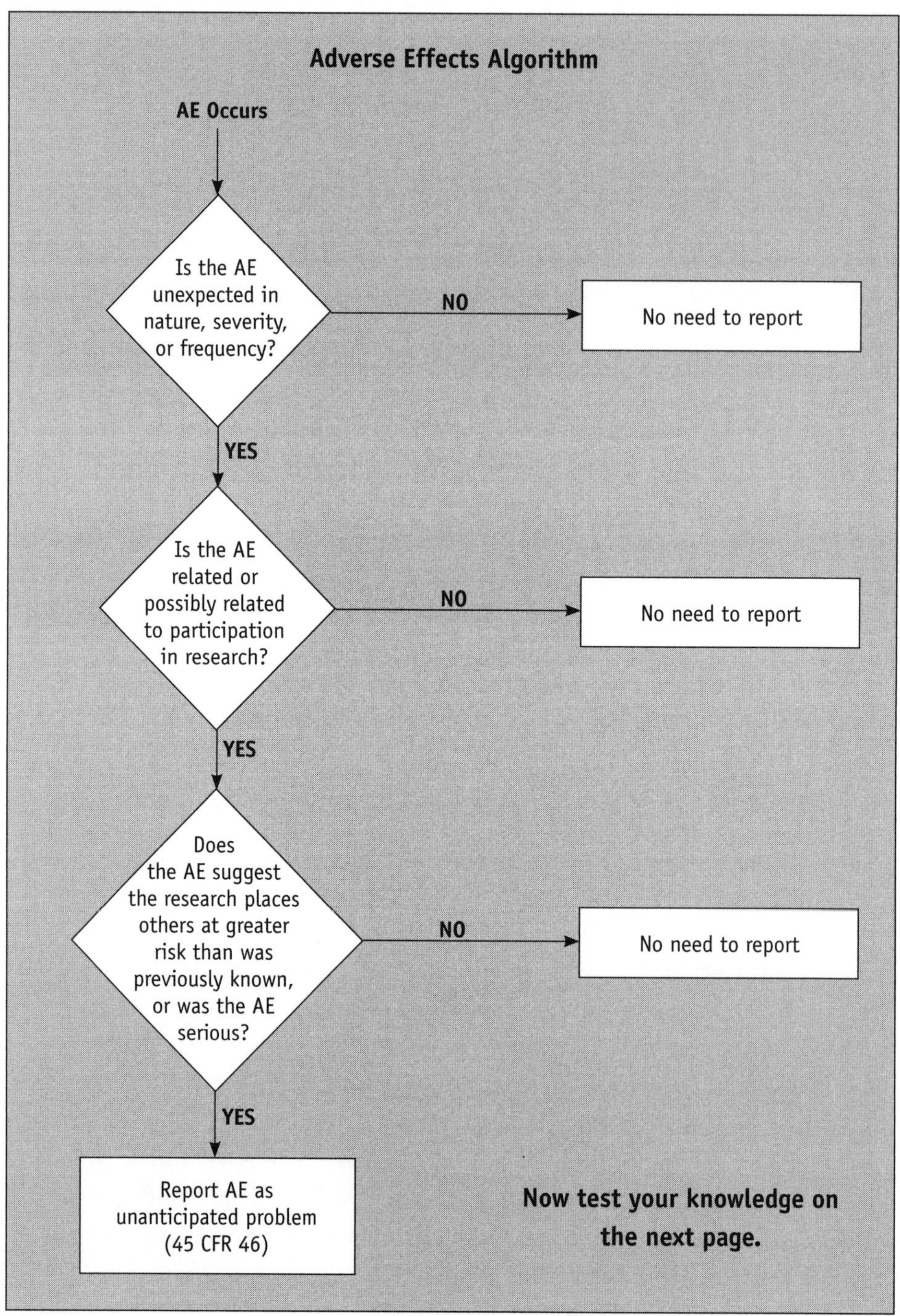

Test Your Knowledge![37]

Do you report the following?

a. The Investigator's Brochure lists elevated liver transaminases. Your volunteer develops hepatic necrosis.

b. Your volunteer develops angiodema or Stevens-Johnson syndrome

c. A patient with cancer dies during trial participation.

d. A volunteer develops a tendon rupture.

e. An elderly subject falls and breaks a hip.

f. Volunteers' "data are stored on a laptop computer without encryption, and the laptop computer is stolen from the investigator's car on the way home from work."[38]

g. A volunteer on a study testing "the safety and efficacy of a new investigational anti-inflammatory agent for management of osteoarthritis develops severe abdominal pain and nausea one month after randomization. Subsequent medical evaluation reveals gastric ulcers." The consent form notes a "2 percent chance of developing gastric ulcers."[39]

Answers[40, 41]

a. Yes. "Hepatic necrosis would be unexpected (by virtue of greater severity) if the investigator brochure only referred to elevated hepatic enzymes or hepatitis." (FDA)

b. Yes. "A single occurrence of a serious, unexpected event that is uncommon and strongly associated with drug exposure (such as angioedema, agranulocytosis, hepatic injury, or Stevens-Johnson syndrome)" should be reported. (FDA)

c. No, but debatable. This is not "unexpected" unless "the event rate is higher in the drug treatment group compared to the control arm" (FDA) but is a worrisome blind spot from my perspective. See "Who's Minding the Store?" in chapter 8 for an illustrative example.

d. Yes. Even "a single occurrence of a serious, unexpected event that is not commonly associated with drug exposure, but uncommon in the study population (e.g., tendon rupture, progressive multifocal leukoencephalopathy)" should be reported. (FDA)

e. Debatable. If the subject requires hospitalization, the event should be reported. The underlying question is why the subject fell. Did the subject become dizzy and lose balance, a known side effect of quinolones? Did he or she develop an arrhythmia from a drug interaction? Or did the subject trip on an obstacle because he or she wasn't paying attention?

f. Yes. This was unanticipated and "placed the subjects at a greater risk of psychological and social harm from the breach in confidentiality of the study data than was previously known or recognized." (OHRP)

g. No. It was not more severe or frequent than expected by an individual investigator. This again requires the sponsor to carefully gather and analyze data across multiple sites and report if the incidence of a problem is more frequent or severe than anticipated. For prompt analysis and reporting to the IRBs to occur, a certain leap of faith is required unless a strong DSMB is in place.

Be forewarned! SAEs usually occur on Friday nights, especially at the beginning of a holiday period. Despite this aggravation, I have always maintained a low threshold for calling in SAEs, and I follow up aggressively if I think this is possibly a previously unreported event.

The True Story of "Chicken Man"

Once there was a quinolone study. Now, quinolones, as a general class of drugs, are known to produce central nervous system side effects, such as hallucinations, insomnia, and headaches, in addition to oddball reactions, like sunburn. So these potential adverse reactions were described in the informed consent agreement, and Mr. H. agreed to participate in the trial.

On the day after enrollment, I went to visit him on my rounds and, as is my custom, I asked him if he had any new problems. With a perfectly straight face, he said that he had thought he was a dog and wanted to run after cars. The next day, he said he wanted to have sex with a chicken!

The third day, Mr. H. had asked the nurses to alert him when I was about to arrive. When I walked in and, bracing myself, asked him if there was anything new, he blew fake feathers out of his mouth at me and started clucking and flapping his arms.

"Chicken Man" was a delight to care for in the brief time that our friendship had to develop. He had a wonderful sense of humor and loved joking with people. I still think of him often and am sorry I wasn't able to know him better.

As a joke in his tradition, we wrote up a mock SAE form for the pharmaceutical company, wanting to share this delightful tale with them. Don't try it. Company regulatory personnel are a humorless lot!

Safety Reports

The most difficult study reports to track are the IND safety reports and local adverse events reports to the IRB. On worldwide studies in particular, one could drown in the IND reports submitted to the IRB. In this case, using a central IRB is much easier than using a local one, as the sponsor will submit the necessary reports directly to the IRB for you, and the IRB will automatically inform the study sites if any changes are necessary. In contrast, with a local IRB, the site investigators must submit each safety report to the IRB. Furthermore, it is imperative that the site receive a letter back from the IRB that acknowledges receipt of the information and explains whether any action is necessary. Budget extra administrative time for a worldwide study!

Maintaining the regulatory documents and CRFs for a trial is like picking up your room when you were little—not much fun, but easier to do a bit at a time as you go along. It's extraordinarily tempting to procrastinate on the "administrivia" and then be faced with a mountain of regulatory documentation. Your mom was right: do it now. The same upkeep rule applies to the CRF and queries. The source documents and the CRF should tell a story about what happened with a patient. It is much easier to fill in any gaps while everyone remembers the patient (and before changes occur in study personnel) than later.

Figure 6.2 shows the ebb and flow of the endless cycle of reports and regulatory documents that pass through a study site office. It's not so hard to play this game—you just need to make sure the cycles are completed. You can get help with this by using the "IRB Communications Checklist" and "IRB Communications Log" available at http://conductingclinicalresearch.com.

Are you thinking (wishing) that the end is in sight? We're getting there—almost. Hang on.

Study Closing

On reaching the study closing point, you are likely either to feel, "Thank goodness it's over" or to wonder, "When will I see you again?" depending on the sponsor company or its monitors. For the most part, this phase should simply involve tying up loose ends. As noted earlier, at the end of the study the CRA (monitor) will come for a closeout visit, which is like a recapitulation of the initiation visit, in reverse. At this time, the monitor will conduct a drug inventory and accountability check and, usually, help prepare the leftover stock for return to the drug company. (See the "Study Closeout Checklist" at http://conductingclinicalresearch.com. The sample "Drug Accountability or Dispensing Log" will help you track drug supplies during the course of the study.) Again, logs must be filled out to document everything for the government.

View from the Trenches

Sponsor-Site-IRB Communications

There is a rather rhythmic flow of paper cycling through the study site office. If the drudgery of the paperwork weren't so oppressive, one could almost appreciate the cyclic rhythms as a natural "life cycle." For example, the sponsor will send an IND safety report about an adverse event that was noted in, say, Latvia. My coordinator dutifully adds it to my pile of daily mail and reports to review. I initial the report and decide on its level of urgency in transmitting it to the IRB. I toss it back to the appropriate pile on the coordinator's desk. She gathers up the IND safety report and other reports, copies them, and submits them to the IRB. The original paper is filed in the official regulatory binder. A cover letter must be generated for the IRB, listing each report and requesting acknowledgment of receipt, as well as asking whether the IRB requests any action be taken because of the possible new AE finding. The cover letter comes back to my pile for signature. The IRB then sends the appropriate mirror-image letter back, and this also is filed. If I'm lucky, my coordinator will bypass my pile this time and just file the thing.

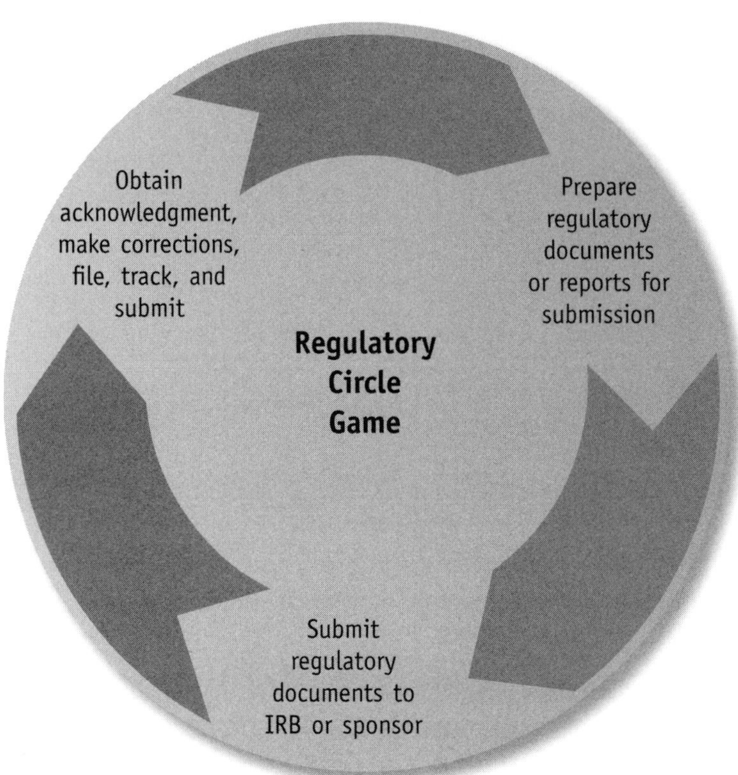

Figure 6.2 Regulatory circle game

Activities at the closeout visit include

- Checking regulatory documents and procedures. Are all the IRB approvals and acknowledgment letters in place? The final report to the IRB and the sponsor must be completed and filed, along with documentation of its receipt by the IRB.
- Checking that regulatory documents are complete and current.
- Checking that IND reports have been submitted. Do you have acknowledgment from the IRB documenting receipt?
- Reviewing outstanding CRF queries or edits. Grit your teeth and just try to be quickly done with one of the most unpleasant tasks on a study. Neither the sponsor nor the CRA is allowed to make changes to the CRF without your permission, so you have to do it. Remember, your final grant payment is dependent on this step.

- Checking the study drug inventory and returning the remaining study drug.
- Checking storage of CRFs. Remember that CRFs must be kept almost in perpetuity. As you prepare them for interment, it would be useful to mark each box with the name and date of the study and how long the CRFs must be retained. Before you consider off-site storage or disposal of records, prepare a log of all the study participants, including their names and study subject numbers, and save this log. I also try to keep samples of consent forms or particular study aids that might be useful in the future.

The International Conference on Harmonisation (ICH) requires study records to be retained for 2 years after the last trial is completed; the FDA requires 2 years retention after NDA approval or discontinuation of the IND. Given that studies go on seemingly forever, retention can be a very long time. Realize that the record retention period may be driven by drug company standard operating procedures (SOPs) rather than by the ICH guidelines or FDA regulations. Different sponsors have different requirements, but they generally average 15 years. Check with each sponsor and try to get the answer in writing.

KEY POINT
Informed consent forms are critical. Consider keeping a second copy of them off-site.

Double-check that all of your informed consent forms, in particular, are complete and available for inspection. These and the IRB approvals and communications are critical for your well-being.

At study closeout, you will need to send a report to the IRB summarizing your study enrollment and outcomes, with a special note of adverse events (see the sample "Study Closure Report to the IRB" at http://conductingclinicalresearch.com). The CRA will want to ensure that all AEs—and especially, all SAEs—have been reported both to the IRB and to the sponsor company. Again, this is like a boomerang—if a letter goes out to the IRB, one must come back from the IRB, acknowledging whatever you sent.

The CRA will check that all regulatory documents are in order and then send a bothersome letter citing any "deviations" or "protocol violations" found. You will receive numerous queries or requests for clarification from various reviewers and data analysts that must be answered before the trial database can be "locked" for final analysis. The number of queries is in part dependent on the quality of the CRF design. If the CRF is well designed and consistent in format, fewer errors will emerge to generate queries. Again, the CRA will pressure the site team to resolve the queries, holding final grant payments until this has been done as an additional tool of persuasion. Make sure you budget for query resolution time.

Conclusion

You now have a good technical grasp of the logistical details involved in conducting clinical trials. These details are important, but they pale in comparison to the underlying basis for the trial. The critical issues relate to whether the study questions and design are sound and, most importantly, to the ethics of the study. Before moving on to the ethical issues you are likely to encounter, we'll look at some of the broader issues facing the pharmaceutical industry and the problems hampering drug development.

CHAPTER 7

Perspective on the State of the Industry

> Change does not necessarily assure progress, but progress implacably requires change.
>
> —HENRY STEELE COMMAGER

In earlier chapters, we have focused on an overview of the logistical aspects of drug development and clinical trials and how investigative sites can prepare to succeed in this field. A significant shift has occurred in the clinical trial industry in the past few years, influenced by changing demographics, the regulatory environment, and globalization. This chapter provides the framework for understanding the underlying issues facing the industry.

Costs of Clinical Trials

In order to gain a better perspective on the drug development industry, it will help to have some understanding of the costs of conducting clinical trials. Did you know the following facts?

- Historically, it has taken an average of 12–15 years for a new drug to be brought to market. Although there is now a "fast-tracking" approval path for AIDS and cancer drugs, the process still takes several years. According to Tufts Center for the Study of Drug Development (CSDD), the clinical testing phases and approval times have dropped from 9.2 to 6.9 years since 1992, when the Prescription Drug User Fee Act was implemented, using the fees generated to hire more reviewers to speed the process. However, the time required for clinical development has outstripped this, resulting in a steadily increasing total time to bring a drug to market, particularly for biopharmaceutical drugs such as monoclonal antibodies and recombinant proteins.[1] Between 2002 and 2004, the approval times again increased due to lengthier clinical testing, averaging 8.5 years.[2]

- According to Tufts CSDD, of all the candidate drugs that start out, only 1 of 1,000 makes it beyond the animal-testing phase to human testing, and only 1 in 5 to 1 in 10 of the drugs that make it this far is then approved.[3] Even the more optimistic NIH comments that "unfortunately, the success rate in this preclinical process is low, with 80 to 90 percent of projects failing in the preclinical phase . . . Drug developers colloquially call this the 'Valley of Death.'"[4]

KEY POINT
About 80 to 90 percent of projects fail in the preclinical phase.

- Only 3 in 10 drugs have recouped or netted more than their development costs on the market.[5] So these three drugs must recover the cost of all of the failures for each manufacturer.
- The major annual costs for a large sponsor include
  - \$150–\$200 million for investigators
  - \$50–\$100 million for CROs
  - \$10–\$15 million for central laboratories (special studies)
  - \$8–\$12 million for monitoring[6]
- A new drug's time under patent has markedly decreased due to the longer time needed to bring the drug to market. Keep in mind that while a drug patent is granted for 20 years, 12–15 of those years are lost to the clinical trials phase, leaving only a relatively brief window in which to recoup the development costs.
- A typical New Drug Application "requires nearly 70 studies that consist of, on average, 90,650 pages, and requires an overall investment of \$359 million."[7] The regulatory process itself, preparing both the IND and NDA, represents only 3 percent of research and development costs, but this translates to \$24 million just for this step.[8]
- Delays in completing the approval of a new drug cost from \$684,931 to \$1 million per day.[9]

- In 2000, companies invested more than $26 billion for new drug development.[10] Since then, investment has more than doubled, growing to $50–65 billion in 2008.[11]
- Per-patient grant costs increased 33 percent from 1991 to 1994. This is primarily because drugs are increasingly aimed at difficult-to-treat disorders, such as AIDS, multiple sclerosis, and other immune problems.[12] Although the spending for research and development increased sixfold between 1980 and 2000, the pipeline for new drug development was disproportionately small and almost plateaued, with relatively few new drugs reaching market, in part due to the increasing complexity of the target illnesses.[13]
- According to the widely cited Tufts CSDD, the estimated cost of bringing a new drug to market rose from $802 million to $1.38 billion.[14] These controversial figures have received support from some healthcare analysts, but these analysts used the same methodology with different source data.[15] Not everyone agrees.

The consumer group Public Citizen, noting several flaws in the Tufts analysis, estimates the development costs to be only $110 million. Public Citizen has challenged the Tufts figures because

- The drugs analyzed in the report did not include any drugs that received government funding for development, yet many major drugs do receive federal support, defraying development costs.
- The study did not account for the 34 percent tax deduction the drug companies take for their research and development costs.
- The study included the expenses of project failures and other adjustments.
- The Tufts figures include opportunity costs (the estimated return on the candidate drug compared to the anticipated return on an alternative); the Public Citizen estimates do not.[16]

The Tufts figures also have been challenged by other economists and healthcare experts.[17]

Thus, depending on the underlying interests of the opposing groups—pharmaceutical companies versus public interest groups—drug development cost figures will be widely disparate.

But even if the figures are taken with a grain or two of salt, research and development costs still rose by a factor of 2.5 between 1991 and 2001 in inflation-adjusted figures, and another 60 percent between 2001 and 2006,[18] with the bulk of the increase occurring in the clinical trial phases.[19]

The cost of research and development varies both with the phase of clinical trial and by indication. For example, 2002 CenterWatch data show that nonclinical aspects of synthesis, formulation, and process development accounted for 21 percent of costs. Animal toxicological and safety testing and initial pharmacologic testing represented 16.2 percent of development costs. Clinical trial costs were an additional 35.9 percent of the total.[20]

The variations in expenditures for different indications are quite interesting. They were largely attributed to differences in trial durations and probabilities of success. For example, successful asthma drugs have higher development costs than do drugs like Viagra. Drugs for cancer and rheumatologic conditions are also at the high end of the scale for expected development costs.[21]

The proportion of total research and development funding ranged from a low of 3 percent for biologicals and 4 percent for respiratory illnesses to a moderate 12 percent for infectious diseases and cardiovascular ailments and to a high of 23–24 percent for central nervous system diseases and cancer.[22] Some of the increasing cost of research and development is due to the increasing complexity of technologies and trials. More complicated diseases are being studied, and patients are often more ill. Both factors make volunteer recruitment and retention more difficult and costly. In addition, more procedures are being required, which increases investigator and clinical trial staff time. These changes are clearly illustrated by the Tufts data: between 1999 and 2005, the number of procedures per protocol increased from 96 to 158 (65 percent), trials were 70 percent longer (780 days), and staffs' work effort increased 67 percent. At the same time, enrollment dropped by 21 percent (to 59 percent) and volunteer retention dropped 30 percent (to 48 percent). In sum, researchers are working longer on more complex studies, which makes it more difficult to recruit and retain volunteers—and all for lower reimbursement.[23, 24]

This increase in research and development costs is leading some pharmaceutical companies to refocus their research priorities and to bow out of investing in research on many antibiotics, which are taken only for short periods, or on diseases with limited populations of patients. The latter, known as orphan drugs, are for illnesses that affect fewer than 200,000 Americans (or, in Europe, fewer than 5 in 10,000 people). (Companies do receive tax credits as incentives to develop drugs for such small target populations.) Instead, most companies are focusing their efforts on treatment for common chronic illnesses, such as hyperlipidemia, hypertension, and diabetes.[25] For example, Pfizer's Zithromax, the best-selling antibiotic, is usually taken for only 5 days. It generated $2.01 billion in 2003. In contrast, the company's anticholesterol drug, Lipitor, which must be taken daily for years, generated $9.23 billion in sales.[26] The "net present value," a measure of return on future investment, shows that if antibiotics are given a value of one, cancer drugs will have a value three times greater and drugs for musculoskeletal pain a value eleven times greater.[27] As Dr. Stuart Pocock of the London School of Hygiene and Tropical Medicine so aptly put it, "Companies put huge amounts of money in trials, which have to be directed toward what stands a chance of being in their interests. And their interests are, in general, in danger of being in conflict with what are society's interests."[28]

Innovative Types of Trials

In January 2006, in an unprecedented move, the FDA released new guidelines designed to boost drug development. Only 20 new drugs were approved in 2005—little more than half of the previous year's number—with again lengthening approval times due to more prolonged clinical trial requirements. Recognizing that only 1 in 5 to 1 in 10 candidate drugs will pass the clinical trial phases, the FDA is working to streamline the drug research and development process under an umbrella known as the Critical Path Initiative.

Interesting innovations are occurring. One is allowing "exploratory IND studies" instead of traditional phase 1 studies: testing much smaller doses of drugs in smaller numbers of volunteers, carefully evaluating the pharmacokinetics and pharmacodynamics of the drug, and projecting what might happen with larger doses. These new "phase 0," or "microdosing," clinical studies will use less than 1⁄100 of the expected active dose of a new drug (to a maximum of 100 micrograms), which will be given to only 8–10 volunteers. Because of advances in assaying and imaging techniques, the companies would still be able to study the PK and PD of these tiny amounts. The use of small doses might enable researchers to more readily select among several candidate drugs, based on the PK and PD data, before committing to larger human trials.[29, 30] Phase 0 trials are particularly applicable for cancer trials and came from the recognition that few new oncologic agents made it through early clinical testing because of toxicities. The Division of Cancer Treatment and Diagnosis (DCTD) and the Center for Cancer Research NCI Experimental Therapeutics (NExT) program formed a collaboration to expedite studies of new compounds targeted toward specific sites or mechanisms of action. Exploratory IND studies are valuable for developing biomarker assays that may assess the efficacy, mechanism of action, and toxicity of promising targeted treatments before investing in costly large trials.[31] Since 70 percent of compounds for new cancer therapeutics fail costly phase 2 trials, it's important to try to identify the most promising candidates early in testing.[32]

The advantages of a microdosing approach are described by the NCI.[33] Abbott's ABT-888 was the first compound to undergo phase 0 testing. The drug was tested in only 14 volunteers, and studies focused on the drug's mechanism of action. The entire trial, from initiation to data analysis that confirmed proof of concept, took less than 6 months. ABT-888 is undergoing testing in phase 1 trials; it is a model for phase 0 testing and exploratory INDs.

The new exploratory IND guidance[34] will also make it much easier for small biotechnology companies, the National Institutes of Health, or academic medical centers to economically manufacture small amounts of drugs for the limited human testing in phase 0.

The benefits of earlier, exploratory testing are not limited to oncology trials. For example, in May 2009, the NIH launched an important integrated drug development pipeline to produce new treatments for rare and neglected diseases under an initiative called the Therapeutics for Rare and Neglected Diseases (TRND) program. This is important because industry has been reluctant to invest in such drugs, which are not as profitable as others it prefers to focus on. The intent is for the NIH's TRND program to bear the burden of the difficult preclinical work. If a successful compound is identified, TRND will work with private industry to test the therapy in patients. The NIH project will also devote some effort to improving the actual drug development process, creating new approaches that can then be shared across the organization's divisions.[35]

The FDA is also leaning toward allowing greater use of surrogate markers in determining efficacy. Such end points have already been used in assessing efficacy of anti-AIDS drugs, substituting drops in viral loads or increases in CD4 (helper T cells, which reflect the condition of the immune system) counts for mortality data. Similarly, new imaging techniques, such as PET (positron emission tomography) scans or assays for blood levels of tumor markers, may show early response to drugs for cancer.

The use of biomarkers is not entirely without controversy. For example, the FDA received harsh criticisms for its approval of Avandia (rosiglitazone), a drug for diabetes. The drug received approval, in part, on the basis of the surrogate marker of better glycemic control (lower blood sugar). However, further studies suggested that rosiglitazone is associated with an increased risk of myocardial infarction. So care needs to be taken when extending favorable biomarker outcomes to presumed clinical outcomes.[36, 37, 38] Similarly, the use of surrogate markers leaves unanswered the question of whether these drugs improve either survival or quality of life, particularly for cancer.

Phase 0 studies have also been criticized because microdosing enables small amounts of drugs to be given to volunteers before a true informed consent can be given since many of the former animal safety study requirements are markedly reduced. On the other hand, experience with the first successful phase 0 trial showed that volunteers accepted participation out of a sense of altruism.[39] Other critics also note that pharmacokinetics in healthy volunteers may not match those in cancer patients.[40]

Microdosing has not yet achieved widespread acceptance, but its promise—that of focusing drug development efforts on the most promising candidates—is likely to ensure continuing interest in this path.

Another relatively recent innovation is that of "adaptive clinical trials." Derek Lowe provides a great reason for this type of trial design: "In too many cases, the chief result of a trial is to show that the trial itself was set up wrong, in ways that only became clear after the data were unblinded." Adaptive trials attempt to avoid this problem by allowing staged protocols, with interim decision points and predetermined end points, which then lead to a new sequence of study. It sounds like a statistician's nightmare to design well, but it allows the trial to be modified based on what is learned along the way.[41, 42, 43] This seems eminently reasonable, though the approach has come under criticism largely because of blinding issues.

Each of these attempts to develop a novel, improved clinical trial design is undertaken with the intent to expedite drug and medical device study and approval.

The use of surrogate biomarkers, as was seen with the acceptance of HIV viral load and CD4 counts as evidence of efficacy, reflects another shift at the FDA and in study design—that of encouraging collaboration among typically rival pharmaceuticals. For example, Merck's sharing of its protease data greatly expedited the development of protease inhibitors, an entire class of new, lifesaving drugs.[44] Similarly, in 2006, a collaborative public-private partnership, the Biomarker Initiative, was formed among the Foundation for the National Institutes of Health (FNIH), NIH, FDA, and the Pharmaceutical Research and Manufacturers of America (PhRMA).

The Critical Path Initiative includes several programs designed to expedite the drug study, manufacturing, and approval process. These programs include a greater emphasis on collaboration, modeling, and tools:

- Animal models of human disease
- Development of biomarkers
- Bioinformatics, including computer-model-based drug development, electronic data capture, and data mining[45, 46, 47]
- Predictive Safety Testing Consortium between industry and the private Critical Path Institute
- International Serious Adverse Events Consortium (SAEC)

Comparative Effectiveness Research

Given soaring healthcare costs, enormous budget deficits, and the strained economy, the focus of proposed research has recently shifted to a more controversial type of trial design, that of comparative effectiveness research (CER). While earlier types of trials usually centered on establishing the efficacy of a drug or device compared to a placebo (a noninferiority trial), the new focus is on comparing the effectiveness between available therapies. This research is a congressional mandate as part of the American Recovery and Reinvestment Act (ARRA) of 2009. The legislation defines CER as covering "research that compares the clinical outcomes, effectiveness, and appropriateness of items, services, and procedures that are used to prevent, diagnose, or treat diseases, disorders, and other health conditions." The law directed the Institute of

Medicine to make recommendations for national priorities for CER funding—which it did in a remarkably short time.[48]

The current drug and device development processes focus on noninferiority trials, which have a lower threshold for success than do direct, head-to-head comparisons between products. As Stanford researchers recently noted, "Developers face few incentives to conduct active-comparator superiority trials and understand that they benefit from the unacknowledged deficiency of evidence. The development or marketing of me-too drugs and devices may provide a greater return on investment than research aimed at true clinical innovation."[49]

Not surprisingly, the CER plan has come under attack by pharmaceutical companies, despite the assurance, for now, that the research will not be used to restrict physicians' prescribing choices based on cost-effectiveness data.[50] Others are concerned that, rather than supporting rational healthcare decision making, the CER initiative is the first step down the slippery slope toward healthcare rationing.[51, 52] An interesting proposal—intended to close the evidence gap and more directly benefit prescribers and consumers—is to have the FDA require comparative effectiveness labeling on its products to make the benefits and risks of each product clearly evident.[53, 54] This debate over whether to provide labeling information reminds me of the attempts to block unit pricing and nutritional labeling on products at the grocery store.

With each of these recently adopted innovations and new ones under consideration, there are two factors to be weighed—what is in an individual's interest versus what may be best for society's interests. It will be interesting to watch this debate evolve.

In addition to the costs of drug development, a number of logistical impediments lie in the path of developing a successful new medicine. Let's examine these roadblocks in more detail.

"Breaking the Scientific Bottleneck"

Clinical research has aptly been described as the "neck of the scientific bottle." All scientific discoveries have to traverse this process before they can be of benefit to people. An overview of the major problems facing clinical research—and recommended solutions—is thoughtfully described in "Breaking the Scientific Bottleneck," a summary of a Clinical Research Summit.[55] The problems cited in that report and by others include the following:

- Clinical research is neither well understood nor valued by the public. While the research and development pipeline is currently growing, the pool of investigators is not keeping pace. Also, many of the drugs in development are for similar treatment indications, which further increases the competition for both investigators and patients. This is a significant factor contributing to the recent shift of study sites to countries other than the United States.[56]
- The cost of carrying out clinical trials is considerably lower outside the United States—40 percent lower in Canada, 60 percent lower in Poland, and 70 percent lower in South Africa, for example.[57]
- Insufficient numbers of physician investigators exist and too few are being trained. In part, this growing void is due to the debt burdens faced by young medical graduates, which discourage them from undertaking the length and rigors of the training in research (see chapter 10).[58] In part, emphasis has been placed less on training in research and more on the pragmatics of delivering cost-effective care for a managed care environment.
- An estimated 56,000 investigators are required worldwide with a 15 percent investigator shortfall expected by 2005.[59] The number of foreign researchers registered with the FDA has been growing rapidly—from 5 in 1991 to 453 in 1999 in South America, from 1 to 429 in eastern Europe, and from 2 to 266 in southern Africa. This trend is continuing through this decade.
- In 2007, there were more than 26,000 investigators globally.[60] The proportion of U.S. principal investigators decreased from 96 percent of the total global pool of FDA-regulated investigators in 1990 to 54 percent in 2007. During this period, while the number of U.S. investigators decreased 3.5 percent annually, there was a corresponding 13.5 percent annual increase in the number of foreign investigators.[61] More specifically, particularly rapid growth was noted in Russia, Poland, Bulgaria, and Romania in 2008. South Korea, Taiwan, and India were the hot growth spots in Asia. The notable exception was China, which showed a 30 percent drop in PIs signing Form FDA 1572s from the previous year.[62]

KEY POINT
Opportunity: 30,000 investigators are needed to conduct clinical trials.

- Similarly, there has been a shift in study patient demographics. In 1994, Eli Lilly and Company had 590 subjects in Africa, the Middle East, and central and eastern Europe; in 2000, 7,300 were anticipated.[63]
- Many trials lack adequate enrollment. An estimated 19.8 million patients were needed to fill industry-sponsored trials in 2005, up from 2.8 million people in 1999.[64] Overall, only 1–2 percent of the U.S. population participates in a clinical trial in a given year. Yet an average of 3,900 patients are required per NDA, and this requirement is increasing 7–10 percent per year.[65] Even among cancer patients, less than 4 percent participate in clinical trials.

KEY POINT
Approximately 19.8 million patients were needed for trials in one year.

- Data are lacking on sponsorship and funding of clinical research. Different sources may be unaware of research being undertaken as there had been until recently no central registry of trials, leading to inefficient duplications rather than effective partnerships.
- Insufficient funding exists for some types of clinical research, especially for research on the natural history of diseases and for collaborative research between basic scientists—who do bench (laboratory) research to understand the underlying mechanisms of disease or action—and those who do clinical research.
- Insufficient emphasis is placed on transferring and incorporating research findings into clinical practice.
- Collaboration among different disciplines and research groups is normally lacking.
- No comprehensive, credible national plan for clinical research exists.[66]

The stagnation in clinical research and the translation of bench discoveries to useful products is striking. From 1993 to 2003, U.S. research and development spending increased 2.5 times while both the number of new drugs (new molecular entities, or NMEs) and the new Biologics License Applications (BLA) showed a striking decline. The report of the Association of American Medical Colleges and FDA conference echoes the findings of the prior Clinical Research Summit and extends recommendations for improvement.[67]

Significant changes have occurred in the clinical trial industry in the past 5 years, many attempting to relieve the bottleneck—not all successfully.

The most time-consuming activities are patient enrollment (23 percent of the trial time), treatment (21 percent), study design and protocol development (17 percent), and site selection (9 percent).[68] Following is an overview of the bottleneck highlights.

Investigator Turnover

Earlier, I noted that insufficient investigators are being trained. A related serious problem is the high turnover in investigators. In part, this is due to a lack of "institutional memory" that accompanies the turnover in personnel at the sponsor and CRO companies. It also appears to reflect an attitudinal shift, where many companies seem to view investigators as readily available commodities or interchangeable parts, rather than long-term partners. This is a shortsighted approach. For one, at the same time as trials have grown increasingly complex, the pool of experienced investigators (those who have conducted more than five studies) has markedly decreased to only 16 percent. The remaining 84 percent have experience with fewer than five studies, meaning that they are unlikely to have become truly proficient at this specialty.[69] It reminds me a bit of my medical training, where we were irrationally on the worst schedules with the most sleep deprivation when we were taking care of the most seriously ill patients in the ICU or a high-volume emergency room.

Wouldn't you want to retain the most experienced investigators for complex protocols? Yet in the current climate, there seems to be no incentive for good performance and a good investigator is likely to be undervalued because there is a steady influx of new ones.[70]

Cutting Edge notes other long-term advantages for a sponsor cultivating partnerships with experienced investigators who are "driven primarily by the science." "Physicians excited about a treatment will help sell and market the value of the trial by illuminating the potential impact of the drug being tested . . . more than anything, establishing a personal relationship with an investigator through a long association helps to ensure successful trials. A strong relationship, as well as promise of more research further down the pipeline, is a strong incentive for investigators to give a company's trial the attention and devotion necessary."[71]

As we saw in "Win-Win Relationships" in chapter 3, some automakers—and the occasional enlightened sponsor personnel, are realizing the financial benefits of collaborative partnerships. Hopefully more sponsors will attain enlightenment—or enlightened self-interest.

Volunteer Retention and Recruitment

As noted earlier, the participation rate, even in cancer trials, is less than 5 percent. The initial hurdle, of course, is communication with potential volunteers. A general lack of awareness exists about the need for and benefits of clinical trial participation, and less than 4 percent of the public participates in research. In part, this is likely due to sensational news about studies gone awry and the use of human "guinea pigs." According to Harris Interactive, a whopping 81 percent of the general population say that they have never had the opportunity to participate in a clinical study. The majority of those that have had the opportunity have enrolled.[72] And 81 percent of people in the United States are not aware that there are human subjects protections such as institutional review boards.[73]

But mistrust of clinical researchers has markedly increased, not without some justification. "From 1996 to 2002, the percentage of the public who distrusted information received from clinical research professionals increased from 28% to 75%."[74] Similarly, the OIG noted a tenfold increase in complaints against sites.[75]

Increasingly restrictive enrollment criteria can be barriers to recruiting volunteers. While the number of exclusion criteria remained fairly constant from 1999 to 2005, the number of inclusion criteria increased almost threefold and has made it considerably more difficult to recruit volunteers.[76] Enrollment rates dropped from 75 percent between 1999 and 2002 to 59 percent between 2003 and 2006.

Similarly, volunteer retention dropped from 69 percent to 48 percent between these two study time periods. The retention rate may have worsened because of the rise in the average number of procedures required for completion from 89.8 to 150.5. Or it may reflect the increased number of adverse events and serious adverse events seen in the second period—but that may, in turn, reflect the growth in trials focusing on treatments for chronic diseases and on biologic agents, which generally target more serious illnesses, such as Crohn's disease and rheumatoid arthritis.[77]

Protocol Design

As noted earlier, trials have been increasing in complexity, and sponsors have had to respond to the resultant difficulty in recruiting and retaining volunteers and investigative staff. Pharmaceutical sponsors are working both to reduce costs and to increase their productivity through innovations in protocol design, such as microdosing and adaptive trials. They are also attempting to streamline the protocol requirements themselves. As the Tufts CSDD data showed, between 1999 and 2005, there was a 6.5 percent annual growth in the number of unique procedures per protocol as well as an 8.7 percent annual growth in the frequency of the protocol activities. There is slowly increasing recognition that the bloated activities and subsequent data collection need to be trimmed to focus on essentials.[78]

Cutting Edge has noted that sponsors often gather 5 to 10 times more data than is necessary—and that subsequently delays and costs accrue due to the need to process, clean, and analyze the extraneous information. Proposed solutions include working more closely with biostatisticians and regulatory agencies to identify essential information earlier in the process.[79]

Transparency

The problem of lacking data on the sponsorship and funding of clinical research has been greatly improved. One of the driving forces was the realization that many significant data results were being buried and that the reporting of negative trials was lacking—sometimes because they were perceived to be of little interest and other times because of restrictive publication clauses in contracts that prevented investigators from reporting trial findings without sponsor approval.

As we'll see in chapter 8, the marked evidence bias began to change in 2005 when the International Committee of Medical Journal Editors (ICMJE) announced that registration in a public trials registry would be a requirement for having publication privileges in the editors' respective journals. Further, as part of the FDA Amendments Act of 2007, Public Law 110-85 was put in place, legally requiring registration of drug and device trials to be submitted to the FDA and detailing specific required elements.[80]

Electronic Data Capture

All the data that are generated need to be captured and transmitted to the sponsor for verification and analysis. This step has been traditionally done by hand, with laborious transcription of the data to paper-and-pen case report forms that are completed and submitted. There is increasingly a move toward electronic data capture (EDC), which makes a certain amount of sense. In theory, EDC is a wonderful innovation and greatly reduces costs for the sponsor. The cost per page is reduced by 80 percent with EDC, errors are reduced by 90 percent, and time to database lock is markedly shortened. A report by Forrester calculated operational savings of almost $350,000 in a phase 2 trial and more than $6 million for a typical phase 3 trial.[81]

Real-time data allow shipping of limited supplies to sites that are actively enrolling patients or automation of similar processes. Early decisions can be made because the data are more readily accessible for analysis in a timely fashion, particularly useful on an adaptive trial. For the sponsor, EDC also reduces labor and costs and helps with project management, as information is immediately available regarding enrollment, protocol deviations, dropouts, and adverse events.

E-source documents may be the wave of the future if standardization occurs and mechanisms are worked out for linking these to electronic medical records. An e-source document has the advantage of generally being recorded more contemporaneously. Screen prompts can be a tremendous boon in verifying eligibility for participation, particularly in verifying concomitant medication exclusions. Prompts also can help ensure that fewer data are missed. Another advantage is that of providing a better audit trail. The FDA wants data that can be described by the acronym "ALCOA": attributable, legible, contemporaneous, original, and accurate. EDC certainly is better than hastily hand-scribbled notes. Also, patient compliance with EDC diaries (aka patient-reported outcomes [PROs]) was 94 percent, compared to 11 percent with paper diaries, and was much more timely.[82]

However, the problem with EDC, in my experience, is that a study site may be burdened with additional transcription of source documents or be stymied by glitches in the computer program that block further data entry or require input of misleading information to get beyond a particular screen. There is no standardization, and sponsors often require dedicated laptops with different programs, and sometimes even dedicated phone lines, which can be cumbersome, as well as enormously wasteful.

These challenges have been confirmed by others. For example, "With one recent study, the site had to enter data on 46 separate pages for every neurological exam done by the investigator. Each exam took only ten minutes, but data entry took a whopping 90 minutes." The site coordinator reported, "We almost quit recruiting for the study because we were losing money."[83]

RapidTrials' Lisa Meyerson and Tracy Harmon Blumenfeld note,

Keep in mind that sites working simultaneously on multiple studies are often working with a series of tools and systems that are unique to each sponsor or study. One site recently reported using seven unique technologies—interactive voice recognition, document management, EDC system, e-diary, ECG system, central lab, and patient recruitment—over the course of one study.

If a site is participating in five studies, each requiring seven systems, then it is possible that a single study coordinator may be expected to access 49 different technologies, each with a different user name, password, navigation, hotline, and training program. Once the study is complete, they may never use the systems again. Forced to prioritize their time, it is reasonable to expect that study coordinators will favor user-friendly studies with low operational and technology hurdles, even if that means turning down trials of drugs with greater lifesaving potential.[84]

And, as with paper case report forms (CRFs), data entry is not standardized; unfortunately, each company has specific and unique requirements for inputting information.[85] With EDC, errors may be less immediately evident, and you may be blocked from going further or generating queries if data are entered incorrectly. Data entry tends to be batched more than with paper CRFs, so it can be more difficult, time-consuming, and frustrating for coordinators to go back, find missing data, and correct any errors.[86]

KEY POINT
EDC is good for sponsors but not for sites.

Data errors could be greatly reduced by well-designed electronic source documents and CRFs. Second to patient enrollment, reducing data errors is a major concern cited by sponsors.[87] Hopefully, efforts like those of the Clinical Data Interchange Standards Consortium, which is developing a set of global standards, will reach fruition. EDC holds promise for the future; it is not yet ready for prime time.

Standardization

Currently, each sponsor CRO develops its own set of report formats, which sometimes differ significantly even on trials from the same company.

One very welcome change is that of attempting to standardize protocol and CRF elements. A tremendous amount of time and energy is wasted on reinventing the wheel and learning multiple new formats. For example, something as simple as dates can have multiple alternative formats:

5/26/2009, 26May2009, 26May09, and 5/26/09—or even 26/05/09, if you are European.

Now, particularly on government trials, modules and templates are being developed to simplify and standardize processes.

One illustrative example of the benefits of standardization is eDISH (electronic tool for drug-induced serious hepatotoxicity). The eDish tool takes abnormal liver test results from all the patients exposed to a drug and displays the data visually, enabling the user to tell at a glance if hepatotoxicity is likely and to easily identify and further assess cases of possible concern.[88]

A neat new program is the Federal Investigator Registry of Biomedical Informatics Research Data (FIREBIRD), which is a software application that supports electronic submission of clinical trial investigator information to trial sponsors and regulatory bodies. So now, you won't have to laboriously complete a zillion forms for different sponsors and regulatory agencies. If you don't have security concerns about putting all of your information on-line, you can now "create and maintain a profile of professional information, and can complete and sign an investigator registration packet which includes the FDA Form 1572, CV, Financial Disclosure Form, and other sponsor required forms." This will all be kept in a handy niche in cyberspace, ready to be submitted to the sponsor of your choice. FIREBIRD is the first module from a partnership between the FDA and National Cancer Institute to create an electronic infrastructure for clinical trial support.[89] You can learn about other tools like these in appendix B.

A number of suggestions have been proposed to help expedite drug development. For example, at the 2002 IDSA/PhRMA/FDA Working Group Meeting, representatives from the Infectious Diseases Society of America, Pharmaceuticals Research and Manufacturers of America, the FDA, the CDC, and the National Institute of Allergy and Infectious Disease (NIAID) generated the following suggestions, which were presented in a letter to the commissioner of the FDA:

- *Define guidelines for new drug development . . .*
- *Develop a clear-cut process for clinical trials that target specific bacterial pathogens (e.g., S. aureus) in addition to a specific infectious disease (e.g., pneumonia) . . .*
- *Develop and apply scientifically valid surrogate end points of efficacy . . .*

- *Explore designating new antibacterials as "orphan drugs" . . .*
- *Waive user fees for antibacterial new drug applications.*
- *Use valid pharmacokinetic/pharmacodynamic data, supported by appropriate animal model data, to allow smaller clinical trials of higher quality.*
- *With tighter controls, reduce the number of efficacy studies required for each additional indication.*
- *Restore patent protection for antibacterials equivalent to the time required for the FDA to review new drug applications.*
- *Consider other intellectual property protections to foster new R&D, including those successfully implemented for pediatric drugs.*[90]

The letter goes on to recommend the following:

- Tie patent extension to reinvestment in research and development.
- Study appropriate antibiotic use.
- Conduct placebo-controlled trials for illnesses thought to be largely viral in etiology, such as chronic bronchitis and sinusitis, rather than comparing two drugs. (If a patient's condition worsened significantly, then he or she would be dropped from the trial and provided with other interventions, just as in more traditional clinical trials.) These trials would prove whether antibiotics are necessary for such illnesses or not; hopefully, this would result in limiting antibiotic use and thus slow the development of resistance.[91]

The FDA has otherwise attempted to standardize the drug evaluation process. It has established requirements for studies for specific indications, and it helps provide guidance in protocol design through meetings with the sponsor.[92] Unfortunately, some people complain that increased interaction with the FDA regarding protocol design increases the development and start-up time. On the other hand, I would expect that having more FDA input early on ultimately reduces development time because companies know and can plan for the FDA's detailed expectations. Some sponsors conclude, however, that the increased stringency of the FDA "mandating more specific patient populations for more refined end points" is more problematic because it seriously restricts the patient pool, making it "impossible to find a significant number of patients at a moderate number of sites."[93]

But despite the attempts at standardization, many impractical trials are still proposed. Other trials ultimately produce no useful information because of flaws in protocol design.

The nature of large trials virtually guarantees huge costs. For example, one major problem on long-term studies has been that too many unexpected and uncontrolled variables occur during the course of the trial. Occasionally, this type of flaw may be fatal to the drug company, given the extraordinarily competitive nature of the industry. And the FDA's rejection of a trial's data can do much more than devastate the company involved. It can have ripple effects on other companies and even entire industry sectors and then stocks. A recent illustrative example is that of ImClone, the subject of much recent adverse publicity and now the target of many class action suits, investigations, and other unwanted attention. ImClone had a promising new anticancer drug, Erbitux, in its pipeline—so promising that it was accepted on the FDA's fast track for approval. Bristol-Myers Squibb bought $2 billion worth of ImClone stock based on the promising future of this drug. In December 2001, the FDA declined to accept ImClone's data, saying that the protocol design was flawed and that, therefore, the company had not proved the drug's efficacy. Stocks crashed, and some analysts are saying this incident has shaken the entire biotech industry.[94]

If a research design is seriously flawed, the FDA may not accept the data, either calling instead for further studies or simply rejecting the NDA. Even if the NDA eventually receives approval, the review process for the application can easily take 2–3 years.

View from the Trenches

I have been a Principal Investigator on most of the major sepsis protocols in the past 8 years. Each trial failed to show a statistically demonstrable benefit to the use of the study drug compared to a placebo in addition to standard care. In part, it appears that this failure was because each trial had slow enrollment. (Because sepsis is an uncommon event, it required approximately 18–24 months to accrue the requisite number of patients.) It appears that advances in supportive care during the enrollment period resulted in enough improvement in the patients' conditions to wipe out any evident differences between the active study drug and placebo groups.

Administrative Delays

Getting started with your study isn't as simple as it used to be. Although it's relatively easy to control factors in your own practice, outside agents may throw a monkey wrench into your plans. Besides patient recruitment, the historical bottleneck in study completion, the IRB is often blamed for delays in study start-up, prompting some to favor use of a central IRB.

Recent research, however, shows that IRBs are not the major culprit—in fact, delays are now the most severe in the contracting and negotiating process.[95] Budget and contract negotiations involve multiple parties including the CRO, investigator, IRB, insurance providers, multiple vendors (lab, radiology, send-outs, etc.), and billing and legal departments. Process mapping of the Vanderbilt University Ingram Cancer Center and its community affiliates network illustrates the complexity of the process and shows that the university approval process requires 20 steps and 13 decision points versus 17–30 steps and 4–16 decision points at the community study sites. Similarly, many more participants and steps were involved in the approval process at the university than at the community sites, as one would expect. The median time to open an oncology trial was 178 days, with almost 100 days being consumed by negotiations.[96] Start-up times tend to be even longer overseas, averaging 182 days in western Europe, 207 days in eastern Europe, and 262 days in Asia, compared to 37 days for U.S./Canadian sites using a central IRB and 107 days for those using a local IRB.[97]

KEY POINT
Contracting is the major administrative hurdle.

Shift in Growth

As of 2008, before the global economic slump, the clinical trial industry was thriving, measured by the number of active commercial IND applications: 5,700, up 20.2 percent over the prior year. Oncology remained the most active therapeutic area (14.7 percent of trials). Pain and rheumatologic indications showed the greatest growth. Trials of anti-infectives also grew, particularly those for viral infections, special pathogens, and transplant-related infections. Similarly, clinical trial starts (newly initiated programs) rose from 441 in 1998, with a decline and plateau that extended through 2003, to 795 in 2008. Biologic drugs regulated by CDER (not vaccines or cell/gene therapies, which are regulated by CBER) showed a much more modest growth.[98]

The good news is the growth in trials. The bad news—for the United States—is that much of the growth is occurring overseas. Let's look at why.

Where Have All the Trials Gone?

One of the marked changes in the few years since the first edition of this book is how much clinical research has shifted overseas. Let's look at what is driving the shift and some of the implications of the move.

KEY POINT
More than half of sites are located outside of the United States.

The current climate for clinical trials was reviewed in the *New England Journal of Medicine* in 2009.[99] Duke University researchers reviewed 300 trials reported in the *Journal of the American Medical Association, Lancet*, and the *New England Journal of Medicine* from 1995–2005 and found that by 2005, fully 56 percent of sites were located outside of the United States; one-third of trials were done solely outside of the United States. The number of U.S. trials decreased by 10 percent over that decade.

One common misconception is that the FDA requires studies of drugs to be marketed in the United States to actually have been done in the United States. There is no such requirement! The FDA once required foreign research to be done under an IND application or under Declaration of Helsinki standards but the Helsinki requirement was abandoned by the United States in 2008.

The Duke study also showed a large increase in the number of countries doing trials, corresponding to the large increase in the number of subjects needed to keep pace with research, from 215 to 661 per study over that decade. Large phase 3 trials can easily require 4,000 patients.[100]

The corresponding shift in investigators shows a similar trend: between 1990 and 1999, the number of non-U.S. investigators increased more than 300 percent. There was an average 13.5 percent annual increase in overseas investigators versus a 3.5 percent annual decrease in the United States.[101]

The steady decline in U.S. investigators can be attributed to several major factors. The first is a lack of exposure to clinical research during training. The second is the enormous time commitment and growing administrative and regulatory burden, which makes it hard to retain clinicians as physician investigators. In 2000, 45 percent of all PIs decided to quit after their studies ended, compared to a 27 percent turnover rate a decade earlier. In addition to the growing regulatory and administrative burdens, the work effort and complexity of trials have markedly increased while compensation has decreased to a profit level of just 2 percent.[102, 103, 104, 105] When asked about reimbursement for conducting clinical research, I used to respond, "Beats Medicaid." I'm a bit less confident with that response now.

In my own experience, it's more difficult to remain successful as a researcher in a community hospital setting because of the marked cutbacks in hospital support staff. I used to be able to rely on the help of staff nurses, lab personnel, and ancillary support, rather than needing a coordinator to personally do every procedure. In the recent climate, the workload on everyone has been greater, resulting in more errors, and staffing cutbacks have resulted in many services being available only from 7:00 a.m. to 3:00 p.m. Monday through Friday. It is nearly impossible to conduct inpatient trials in such an atmosphere.

While the United States is still the most desirable country for clinical trials, especially because of our infrastructure and regulatory climate, China is a close second, as figure 7.1 shows.[106]

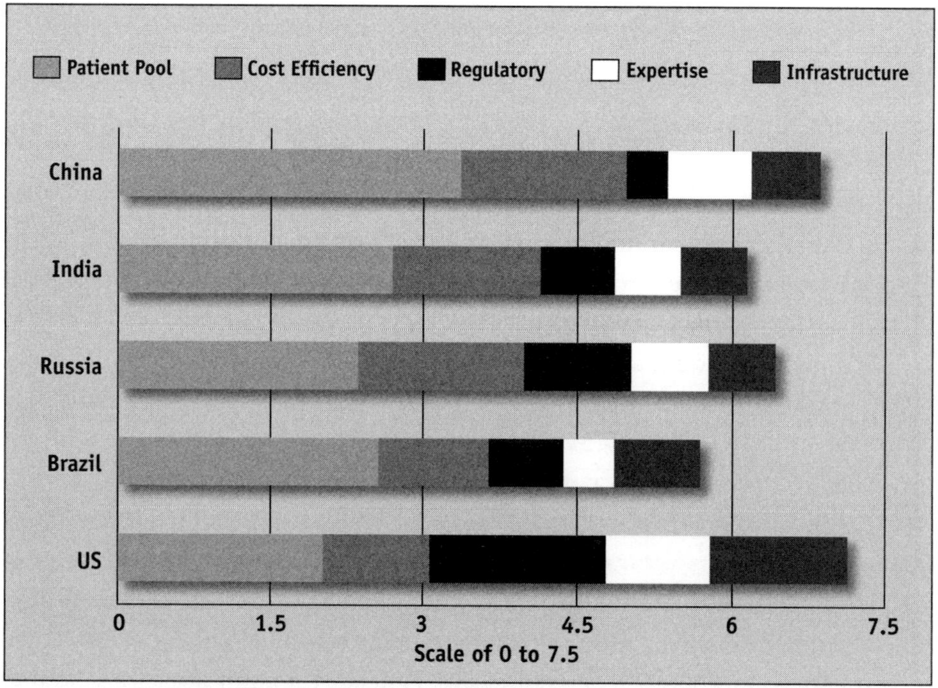

Figure 7.1 Country attractiveness index (Adapted from A. T. Kearney; used with permission.)

What is driving the shift overseas? Access to patients. The number of patients needed for trials rose from 2.8 million in 1999 to 19.8 million in 2005.[107] A quick look at a graph of the world's population shows us that the 19.8 million is a significant chunk of the U.S. population (300 million) but a much smaller proportion of the population of China (1,300 million) or India (1,150 million).[108]

Not only do studies need more volunteers overall, but they increasingly need large numbers of patients with specific conditions. Companies clearly can't find large volumes of patients in the United States—if those groups existed, only 1–2 percent of patients here participate in trials. Given the smaller population in the United States and the low participation rate, sponsors are forced to go overseas. In Asia, for example, Wyeth has identified "phase II super centers" with up to 9,000 outpatient visits a day.[109] It is also common overseas to have specialized hospitals focusing on heart disease, diabetes, and so on; such centralized and specialized care centers are unusual in the United States.

Inclusion-exclusion criteria are also much more restrictive now, making identifying patients who meet enrollment criteria a herculean task. Another huge logistical advantage overseas is that many people there are "treatment naïve," not having received prior therapy for the condition, and are less likely to be taking other medications that might confuse the outcome data and be enrollment exclusions.

KEY POINT
"Toto, I've a feeling we're not in Kansas anymore."

In addition, efforts are being made to do testing in different ethnic and racial groups because outcomes may be different. The cancer drug Iressa, for example, has been found to be effective in Asian populations but not in the United States.[110] Japan is the second largest consumer of pharmaceutical products, so there is considerable competition for study patients in that country. Interestingly, Brazil has the largest population of Japanese outside of Japan. This makes it a convenient site for some sponsors because the competition for Japanese patients there is not as great, and the data will still be acceptable under the guidelines of *ICH Topic E5: Ethnic Factors in the Acceptability of Foreign Clinical Data.*[111]

Another example is that approved doses of drugs in the EU, United States, and Japan are different in about one-third of cases; the Japanese doses are generally lower (e.g., for the cancer drug capecitabine or the antibiotic telithromycin). Similarly, the frequency of adverse drug reactions (ADRs) varies in different regions, with Japan again having more ADRs due to some medications (e.g., the antirheumatic leflunomide causing more interstitial pneumonia) than Europe or the United States. The Japanese FDA equivalent, the MHLW/PMDA (Ministry of Health, Labour and Welfare/Pharmaceuticals and Medical Devices Agency) therefore specifically requires data obtained in Japanese patients to support drug applications.[112]

As noted previously, slow recruitment causes 85–90 percent of the delay in trials, and the delays are enormously costly. Thus, sponsors will focus their resources in areas with rapid recruitment potential—such as Russia and the Ukraine, where recruitment may be 10–25 percent higher than in the United States.[113] And we know that money drives most everything now. Trials in Russia are 60 percent less costly than in the United States; China, 50 percent less; and India, about 45 percent less.[114]

Besides the lower direct costs of clinical trials overseas, the potential markets in India, China, and developing countries are huge, so placing trials overseas is one way of grooming the market, or "greasing the wheels," in the vernacular.

The major concerns about the industry's move overseas are that some countries may have far fewer resources with which to successfully complete trials. For example, the Drugs Controller General of India (similar to the FDA) has very limited staff: three pharmacists, no medical doctors.[115] There are marked limitations on procedures for protocol and informed consent review, the availability of trained IRB members, quorum requirements, monitoring, and independence—not unlike some places in the United States.[116]

On the other hand, conducting trials in the United States presents considerable problems, the biggest of which are the difficulty in recruiting patients and the low volunteer rate, which is even less than 5 percent for cancer trials. The United States also has a smaller pool of subjects and heavier competition for patients because the country has more drugs in development, tighter and more restrictive inclusion-exclusion enrollment requirements, and requirements for larger trials. Furthermore, the United States is now saddled with HIPAA, which has made identifying and recruiting patients much more difficult and expensive.[117] Cultural differences also come into play. The United States has more mistrust of pharmaceutical companies and physicians, fewer risk-tolerant patients, and a more litigious climate.

Costs are the driving factor. The direct costs of conducting trials in the United States are much higher than costs in most other countries, Germany being the notable exception. Wages and employee benefits, often 30 percent of a worker's base pay, are a significant factor.[118] Administrative costs are also much higher in the United States; increasingly, sites even need to hire a designated person to reconcile billing to ensure that Medicare or third-party payers are not inadvertently billed, which could lead to charges of fraud and hefty penalties.[119]

The standard of care has been generally higher in the United States than in many foreign countries, leading fewer people to participate in trials as a way of obtaining better access to care; in fact, many health insurance policies prohibit participation. Given the explosive growth in the ranks of the uninsured, this dynamic will likely change.

The final criticism of the shift in trial placement relates to regulatory and ethical concerns. The regulatory climate and IRB review processes are different overseas. Some complain that there is little information on foreign IRBs and no oversight, and it is difficult to audit foreign PIs. IRB protocol review may differ regarding emphasis on participant protections; more ethical issues may be raised regarding patients' levels of understanding and education, calling into question the adequacy of informed consent and the voluntariness of the participation.

Efforts are being made to reverse this trend, with the push for translational science awards and increased support for training in clinical research. Efforts are also being made to improve the research infrastructure overseas.

Overseas Drug Manufacturing

In addition to concerns about drug development being shifted overseas, a related problem is that of drug manufacturing. A growing worry is that critical ingredients for many drugs are exclusively produced overseas, largely in China and India. These include the commonly prescribed medications penicillin, prednisone, and metformin. The overreliance on outsourcing important medications raises obvious security concerns.[120]

An additional growing worry is that of counterfeit drugs. It's estimated that "around 1 per cent of drugs in developed countries, and 10–30 per cent of drugs in developing countries, are counterfeit; in regions of Southeast Asia, the proportion of counterfeit antimalarials is even higher," posing a tremendous public health problem.[121]

Conclusion

We've examined some of the deeper problems facing the drug development enterprise. This lays the foundation for a better understanding of the most interesting and challenging aspects of trials, which are addressed in the next two chapters. Chapter 8 reviews basic ethical principles and introduces the topics of vulnerable populations and conflicts of interest. Chapter 9 is more challenging and controversial, exploring the interface of society, politics, and research.

CHAPTER 8

Ethical Issues in Human Subjects Research

The first step in the evolution of ethics
is a sense of solidarity with other human beings.
—ALBERT SCHWEITZER

The issue of ethics in clinical research has received a great deal of press coverage, most of it unfavorable.[1] In this chapter, we'll first review briefly how and why research became regulated and then look at some of the ethical issues confronting researchers. An excellent overview of the ethical aspects of research is available on the NIH's Office of Human Subjects Research Web site.[2] The following historical background is abstracted largely from that site, with permission. This tutorial should be mandatory for coordinators and investigators and should, in an expanded form, be incorporated in medical school curricula.

Some ethical principles, such as the need for informed consent, seem to be clearly the right thing to do. Some activities, such as the Tuskegee experiment (see below), are clearly wrong. The vast majority of ethical concerns, however, are less clear and raise many controversial questions, which will be discussed in this chapter.

For those readers who may be interested, a supplemental overview and further resources relating to the controversies surrounding the politics of research are provided in chapter 9. That section is intended purely to raise awareness of these interesting ethical debates. It is, of necessity, more difficult and thought-provoking reading and is not necessary for learning to conduct clinical trials sponsored by pharmaceutical companies—but it is background material that I wish I had known about earlier in my career.

Historical Context

"Medical research," as it was euphemistically called, first came to considerable, undesirable attention during World War II, when the Nazis tortured many of their victims under the guise of conducting research. In 1946, 23 doctors were indicted; in 1947, at the Nuremberg trials, 7 of these were sentenced to death and 16 were imprisoned. The verdict included a section on "Permissible Medical Experiments," subsequently known as the "Nuremberg Code." This code for conducting research required that participants' consent be voluntary and that the risks to those individuals should be understood and weighed into their decision to participate.

Other ethical lapses were occurring concurrently in the United States. Perhaps the best known is the Tuskegee experiment, conducted between 1932 and 1972, in which men (mostly African Americans) with syphilis were observed, without medical intervention, to study the natural history of the disease. The participants were subjected to spinal taps after being misinformed that they were receiving "special free treatment" when in fact they received no treatment. By the mid-1940s, the death rate among these men with syphilis was noted to be two times higher than that of a control group. Even though penicillin was available at that time and had been found to be effective for treating syphilis, the infected men were neither informed of its availability nor treated to cure their infection. By the time the study was ended in 1972, 28 of the 399 "subjects had died of syphilis, 100 others were dead of related complications, at least 40 wives had been infected and 19 children had contracted the disease at birth." In 1973, a class action lawsuit was settled, with the government distributing about $10 million to survivors and families.[3]

Earlier experiments had been performed on prisoners and, during World War II, conscientious objectors. The military also conducted radioactivity, germ warfare, and hallucinogenic drug testing.

Similar unethical studies were conducted in the 1960s, when some hospitalized patients were subjected to "treatments" without their knowledge or consent. In another case, the Willowbrook Study, mentally disabled children could receive access to treatment they needed only if their parents agreed

The Nuremberg Code[4]

1. The voluntary consent of the human subject is absolutely essential. This means that the person involved should have legal capacity to give consent; should be so situated as to be able to exercise free power of choice, without the intervention of any element of force, fraud, deceit, duress, overreaching, or other ulterior form of constraint or coercion; and should have sufficient knowledge and comprehension of the elements of the subject matter involved as to enable him to make an understanding and enlightened decision. This latter element requires that before the acceptance of an affirmative decision by the experimental subject there should be made known to him the nature, duration, and purpose of the experiment; the method and means by which it is to be conducted; all inconveniences and hazards reasonable to be expected; and the effects upon his health or person which may possibly come from his participation in the experiment. The duty and responsibility for ascertaining the quality of the consent rests upon each individual who initiates, directs or engages in the experiment. It is a personal duty and responsibility which may not be delegated to another with impunity.
2. The experiment should be such as to yield fruitful results for the good of society, unprocurable by other methods or means of study, and not random and unnecessary in nature.
3. The experiment should be so designed and based on the results of animal experimentation and a knowledge of the natural history of the disease or other problem under study that the anticipated results will justify the performance of the experiment.
4. The experiment should be so conducted as to avoid all unnecessary physical and mental suffering and injury.
5. No experiment should be conducted where there is an a priori reason to believe that death or disabling injury will occur; except, perhaps, in those experiments where the experimental physicians also serve as subjects.
6. The degree of risk to be taken should never exceed that determined by the humanitarian importance of the problem to be solved by the experiment.
7. Proper preparations should be made and adequate facilities provided to protect the experimental subject against even remote possibilities of injury, disability, or death.
8. The experiment should be conducted only by scientifically qualified persons. The highest degree of skill and care should be required through all stages of the experiment of those who conduct or engage in the experiment.
9. During the course of the experiment the human subject should be at liberty to bring the experiment to an end if he has reached the physical or mental state where continuation of the experiment seems to him to be impossible.
10. During the course of the experiment the scientist in charge must be prepared to terminate the experiment at any stage, if he has probable cause to believe, in the exercise of the good faith, superior skill and careful judgment required of him that a continuation of the experiment is likely to result in injury, disability, or death to the experimental subject.

to the children's participation in a study in which the children were infected with the hepatitis virus.[5] (The children were in an institutionalized setting where there was a very high likelihood of them contracting hepatitis on their own.) This kind of coercion is frowned upon today. Nonetheless, it does clearly persist, as indigent patients in particular may find that clinical trials offer their best source of treatment or their only access to expensive treatments. While a consent process is now in place, discerning readers might question the voluntariness of the participation in some circumstances.

In 1964, the World Medical Association, in a somewhat tardy response to the Nuremberg horrors, formulated the Declaration of Helsinki.[6] This code differentiated between therapeutic and nontherapeutic research. It, too, required informed consent, but it expanded this practice to allow for surrogate consent when the research subject was incapable of providing the consent (because of physical or mental incompetence). The Declaration of Helsinki and the subsequent *Ethical Principles and Guidelines for the Protection of Human Subjects of Research* (the "Belmont Report")[7] form the basis for most of the FDA and ICH good clinical practice guidelines.[8] In 1974, federal regulations expanded consent requirements, allowing surrogate consent from a legal representative but adding protections for subjects by requiring the participant's "assent" in the case of a consent from a surrogate. (Assent is the willingness to participate indicated by an individual who is not entirely competent in a legal definition.)

The Tuskegee experiment first became publicized in 1972. In response to the public outrage over how the study was conducted, the Department of Health, Education, and Welfare (DHEW) examined the issues. As a result, in 1974 Congress passed the National Research Act, requiring institutional review boards to review all DHEW-funded research and creating the National Commission for the Protection of Human Subjects of Biomedical and Behavioral Research, which issued guidelines that continue to serve as the ethical foundation of human research design.

Just as Tuskegee became synonymous with unethical concerns involving race, the case of Jesse Gelsinger has come to symbolize concerns about financial conflicts of interest. This 18-year-old boy was the first patient to die because of a gene therapy experiment. He was born with an error of metabolism that limited his ability to eat and to metabolize protein. Most people affected with this ornithine transcarboxylase deficiency (OTCD) die in infancy. Although Jesse had a milder form of the illness, controlled with medications, he altruistically volunteered for this trial. The goal of this experiment was to replace the defective gene with a normal one, delivered into his cells by an adenovirus. A few days after receiving the treatment, Jesse died of progressive failure of multiple organs. Subsequent investigation raised questions about the adequacy of his consent, whether serious and relevant safety information had been withheld, and whether the investigators were influenced in enrolling Jesse on this trial by financial interests. The result has been some tightening of safety review measures and increased education for researchers regarding conflicts of interest.[9]

Before we delve into the ethical issues you are likely to encounter, we'll orient you with a historical review of developments in medical ethics (table 7.1).

Table 7.1 Ethical development milestones

Year	Event
1932–72	Tuskegee experiment on syphilis
1939–45	Nazi experiments
1944–74	Human radiation experiments by U.S. government
1946	Nuremberg trial of doctors responsible for the Nazi experiments
1947	Nuremberg Code outlining ethical principles required for research
1948	United Nations adoption of Universal Declaration of Human Rights
1953	NIH policy, the first U.S. federal policy introducing independent reviewers to examine research, forerunners of the IRBs
1963–66	Willowbrook Study, involving hepatitis research on mentally retarded children, raising issues of access to care, consent, and coercion
1964	Declaration of Helsinki international agreement on recommendations for the ethical conduct of medical research
1972	Public exposure of Tuskegee syphilis study
1974	First federal protections for human research participants
1979	Belmont Report promoting three principles for research
1980	Food and Drug Administration regulations (see *Code of Federal Regulations,* Title 21, part 50)
1982	Council for the International Organizations of Medical Sciences (CIOMS) publication of the *International Ethical Guidelines for Biomedical Research Involving Human Subjects* addressing ethics and conduct of research in developing countries, cultural differences, subject recruitment, informed consent, and external review
1985	U.S. Public Health Service Task Force on Women's Health Issues encouraging inclusion of women in research
1990	Society for Women's Health Research

Year	Event
1991	Adoption of Federal Policy for the Protection of Human Subjects, aka Common Rule, applying ethical standards of the Department of Health and Human Services (45 CFR 46, subpart A) to research supported by agencies of the federal government, including the departments of Agriculture, Energy, Commerce, Justice, Defense, Education, Veterans Affairs, Transportation, Health and Human Services, and Housing and Urban Development, National Science Foundation, NASA, Environmental Protection Agency, Agency for International Development, Social Security Administration, CIA, and Consumer Product Safety Commission
1993	Public exposure of U.S. human radiation experiments
1993	NIH Revitalization Act mandating inclusion of women and minorities in research
1993	NIH Office of Research on Women's Health
1994	Advisory Committee on Human Radiation Experiments, convened by President Clinton to investigate the government's radiation experiments during the period of 1944–1974, involved intentional radioactive releases, and made recommendations to ensure this type of action would not be repeated
1995	National Bioethics Advisory Committee, established "to promote the protection of the rights and welfare of human participants in research, to identify bioethical issues arising from research on human biology and behavior, and to make recommendations to governmental entities regarding their application"[10]
1997	Food and Drug Administration Modernization Act (FDAMA) requiring the FDA, NIH, and pharmaceutical industry to develop guidance on the inclusion of women and minorities in trials
1998	Pediatric Studies Rule passed by Congress, stipulating that new drugs for children must include specific pediatric labeling information
2000	Further publicized ethical abuses prompting establishment of the Office for Human Research Protections (OHRP) within the U.S. Department of Health and Human Services; replaced the NIH Office for Protection from Research Risks (OPRR) and expanded it to include responsibility for all 17 federal agencies included under the Common Rule regulations

Ethical Principles (the Belmont Report)

In 1979, after 5 years of work, the National Commission for the Protection of Human Subjects of Biomedical and Behavioral Research published its report, *Ethical Principles and Guidelines for the Protection of Human Subjects of Research*, generally known as the "Belmont Report." This report concluded that all clinical research should meet three general principles of respect for persons, beneficence, and justice.[11]

Respect for Persons

The first Belmont principle is respect for persons. This basically refers to an individual's autonomy, or right to make decisions for himself or herself based on a review of available information. In other words, the individual is given enough information about the risks and benefits of a trial to make a decision about participating. This principle is expressed in the elements of the informed consent, which requires that

- Information necessary to make a decision must be presented—that is, the risks and benefits, if any, of participation.
- The information must be presented at a level that can be understood by the patient or study subject.
- Participation must be voluntary.

This last criterion, assuring voluntariness, is perhaps the most difficult of these parameters to meet, as it requires that the subject's consent must be free of coercion or pressure. For example, perceived authority is (or used to be) inherent in a doctor-patient relationship, with the patient generally relying on the physician to make decisions and deferentially opting to respond, "Whatever you think is best, Doc." In this setting, it is imperative that the volunteer not be urged to participate if she or he would prefer not to.

Beneficence

The second Belmont principle, beneficence, requires that a study should not only meet the maxim "First, do no harm" but should also provide some benefit to the subject. One of the interesting dilemmas here is whether the benefits outweigh the risks. Who decides? Does the volunteer, does the IRB, or does some well-meaning but paternalistic governmental agency? A prime example of this dilemma is the issue of living donors, particularly for adult liver transplants, which at this time are new and experimental. Does the healthy donor have the right to consent to a potentially life-threatening procedure to benefit another person? Donating brings no physical benefit to the donor, and it carries significant medical risks. Are the perceived psychological benefits (altruism, helping another person specifically, and advancing knowledge generally) to be accepted? Or does pressure from the intended recipient or other family members create too much underlying coercion?[12]

The other half of the principle of beneficence "requires that we protect against risk of harm to subjects and also that we be concerned about the loss of substantial benefits that might be gained from research."[13] This means that researchers should avoid being too paternalistic (with well-intentioned safeguards), preventing patients access to therapies that some might view as too risky and thus depriving them of any possible benefits from the treatment. AIDS activists used this principle to challenge the lack of access to potential AIDS therapies in the 1980s. In 1987, the FDA expanded the use of experimental drugs to include treatment of serious and life-threatening illnesses because of the pressure brought to bear by these activists. This topic is currently a source of contention in studies involving foster children and pregnant women.

Justice

The third Belmont principle is that of distributive justice, meaning that the risks and gains from research participation should be equitably distributed among different populations. Historically, this has been interpreted to mean that classes of vulnerable patients, such as the indigent, the institutionalized, the disabled, minorities, pregnant women, and children, would not be subjected to risks because they were readily available or defenseless (as in the Tuskegee experiment). At the same time, an obligation to help vulnerable subjects means that this protection must be balanced with attempts to study some of these same populations to determine whether they have unique needs. For example, it is now known that women metabolize drugs differently than men do. So while one might want to protect women (especially if pregnant) from drug toxicities, excluding women from trials might also prevent them from benefiting by having the drugs prescribed in the most efficacious manner. Brief examples of research on vulnerable populations follow.

Vulnerable Populations: Military

Despite the Nuremberg Code's development at the end of World War II, between 1944 and 1979 the U.S. government conducted its own human experiments on the effect of exposure to hazardous materials without the awareness or informed consent of the participants. These experiments were conducted with a variety of radioactive, chemical (toxic and hallucinogenic), and biological agents. In the 1940s, for example, 60,000 military personnel were used to test the chemical agents mustard gas and lewisite. In some cases, the study subjects experienced coercion from their superior officers, and in others, they were threatened with imprisonment in Leavenworth Penitentiary for refusal to "volunteer." The secrecy of the studies and subsequent denial by the Department of Defense also deprived many of the subjects of appropriate medical follow-up care and compensation.[14]

Between 1951 and 1969, a variety of open-air tests using biological and chemical agents (including Venezuelan equine encephalitis virus and the nerve gas agent VX) were conducted at the Dugway Proving Ground in Utah. From 1940 to 1962, atomic weapons tests were conducted in the South Pacific, New Mexico, and Nevada, exposing thousands of people to radioactive fallout. Further intentional nuclear releases were conducted in Oak Ridge, Tennessee; Los Alamos, New Mexico; and Hanford, Washington, to study the effects of fallout. According to a 1994 Congressional review, the Department of Defense "has demonstrated a pattern of misrepresenting the danger of various military exposures that continues today," in addition to committing a variety of other abuses.[15]

Bartering Blood for Brainpower

I believe the following case illustrates violations of both the first and second Belmont principles of respect for persons and beneficence.

Some time ago, a young patient I knew had an unusual medical problem. She was told that she had a serious pituitary and hormone imbalance and that she would probably never be able to bear children. Her doctor wanted her to see a leading specialist in this area, "Dr. Stratosphere," (Dr. S.). Unfortunately, there was no way to get an appointment with him. Her primary care physician, "Dr. Worshiper of Stratosphere," felt inadequate and useless in dealing with the patient's condition, as it was beyond his experience. So he strongly urged (translation: coerced) her into becoming a volunteer in Dr. S.'s clinical research center so that she would gain access to expertise and a medical opinion while being studied. The patient was not happy about this. She was actually terrified of one of the medications she was to be given but went along with taking it, having been told that there was no other way to see Dr. S. and that her response to the medication might help the doctor make a diagnosis and answer the question of infertility. As it turned out, she never did get an evaluation or an opinion from Dr. S. as the "access" was only to his coordinator, who simply administered medications, made routine observations, and drew lots of blood. So no medical benefit was gained, even though that was what the patient was seeking (while bartering her blood and cooperation).

The patient was not presented with true informed consent, and the setting was coercive, with pressure being applied from her doctor and superior. The patient received no benefit because the research was in the study of human physiology, without the clinical application that was implied—all illustrating violation of the Belmont principles.

The Department of Energy has also conducted unethical radiation experiments on civilians without their knowledge, using plutonium injections as well as irradiation. This was brought to the public's attention by *Albuquerque Tribune* reporter Eileen Welsome in 1993, which resulted in an official review known as the "ACHRE Report" (Advisory Committee on Human Radiation Experiments), the following year.[16] Although most of the tested population showed no ill effect, this report did blame the government for lapses in ethics and judgment because the radiation exposures were conducted without the subjects' consent. The report noted that subjects also had no redress for the wrongdoing, given the government's actions "to keep the truth from them." The ACHRE commission recommended that the government issue apologies and compensation to those affected by the experiments, and it stressed the need for further human subject protections. Individual apologies were issued by President Clinton in 1995, and compensation was provided to the families of the plutonium injection subjects.[17] The ACHRE Report concluded, "The greatest harm from past experiments and intentional releases may be the legacy of distrust they created."[18]

A different pattern of military study emerged between 1954 and 1973 during Operation Whitecoat. Seventh Day Adventists volunteered to be exposed to biological agents or trial vaccines in lieu of active military service. These 2,300 conscientious objectors were exposed to live infectious agents, including tularemia, Q fever, and anthrax.[19] Perhaps they were truly selfless. Perhaps the risks were not as apparent then as they are now, decades later. We would like to think those were different times. However, a similar debate might be argued in the future about current trials of vaccines and agents being developed to counter terrorism.

Vulnerable Populations: Children

A recent example of the growing use of another vulnerable population is a shift to studying drugs in children. While a necessary endeavor, this area is fraught with ethical dilemmas. On the one hand, children have unique needs and cannot simply be considered "pint-sized people." On the other hand, children may be less capable of understanding risks and the consequences of their actions, given their educational experience, emotional maturity, and limited life experiences, than are many adults. Finally, because they are minors and in a dependent relationship with their adult caretakers, children are more susceptible to coercion. Because of these factors, they are considered to be vulnerable research subjects.

In 1997, under the FDA Modernization Act, Congress offered pharmaceutical companies large incentives to do pediatric testing, in recognition of the unique characteristics of children. Congress gave the manufacturers an extra 6 months patent protection and exclusive marketing in exchange for testing specific drugs in children. The Pediatric Studies Rule, passed by Congress and published in 1998, required that new drugs that will be commonly used or important for treating children include specific pediatric labeling information.[20]

To better direct this new line of research, the Institute of Medicine sponsored a roundtable in 1999, called Rational Therapeutics for Infants and Children, to explore the direction such research should take. One 1994 survey examined the 10 drugs most commonly prescribed for children that lacked pediatric labeling—these drugs were prescribed more than 5 million times. Three were for asthma; albuterol inhalers alone were prescribed more than 1.6 million times. Other medications included ampicillin, antidepressants, and Ritalin.[21] However, the Pediatric Studies Rule testing requirement was subsequently challenged in court in a typical "industry versus regulatory" battle. In 2002, a U.S. District Court ruling barred the FDA from enforcing it, saying the FDA had exceeded its statutory authority.[22] Consequently, drugs will continue to be given to kids without adequate studies supporting their specific safety and efficacy in children. How does striking down the Pediatric Studies Rule balance with the principle of distributive justice?

Fortunately, increased recognition of the unique needs of this population is resulting in slow improvement. Under the Best Pharmaceuticals for Children Act of 2002 (BPCA 2002), the NIH delegated to the director of the Eunice Kennedy Shriver National Institute of Child Health and Human Development (NICHD) the authority and responsibility for pediatric drug development. The NICHD responded with a priority list of drugs including antibiotics (azithromycin, ethambutol, rifampin, acyclovir), diuretics (furosemide), antihypertensives (hydrochlorothiazide), antidepressants (bupropion), and anticancer agents (methotrexate, vincristine).[23]

The BPCA was reauthorized in 2007 under the FDAAA, extending both research and patent and marketing exclusivity rewards. Under the Pediatric Research Equity Act, drugs for pediatric use are required to have testing earlier in the overall development process, rather than waiting for extensive testing in adults. Postmarketing surveillance for a year also became required.

Studies conducted under BPCA showed that prior dosing—done by guess and by gosh extrapolations—really put children at significant risk. Consequently, 87 percent of drugs approved for pediatric use had subsequent changes in labeling. The studies showed significant differences in absorption, distribution, metabolism, and elimination of drugs, varying with both the age and sex of the patients. (Note: Pediatric studies are all done for treatment; they are never done with healthy volunteers.)[24, 25] No predictable pattern was seen in the required dosing changes; some doses were ineffective, others initially toxic. Fully 20 percent of the trials showed no efficacy in children, and another 20 percent revealed new side effects that were previously unknown.[26] For example, five studies in children showed that sumatriptan, a very effective treatment for migraines in adults, not only didn't work in kids but led to serious side effects, such as stroke and loss of vision.[27]

It is appalling to me that in 2002, the industry successfully opposed studying drugs in the very population that would be exposed to them and that this decision was upheld by the U.S. District Court. At least pediatric studies are finally beginning to receive the attention they deserve even if it's not for the right motive.

Some pediatric trials continue, and attempts have been made by the American Academy of Pediatrics and the International Conference on Harmonisation to develop ethical guidelines for studies in children. Recommendations for pediatric trials include the following:

- Ideally, the pediatric subject should have the potential to benefit from participation in the trial.
- The study must take into account the unique characteristics and needs of children and their special needs as research subjects.
- The study design should also take into account racial, ethnic, gender, and socioeconomic characteristics of the population being studied.
- The research and procedures should be explained to the subject in age-appropriate language.
- Children aged seven and older should assent in addition to full informed consent being obtained from their parent or guardian. The children should

also understand that they can withdraw from the study except in life-threatening circumstances.

- Placebo-controlled trials are acceptable only if there is no approved or adequately studied therapy for the condition being studied.
- Studies for less serious conditions, or symptomatic treatment, should include "early escape" or discontinuation criteria.
- Discomfort and distress should be minimized. For example, the number of blood draws should be minimized by the use of indwelling catheters, placed under topical anesthesia.
- Caregivers should be trained to assess for adverse events.
- Compensation should be "token," so as not to be coercive.[28]

The controversy over pediatric trials is epitomized by studies in HIV-positive foster children. On the one hand, researchers felt that the trials were in the children's best interests as the children received expert care and access to drugs that were believed likely to benefit them. On the other, while the foster children had a guardian, they had no independent advocate. One group argues that foster children are too vulnerable to participate in such trials; others, that it is unethical to withhold the potential for benefit from these children.[29] What is generally overlooked in this dispute is that all HIV-positive children in New York City were offered these trials, not just foster children, and no other approved treatment existed at the time. Wouldn't it have been more unethical to deprive the foster children of the expected potential benefits of these drugs?[30]

Special Populations

Four unlikely groups of people have been notably absent from many clinical trials—teenagers, the elderly, obese patients, and minorities. These groups are special in that they fall through the cracks and are excluded from many clinical trials by design. They are (arguably) not considered "vulnerable" populations, however, as that term is typically applied to those who are defenseless or more susceptible to coercion and to those who are unable to give informed consent.[31]

Teens and Young Adults

In a 2008 British report, recruitment into cancer trials included 51 percent of 10-to-14-year-old patients but dropped to 25 percent of 15-to-19-year-olds and only 13 percent of 20-to-24-year-olds.[32] Yet cancer is the primary cause of disease-related death in the 13-to-24-year-old age group in England, and inclusion in cancer trials has been shown to significantly improve survival.[33] Similar patterns have been shown in the United States.[34]

Adult trials traditionally exclude those below age 18, and pediatric specialists tend to focus more on younger kids; older teens tend to fall between the interests of the two specialties. Specialized cancer centers with multidisciplinary teams focusing on 0-to-18-year-olds have been proposed as a solution (though this would still leave young adults out in the cold). Perhaps teens and young adults should be considered a minority group for outreach efforts in clinical trials.

Elderly

Similar problems have been seen regarding enrollment of elderly patients. A review of cancer patients from 1995 to 2002 showed that the proportions of the overall cancer trial populations aged 65 and older, 70 and older, and 75 and older were 36 percent, 20 percent, and 9 percent compared with their representation in the cancer population of 60 percent, 46 percent, and 31 percent, respectively.[35] Barriers to participation include

- Age restrictions in inclusion-exclusion criteria (many trials specify ages 18–65, for example)
- Comorbidities (elderly average five morbidities) and concern that these will confound the results
- Polypharmacy (20 percent of nursing home residents use 10 or more drugs daily), which increases the risk for drug interactions
- Declining renal and hepatic function associated with aging
- Informed consent issues
- Physician attitudes[36]
- The aversion sponsors and investigators have to patients dying during clinical trial participation and the lack of accountability for adverse events or deaths (see "Who's Minding the Store?" later in this chapter)

The end result is that for many indications—and not for just oncology trials—no evidence-based guidelines are available for treatment of elderly patients. This may soon change—the ICH recently issued a new set of guidelines regarding studies in geriatric populations, and the FDA issued its draft guidance late in 2009.[37] Stay tuned.

Obese Patients

Huge numbers of markedly obese patients live in the United States. While I have seen little literature on this topic, one thing I have been acutely aware of in my own practice is the lack of data on treating the morbidly obese.

For example, a weight over 300 pounds is a common exclusion criterion on many trials. So again, there is little evidence-based medicine and a considerable problem knowing how to dose obese patients with a variety of medications. Little pharmacokinetic or pharmacodynamic information is available, and much of that is limited to healthy volunteers.[38]

Accurate physical examination is near impossible at times. Many patients are too obese to have diagnostic imaging studies, especially CAT scans or MRI scans, reducing us, it seems, to veterinary medicine. Various recipes exist for drug dosing in obese patients—some based on ideal body weight (IBW), some on actual body weight, and some based on witchcraft (somewhere in the middle between IBW plus a percentage of the excess weight).[39]

KEY POINT
Requirements for ethical research: Is the study asking a valid and important question—is it important enough to warranty any risk?

The concern about the lack of evidence is particularly timely, given that serious illness and deaths from Influenza A H1N1 are disproportionately affecting the obese. Some studies have been proposed, such as Oseltamivir Pharmacokinetics in Morbid Obesity (OPTIMO), but are just getting started.[40] Given the unfortunate change in patient demographics in the United States and the epidemic of obesity here, clinical trials focusing on this population would be most welcome.

Minorities

We have seen an increasing push to enroll minorities in clinical trials, in part because of ethnic differences in responses to some medications and in part to reduce health disparities. While the NIH Revitalization Act of 1993 encouraged this, little infrastructure or support was provided. Barriers to enrollment include language, cultural, and educational factors (see the "Health Literacy" and "Cross-Cultural Issues" sections in chapter 5).

Individual Research Practice: The Nature of the Beast

Ethical dilemmas are inherent in the process of conducting clinical trials, in part because of the structure of the relationships between the individual parties and their competing (and sometimes conflicting) interests. A brief overview is well presented by Cullen Vogelson in an article in *Modern Drug Discovery*.[41] His description certainly parallels my experience, with the most obvious conflicts relating to grant payments.

Volunteer recruitment is another area that demands difficult choices. This is often due to the pressure to identify patients and meet enrollment targets, which leads to the temptation to enroll marginally qualified candidates.

Choices must also be made when classifying adverse events as "unrelated" or "possibly related" or "probably related" to an investigational drug. Sometimes objective criteria exist for assessing the severity of the reaction. Guidelines for attributing causality are usually less clear.

As a Principal Investigator, you must make decisions about to whom you delegate responsibilities and how you supervise your subinvestigator or coordinator. While this may not initially appear to be an ethical issue, the decision can have a major impact on your patients. (See the 2007 FDA guidance regarding the supervisory responsibility of investigators.)[42] Errors in judgment may also influence your continued ability to conduct clinical trials, especially if an audit should be called due to a serious adverse event.

While the focus has usually been on financial conflicts of interest (COIs) in clinical trial conduct, other pressures might also introduce bias. The Institute of Medicine just issued a new report in which it defined COI as "a set of circumstances that creates a risk that professional judgment or actions regarding a primary interest will be unduly influenced by a secondary interest." These circumstances extend to professional advancement and pressure to publish or extending friendship to family, colleagues, or students, among others.[43]

These issues are identified here because most of the discussions in the available literature regarding individual researchers and ethics are devoted to financial conflicts of interest rather than to these decision-making factors.

Financial Pressure and Conflict of Interest

Considerable attention has been paid to conflicts of interest among private individuals conducting research for pharmaceutical companies. Investigators

View from the Trenches

I have some reservations about a particular class of antibiotics as my experience has been that my elderly patients commonly experience worsening confusion, light-headedness, or insomnia when they take them. My colleagues don't often identify these side effects. Perhaps the difference is that I actively look for new symptoms because of my clinical research experience; my colleagues tend to dismiss such symptoms as due to age, illness, and the stress of hospitalization rather than to a medication. So if a patient could be enrolled on a protocol with one of these agents that I have reservations about, do I offer him or her the drug because it is likely to be prescribed by the primary physician anyway, or do I withhold offering it because of my own experience and concerns? What if the patient is indigent or the study offers significant perks for the patient?

are required to complete financial disclosure forms for every trial in which they participate. We are now also required to disclose relationships with sponsors when submitting articles for publication and when making presentations. Surprisingly, at the same time that disclosure requirements for the private physicians were made much more stringent, those for the government physicians and researchers (at the federal level) were loosened, as outlined below.

Previously, government sponsored research at the National Institutes of Health was considered purely motivated and untainted by commercial interests. Margaret Heckler, former Secretary of Health and Human Services, described it as "an island of objective and pristine research, untainted by the influences of commercialization."[44] A recent exposé notes that this isolation from commercial influence is no longer the case but that abuses have been few.[45] In the 1980s, in part due to pressure to translate basic bench research into treatment for patients, research collaborations between the government (NIH) and industry became acceptable. In fact, as Evan DeRenzo explains, "the quest for more and tighter public-private collaborations produced a gold rush mentality. Virtually every government agency and university set up a Technology Transfer Office or its equivalent. The pressure to conduct 'translational' research, the buzz word for moving research from the bench to the bedside, was palpable" and was fueled by Congress.[46]

Legislation enacted in the 1980s fueled the collaboration between government and industry, which eventually resulted in some of the later financial COI charges. For example, the Bayh-Dole Patent and Trademark

Laws Amendment Act of 1980 allowed academic institutions to have the intellectual property rights when carrying out government-funded research, thereby receiving the patent and licensing funds and ongoing royalties. Similarly, the Small Business Patent Procedures Act of 1980 altered prior policy by granting exclusive licensing of patent rights to small businesses and universities, among others. Further legislation also encouraged technology transfer and provided antitrust protection. Such collaboration is good in that it encourages more rapid technological advances. But it does not come without its own costs—those of fueling competitiveness rather than collaboration and shifting many investigator and sponsor resources away from basic science to potentially more lucrative lines of research.[47]

In 1995, Dr. Harold Varmus, then the director of the NIH, rescinded the longstanding policies that prohibited investigators from accepting consulting fees or stock from industrial trial sponsors. Annual limits on work and revenue from outside the NIH were also removed. Requirements for reporting potential financial conflicts of interest were gutted, allowing bypass of public disclosure requirements that are required of investigators in the private sector.[48] A *Los Angeles Times* report outlined some of the implications that evolve from these close relationships. The collaboration may raise some understandable concerns about influence on

- Directions that research may take
- Interpretation of data
- Reporting of adverse events
- Awarding of grants

Given the climatc and the push for new products, it's no great surprise that ethical lapses occurred. The pendulum has been swinging back. The NIH now requires fairly stringent reporting, including reporting of salary or stocks totaling more than $10,000 for a related company.[49] Unfortunately, it appears that there is still little oversight, and researchers from the NIH and universities that receive federal grants still have frequent financial conflicts of interest, particularly related to equity interests.[50, 51, 52]

A particularly hot issue is to what degree financial interests should be disclosed by investigators to prospective research participants. Surprisingly, the impact of such disclosure varied. In one study, 5 percent of volunteers said they would not participate because of an investigator's equity interest. Others viewed that investment as a plus, feeling the PI would work harder or believed more strongly in the potential benefit of the intervention. The typical per-patient payment to investigators did not generate concern. One issue is whether the disclosure might distract from discussion of more immediate risks and benefits. The desire for disclosure rose with the level of risk of the study. Overall, some disclosure was viewed favorably, as improving trust, but was felt to be better if limited in detail.[53]

In addition to the ethical questions, there have been lawsuits related to lack of disclosure of financial conflicts of interest as well as other lapses in informed consent and study conduct, as outlined in the table in appendix A.

Obviously, the primary goal of a drug company is to make money, to support its day-to-day operations, and to meet its investors' expectations. Thus, the primary focus is to develop not only a good and useful drug product but to do so efficiently and rapidly and to maximize profitability (see "Costs of Clinical Trials" in chapter 7). Enormous pressure is placed on the CRAs and the study site to rapidly deliver evaluable patients. As with any business endeavor, this pressure then tempts the site's team to cut corners.

Individual sites often experience pressure to enroll borderline patients, frequently in the form of financial concerns for the site team or the investigator. After all, the site has to meet overhead and salary expenses. In many academic centers, the income from drug study protocols also pays for equipment or personnel for the department that generates the funds. Thus, pressure may be particularly high on some academically oriented investigators to enroll borderline patients. This pressure may come either directly from their superiors or from the desire to be one of the lead investigators on a trial. Prominent positioning on a trial is often rewarded by prestige and financial benefits for the department as well as by coauthorship on publications. These rewards in turn determine rank and tenure. In addition, if a study site is

View from the Trenches

Only once can I recall receiving pressure regarding how I classified an adverse event, and I believe that was primarily because of an honest difference of opinion between the sponsor's physician and me. All of the sponsors I have worked with actively strive to have PIs conscientiously report any potential adverse event and audit aggressively so as not to overlook any.

not competitive in enrollment, it risks being closed, an event that may also damage the site's prospects for future trials.[54]

The type of grant structure can also sometimes lead to ethical dilemmas in the form of temptations to enroll borderline subjects. For example, you would be wise to avoid bonuses for reaching specific target benchmarks in a study. Incentive clauses in contracts appear to be offered less frequently and are less often a problem than they once were, but when considering undertaking a study and negotiating a grant, you need to evaluate the pressures inherent in the structure of the grant and any bonuses. The contract and grant payments can be structured in ways that either increase these temptations or reduce them. Try to get the grant structured to minimize these ethical pressures on your site. This can most comfortably be done by staying with a simple fee-for-service arrangement. Other suggestions are noted in the sidebar, "Proposal for Investigator Grants."

View from the Trenches

Proposal for Investigator Grants

Having experienced pressures from the structure of grants, I would propose that the pharmaceutical industry make the following changes in grant payment schedules in order to reduce the financial pressure to cut corners. I believe these changes would go a long way in reducing any ethical concerns prompted by such enticements. Instead,

- **Pay a reasonable amount for the effort and expense of screening patients for enrollment, rather than basing all payments on enrollment numbers. This would reduce the temptation to enroll "marginal" patients, as the grant per patient wouldn't be "all or nothing."**
- **Structure the grant to better reflect the amount of effort, stress, and skill required to conduct a study well and to get good, "clean" (complete and accurate) data, rather than simply responding to the number of subjects who complete the study. No incentive in the system exists now to reward obsessive compulsive worriers, such as myself, who hover over our patients, mindful of our added responsibilities in the research setting. Nor is there any incentive for experience or accuracy. In fact, since grants are now fairly uniform across the study sites for a given trial, it is in the site's financial interest to have the least trained, lowest paid individual on the team perform the study activities. (I suppose that is why so many eyebrows are raised when sponsors learn that I conduct, with rare exceptions, all the study evaluations myself.)**

Continued on next page

Other Pressures

Just as pressures on individual study sites tempt investigators to take shortcuts, similar pressures are brought to bear on pharmaceutical companies, leading to the temptation to cut corners and raising ethical concerns. The intense pressure to recruit patients has been outlined by the U.S. Department of Health and Human Services Office of Inspector General in a report called *Recruiting Human Subjects: Pressures in Industry-Sponsored Clinical Research.*[55] This report analyzes some of the elements fueling the changes to the clinical trials environment. As we noted in "Costs of Clinical Trials" in chapter 7, these elements include the following issues:

- Higher drug development costs result in a push for more rapid turnaround times for testing and approval.
- A larger pool of subjects is required because more drugs are in development and more subjects are needed for each trial. (There were 3,278 drugs

Continued from previous page

- **Eliminate bonuses for rapid recruitment or for specific numbers of patients enrolled. Note that these incentives may not all be strictly financial and may include coauthorship or, less commonly, travel. Such bonuses put undue pressure on a site to enroll borderline patients. Again, I suggest bonuses based on the quality of work, awarded to the site that reports serious adverse events the most thoroughly or receives the fewest data queries, for example. The current bonus system is simply too tempting and coercive. Per-patient grant payments should be adjusted to be more fair (or even generous).**
- **Structure grant payments so that there is no disincentive for dropping a patient from the trial. Again, I have a low threshold for dropping study patients from the trial if they are not getting better as rapidly as I would expect them to with an alternative agent or if I feel they are experiencing a significant side effect. I actively look for side effects of medications in all of my patients (study and nonstudy). I do this because it is the right thing to do and I need to sleep at night with no regrets for what I have done to a patient. At the same time, I am aware that in many cases dropping a patient from a study will mean a significant financial loss for my practice. This is why I try to structure grants so that if a patient drops out because of a problem with the study drug, we still receive full payment. (It is actually much more work to report a patient who experiences a serious adverse event than a patient who completes the study uneventfully.) If the patient drops out or is unevaluable because of an error at my site or because he or she was lost to follow-up, suggesting that the patient wasn't screened as well as one might have liked (or that the patient lied), then there is a financial penalty for the site.**

in preclinical studies in 1998 compared with 2,585 in 1995.) Patients' cases are often more complex because chronic illnesses, rather than acute ones, are increasingly targeted for studies, given that they are far more profitable. Because of this complexity, fewer patients are likely to be evaluable or to complete the studies. Longer trials are required to evaluate long-term safety and efficacy. And current attempts to look for gender or racial differences in clinical trials may also result in the need for more subjects.[56]

- A push for finding more efficient study sites is underway. This push fuels a shift to private practice and new investigators.
- Pressure is exerted to find patients who meet unrealistically restrictive entry criteria. This situation is aptly described as the "curse of poor protocol design." In one example, only 9,700 patients were found to meet the definition for the study indication, insomnia, out of a database of 1.8 million. Of those 9,700, only 581 would have met all the inclusion and exclusion criteria for enrollment.[57]

Another ethical issue has been raised: whether an individual investigator's access to trials influences whether or not a specific manufacturer's drugs are available on a hospital's formulary (the list of drugs that may be prescribed in that hospital). This influence seems unlikely, both because most doctors are reasonably ethical and because formulary decisions are made by groups of people, generally including physicians, pharmacists, and administrators. (The formulary committee's primary consideration is drug cost rather than efficacy, though efficacy is weighed into the equation.)

Some people are concerned that the investigator-sponsor relationship might alter a physician's prescribing patterns. Some studics are in progress looking at whether there is a correlation between a physician's participation on a trial and his or her subsequent prescribing practices. Such a correlation does not necessarily translate as the result of undue influence by the financial benefits of having conducted research for a pharmaceutical company. A more likely explanation is that doctors prefer to prescribe drugs they are familiar and comfortable with and in which they have confidence. Through participation as a researcher, one inevitably gains experience and knowledge about the drugs used on a trial. Oftentimes that knowledge is an advantage for the sponsor; occasionally, it is not.

Whose Body Is It? Tissue Ownership

The explosion of research in proteomics (protein and enzyme structure and function) and genomics (gene expression and function), potentially very valuable especially for diagnostics and treatments for cancer, heart disease, and other chronic diseases, has led to valuable discoveries with great commercial value. Squabbles over ownership of tissue or blood samples or other genetic material have predictably followed.

Several prominent cases illustrate some of the problems. The first is the sad tale of John Moore, a man with hairy-cell leukemia, well-told in Rebecca Skloot's excellent article "Taking the Least of You: The Tissue-Industrial Complex." After Moore underwent an appropriate treatment of having his spleen removed, his physician, David Golde of the University of California, Los Angeles, insisted that Moore return for frequent follow-ups for removal of blood, bone marrow, and other tissues. After years of this, Moore expressed concern over the expense of travel from Seattle to UCLA; Golde then reportedly offered to pay for his trips and lodging.

Seven years after the initial surgery, Moore was presented with a consent form stating, "I (do, do not) voluntarily grant to the University of California all rights I, or my heirs, may have in any cell line or any other potential product which might be developed from the blood and/or bone marrow obtained from me." Moore refused, became suspicious about Golde's persistence in seeking this consent, and hired a lawyer. Imagine their surprise when they discovered that Golde had filed a potentially lucrative patent on the "Mo" cell line! The potential licensing of Mo was estimated to reach $3 billion.[58]

In a landmark case, Moore sued Golde and UCLA on a number of grounds, including breach of informed consent and "conversion (using or controlling someone else's property without permission)." A series of judgments and appeals followed. Moore lost the initial suit. In round two, "in 1988, the California Court of Appeal ruled that a patient's blood and tissues remain his property after being removed from his body. The judges pointed to the Protection of Human Subjects in Medical Experimentation Act, a 1978 California statute requiring that research on humans respect 'the right of individuals to determine what is done to their own bodies.' They ruled: 'A patient must have the ultimate power to control what becomes of his or her tissues. To hold otherwise would open the door to a massive invasion of human privacy and dignity in the name of medical progress.'"[59]

Golde appealed to the state supreme court and, in an unsurprising victory for business, won in 1990. Even though the court agreed that there had been a lack of informed consent and a breach of fiduciary duty, it denied that Golde's gains were "ill-gotten."[60] The court ruled that "Moore couldn't own his cells, because that would conflict with Golde's patent. Golde had 'transformed' those cells into an invention. They were, the ruling said, the product of Golde's 'human ingenuity' and 'inventive effort.'"[61]

Furthermore, "the court said that ruling in Moore's favor might 'destroy the economic incentive to conduct important medical research.' It worried that giving patients property rights would 'hinder research by restricting access to the necessary raw materials' and create a field where with every cell sample a researcher purchases a ticket in a litigation lottery.'" The supreme court refused Moore's appeal.[62]

Some, including legal expert Lori Andrews, argue that instead of fueling research by providing lucrative financial incentives, this ruling actually made scientists less likely to share samples or work collaboratively[63]—which we see to this day (e.g., in HIV and Influenza H1N1 research). The notable exception to this occurred during the SARS epidemic, which was stopped only because of an unparalleled degree of cooperation.

I agree with Andrews's arguments—and even more so with ethicist E. Haavi Morreim's assessment about the patient's treatment: "Moore was exploited, completely without his knowledge or consent, for others' ulterior gain. Yet this dignitary offense is not typically deemed a compensable injury under malpractice law."[64]

The other closely watched case is that of *Washington University v. Catalona*, decided in 2008. Dr. William Catalona, a prominent prostate cancer surgeon at Washington University, collected over 30,000 tissue samples with his patients' permission. He used them for research, including developing the prostate-specific antigen (PSA) test widely used now for diagnosing prostate cancer.

After increasing tensions with the university, Catalona moved to Northwestern University and asked his patients if he could transfer their tissue samples there. Six thousand patients requested transfer of their specimens to Northwestern. Washington University not only denied these requests but sued to prevent Catalona from even contacting other patients to seek their permission to transfer samples. It claimed, as many employers do, that employees have no rights to intellectual or other property. Patients jumped into the fray, claiming their ownership rights to their tissue and the right to control the use of their tissue—in this case, specifying that it was for Dr. Catalona's research, not for that of the university at large.

Washington University claimed that the tissue was a donation to the university and could be used as the institution saw fit (in this case to profit from its sale), as long as it was anonymized (unlinked from any identifying information or medical records). It also noted that patients retained the right to have their tissue destroyed, per the informed consent.

Dr. Catalona and his patients lost in court on the first round; they appealed and lost again, with the eighth circuit appeals court viewing the tissue as a "free and generous gift" to Washington University. In one final stand, "Dr. Catalona asked the Supreme Court to rule that the Common Rule prohibited the university from asking the research participants to waive their ownership rights, and therefore the research participants still owned the samples and could direct their future disposition."[65] The Supreme Court justices declined to hear the case.

So what's the take-home message from the lawyers? Be careful in your consent wording to specify ownership of tissue. State that it is a donated gift to a specific party (specify whom) and that its use for future research is allowed. "Language that appears to waive the subject's rights should be carefully reviewed in light of the Common Rule's prohibition against exculpatory language."[66]

While the lawyers seem focused on property law, some ethicists are debating how these rulings fit in with the principles of autonomy, respect for persons, and collective public interests.[67] Similarly, what happens if retention of tissue conflicts with cultural or religious beliefs or, as noted by Catalona, if tissue samples are needed by patients in the future for their own care?

Business versus Patients

While I understand some of the logistical difficulties in transferring specimens (and, in this case, the university's claim regarding employer-employee relationships), the common theme in the cases I reviewed is that business interests trump patient interests—and I suspect that many patients might be less altruistic in the future.

Because of concerns raised by such cases and patients who were upset that tissue specimens at the NIH were being shared with pharmaceuticals, various rules have been implemented. In 2005, the NIH developed the NCI

Best Practices for Biospecimen Resources, including informative sections on ethical, legal, and logistical issues.[68] It and the related Cooperative Human Tissue Network (CHTN) state that the recipients "shall not sell any portion of the tissues provided by the CHTN, or products directly extracted from these tissues (e.g., protein, mRNA, or DNA). The recipients also must agree that they shall not transfer tissues (or any portion thereof) supplied by the CHTN to third parties without prior written permission from the CHTN."[69]

One interesting problem is that, while the best practices proposal allows for possible options, such as tiered donation on informed consents (allowing donation for X but not Y in future research) and consent for future unspecified research uses, HIPAA precludes donations that are not for a specific research purpose.[70, 71] We're going through the looking glass again, I'm afraid.

Patents versus Public Health

The patenting and ownership mania is growing to even more disconcerting extremes, with successful attempts to patent even observations about natural processes. For example, Metabolite licensed a patent on a procedure to measure homocysteine levels and correlated the results with vitamin deficiencies, concluding that elevated levels were likely due to a B vitamin deficiency. Each time LabCorp, a major lab testing company, used the test, it paid a royalty to Metabolite. LabCorp then began to using a competitor company's test instead but provided the interpretation of the test results. In *Metabolite v. LabCorp*, "the Court of Appeals for the Federal Circuit held that LabCorp induced infringement of that patent (and thus was liable for over $2 million in damages) based on the publication to physicians of a law of nature—the relation between levels of homocysteine and vitamin deficiency."[72]

A more widely known issue relating to ownership is the battle over pharmaceutical companies' patents versus the health needs of large populations, particularly in developing countries. This first received considerable publicity regarding access to HIV medicines in sub-Saharan Africa, the region most seriously affected with AIDS (more than 70 percent of affected people resided there in 2001), where drug prices made treatment impossible.[73]

In 1994, the World Trade Organization made the Trade-Related Aspects of Intellectual Property (TRIPS) Agreement, which provided intellectual property protection. Some considered compulsory licenses, in which the government can force the patent holder or manufacturer to grant use to others, a means of ensuring access. TRIPS was challenged in 1997 by the South African

Medicines and Related Substances Control Amendment Act, which would have allowed the government to use generics.

True to form, the pharmaceutical companies sued the government of South Africa. In this case, activists successfully mounted protests and PhRMA's suit was dropped. Shortly thereafter, the South African government began providing antiretroviral treatment on a massive scale.[74]

Other cases illustrate the clash between patents and public health. For example, with the anthrax scare, many were unhappy with Bayer Corporation's sole ownership of the drug of choice, Cipro, and the U.S. government considered compulsory licensing to enable increased production (and lower cost) of the antibiotic from generic manufacturers. David Resnik and Kenneth DeVille proposed five conditions for such an action to reasonably override intellectual property rights: national emergency, absence of alternative inventions, failure of good-faith negotiations, fair compensation for loss, and time limitation.[75]

Another timely example is that of flu-related patents. In one case, a group of scientists was able to resurrect the deadly Spanish influenza virus using tissue from a well-preserved victim of the 1918 pandemic, raising a number of ethical and security questions as well. One issue that these scientists didn't have to deal with was ownership of the tissue or consent from the victim or his descendents for "future use" research. In another case, the U.S. government applied for a patent for a "bird flu" vaccine in 2006. One of the troublesome aspects of this is that the government used samples from Indonesia, Thailand, Hong Kong, and South Korea that were sent to the WHO Global Influenza Surveillance Network by Indonesia and provided to support public health. Such global networks work only in an atmosphere of trust and collaboration—and will clearly fail if proprietary claims are made on donated samples intended to be shared for research rather than profit.[76]

We have recently had an example of the consequences of patenting flu vaccines. Indonesia has had a high number of deaths from Influenza H5N1 (avian flu). In 2007, it stopped sharing virus samples with WHO, wanting to stake a claim to intellectual property rights associated with possible vaccine development and to protest that vaccines are often unaffordable in developing countries. As of November 2009, Indonesia was still trying to negotiate a compromise with WHO regarding virus sharing and "material transfer" to pharmaceutical companies, which would allow them to develop a vaccine commercially. In the meantime, Indonesia and other developing countries are waiting for donations of the Influenza H1N1 vaccine as a demonstration of wealthier countries' commitment to some level of equity and access to medicines essential for public health.[77]

Patient-Prompted Ethical Issues

Ethical dilemmas are also prompted by patients. Probably everyone in the medical field has had experience with patients who lie about their medical histories or problems or who simply forget significant but remote details. When an investigator enrolls a patient in a trial, the investigator has to rely on the patient to provide an accurate and complete history. Sometimes old records are available; more often, they are not. Particularly common issues that patients lie about are histories of seizures, alcohol or drug use, and psychiatric problems. Yet each of these, if known, could influence an investigator's decision as to whether to pass a given patient through screening to enrollment in a trial.

Occasionally, patients may lie to gain access to medical therapies that would not otherwise be available to them (because they meet some excluding criteria or are on a conflicting medication). Sometimes, patients have a financial motive for participating in addition to the access to free care, although this is rare for therapeutic trials with ill patients. It is also minimized by making reasonable payments to cover patients' time and trouble in participating (e.g., gas, parking, taxi fare), rather than excessive participation fees that might be unduly tempting or coercive. More often, patients who lie want the extra attention they receive by participating or the access to possibly better therapies.

Ethical concerns about patients involve two other aspects of the PI-volunteer relationship. One occurs when the PI is also the patient's personal physician, a delicate balancing act. Although a physician's loyalty to his or her patient should be utmost, this is not always compatible with the requirements of a protocol. Surveys have shown that patients are more likely to participate in a study if their physician is the PI. Physicians have to be very careful to respect that trust.

Another wrinkle in the PI-patient relationship is that sometimes physicians so intensely want to help their patients that they are willing to bend the enrollment criteria for a trial so a patient can have access to a potentially lifesaving drug, even if this compromises the accuracy of the trial. A recent survey showed that almost 64 percent of respondents thought that researchers should deviate from the protocol to improve subjects' care. Of the 69 percent of respondents who reported having had a patient ineligible to participate in a trial but for whom they believed the trial would be beneficial, 22 percent recruited the patient anyway. And of the 36 percent who said one of their patients had met termination criteria but seemed to benefit medically from the trial, 9 percent reported that they kept the subject in the trial.[78, 79]

Drs. Stephen Straus and James Wilson, both of whom had volunteers die on phase 1 trials, note that investigators are inherently enthusiastic and optimistic about their trials or they could not overcome the hurdles they encounter in their research and sustain their effort.[80, 81] Wilson adds, "This dual role/relationship [of physician and investigator] may confuse research with clinical care and puts the investigator in a position to heavily influence the patient's/subject's decisions."[82]

Adverse Events: Related Ethical Issues

Cullen Vogelson raises the point that investigators and coordinators are notorious for underreporting minor adverse events, especially those they feel are unimportant or not attributable to the study medication.[83] While this claim of underreporting is probably true, the oversight may be attributed to different motives. This issue reflects neither wanton or cavalier disregard for adverse events nor sloppiness at the investigative sites. The issue is more likely to reflect differences in perspectives. Many investigators understand how important it is not to suggest potential side effects to the patient beyond

View from the Trenches

The most bizarre and difficult patients to care for are those with Munchausen syndrome, who feign or create illness to obtain medical attention. This can be carried to extremes. I have had patients who injected themselves with substances deliberately to cause infections and patients who have sought and even undergone repeated surgeries (usually exploratory abdominal ones). The individual I was most duped by sought invasive procedures, claiming to have AIDS when in fact he didn't. He had studied the symptoms and medications and knew more about the illness and workup at that time than I did. Eventually, I learned that he went from state to state repeating this scenario.

having already told them, as part of the informed consent process, that certain symptoms have been known to occur with the drug in question. Further, investigators instruct their patients that it is important to report anything new that they experience while participating on a trial. When you see patients for their visits and examinations, you ask them if they have had any new problems. You do not, however, ask them if they have experienced symptom X because that might bias their response. Sometimes an investigator will initially miss an adverse event in this way and then become aware of it by looking at the nurse's notes or noticing that certain medications were administered (e.g., a painkiller). The physician can then ask the patient for what symptom he or she sought the medication. Patients often will tell a nurse one thing and a doctor another or not remember to mention something at a particular visit but bring it up at a later visit.

Furthermore, CRAs monitor each site regularly, every 1–2 months on active studies with steady enrollment, and one of their major focuses is, in fact, taking note of adverse events, be they new symptoms or changes in lab test results. This monitoring provides a safety net for catching adverse events, and data analysis provides another. Queries are generated when an as-needed medication, such as acetaminophen, is listed without a corresponding diagnosis in a patient's medical history. The site then has to review the medical record to resolve the discrepancy.

Practically and ethically speaking, attributing causality of an adverse event is no easy matter. Particularly with critically ill patients who are on multiple medications, it is extraordinarily difficult to decide if a change is due to underlying illness, medication interactions, or new complications of the disease. This is why we have computers and multivariate analysis.

A separate issue concerns adverse event reporting. No deterrent exists for reporting an AE, but there is inherently, perhaps, a disincentive, in that each AE generates yet more work and another report. However, these AEs (headache, nausea, etc.) are undoubtedly going to be picked up by the CRA monitoring the study data, and paperwork will need to be completed then. This, again, is more costly to the site, both in time and aggravation, in that someone must review the patient's course on the study to complete the necessary forms. It is simply easier—less annoying and less work—to track this information as you go along and report it with the initial CRF.

Significant penalties can be incurred for failing to report a serious adverse event, and SAEs are defined in unambiguous terms. If such a failure reflects a continuing pattern, the FDA might put sanctions on the investigator's or the sponsor's ability to continue conducting trials. Investigators are required to notify the sponsor of an SAE within 24 hours of becoming aware of it. Most often, sponsors do not try to influence the investigator's attribution of causality. Occasionally, pressure is put on the investigator to not call an SAE "probably related" to the study med, but this is a rarity. Most medical monitors and researchers are ethical physicians, conscientious and concerned about a drug's safety, and they would, no doubt, value those concerns above pressures to promote the drug. However, this is apparently not always the case, as illustrated by the following exception.

In gene therapy trials in particular, serious adverse events have been grossly underreported. Most surprising and disturbing are some apparently active attempts to hide serious adverse events and deaths. As LeRoy Walters, the former chairman of NIH's Recombinant DNA Advisory Committee and former head of the Kennedy Institute of Ethics at Georgetown University, commented, "Probably the clearest evidence of the system [to protect research subjects] not working is that only 35 to 37 of 970 serious adverse events . . . were reported to the NIH" as required. "That is fewer than 5 percent of the serious adverse events."[84] In such cases, a "clinical hold order" may be issued by the FDA to the sponsor, requiring suspension of an ongoing investigation and financial or other sanctions against both the investigator and sponsor.

Multiple levels of safeguards are in place at the level of the individual investigative site conducting clinical trials for pharmaceutical companies. For example, the sponsor requires the Principal Investigator to review all of the laboratory tests and assess whether changes in test results are study drug related or not. The magnitude of the change is assessed in addition to the attribution. New symptoms, such as nausea, diarrhea, or rash, are similarly assessed. The sponsor also sends a monitor regularly—often every few weeks—to review every scrap of data that the site has captured and to then discuss every new finding with the coordinator and the investigator. Simultaneously, lab test results, EKGs, and other reports are submitted to the sponsor. An individual site is likely to have limited experience with a given drug; it would be unusual for an investigator at an individual site to be able to detect a pattern of significant side effects. It is in fact up to the sponsor's team, with its vast analytical resources, to carefully analyze these reports, gathered from multiple sites, and it is up to the sponsor and the

FDA to see if any systematic and/or significant new findings are attributable to the experimental drug.

Data Safety Monitoring Boards

As clinical trials have grown larger and more complex, Data Safety Monitoring Boards (DSMBs) have taken on increased importance and are therefore also receiving increased regulatory attention. As mentioned in chapter 1, the primary responsibility of these committees is to identify safety issues as rapidly as possible. Secondarily, they evaluate data at regular intervals to determine if a trial is worth continuing or if it should be stopped for futility. Interim analyses are kept confidential to not bias the study, unless there is a notable finding. Sometimes DSMBs find that a trial's objectives have been met, allowing the trial to be stopped early, or find similar unexpected successes. This was seen most recently with Pfizer's Sutent (sunitinib), a drug shown to be efficacious for pancreatic cancer.[85]

DSMBs monitor enrollment, comparability of the treatment groups, protocol compliance, and data quality to assess differences in outcomes and adverse events. Independent DSMBs are critically important in looking at trials with an expected high morbidity or mortality (such as sepsis trials) or high-risk procedures, or in comparing rates of serious toxicity between treatment groups. Monitoring by DSMBs is also important for studies involving use of vulnerable populations, multicenter studies, and studies involving new science, such as gene therapies. It is not generally needed or used for short-term trials where no significant safety or efficacy issues are expected. It is required for all NIH phase 3 trials.[86]

Some of the push for using a DSMB came from failures of IRBs in providing adequate oversight. But using a DSMB introduces its own set of problems: increased cost, group composition, and conflict of interest issues. Selecting independent members where a limited pool of people with adequate expertise is available, without running into conflict of interest complaints, can be quite difficult.

Standards have been recommended for the composition of DSMBs and for conduct of the committee. For example, people with obvious financial conflicts of interest should not be selected, and members should ideally come from outside the institution or sponsor.[87] Members should have no COI by career involvement, involvement in regulatory issues that might affect the product, or publication or authorship rights. Other problems can arise from conflicts between concerns noted by a DSMB and the subsequent response from the sponsor. Such conflicts were illustrated in the Merck Vioxx studies and ultimately (and unfortunately, from my perspective) led to Merck's withdrawal of Vioxx from the market in 2004.[88, 89]

Publication Ethics

Two areas of publication are pertinent to clinical investigators: publication bias and ghostwriting. The key warning, with both, is that as much as coauthorship is an often-sought goal, it also requires care so as not to hurt you or your reputation.

Ghostwriters in the Sky

What seemed innocuous previously were the offers of help from sponsors regarding manuscript preparation, not unreasonable given the enormous time commitment and complexities involved in the process. It was pretty common to have help in compiling the statistics or writing the materials and methods section and some background material, with the author then writing the conclusion and signing off as to the veracity of the submission. A recent review of articles published in 2008 revealed that 7–11 percent of those published in top medical journals had ghostwriters, described as "unacknowledged research or writing contributions by people other than the author."[90]

Now the International Committee of Medical Journal Editors has rather draconian requirements. If you want your data published in a prestigious journal, you face additional hurdles of having to agree to a gag order and having your results "quarantined" prior to publication. (This means you are not allowed to present your results anywhere prior to the article's debut in the prominent journal.)

Additional complexities might trip up the unwary. For example, the FDAAA "mandates the posting of summary results data for certain trials in ClinicalTrials.gov. Thus, the ICMJE will not consider results data posted in the tabular format required by ClinicalTrials.gov to be prior publication. However, editors of journals that follow the ICMJE recommendations may consider posting of more detailed descriptions of trial results beyond those included in ClinicalTrials.gov to be prior publication."[91] This hardly seems to be in the public interest.

Be similarly careful to avoid conflict of interest bias charges if you are presenting data at a meeting or serving on a panel forming practice guidelines. Because of the law of unintended consequences, it can be hard to find any experts meeting the current political correctness purity tests.

In a prescient 1993 commentary, "Conflict of Interest: The New McCarthyism in Science," Kenneth Rothman warned about overemphasizing author affiliations over a paper's scientific merit. Laurence Hirsch, in an excellent review, notes that despite concerns about COI, even an analysis by Public Citizen was unable to demonstrate a relationship between COI and FDA drug advisory committee member voting patterns—nor did it find that "conflicted" members would have changed the outcomes.[92]

Publication Bias

Considerable attention has been placed recently on the fact that negative findings or adverse results often go unreported. For example, one group of researchers identified all the efficacy trials included in NDAs for new drugs approved by the FDA in 2001 and 2002 and then reviewed related literature. Unsurprisingly, "trials with favorable outcomes were nearly five times as likely to be published as those without favorable outcomes."[93] In part, this is because the nonfavorable findings may be viewed by the researchers as "uninteresting"; in part, it reflects clinical trial agreement clauses that prohibit publication without the sponsor's approval (as in the Betty Dong affair described in chapter 3). Conflicts of interest leading to reporting and publication bias have received considerable attention (e.g., for Merck's Vioxx and Pfizer's Celebrex). At least one of the major articles on selective reporting appeared in *JAMA*.[94]

In a 2004 study by *JAMA*, cherry-picking of trial results was found and further reported with the provocative solution of "Sarbanes-Oxley for professors." In a *Wall Street Journal* article, Anne Wilde Mathews quotes Douglas Altman, author of the *JAMA* study, as saying, "It was a shock to find that what we thought was the most reliable information wasn't." Further, Catherine DeAngelis, *JAMA*'s editor in chief, stated, "We were burned very badly."[95]

Because of the news of frequent reporting biases, the World Health Organization has called for standards in the reporting of clinical trial results.[96] Similarly, the Consolidated Standards of Reporting Trials (CONSORT) group of researchers, methodologists, and medical journal editors has produced a series of recommendations for reporting results of randomized clinical trials "facilitating their complete and transparent reporting, and aiding their critical appraisal and interpretation."[97]

The expression of concern from DeAngelis has a certain irony now. In brief, Jonathan Leo wrote a letter to *JAMA* in 2008 reporting that a study of Lexapro in stroke patients published in *JAMA* failed to disclose a conflict of interest of an author. After receiving no response, Leo wrote to the *British Medical Journal*, which published his letter. A quite scandalous catfight followed, which included publication of an editorial (coauthored by DeAngelis) accusing Leo of sparking an unfair rush to judgment. In an astonishing demonstration of an ethical lapse, *JAMA* subsequently removed the editorial from its Web site. As ethicist Udo Schuklenk explained, "a) *JAMA* has excised its first publication from its website as well as biomedical data-bases (I have no idea how the latter feast [sic] was achieved). No retraction notice was published, no erratum of any kind. As one of my colleagues pointed out: what does this mean for the substantial commentary (overwhelmingly critical in nature) that was published in various fora on this now non-existent article?" Fortunately, he provides links to the article to demonstrate his point.[98] Another blogger aptly describes this incident as *JAMA* having dropped the inconvenient article down an Orwellian "memory hole."[99]

The move toward reducing publication bias by having clinical trial registries and publication standards is most welcome. These changes should result in less biased reporting and increased information about negative trials and adverse outcomes. Also welcome would be more open journals such as those of the Public Library of Science, rather than the subscription-only journals that obstruct transparency and make evaluating trials, researching, and writing an unnecessarily arduous practice.

Practice Guidelines

Practice guidelines are recommendations from specialty societies' panels of experts regarding the best treatments for specific conditions. While intended to be educational guidances, they are increasingly used prescriptively as standards of care in a legal context. These expert committees often, and perhaps unavoidably, appear to have conflicts of interest.

The majority of researchers on these panels have likely received grant money, consulting fees, or similar compensation from pharmaceutical sponsors. One report, reviewing more than 200 guidelines, states, "more than one third of the authors declared financial links to relevant drug companies, with around 70% of panels being affected."[100]

It's not surprising that many guidelines tend to encourage use of patented drugs rather than less expensive generics. I don't believe the motivation is all financial, however. There is strong peer pressure to demonstrate that you are up to date with literature and advances by using the latest drug. The barrage of advertising and attention that new drugs receive undoubtedly contributes as well. And so does a sincere belief that the new drug has benefits over the older one, whether real or imagined, as well as the shorter period in which to have recognized adverse outcomes.

COIs affect practice guideline recommendations for a wide array of conditions, including diabetes, hypertension, hyperlipidemia, and psychiatric conditions.[101] The effects of these COIs are problematic in that they enormously increase the costs of drugs (especially those subsidized by the public via Medicare or Medicaid) and shape pharmaceutical pipelines in ways that are counterproductive for society as a whole.

Off-Label Uses

An additional problem is the off-label promotion of drugs (aka deceptive marketing) and the enormous cost of unproven and unnecessarily expensive medications. Two companies made headlines in 2009, though others have had similar ethical lapses. Eli Lilly, for example, entered into a $1.415 billion settlement with the Department of Justice in January 2009 over its off-label promotion of Zyprexa (a drug for schizophrenia) for dementia.[102] Similarly in September 2009, Pfizer pled guilty to off-label promotion of Bextra as well as three other drugs and paid $2.3 billion in fines and penalties.[103] Both of the named drugs have significant risks; Bextra was removed from the market in 2005.

Do these fines sound like significant recompense? No way! Given that about 15 percent of all drug sales in the United States are for off-label uses and that the companies enjoy huge profits, the fines are small potatoes—just the cost of doing business.

In the case of Pfizer's Neurontin, for example, "Pfizer took in $2.27 billion from sales of Neurontin in 2002. A full 94 percent—$2.12 billion—of that revenue came from off-label use." Neurontin's off-label use made it even more profitable than Pfizer's blockbuster Viagra for several years. It has earned more than $12 billion in revenue.[104]

These are just some of many such examples, risking patients' health for profits. Yet apparently the government has not pursued felony cases against the parent companies because they, like Wall Street banks, are considered "too big to fail"; felony convictions would preclude the companies from being reimbursed by federal programs such as Medicare and Medicaid, potentially causing them to fail.[105] Instead, the settlements are made through the parent companies' subsidiaries.

So the companies and investors are making huge profits at taxpayers' expense via fraudulent claims to public programs. Yet if I even waive the copay for an indigent Medicare patient, I could be charged with violating the same False Claims Act that Big Pharma has violated. Do you think that would be similarly brushed aside?

Ironically, at a recent FDA course I attended, a lecturer from Pfizer repeatedly focused on the "partnership for public health" with clinical investigators. There seems to be a bit of a disconnect.[106]

IRB-Related Ethical Issues

In several well-publicized occurrences, IRBs have failed to act as safeguards for patients on clinical trials. Several contributing factors come into play in different settings. IRB members do the best they can; they are generally volunteers (rather than being paid for their time), have little or no formal training, and, until recently, have had no uniform standards to guide them. The U.S. Department of Health and Human Services Office of Inspector General examined these problems and made several recommendations in 1998, emphasizing ongoing education in ethics and federal oversight as well as oversight from a Data Safety Monitoring Board equivalent for multisite studies.[107] Particularly for smaller institutions, the IRB staff simply does not always have the requisite expertise to carefully evaluate the risks and benefits of a proposed protocol. Efforts are being made to correct these problems. For example, since 1974, Public Responsibility in Medicine and Research, the Association for the Accreditation of Human Research Protection Programs, and the Council for Certification of IRB Professionals have provided an accreditation system for programs.[108]

The AAHRPP accredits institutions and investigators as well as IRBs. Accreditation is based on an evaluation of an organization's structure and processes and an assessment of whether consistent regulatory, legal, and ethical procedures and requirements are in place; specific outcomes or decisions are not evaluated. In April 2009, Pfizer became the first pharmaceutical company to receive AAHRPP accreditation, sought in apparent response to an "erosion of public trust" following highly publicized lawsuits over its Celebrex and Trovafloxacin drugs.[109]

A recent scandal surrounding an IRB further highlights the need for better standards and responsibility. Coast IRB had approved a product called Adhesiabloc, developed by Device Med Systems. There was one little problem: in March 2009, reports noted that "the company approved the methodology for a fake clinical trial of an equally fake surgical gel produced by a fake company that Congress and the Government Accountability Office had set up" in an impressive sting operation.[110] Subsequent counterarguments were made that perhaps the sting itself was illegal, but the denouement was that Coast IRB was forced to close, disrupting some trials in the transfer to other IRBs.[111] Western IRB and others were the lucky beneficiaries. If you enjoy watching scandals unravel, this episode makes a good read.

What is not often discussed is the existence of inherent conflicts of interest for IRBs similar to those for investigators. Conflicts are most commonly financial. For example, commercial IRBs are paid directly by the drug company sponsor and therefore would not, presumably, want to "bite the hand that feeds it." Nonfinancial ethical conflicts may be due to excessive personal involvement or prejudgment by the experts on the board.[112] Conflicts may arise when there is a personal or collaborative relationship between the investigator and the IRB member. Increasingly, competition may exist between the PI and IRB members. IRB members should recuse themselves from committee participation under such circumstances where there is a conflict of interest.

In a rather scathing article, the relative merits of commercial versus local IRBs are debated.[113] Western IRB, founded in 1977, is mentioned as overseeing more than half of all new drug submissions to the FDA. It is highly regarded by many and has AAHRPP accreditation but has had lapses, including a suit for approving a placebo-controlled study of a drug for psoriatic arthritis. It also oversaw trials with the infamous Robert Fiddes—often used as a poster child for education about fraud—and other trials in which investigators were charged with lying to the FDA and endangering subjects' lives.

According to a *Bloomberg Markets* report, "about 60 items are considered at each meeting, giving members an average of four minutes to discuss each issue. The meetings and their minutes are closed to the public."[114] In defending Western IRB and other commercial IRBs, Ezekiel J. Emanuel, chair of the Department of Clinical Bioethics at the NIH, notes that the for-profit IRBs actually have a better OHRP inspection record than IRBs of not-for-profit institutions.[115] While I agree that the issue should not be "For-Profit Bad, Not-for-Profit Good," the volume of studies and resultant level of oversight are quite disconcerting.

Another irony in all of this is the Form FDA 1572 obligations that places responsibility on an investigator to ensure that the IRB "complies with the requirements of 21 CFR part 56" and will provide continuing review for the clinical investigation. How, exactly, are we supposed to do that?

While conflict-of-interest debates generally focus on individual practice settings, the potential for conflicts is equally strong at academic institutions. These university settings receive both income and prestige from their ongoing studies and expect IRB support, with subject protection, too. The institution can tout that it is providing state-of-the-art medical care and that it has been selected as a research site over its competitors by a leading pharmaceutical company.[116] In such an environment, an IRB must make concerted efforts to act independently and dispassionately.

As with for-profit IRBs, academic institutions now receive significant financial support from the pharmaceutical sponsors through their review fees. The volume of studies reviewed is similarly inappropriate. In fact, criticisms following Ellen Roche's death during a Johns Hopkins trial noted that one IRB, meeting every other week, was responsible for 800 new proposals and annual reviews. The analysis also noted that the university's culture viewed the oversight process as a barrier to research rather than a safeguard.[117]

Unanticipated Risk in Clinical Trials

Perhaps no case better illustrates the confluence of bad decisions than the TeGenero trial in 2006, in which six healthy volunteers sustained serious, life-altering injuries. Several reviews provide an excellent dissection of the case.

Norman Goldfarb accompanies his review with a copy of the trial's informed consent. Both should be studied by all interested in research ethics.

In the TeGenero trial, healthy volunteers were given a new type of monoclonal antibody drug, which acted on their immune systems, as part of a first-in-human study. All eight volunteers were given rapid IV infusions of the investigational drug or a placebo over a period of about an hour. Within hours, the six men who received the active drug became progressively critically ill, with "cytokine storm" syndrome causing multiorgan failure, and were transferred to an intensive care unit. Miraculously, none died.

Important lessons were learned from this disastrous trial and are detailed in the table in appendix A. The initial question asked was why "an agonist drug [one that boosts response] targeted at compromised immune systems was given to individuals with intact immune systems."[118]

Reviews by the Medicines and Healthcare products Regulatory Agency (MHRA) found no significant deficiencies in good clinical practice (which others might argue with), good laboratory practice and animal testing, or good manufacturing practice and appointed a special expert group (the Duff commission) to provide further direction. Of special note, in terms of what the group felt was done right, was that testing had been done in animals and that "at a dose that was numerically 500 times larger than that given to human volunteers, cynomolgus monkeys did not develop a cytokine release syndrome."[119]

The MHRA concluded, "TGN1412 is a new class of monoclonal antibody . . . In this case the resulting activity seen in humans was not predicted from apparently adequate pre-clinical testing. This . . . raises important scientific and medical questions about the potential risks associated with this type of drug and how to make the transition from pre-clinical testing to trials in humans."[120]

The Duff commission identified

> *factors that should raise the level of caution for first human exposures to new agents. These include:*
>
> - *any agent whose effects might cause severe physiological disturbance to vital body systems;*
> - *agonistic or stimulatory actions;*
> - *novel agents and novel mechanisms of action where there is no prior experience;*

- *species-specificity of an agent making pre-clinical risk-assessment in animal models difficult or impossible;*
- *the potency of an agent, eg compared with a natural ligand; multifunctional agents, eg bivalent antibodies, FcR binding domains;*
- *cell-associated targets;*
- *targets that by-pass normal control mechanisms;*
- *immune system targets;*
- *targets in systems with the potential for large biological amplification in vivo.*[121]

Others are less gentle in their criticism, particularly noting that inadequate emphasis was placed on published reports indicating that monkeys show a much lower response to T cell activating agents than do humans, that dosing should have been based on pharmacologic data (rather than toxicity), and that inadequate attention was give to the "acute mitogenic [causing cell division] activity of the antibody."[122]

Michael Goodyear observes that early trial registrations might provide a level of transparency that would avoid this type of disaster—yet there is strong resistance to registries, particularly for phase 1 trials, because of industrial competition, where secrecy is preferred to help maintain an advantage. He appropriately concludes, "Phase I trials in healthy volunteers raise special ethical issues when the benefits are non-existent and the risks are high."[123]

While this was a highly visible, dramatic case, it was atypical, being a phase 1 study that injured healthy young volunteers. Many procedural and ethical lapses occurred, in both study design and implementation. Of particular note is the ill-advised decision to give a first-in-human drug, especially one that is an immunomodulator, at 10-minute intervals, rather than spacing administration to new volunteers days, if not weeks, apart, after clinical and lab data were assessed.

Further questions were raised about the level of expertise of the IRB and the investigators. The consent was at a college-graduate level and contained phrases that tended to downplay risk. Large inducements were offered in the advertising and payment: "The TGN1412 study's subject recruitment posting at www.drugtrial.co.uk stated, 'You'll have plenty of time to read or study or just relax—with digital TV, pool table, videogames, DVD player and now FREE

Internet access! You can even just catch up on some sleep!'"[124] "For your time, and to compensate for any inconvenience, a payment of £2000 will be made on completion of the study."[125] Other problems included coercive clauses regarding payment for participation, lack of protection regarding payment for care related to subject injuries, and lack of access to the ethics committee.

Later in this chapter, we'll look at a more familiar example, one you might readily encounter in your own practice.

While a number of the decisions in the TeGenero case illustrate significant errors in judgment, sometimes bad things happen even when everything was done correctly. The 1993 trial of fialuridine (FIAU), again representing a new class of drugs, shows that clinical trials can have tragic and truly unanticipated risk. In that phase 1 trial, headed by NIH experts Drs. Stephen Straus (a NIAID virologist) and Jay Hoofnagle (a hepatologist and director of the Division of Digestive Diseases), five patients receiving the new antiviral drug as treatment for their hepatitis B died and two required liver transplants. The finger-pointing and political fallout from these deaths are discussed in "Politics of Research: The FDA" (chapter 9). Let's look at the IOM conclusions and also the more human impacts on the researchers and their work.

The IOM reports that when the first patient died with an unusual presentation of systemic lactic acidosis and hepatic steatosis (later classified as FIAU syndrome), extensive review occurred but no conclusion could be reached as to the role of the drug, given the patient's other health problems. When the second patient was hospitalized with lactic acidosis, Dr. Adrian DiBisceglie, chief of the Hepatitis Study Section, promptly drove to Virginia (80 miles each way) to personally investigate. The IOM committee commended the investigators for the way they "promptly recognized the syndrome of FIAU toxicity in the second patient" and stated that "their subsequent response to the crisis was exemplary."[126]

Besides vindicating the physicians and NIH process, the detailed report of the IOM investigation puts the patients' deaths in considerable context. First, the investigators note that serious adverse events on phase 1 trials are very rare, citing a prisoner study where a "clinically significant medical event occurred once every 26.3 years of individual subject exposure. In 805 protocols involving 29,162 prisoner subjects over 614,534 days, there were 58 adverse drug reactions, of which none produced death or permanent disability. The only subject who died did so while receiving a placebo." Another cited study concluded "that the risk of either disability (temporary or permanent) or of fatality was substantially less than the risk of similar unfortunate outcomes in similar medical settings involving no research."[127]

In this case, the deaths were subsequently found to be due to a novel mechanism, through interference in mitochondrial DNA by the drug, with no toxicities having been seen in the animal testing phases. "It can be anticipated that novel drug toxicity appearing for the first time in humans and not predicted by animal models will occur again in the future because it is an inherent risk of all new drug development programs. An appropriate response to such an event is to learn the mechanism of the toxicity and devise new predictive models."[128]

The IOM concludes with an interesting observation on the dangerous consequences of assuming that all calamities are preventable and the result of carelessness or greed. The blame game "has the effect of reinforcing the erroneous public perception that new treatments can be developed and tested free of risks."[129] And this jeopardizes the future of clinical research itself—as scientists note that the scapegoating jeopardizes their reputations, careers, and livelihoods, prompting many to choose safer and more financially rewarding career paths. This is a huge societal loss.

Recounting the toll of these deaths from an accused investigator's perspective, Stephen Straus reaffirms the committee's concerns. I found his essay both enlightening and poignant and would highly recommend it to any budding researcher.

Straus reviews the motivations that draw physicians to research, tellingly noting, "We conduct clinical research for the same reasons that subjects participate in them: we are inveterate optimists." After recounting the background that led to the trial, the deaths, the soul-searching, and the investigations, Straus turns to the personal and professional toll. He notes that hepatitis drug development stopped during the 2 years of the investigation. Several prominent careers nearly ended. He also comments that had he done the trials alone or been less obsessive in his recordkeeping, the outcome for him would likely have been worse. While he still conducted clinical research, he never again undertook a phase 1 study. Despite all, he continued his research and mentoring, delivering a moving lecture on the topic of unanticipated risk and his own experiences on November 13, 2006.[130] Dr. Straus died of brain cancer 6 months later.

Who's Minding the Store? A Case Study

Numerous and sometimes apparently conflicting factors must be carefully weighed in considering the ethical issues of a given patient's participation in a trial, compounded by the varying interests, motives, and perspectives of the parties involved. The following unfortunate case study illustrates what some of the ethical issues are and what can go wrong.

Mrs. G. died a few months ago. She was diagnosed with cancer about 15 months before, after a delayed evaluation by her primary care doctor. Waiting for tests to look for metastases caused more delays, then a series of scheduling problems at Big U and a misadventure with anesthesia both delayed surgery that was intended to be curative. It seemed as though almost everything that could go wrong did, except that Mrs. G. and her family met some overall pleasant and competent doctors and nurses. Finally, Mrs. G. underwent the major surgery, a lung resection, which was painful but otherwise uncomplicated, with the belief that this would eradicate her cancer. A short time later, on a routine follow-up visit, she was found to have metastatic disease that had not been recognized preoperatively. (Things like this are not always apparent at the time, in fact, but appear obvious with 20-20 hindsight.) Mrs. G. then received an attempt at chemotherapy with a relatively nontoxic drug, which failed. At the same time, she was randomized to participate in an oncology trial that compared chemo with special supportive hospice care to chemo alone. Fortunately, she received extra support from the trial program, which enormously improved her spirits and her quality of life. She thrived on the extra TLC and very much appreciated the added attention from the support staff that came to visit her.

When the first chemo failed, Mrs. G. surprisingly wanted to try an experimental chemotherapeutic agent, though she was blessedly asymptomatic from the cancer. She didn't fit into any trial in her community but was able to receive the experimental medicine on a "compassionate use" basis through a treatment IND. This provision for access to investigational new drugs is occasionally made for patients with serious or life-threatening diseases who don't fit precise protocol requirements but might benefit from the investigational medicine. When a patient receives medication as a compassionate use indication, there are, nonetheless, informed consent, clinical evaluation, and FDA reporting requirements—similar to those expected for a full-fledged trial.

On this investigational chemotherapy, Mrs. G. developed severe vomiting and diarrhea and general malaise.

The Ethical Issues and Dilemmas

The oncologist investigator, the PI of the chemo trial, initially did not order much lab work. When he did, the results showed that Mrs. G. was profoundly dehydrated and was going into renal failure. So, one might ask the following questions about this case:

- What does hospice and comfort care encompass? Where does an investigational chemotherapy component fit with the philosophy of hospice?
- If a hospice patient is receiving an experimental medication, how much lab monitoring should be done, since blood draws hurt, to watch for potential toxicities from the investigational med? Should the monitoring requirements be different for patients with an end-stage illness?
- How might or should the monitoring requirements have been modified when the patient developed an adverse event—in this case, severe diarrhea?
- What would have been an appropriate response to the seriously abnormal lab test results, when they were found?

In fact, the PI doctor's response to Mrs. G.'s abnormal lab results was essentially to do nothing. She was given a small and inadequate amount of IV fluids, which were then stopped with the rationale that she was a hospice patient and therefore was to receive only supportive care. The doctor felt the IV replacement therapy was too aggressive. So then,

- Why offer chemotherapy to a patient in hospice if you are not otherwise going to provide supportive care?
- If the patient suffers a complication from the chemotherapy, is there not an obligation to attempt to remedy that complication, at least by simple measures?
- Who should make the assessments and therapeutic decisions? How much weight should be given to those of the nurse, who is making the daily patient evaluations and is extremely familiar with the patient, versus

those of the physician who is the "Principal Investigator," responsible for the trial but in this case not involved on a day-to-day basis?

Mrs. G.'s family discussed these issues with her nurses and physicians. The hospice doctor was kind, but he refused to treat the dehydration as he felt IV fluids were not an appropriate part of hospice care, which should be limited to comfort care—yet this patient was on an investigational chemotherapeutic drug. On the other hand, this doctor later gave Mrs. G. frivolous and worthless antibiotics, which not only represented "futile care" but caused unpleasant side effects. (I say "worthless" because the antibiotics were not necessary, in that they could not change the outcome of her illness.)

The PI of chemo was not terribly responsive to the family's attempts to communicate and to understand either the cause of Mrs. G.'s deterioration or whether any simple measures might be helpful. When asked about the dehydration and renal failure, he told them that there was no requirement on this protocol for any lab monitoring. I found this astonishing.

- Is it appropriate to use antibiotics for patients with no outlook for recovery when this use contributes to the enormous problem of emerging antibiotic resistance (aka "superbugs") that threatens the entire community? Does it make sense to give these drugs when they often cause unpleasant side effects?

- Requirement or not, is there not an ethical or moral obligation to follow up on side effects, or adverse events, especially when they are clearly related to the investigational medicine?

The other astonishing comment was the circuitous argument from the PI that he had not reported renal failure as an adverse event because it had not been previously reported in the Investigator's Brochure as an adverse event. With that line of reasoning, we would never discover anything!

The suggestion was made to the involved physicians that they reassess their approach (which is by no means unique) to treating oncology patients in clinical trials. "No code" should not mean "no treatment" for readily treatable problems or symptoms. Conversely, it seems barbaric to continue to treat many patients, for whom "comfort measures" are a more appropriate and humane response. Perhaps the patients should be more explicitly involved in addressing these issues. When I discuss treatment options with my own patients I try to be mindful of the *House of God* adage, "They can always hurt you more."[131]

Next, Mrs. G.'s family weighed their options as to whom to call—not to be vindictive but rather to use this situation as an educational forum in the old tradition of candid M and M, or morbidity and mortality, conferences. Should they call the local IRB? The pharmaceutical company? Perhaps the watchdogs at the FDA? Since the family's intent was to see that such events didn't happen to someone else, rather than to be downright malevolent, they concluded that they would try addressing the issue with the drug company sponsor and asked me to do so on their behalf.

After numerous calls trying to sort out the players, I was able to speak with a physician at the sponsor company, "Maker of False Hopes, Mfg." The medical monitor was reasonably polite and told me that there was in fact no requirement on the protocol for any lab work to be done. And this protocol had been designed with the guidance and approval of the FDA! I asked for a copy of the informed consent form, which was refused. The head doctor did say that the drug company had added a statement to the consent form stipulating that patients should report diarrhea to their doctors, putting all the onus on the patient. I requested that the sponsor send a note to investigators suggesting that they check for renal failure or electrolyte abnormalities in patients with severe diarrhea, but the head doctor declined to do so, saying these observations were at the discretion of the individual investigator.

As a clinical investigator myself, the most astonishing thing I was told was that there was no requirement in this protocol for the investigator to report adverse events, except SAEs, as the sponsor was collecting these data on its other, "real" (therapeutic investigational, rather than compassionate use) trials. So here we had a patient who developed renal failure, a previously unreported symptom, not reported now because there is no regulatory requirement to do so and because the PI had not seen the symptom previously reported. This makes no sense to me. And the patient, who had now suffered miserable toxicities that ruined her quality of life, died. Mrs. G.'s death also was not reported as an SAE because it was attributed to her cancer and not to possible acute renal failure from the experimental drug. The FDA, charged with patient and drug safety, allowed a protocol to go forward with no lab monitoring requirements and no reporting requirements except SAEs—and death of a hospice patient is not considered an SAE.

Going back a step in our discussion, one might have asked how and why this patient's symptoms progressed to the point of acute renal failure. When Mrs. G. developed recurrent vomiting and diarrhea as well as progressive weakness, I would have expected the PI to have ordered basic lab tests drawn—electrolytes, BUN, and creatinine at a *minimum*—to assess the cause and severity of the new symptoms. At which level—the PI, the local IRB, the drug company, or the FDA—were the "system errors," as they are euphemistically called, occurring? Where was the accountability and responsibility?

Many patients, those with cancer in particular, are aggressively lobbying the pharmaceutical companies and the FDA to fast-track drugs to make them available for patients with few other options. Should patients in such circumstances be allowed to try anything and to grasp at straws, or should there be a restraining influence somewhere along the line? Many patients are willing to assume any risk. Who ensures that appropriate safeguards are in place?

This is but one case—one sad example—of the many ethical issues that arise in a patient's care. The care Mrs. G. received was disappointing, as it did not meet my expectation for the minimal standard of care on any of my own patients. If a patient is participating in my clinical trials, I look for potential complications of the investigational medication even more keenly than I do with nonstudy medicines. In this case, I probably would have ordered a serum lipase and liver enzyme tests, too, to look for toxicity that might have caused Mrs. G.'s nausea and vomiting.

I want to reiterate that I am happy that Mrs. G. had the opportunity to participate in a trial because that is what she wanted to do. (Despite my reservations, I stayed out of this decision and told her that it was for her to weigh the risks and benefits for herself.) However, I am unhappy with the lack of oversight and responsibility shown by her doctors and the drug's sponsor. Our first obligation must be to keep in mind the maxim "First, do no harm."

Conclusion

As you can see, one must consider many complex ethical issues in designing and conducting clinical trials. While this chapter has offered questions for the investigator to consider and some approaches by which to counter some of the potential problems that you are likely to face, many of these dilemmas are not readily resolved. The debates over the balance between the demands of distributive justice and protections for vulnerable populations are particularly timely. This issue was illustrated by the examples of HIV treatments for pregnant women and foster children. The case of Mrs. G. illustrates ethical questions that almost any physician is likely to encounter on a regular basis. In addition to the Belmont principles, increasing attention has been focused on other requirements for ethical research: that a collaborative partnership be developed with the community being studied, that subject selection be fair, and that the study have social value and scientific validity.[132] The next chapter will place these day-to-day concerns in a broader context and supplement that with an overview of related societal and political issues.

CHAPTER 9

Society and Politics

> Ethical axioms are found and tested
> not very differently from the axioms of science.
> Truth is what stands the test of experience.
>
> —ALBERT EINSTEIN

There is no question that research is political. From which questions are asked, to setting the research agenda, to allocating and distributing grant monies, decisions are based on the social context and political climate of the times. A number of specific social and political issues impact the direction of research, the specific topics studied, and the populations included. These include gender and racial disparities as well as the growing influence of religion on research. The following sections provide an overview of the evolution of thought and of the arguments regarding these more nuanced topics, which remain unresolved. Examples are provided to illustrate the difficulties in each of these areas and to pique your interest in reading more. These subjects are provocative and contentious. At the same time, they provide a different and important perspective for your consideration as you enter the field of clinical research. I hope you will find this area as interesting and challenging as I do.

Politics of Research: The FDA

Before we delve into the discussion of some specific problems affecting research ethics, it is important to put this in the context of the politicization of the FDA, under the recent Bush administration in particular, which led to the characterization of the "broken FDA."

During that period access to healthcare information, health services, and medical research became limited by two growing trends: the infusion of increasingly restrictive religious doctrines and the implementation of ideology-driven—rather than scientific, evidence-based—public policies. Initially, access to science-based information was limited through censorship and even distortion in government sources (e.g., data regarding the efficacy of condoms in preventing HIV infections and STDs were removed from the CDC's Web site).[1, 2]

Ideologic shifts were also demonstrated by resource allocations. For example, HIV prevention programs at the CDC were reduced by $4 million while funding for abstinence-only programs rose from $20 million to $167 million, despite the lack of evidence of effectiveness, in contrast to the previous peer-review, scientific-merit-based process of NIH grant funding.[3, 4, 5, 6, 7, 8, 9]

The trend away from evidence-based medicine affects healthcare practitioners in numerous areas, ranging from patient education and disturbingly eroding standards of medical care to selection of research topics, grant writing, and the research funding process. Upon her dismissal from the President's Council on Bioethics in 2004 for disagreeing with the administration's stance on stem cell research, Dr. Elizabeth Blackburn, a prominent cancer researcher and one of only three full-time biomedical researchers on the council, wrote, "When prominent scientists must fear that descriptions of their research will be misrepresented and misused by their government to advance political ends, something is deeply wrong."[10] Among her many honors, incidentally, is the 2009 Nobel Prize in Medicine though she was no longer good enough for Bush's council.

Numerous other examples of the politicization of science exist, but for now, we'll focus on the FDA and the impact on drug development and approval.

The FDA has been a rather political entity since 1988, when appointment of the commissioner was changed to require Senate confirmation. There has been ongoing criticism of the FDA, though never to the extent of the past few years. Part of the concern is apparently related to instability at the FDA, given the frequent turnover in commissioners. Ironically, this situation has worsened since the 1988 Food and Drug Administration Act, with the position of FDA commissioner going vacant for an average of 2.5 months before to 17 months since and the resultant problems at the agency from lack of leadership.[11]

A brief history of the FDA commissioners and other key persons over the past 20 years illustrates politics at work in the FDA.

David Kessler (commissioner, 1990–1997) took a great deal of heat for trying to have the FDA regulate tobacco products and for trying to gain approval for RU-486 (mifepristone). (He lost on both counts.) He was also notable for being appointed by President George H. W. Bush and retained by President Clinton.

Jane Henney (commissioner, 1998–2001), also appointed by Clinton, authorized FDA approval of RU-486. She was, not surprisingly, ousted when George W. Bush took office. She also tried to change business as usual by filling positions with career appointees rather than political ones, actively demonstrating her goal of "leading policy and making enforcement decisions based on science, not on political whims."[12]

An infamous nominee for chairing the FDA advisory panel on women's health policy was Dr. W. David Hager, an obstetrician-gynecologist. He had helped prepare a "citizens' petition" calling for the FDA to reverse its approval of RU-486. He was perhaps more widely known for his reported refusal to prescribe contraceptives to married women and as author of a book that "recommends specific Scripture readings and prayers for such ailments as headaches and premenstrual syndrome."[13] After the outcry of critics, he was not appointed chair of the advisory panel but did serve on it in 2002–2005, despite bipartisan opposition.[14]

Mark McClellan (commissioner, 2002–2004) was an economist appointed by George W. Bush. McClellan reportedly had decided against approving Plan B for emergency contraception even before his staff completed its analysis.

Lester Crawford (commissioner, July–September 2005) was a veterinarian also appointed by George W. Bush. His term is perhaps best remembered for three features: the audacity of a vet making decisions about women's health and reproduction, his vehement opposition to Plan B's approval, and the criminal charges against him for false reporting about holdings relevant to his appointment (that he and his wife owned stocks in food, beverage, and medical device companies that he was in charge of regulating).[15] No conflicts of interest there! He got off with probation and a fine.

Another casualty of Crawford's brief and divisive tenure at the FDA was Susan F. Wood, who resigned as assistant FDA commissioner for women's health and director of the Office of Women's Health because of the politicization of the agency—specifically, having the approval of Plan B emergency contraception denied, despite scientific evidence of the pill's safety and recommendations from the FDA's own advisory committee.[16]

Andrew C. von Eschenbach (commissioner, 2005–2009) had been the head of the National Cancer Institute before being appointed as FDA commissioner. At the FDA, he was criticized for not approving Provenge for prostate cancer, despite the recommendation of an advisory committee. He is also tied to the decision of the FDA to deny emergency contraceptives over-the-counter status, despite the recommendation of the FDA's advisory group and its own staff members, as well as that of many medical organizations.[17] The FDA had followed advisory committee recommendations in every other case in the past decade. He is also known for reportedly threatening FDA reviewers who disagreed with him. Von Eschenbach's ideologic, rather than evidence-based, decisions were so egregious that on March 23, 2009, the U.S. District Court (*Tummino v. Torti*) ordered the FDA to reconsider its decision blocking access to Plan B. It also ordered the FDA to act within 30 days to extend over-the-counter access to 17-year-olds. The court's conclusions about the FDA's behavior were neither subtle nor kind.[18]

The FDA's ability to function and its reputation have been seriously hurt in the past decade. In a 2006 survey of FDA scientists, about 18 percent responded that they had been asked to exclude or alter information or their report's conclusions for nonscientific reasons. A further 60 percent were aware of cases where industry "inappropriately induced or attempted to induce the reversal, withdrawal or modification of FDA determinations or actions." One-fifth (20 percent) said they had been "asked explicitly by FDA decision makers to provide incomplete, inaccurate or misleading information to the public, regulated industry, media, or elected/senior government officials."[19] Lest you think this survey was markedly biased, even Senator Chuck Grassley, a staunch Republican, commented on the survey report, "The responses of these scientists reinforce the findings of the independent Government Accountability Office, which said the process for reviewing drugs on the market is deeply flawed."[20]

As a result of the politicization, the FDA staff has reportedly become greatly demoralized, interfering with its ability to function and protect the public. FDA whistle-blowers have testified that the agency considers the drug companies its clients, and its decision making furthers the interests of those clients.

Many experienced and valuable clinicians have left the agency, leaving a void. Equally importantly, the FDA has lost considerable respect and authority in the eyes of both the public and important members of Congress.

A recent sign of change was the May 2009 appointment of two well-respected physicians to lead the FDA, Drs. Margaret Hamburg and Joshua Sharfstein. It's too early to tell what will happen under their tenure, but their appointments are encouraging.

From 2001 to 2009, the most obvious politicization at the FDA was related to women's health issues, and especially access to contraception.

Other notorious cases surround the safety of antidepressants for children and adolescents, the safety of COX-2 inhibitors like Vioxx, and the approval of the antibiotic Ketek.

For example, Dr. Andrew D. Mosholder, a senior epidemiologist and whistle-blower at the FDA, was prevented from reporting his findings that children given antidepressants other than Prozac were almost twice as likely to attempt suicide as were those given placebos. His findings were subsequently confirmed by other studies. British health authorities had long before reached the same conclusion and recommended banning all but Prozac for children.[21]

Similarly, Dr. David Graham testified to Congress that his efforts to publish warnings about Vioxx were delayed and that he was subjected to retaliation.[22] Subsequent studies have confirmed the increased cardiovascular risk, and Merck removed Vioxx from the market in 2004. (While I agree with much of Dr. Graham's and others' concerns about COX-2 inhibitors, I feel that a black-box warning to consumers would have been a more appropriate response than having it removed from the market, as it was a uniquely effective drug for many individuals.)

In his withering testimony about the FDA, Graham observes:

> *The organizational structure within CDER is entirely geared toward the review and approval of new drugs. When a CDER new drug reviewing division approves a new drug, it is also saying the drug is "safe and effective." When a serious safety issue arises postmarketing, their immediate reaction is almost always one of denial, rejection and heat. They approved the drug so there can't possibly be anything wrong with it. The same group that approved the drug is also responsible for taking regulatory action against it postmarketing. This is an inherent conflict of interest . . .*

> *The corporate culture within CDER is also a barrier to effectively protecting the American people from unnecessary harm due to prescription and OTC drugs. The culture is dominated by a world-view that believes only randomized clinical trials provide useful and actionable information and that postmarketing safety is an afterthought. This culture also views the pharmaceutical industry it is supposed to regulate as its client, over-values the benefits of the drugs it approves and seriously under-values, disregards and disrespects drug safety.*

The other inherent conflict of interest between the FDA and the pharmaceutical industry is that user fees from the industry account for a large proportion of the FDA's budget (42 percent in 2006).[23] These fees are linked to drug approval and intended to expedite the process. The industry doesn't just hand the money to the FDA—it has very detailed input into how the money is spent—the equivalent, according to one critic, of "putting the fox in the chicken coop."[24]

Finally, the case of Ketek is an illustrative example of why the FDA has lost credibility and respect and what needs to be done to regain both.

In addition to the findings of investigator fraud and fraudulent data having been knowingly submitted by the sponsor, Sanofi-Aventis, to the FDA, Ketek's approval stirred up a hornet's nest of criticism about the FDA and a congressional investigation led by Senator Grassley and Representatives Waxman, Dingell, and Stupak. Dr. Ross, FDA reviewer for Ketek, testified that he had been pressured to soften his findings about liver toxicity due to the drug and threatened by FDA Commissioner von Eschenbach, who said, "If you don't follow the team, if you don't do what you're supposed to do, the first time you'll be spoken to, the second time you'll be benched, and the third time, you'll be traded," according to Ross.

In this protracted battle, questions were raised by Congress regarding the truthfulness of von Eschenbach's testimony and whether he deliberately misled the Subcommittee on Oversight and Investigations.[25] The FDA refused congressional requests for documents related to its approval of the drug, prompting the committee to threaten to hold Secretary of Health Michael Leavitt in contempt.[26] Subsequently, Leavitt agreed to allow the documents to be reviewed, and high drama was avoided.

But the saga continues, with other ongoing investigations and a multitude of reports, seasoned with revelations of occasional scandals. The most recent of these was the FDA's approval of an unsafe knee device, Menaflex, after the agency received "'extreme,' 'unusual' and persistent pressure from four Democratic legislators from New Jersey." What's different? The FDA did some soul-searching about its procedures and admitted that its decision for approval was inappropriately influenced by politics. The FDA even asked for an Institute of Medicine review of its faulty approval process. Perhaps there is hope.[27]

One other historical case of note regarding politics and research is that of the fatalities on the fialuridine (FIAU) hepatitis trial. Not surprisingly, the deaths resulted in a major public outcry, some political grandstanding, and sensational headlines rather than careful investigative journalism. For example, one article was titled "And Then the Patients Suddenly Started Dying: How NIH Missed Warning Signs in Drug Test."[28] Not emphasized was that it can be quite difficult to attribute causality of abnormal liver tests, as can be seen with hepatitis itself or the underlying diseases of the trial participants, which included not only hepatitis B and alcoholism but also HIV with advanced AIDS and concomitant antiretroviral therapy in some. In addition, interfering criticism came from Congress, especially Representative Edolphus Towns.[29] The FDA and NIH began pointing fingers at each other. The FDA, although reportedly closely involved with the trial from the outset, severely (and publicly) criticized the investigators for breaching research regulations, and all received official reprimands via warning letters. The FDA also criticized the inadequacies in consent, errors of judgment, and numerous "protocol violations."[30] The NIH did another investigation, vindicating its staff and thereby raising suspicion of a whitewash. At one point, Dr. Straus contacted the Office of the General Counsel at the NIH and learned that it would not represent the investigators, leaving them to face staggering legal bills.[31]

The IOM was eventually called to referee between the factions. The IOM strongly disagreed with the FDA's "call for worst-case analyses; i.e. assuming that all adverse health events in trial patients, and more importantly in former trial patients, are drug-related." Their bottom-line conclusion was that there was no way these toxicities could have been predicted from animal testing or other screening, particularly in patients with underlying liver disease—that this toxicity was not previously known.[32]

Ultimately, the IOM report, which examined not only this trial but two others with related drugs, exonerated the investigators and also praised them for their attentiveness to their volunteers. The report expressed concern that the "FDA compliance audit was not as informed or balanced as it should have been" and that the official reprimands were made public even before the investigators received their letters. The IOM did have some recommendations for improving the safety of volunteers, including real-time reporting; requirements for training researchers on regulatory and ethical obligations as well as the conduct and design of trials; no-fault compensation for research injury by government, sponsor, or a combination of both; and development of a database from previous IND control groups "to custom match patients in new drug trials with controls from previous trials, matching not only for entry criteria but also for disease extent and severity, concomitant medications and other confounding variables."[33] Disappointingly, many of the IOM recommendations have not yet been adopted, 15 years after they were made.

Politics of Research: Women

Over several decades, a hard-won shift has been achieved in our society's perception of women's health issues and of women's roles in research participation. This change in perception occurred in the broader context of battles and resentment over other gender issues such as pay inequities and abortion rights. For example, it used to be commonly thought that preventing women from participating in research trials protected them. Since the 1960s, this perception has changed and such restrictions are now viewed by many as paternalistic and discriminatory. This shift in perspective was also fueled by a major shift in demographics, which occurred as the baby boom generation reached midlife. Women of this generation were more highly educated and independent than their predecessors. Feminism and the publication of the Boston Women's Health Collective's *Our Bodies, Our Selves* in 1970 further fueled their awareness. As they matured, these women focused their energies on issues that were relevant to their own health, including menopause, breast cancer, and osteoporosis. Their approach to problem solving has been modeled after the successes of AIDS activists and has led to viewing these women's issues in an openly political and societal context, rather than as isolated medical concerns.[34]

One shift in perspective was from viewing institutional restrictions on research participation as protective to viewing them as paternalistic; another shift was from viewing the restrictions as protecting women to viewing them as denying women access to care.

The Belmont principle of justice, which has usually been applied to classes of subjects being exposed to disproportionately greater harm than benefit from trials or being coerced into participation, is now being applied to gender issues. In terms of research, distributive justice is consequently being viewed from the perspective of groups of people being denied access to potential therapies rather than from the historical perspective of groups being subjected to disproportionate risks.

As the FDA notes, women have long been neglected in clinical trials.[35] According to the U.S. Public Health Service Task Force on Women's Health Issues, this "historical lack of research focus on women's health concerns has compromised the quality of health information available to women as well as the healthcare they receive."[36] For example, research in cardiovascular health for women lags decades behind that for men. This oversight occurred even though coronary heart disease is the most frequent cause of death in women and other heart problems account for 2.5 million hospitalizations of women annually as well as 500,000 deaths.[37] Women have been excluded from the major trials on cardiovascular disease, such as the Multiple Risk Factor Intervention Trial (MRFIT) and the Physicians' Health Study. In part, this exclusion was protectionist in origin; in part, it was a result of not wanting to make the studies more difficult to evaluate by having the variables of women's hormonal cycles to take into account. As a result, the role of estrogen in preventing heart disease in women is only now being clarified, decades after the large male trials were completed.[38] Why did this happen?

Most of this oversight was not malicious in intent; rather, much of it was simply cultural in origin. According to an Institute of Medicine report, two types of gender-based assumptions have shaped research agendas and policies. The first is "male bias," or observer bias from the adoption of male perspectives. The second is "male norm," the tendency to view the male experience as the standard or norm for a situation, with female differences being portrayed as "deviant."[39] In the heart studies, the basis of male bias was that the studies were almost exclusively designed and funded by men. The male norm emerged because the investigators did not consider that coronary artery disease affected women at all or that it might affect women differently than it affected men. Thus, trials in women were not planned.

Until recently, medications have been tested almost exclusively in men. This is quite problematic in that gender differences have been found in the effects of some agents, such as certain antidepressants and antiarrhythmics. For example, women are more susceptible to QT prolongation and life-threatening Toursades de pointes arrhythmia than are men. This is notable because a number of antibiotics and other medications may cause this critical arrhythmia as a side effect. Women also may require dosage adjustments, given their typically smaller size than men as well as differences in metabolism.[40] More researchers are recognizing that men and women represent different populations with perhaps unique needs; men and women do react differently to medications and are not interchangeable.

Other consequences of the information deficit regarding women are equally well documented. This deficit affects the availability of diagnostic procedures and effective treatments as well as women's morbidity and mortality. For example, deaths from ischemic heart disease have been declining at a much slower rate for women than for men. Women tend to be diagnosed with heart disease later than men are and are less likely to receive invasive diagnostic procedures. When they do undergo these procedures, including either CABG (coronary artery bypass graft surgery) or angioplasty, they show a higher perioperative mortality rate. These gender differences in mortality are not unique to heart disease. The same pattern has been seen with AIDS, with which women also have a much lower survival rate than do men.[41]

In addition to the scientific shortcoming of assuming but not testing the hypothesis that different populations are alike, some might argue that the systematic exclusion of women from clinical trials is a violation of the third Belmont principle, that of distributive justice and the equitable apportionment of risks and benefits. Women have also borne a disproportionate share of the risks and burden in practice areas such as reproduction because they were the subjects of the bulk of the research on contraceptives and infertility. Women of color bear an even greater proportion of the research risks as many contraceptive studies were done on lower-income minority women, often overseas. (For further discussion, please see "Politics of Research: Race" later in this chapter.) For example, some contraceptive studies were conducted on poor Puerto Rican women rather than on wealthier Caucasian women. The argument for doing this was that Puerto Rico was undergoing a population explosion and therefore had a greater need for effective and affordable contraception for impoverished women. Others view these and similar trials on women of color as eugenics.[42] Applying the principle of distributive justice, this imbalance in research on contraceptives might be considered unjust.[43] Some might argue that women are the primary beneficiaries of research on contraceptives as they bear the burdens of pregnancy and child rearing; others, that they bore all the risks of interventions, which should have been shared by men (or, in the case of birth control pills, by women of greater wealth).

Although the stated intent of excluding women from research trials was to protect them from research risks, this particular view overlooked the possibility that medications might act differently in women given their inherent hormonal differences as well as their monthly cyclical changes in hormone levels.[44] While such protectionism may have been well intended, the result has been an inferior level of care for women. Some have concluded that "researchers must also be careful not to overprotect vulnerable populations so that they are excluded from research in which they wish to participate, particularly where the research involves therapies for conditions with no available treatments."[45] For example, although the rate of AIDS infection rises more rapidly in women than in men and is a leading cause of death of women, attention was not focused on AIDS in women until 1994. Prior to that time, AIDS was considered to be almost exclusively a disease affecting gay men. Delays in diagnosing AIDS in women have contributed to women's lower survival rate compared with men's for this disease, too. Even since AIDS has been recognized as a serious threat to women, research has focused primarily on women's transmission of AIDS to babies rather than women as AIDS victims and sufferers in their own right. This blindness has led to the denial of treatment options available to men and to lags in basic research regarding differences between men and women in AIDS transmission and infection.[46]

History of the Oversight Governing Women's Participation in Research

As noted earlier, the justification for the restrictions on women's participation in clinical trials was a misguided effort to protect women, arising initially out of the Nuremberg Code of Ethics (1949), which was intended to provide protections for research subjects. This code specified that experiments should yield results for the "good of society, unprocurable by other . . . means of study, and not random and unnecessary."[47] In most nonreproductive issues, it was presumably thought that the findings of studies with men could be extrapolated to women. Subsequently, the postmarketing disasters of thalidomide leading to profound birth defects (absence of limbs) and diethylstilbestrol (DES) leading to a rare vaginal cancer further led to women and fetuses being viewed as "vulnerable" populations.[48] In 1977, an FDA recommendation barred women of childbearing potential from participating in phase 1 trials. But in 1985, the U.S. Public Health Service Task Force on Women's Health Issues finally concluded that healthcare for women had been compromised by the lack of research on women's health issues. As a result, the NIH developed a new policy that encouraged the inclusion of women as research participants and suggested that analysis of data should include the examination of differences by sex. At the request of Representative Pat Schroeder and Senators Olympia Snowe and Henry Waxman, the Society for Women's Health Research was founded in 1990. It asked the U.S. General Accounting Office (GAO) to examine whether the NIH was following its own guidelines to increase women's participation in clinical trials.[49]

In 1990, the GAO found that the NIH research and gender guidelines had not been regularly implemented. In fact, in 1991, the Department of Health and Human Services stated, "No pregnant woman may be involved as a subject in an activity . . . unless the purpose of the activity is to meet the health need of the mother and the fetus will be placed at risk only to the minimum extent necessary to reach such needs."[50]

To summarize, until recently the research attention that was directed toward women was largely limited to reproductive issues. Age-related hormonal influences at different stages of women's lives as well as health problems such as osteoporosis and heart disease have been given relatively scant attention.[51] To address these problems a new NIH office, the Office of Research on Women's Health (ORWH) was formed in 1993. The ORWH mandated inclusion of women and minorities in all human research. In 1997, the Food and Drug Administration Modernization Act (FDAMA) required the FDA, the NIH, and drug industry representatives to develop guidelines for the inclusion of women and minorities in clinical trials. Finally, in 1998, the FDA published the Investigational New Drug Application rule, which allows the FDA to refuse an NDA if the safety and efficacy data are not appropriately analyzed by sex.[52] The requirement to allow women to participate in trials was driven by the exclusion of women with life-threatening AIDS-related illnesses from clinical trials due to their being of "reproductive potential."[53]

In 2000, the General Accounting Office found that women were now appropriately included in trials but that data were still not being analyzed by sex—the required information was missing in 85 percent of Investigational New Drug protocols.[54] In 2001, the GAO noted that the FDA was still not consistently assessing research to determine whether or how sex differences affect drug safety and efficacy. The GAO also noted that one in three New Drug Applications still failed to provide sex-specific subgroup analyses.[55]

The 2001 Institute of Medicine report *Exploring the Biological Contributions to Human Health: Does Sex Matter?* made the following recommendations to further define differences attributable to gender:

- Researchers should disclose whether tissue cultures come from males or females.
- In clinical trials with women, researchers should try to note the stage of the menstrual cycle at each woman's study examination to try to determine hormonal effects on toxicity and efficacy.
- Journal editors should encourage data analysis by sex.[56]

Other barriers to women's participation in clinical trials have related to cultural and societal expectations. Recruitment and retention of women in trials have sometimes been more difficult than with men. Partly, this is related to differences in risk-taking behavior. Women are traditionally caregivers for others, both for their children and for elderly family members. Thus, they may be limited in their time and ability to participate in trials, and culturally they are likely to be reluctant to put their personal needs above the needs of others. While women are understandably often reluctant to miss time at work, of necessity saving sick time for when their children are ill, this makes trials with women more difficult to complete successfully; more participants are lost to follow-up or are unable to complete visits. Strategies to improve retention have focused on providing childcare and providing transportation (particularly in inclement weather and for the elderly). Efforts should be made to minimize the time commitment required; flexible appointment times are crucial for retaining women participants.[57]

While some arguments can be made for preferentially focusing on men in trials, there are several counterarguments against limiting women's participation. One is that women use far more health resources than do men, and studies should be based on patterns of healthcare use and types of illness. Another is that women participants have a higher protocol compliance rate than do men.[58]

The good news is that funding for women's health issues is slowly catching up, with the U.S. Congress approving $22 million in 2001 and $37 million in 2002 for the NIH's Office of Research on Women's Health out of a total $23 billion NIH allocation for 2002. Also, representation by males and females is now roughly equal in NIH-sponsored clinical trials.[59] With increased funding and attention to women's medical needs and societal constraints, more rapid progress should be made in reducing the gender information gap. It is important to remain vigilant, however, so that attention to women's needs does not suffer from political influence and again shift into the background.

A Sign of Progress for Women?

Recently, a hopeful example of progress appeared in research on endometriosis, a common and painful gynecologic problem. The incidence of endometriosis is 40–60 percent of women with dysmenorrhea (painful menstruation) and 20–30 percent in women with subfertility.[60]

Despite the fact that endometriosis is so common and disabling to women, little is known about the disease, and women are commonly symptomatically

Pregnancy Discrimination Act[61]

When is discrimination against women not considered discrimination? When the federal appeals court is involved. In a brilliantly circuitous line of reasoning, the majority Republican panel decided that the exclusion of contraceptives from Union Pacific's insurance plans was not discriminatory, as they also excluded condoms and vasectomies. However, the Democratic appointee to the court, Judge Kermit Bye, dissented, perceptively noting that there is an inequality in terms of the medical effect of the lack of coverage since "this failure only medically affects females, as they bear all of the health consequences of unplanned pregnancies."

According to the New York Times, the appellate court stated that "Union Pacific's health plans did not violate the Pregnancy Discrimination Act because contraception is not related to pregnancy." The court brilliantly concluded, "Contraception is a treatment that is only indicated prior to pregnancy . . . Contraception is not a medical treatment that occurs when or if a woman becomes pregnant; instead contraception prevents pregnancy from even occurring."

It is reassuring to know, however, that Rogaine and Viagra will still be covered as medically necessary drugs.

treated with painkillers or oral contraceptives (to suppress their periods) or subjected to hysterectomies. In NIH research funding in 2008, endometriosis ranked 180th, with a $15 million allocation.

A new Center for Gynepathology Research at the Massachusetts Institute of Technology was announced in December 2009, with $10 million in public and private funding, headed by MacArthur genius and biological engineering professor Linda Griffith. Affected by endometriosis herself since age 12 but not correctly diagnosed until age 28, Griffith has undergone nine surgeries (including a hysterectomy) yet still experiences recurrent pain.[62]

Tellingly, "Griffith decided she had to do something to investigate the ailment only when her niece started to have the same debilitating pain and failed to get diagnosed promptly. Griffith wrote detailed letters to her niece's doctor, explaining her disease and its similarities to her niece's symptoms. But the doctor had the same response Griffith's own physicians had when she was a teenager: It was just stress."[63] I find this curious and somewhat sad for a number of reasons. It is a reminder that women's symptoms are all too often dismissed as "just stress" or craziness and that there is still far too much shyness in speaking out about "woman trouble." I am very excited about the coalition Griffith is putting together to research this important problem with the belated attention it deserves.

Politics of Research: Religion

In 1999, 18 percent of community hospital beds in the United States had religious sponsors, of which almost 70 percent were Catholic: religious institutions provided the inpatient care for more than 5.3 million people. Furthermore, 48 (or 8 percent) of these religiously sponsored hospitals are the sole providers of hospital care in their regions.[64] Catholic facilities now account for more than 20 percent of admissions in 21 states and the District of Columbia.[65] Across the country, over the past decade, Catholic health systems have been merging with secular hospitals. In 1998 alone, there were 43 such acquisitions or mergers; 159 occurred over the decade. In many cases, the Catholic health system becomes the sole provider of care in an entire county or region.[66]

Many religious hospitals use their religion's doctrine in determining what services they will or will not provide. Some Baptist and all Adventist and Catholic healthcare institutions do so.[67]

Catholic affiliated healthcare institutions agree to abide by the rules of the United States Conference of Catholic Bishops known as the Ethical and Religious Directives (ERDs).[68] These ERDs include

- Number 4: "A Catholic healthcare institution, especially a teaching hospital, will promote medical research consistent with its mission of providing healthcare . . . Such medical research must adhere to Catholic moral principles."
- Number 28: "Each person or the person's surrogate should have access to medical and moral information and counseling so as to be able to form his or her conscience. The free and informed healthcare decision of the person or the person's surrogate is to be followed so long as it does not contradict Catholic principles."
- Number 52, perhaps the best known: "Catholic health institutions may not promote or condone contraceptive practices . . ."[69]

While no one questions that Catholic (and other religiously affiliated) hospitals do good work, the limitations that sometimes result from the institutionally promulgated religious and ethical policies do have a significant impact on access to medical treatment that is often not acknowledged or given appropriate consideration. This impact extends well beyond the Catholic stance on abortion, which is well known, to other, less obvious issues. Religious restrictions affect access to new technologies, end-of-life care choices, vaccination, risk reduction counseling, and even access to scientific information, as well as reproductive healthcare.

These religious directives have a particular impact on rural communities where the Catholic system is the only source of healthcare. Depending on the nature of the medical problem, the weather and road conditions, and the state of public transportation, it is often not practical or feasible for a patient to seek healthcare elsewhere.

Several less well-publicized threats to research arising from religious beliefs are of growing concern. The first is that of religious restrictions imposed on women's research trial participation, inhibiting women's access to medical advances. For example, a requirement of essentially all research on women of childbearing potential is that the women be using "adequate" contraceptives. Thus, because women may not be counseled on or provided with effective contraceptives at Catholic institutions, they may be excluded from participating in some clinical trials.[70] Currently acceptable phrasing for informed consent forms at many Catholic hospitals states that a woman may be advised that she should not become pregnant while participating on a clinical trial. However, language specifying the type of contraceptive that a patient should use is not allowed. (Samples of acceptable and unacceptable wording are presented in the "Pregnancy and Contraceptive Clauses" at http://conductingclinicalresearch.com.) Because of safety and liability concerns, many trial sponsors will not accept abstinence as an adequate contraceptive method, precluding participation by patients who do not use specified contraceptives.

This impasse results in a blanket limitation on women's access to healthcare in some religious institutions. It might be interpreted as violating the Belmont principles of autonomy and justice, as well as beneficence if the trial is a therapeutic trial. In these cases, the Belmont principles are overridden when one group's religious beliefs are imposed on others, typically without public knowledge, debate, or assent.

The second area of public concern regards access to advances in medical therapy that rely on embryonic stem cells or any other fetal tissue. The ERDs prohibit any use of fetal cells. A variety of therapies are being developed that rely on the use of fetal tissue or stem cells. For example, one treatment under study is for macular degeneration, a leading cause of blindness in the elderly. Another uses fetal tissue to treat Parkinson's disease. Yet another treats diabetes. Each of these will be unavailable in those growing communities where all healthcare comes under religious restrictions. While these issues are not well known, nor often publicized, they are worth noting before you select a site in which to practice and conduct clinical trials.

The third area of conflict between religion, research, and drug development regards vaccine development. Many vaccines have been developed using tissue from fetuses that would otherwise have been discarded. Cells have been continually propagated and used to grow the weakened viruses that are then used for the vaccines. The two most commonly prescribed vaccines were developed on cell lines from the 1960s that have been perpetuated since then. Some pro-life groups, like the Children of G-d, have advocated that children not be immunized with vaccines grown from fetal tissue. A few have gone further, attempting to buy enough stock options in specific pharmaceutical companies to push through a shareholder resolution to block the manufacture of vaccines. So far, they have been unsuccessful.

An attempt has also been made to block further research at Georgetown University—which is a Catholic school—that relies on cultures of fetal tissue. It was deemed not feasible to stop the research because so many ongoing research programs rely on these cell lines. The National Catholic Bioethics Center further rationalizes the research by noting that as the abortions providing the original cells occurred many years ago, it would be more harmful to stop use of these vaccines and cell lines than to continue to benefit from them: "The connection to the abortion was distant and remote enough to say that this in no way encouraged or facilitated further abortions. The good was a proportionally strong enough argument to say, 'Do this.'"[71] Another opinion proposes that it is immoral for parents to deprive their children of vaccinations and that the use of the vaccines does not constitute immoral material cooperation.[72] As an infectious disease physician, I am relieved that the vaccinations will occur; it seems unethical to me to allow children to die from readily preventable infections unless it is their personal choice.

Another concern I have again arises from my experience as an infectious disease physician over too-numerous-to-count years. As clinicians know, feeding tubes, Foley catheters, and similar interventions inevitably lead to increasingly resistant infections in patients. Religiously mandated continuation of treatment may lead to inappropriate and excessive use of antibiotics, resulting in the creation and spread of multiresistant organisms, of particular concern at a time when fewer antibiotics are in the research pipeline and more and more patients are immunocompromised.

In March 2004, Pope John Paul II stated that it is "morally obligatory" to continue use of artificial nutrition and hydration in patients in a persistent vegetative state. In November 2009, the Catholic Bishops revised the Ethical and Religious Directives to formally state, "As a general rule, there is an obligation to provide patients with food and water, including medically assisted nutrition and hydration for those who cannot take food orally. This obligation extends to patients in chronic conditions (e.g., the 'persistent vegetative state') who can reasonably be expected to live indefinitely if given such care."[73] This could have a potentially grave public health impact by fueling the emergence and spread of resistant organisms.

Politics of Research: Race

Many disparities in access to care are based on racial, ethnic, and economic differences. Just as the realization has been growing that there are gender differences in response to therapies, recognition is now emerging that significant racial differences should also be examined.*[74] Because of these differences, in 1994 the NIH mandated that minorities, as well as women, be recruited as subjects for research. One review notes that approximately one-fourth of the U.S. population is made up of "people of color" and that by the year 2050, this proportion will double. However, only 5 percent of clinical trial participants are members of minority groups.[75] Another study found that the proportion of African American participants in trials conducted only in the United States declined from 12 percent to 6 percent between 1995 and 1999.[76] Hispanics were consistently underrepresented relative to their proportion in the population as a whole. Interestingly, this racial disparity in participation was not seen in anti-infective trials but was seen in oncology, pulmonary, and neuropharmacology studies. Subsequent drug labeling reflected racial differences in response to a number of cardiac and renal drugs but not to anti-infectives or chemotherapeutic agents.[77]

A longstanding history of racially related distrust exists among African Americans, in part a legacy of the Tuskegee experiments on black men with syphilis, if not dating back to slavery. A recent study examined the issue of trust and found that African Americans were more likely than Caucasians to believe their doctor would

- Not fully explain their participation in the research (41.7 versus 23.4 percent)
- Expose them to unnecessary risks (45.5 versus 34.8 percent)
- Ask them to participate in research the doctors thought might harm them (37.2 versus 19.7 percent)

---

* For example, in terms of intracellular metabolism of drugs by the cytochrome P450 enzyme, Caucasians are more likely to have abnormally low levels of this enzyme than are Asians. Similarly, African Americans are more likely to experience adverse events such as angioedema from ACE (angiotensin converting enzyme) inhibitors than are Caucasians and also do not respond equally well to beta-blockers, ACE inhibitors, and angiotensin II antagonists.

- Use them as guinea pigs without their consent (79.2 versus 51.9 percent)
- Give them treatment as part of an experiment without their permission (24.5 versus 8.3)
- Prescribe medication to experiment on people without those people's knowledge or consent (62.8 versus 18.4 percent)

The differences noted appeared to be on the basis of race; little confounding was seen as a result of economic status.[78] This mistrust has been recently fueled by adverse publicity regarding trials for treating HIV in children that included foster children. (See "Vulnerable Populations: Children" in chapter 8.) Some of the charges appear irresponsible and sensationalistic, fueled by the rapidity and ease with which rumors now circulate on the Internet. According to *New York Times* reporters Janny Scott and Leslie Kaufman, "All this is happening despite the fact that there is little evidence that the trials were anything but a medical success. Most of the questions have arisen from a single account of abuse allegations—given by a single writer about people not identified by real names, backed up with no official documentation as supporting proof, and put out on the Internet in early 2004 after the author was unable to get the story published anywhere else."[79]

A similar spate of rhetoric is spewing forth in Africa as a result of the adverse publicity surrounding a meningitis trial in Nigeria, which some have sensationally and irresponsibly called the "Nigerian Tuskegee experiment." This sensationalism is now resulting in resistance to polio vaccination and contributing to a resurgence of that disease. As Dr. Chidi Chike Achebe, a Harvard-trained Nigerian physician, perceptively explains, "Finally, it is evident that the vaccine boycott in Nigeria, ill-advised as it clearly was, was informed by a complex interplay of bad science; unclear political and religious agendas; a history of vulnerability and perceived betrayal by government, the medical establishment and big business; and a conceivably genuine, albeit misplaced and ineffective (with possibly catastrophic consequences) attempt by the local leadership to protect the inhabitants of the area."[80]

The most pressing impact of these different racial perceptions is in the area of AIDS/HIV research and care, as HIV infections are running rampant in black and minority communities compared to those of Caucasians. NIH has again looked at factors that contribute to this disparity, including community and societal factors. It emphasizes the need to develop "cultural competency, or the ability to see the world through the lens of a particular culture."[81]

The NIH recommends that healthcare providers have a wider involvement in communities. Healthcare workers should be actively and visibly present at times other than when recruiting volunteers. There is also a need for more minority investigators to become well-trained clinical investigators.

In addition to the question of trust, the NIH notes that, historically, trials and similar interventions often have not resulted in tangible benefits to minority communities. This is another significant deterrent to participation of minority communities in clinical research trials. Examining barriers to care, be they individual, institutional, or cultural, is also emphasized as a way to enable the development of more effective and culturally appropriate interventions.[82]

KEY POINT
"A civilization is to be judged by its treatment of minorities."
—Mahatma Gandhi

One often overlooked barrier to participation is the significant time commitment that many studies require. This disproportionately affects communities of color, which are often economically depressed and thus can less afford the time away from work. Women of color are also often single heads of households, further limiting their willingness or ability to participate in trials given their caretaking responsibilities for children or extended family. On the other hand, in some studies, the financial rewards for participation may be more alluring to people of color.[83]

Other suggestions to help remove these obstacles include targeting culturally appropriate educational programs to the study population and providing cross-cultural curricula for healthcare workers.[84]

Politics of Research: Race and Gender Overlap

One often overlooked area of research ethics involves the intersection of race and gender. This is particularly relevant in terms of developing recruitment strategies and in understanding the reluctance of minorities to participate in research.

Historically, several events have specifically triggered mistrust in research, especially studies involving contraceptives and sterilization in minority women. For example, between 1980 and 1983, fully one-fifth of contraceptive research was conducted in developing countries, such as India, China, Chile, Mexico, and Brazil.[85] Another example is that of oral contraceptive research that was conducted in Puerto Rico. Reportedly, analysis of both uncomfortable and serious adverse events was inadequate in these overseas trials.[86]

A recent debate surrounds the use of quinacrine, an antimalarial agent, for sterilization. Quinacrine causes localized inflammation when instilled into the uterus, resulting in sterilization. It has therefore been used as an inexpensive alternative to tubal ligation in developing countries, prompting some criticism that it has been used coercively and relatively casually, with neglect of larger societal problems. According to a Reproductive Health Technologies Project report, "Little attention was paid to the social and gender inequality that supported higher fertility and left the majority of women with little choice in marriage, sex, and reproduction."[87] Rather than providing increased freedom for women by allowing them some choice over their reproduction, some felt that the quinacrine sterilization was being used to control large populations of women. An extensive discussion of this controversy can be found in *The Quinacrine Debate and Beyond*, the report of the Reproductive Health Technologies Project 2001 meeting. This meeting identified two competing paradigms. The first, called the "technology as neutral paradigm," views technology as neutral. The second, the "technology as embedded into context paradigm," views technology in the context of historical, sociocultural, and political events. In many cases, the basic questions to be asked are, What is the perception of need for the new technology? Who defines the need? Who decides on implementation? Other issues that must be considered prior to implementing such a widespread sterilization program include the following:

- Women's attitudes about contraception and pregnancy, viewed from both a social and a cultural context
- The effect of power inequities between men and women
- Lack of social support for many women
- Coercion by medical providers or government agencies[88]

The use of quinacrine for sterilization has been analyzed from the perspective of the Belmont principles. One of the three principles is that of beneficence. Because quinacrine had been used successfully for treating malaria, its proponents did not consider it to be a new or untested drug and did not undertake safety and toxicity studies on it, although instilling it into the uterus was a new route of administration. The proponents argued that quinacrine provided a safer and less expensive alternative to surgical sterilization and thus would be of great benefit to impoverished women in countries where maternal mortality is high and where few resources are available. However, these researchers did not address other factors that contribute to maternal mortality, which may have provided a safe alternative to sterilization.

Another Belmont principle is that of distributive justice, which requires that the burdens and benefits of research be equitably distributed across cultural lines and populations. In this case, almost all of the women who underwent quinacrine sterilization were low income, poorly educated women of color in developing countries. Thus, the second Belmont principle was not followed.

Respect for persons, granting autonomy, or self-determination, is the remaining Belmont principle. This was violated in the quinacrine study because no explanation of the risks or experimental nature of the procedure was provided and no informed consent was obtained. Hundreds of thousands of women received quinacrine sterilization without adequate information or presentation of alternatives.

Another example of the violation of the Belmont principle of autonomy is the use of reproductive technology as a government or political tool. For example, the U.S. Indian Health Service has been accused of imposing the implanted contraceptive Norplant on Native American women without their consent. Others groups have proposed requiring the use of Norplant as a condition for receiving welfare.[89]

A final theme that emerged from the Reproductive Health Technologies Project 2001 meeting is the need to establish better accountability both in research regarding reproductive health and in the implementation of government or social policies.

Politics of Research: Shifting Studies to Developing Countries

Many U.S. drug companies are looking overseas to conduct their clinical trials, as noted in chapter 7, because the costs are considerably less and pools of potential subjects are more readily available. Recently, 20–30 percent of trials were being done overseas.[90] This shift raises additional ethical issues. Some of the concerns relate to priorities in medical research (and other) expenditures, some to the vast differences in the standard of living between countries, and some to specific human rights questions.

The pace of international trial growth, particularly in India, where the costs are less than half of those in the United States, appears to be increasing. Pfizer is conducting 20 trials there for treating osteoporosis, cancer, schizophrenia, and malaria. Similarly, Eli Lilly and Company is conducting insulin and oncology trials there, and other companies have a growing presence as well.[91]

Conducting trials internationally poses regulatory issues and questions of uniformity of standards. These issues are briefly discussed in chapter 4. That many of the chosen countries are economically underdeveloped raises complex ethical issues.

For example, the issues of race, economics, and justice extend to all countries and raise questions regarding the use of vulnerable communities. These vulnerable populations share several important characteristics:

- Limited economic development
- Inadequate protection of human rights
- Inadequate community and cultural experience with, or understanding of, scientific research
- Limited availability of healthcare and treatment options
- Limited ability of individuals in the community to provide informed consent due to illiteracy and language, educational, or cultural barriers[92]

For example, Harvard researchers came under a great deal of criticism for their involvement in a DNA and gene sequencing study in rural China. The isolated area of Anhui was chosen, as remote areas of this type are thought to provide "purer" genetic material. (Similar studies are ongoing in Iceland.)

Harvard received millions of dollars in grants for this project. The research subjects gave blood samples in exchange for the promise of healthcare that, they say, never materialized. Subjects say they did not receive the promised laboratory test results, follow-up, or discounts on their healthcare expenses. In addition to the funding that never trickled down to the subjects, serious concerns were raised about the voluntariness of the participation. Many of the participants were subject to coercion by local government and Communist party officials: volunteer rates exceeded 95 percent.

Ultimately, as a result of complaints, the U.S. Embassy in Beijing warned "U.S. medical researchers against working in impoverished, rural areas of China where 'healthcare is poor and people are unable to protect their rights.'"[93] An opposing view is that even if the promises had been kept, the political environment or the financial incentives were too coercive for these communities. How does one value the benefits of the research versus the possible impact on the individual?

Relatively little ethical abuse appears to have occurred in the design of clinical trials overseas, given the huge size of the financial stakes. This appears to be because the FDA has required that foreign data, if used to support a New Drug Application, must be collected in a manner consistent either with the Declaration of Helsinki or "with the laws and regulations of the country in which the research was conducted, whichever provides greater protection of the human subjects."[94] Also, if the research includes any funding from the NIH or other part of the Department of Health and Human Services, assurances of compliance with ethical standards must be given to the Office for Human Research Protections (OHRP).

One example illustrating the difficulties of conducting trials overseas involves the 1996 trial of an oral quinolone during a meningitis epidemic in Nigeria. As background, it is important to understand that while meningococcal meningitis is rather rare in the United States, widespread epidemics occur regularly in parts of Africa. In the African "meningitis belt," annual epidemics may infect over 200,000 people at one time.[95] In a 1996 outbreak of meningococcal meningitis, the death rate was higher than 10 percent, with the deaths occurring mostly in children. Of the survivors, 10 percent were left with significant residual mental or physical impairments.[96] So in order to study a new medicine, the sponsor felt that the trials had to be conducted in Africa, where the illness was rampant, rather than in the United States, where only a few sporadic cases occur. It also made logistical sense to explore an oral antibiotic, given that this was an impoverished area.

Some of the decisions made on that trial do appear egregious, such as using an oral antibiotic on critically ill young children and not altering therapy when patients' conditions were deteriorating. The antibiotic had been tested on adults but was, as yet, little studied in children. However, the sponsor was trying to do a hastily planned study during a meningitis epidemic in an impoverished area: this setting might be considered an invitation to disaster. The sponsor had little choice as to locale. (For perspective, my own community's "outbreak" involved three patients, which is fairly typical in the United States.) One might argue that trying an oral agent makes sense in an impoverished area if adequate safeguards are built into the protocol.

The ethical dilemma in this case surrounds the reported lack of such safeguards. No requirement was in place to repeat a spinal tap at 24–48 hours to document effectiveness of the therapy. Nor was there an absolute requirement either to drop patients from the protocol if their conditions were not improving after 48 hours of treatment or to promptly provide alternative antibiotics if a patient's condition was deteriorating. Both practices would be considered standard in the United States. Subsequent concerns were also raised about the protocol design.[97] Such a study is unlikely to ever be repeated. Not mentioned in the general press was the fact that the use of the study drug was not confined to a poor, developing country—pediatric meningitis trials with this drug were also being conducted in the United States by well-respected researchers studying the new options for treating multidrug-resistant bacteria.[98] Update: Further critical information has surfaced since my initial nonjudgmental comments about Pfizer, above. There were significant differences between the U.S. Trovan pediatric meningitis and Nigerian studies. Besides the obvious differences in level of care, higher doses of antibiotic were given in the U.S. study, 100 milligrams per kilogram (mg/kg) of ceftriaxone versus 33 mg/kg per day in Nigeria.[99]

Questions have also been raised regarding the adequacy of the informed consent process in this meningitis trial. Obtaining consent can be difficult in the best of circumstances. Particularly for phase 2 trials, when less is known about the drugs and when they are first administered to ill patients, and for less educated (and often more ill) patients, it routinely takes me 30–60 minutes to explain and review the consent with the patient and family. Perhaps most of us would question the adequacy of informed consent obtained under more difficult circumstances, where probably fewer staff members were capable of explaining the consent, but any perceived inadequacy should be considered in the context of available resources.

In January 2009, a federal appeals court ruled that Nigerian families could sue Pfizer in U.S. courts; Pfizer has appealed this decision to the U.S. Supreme Court, where it is pending.[100] Meanwhile, in Nigeria, officials filed criminal charges against Pfizer and sought $9 billion in restitution; a settlement was announced in July 2009 for $75 million.[101]

Ironically, in the midst of all this and other, unrelated ethics charges, Pfizer became the first pharmaceutical company to receive accreditation from the Association for the Accreditation of Human Research Protection Programs—for its phase 1 clinical research units.[102] Reassuring, isn't it?

Ethical concerns regarding access to care and new therapies are not unique to the 1996 meningitis case but apply to many illnesses. When critically evaluating these concerns, it is important to put them into the context of the local circumstances. For example, according to the Gambia Government/Medical Research Council Joint Ethical Committee, "8 million people die every year in sub-Saharan Africa, 68 percent from communicable, maternal, and perinatal causes compared with 6 percent for those causes among the 7 million deaths in established market economies. In Africa, 23 percent of children die by the age of 15, compared with 1–3 percent in affluent countries; 35 percent of those who reach age 15 in Africa will die by age 60, compared with 11 percent here. Many [sic] contribute less than $10 per head towards the annual health budget."[103] In contrast, the corresponding per capita spending in the United States is $1,059.[104]

KEY POINT
"Statistics are people with the tears wiped away."—Dr. Irving Selikoff

So, one can examine the ethical questions raised by this meningitis trial example from different perspectives. Should the absolute standards of care available in more developed countries be applied across the board, even when adequate resources are not available to achieve these standards in the host country? Or is it perhaps more realistic to conduct trials with reference to the local standard of care? As has been noted, those critical of this latter approach have been rebuked by the Gambian charge that "ethics cannot be owned by affluent countries alone" and that "ethical judgments on studies in developing countries should be made by locally constituted ethical bodies."[105]

Similarly, trials aimed at reducing maternal-fetal HIV transmission in developing countries have come under a great deal of criticism. Again, the intervention may be compared to the local standard, which may be to do nothing or to provide a level of care that appears substandard to us. Harold Varmus and David Satcher rebut the criticisms, arguing, "The most compelling reason to use a placebo-controlled study is that it provides definitive answers to questions about the safety and value of an intervention in the setting in which the study is performed, and these answers are the point of the research."[106]

Recent attempts have been made to reach a consensus on this issue of local versus global standards for the ethical conduct of trials. The Declaration of Helsinki requirements were revised in 2000, requiring uniform standards that provide each participant with the "best current" diagnostic tests and therapy. This has been challenged by several international consensus groups on the grounds that the requirement precludes testing of drugs or interventions that may not be the "best" in the world but are better than the locally available treatments. The international consensus appears to consider such research ethical if it is based on a valid scientific purpose for using a lesser standard, provides social benefits for the local host community, and shows a favorable risk-benefit ratio for the individual research participants.[107]

The Declaration of Helsinki was revised again in 2008. Straightforward and welcome new principles include the following:

- Investigators should disclose potential conflicts of interest to both IRBs and study participants.
- Investigators should report and publish or make public negative findings.
- "Every clinical trial must be registered in a publicly accessible database [i.e., a clinical trial registry] before recruitment of the first subject."[108]

These are valuable additions because of the increased transparency. Studies that lack either safety or efficacy would be readily apparent; no longer would negative results be able to be buried easily. The pharmaceutical industry is understandably unhappy with this development, claiming that it jeopardizes intellectual property rights. Some are proposing to exclude phase 1 trials from this guideline.

Two articles of the declaration have been particularly contentious, however. Article 29 (now 32) discourages the use of placebos except under the following conditions:

- Where no current proven intervention exists
- "Where for compelling and scientifically sound methodological reasons the use of placebo is necessary to determine the efficacy or safety of an intervention and the patients who receive placebo or no treatment will not be subject to any risk of serious or irreversible harm"

Article 30 (now 33) states that volunteers "are entitled to be informed about the outcome of the study and to share any benefits that result from it, for example, access to interventions identified as beneficial in the study or to other appropriate care or benefits." In addition "arrangements for post-study access by study subjects to interventions identified as beneficial in the study or access to other appropriate care or benefits" should be described.[109, 110]

Consequently, as of October 27, 2008, the FDA dropped its requirement that studies—including trials done overseas in support of a US application—must be in compliance with the Declaration of Helsinki. For U.S. approval, studies must now just be in compliance with International Conference on Harmonisation Good Clinical Practice (ICH-GCP) guidelines. A major impetus for the FDA change appears to be concern that the Declaration of Helsinki is subject to change by the World Medical Association, independent of FDA authority, and could thereby be modified to contain provisions that are inconsistent with U.S. laws and regulations. But what does this seemingly minor change really mean, and what are its implications?

ICH-GCP "provides assurance that the data and reported results are credible and accurate, and that the rights, integrity, and confidentiality of trial subjects are protected."[111] As Michael Goodyear explains, "GCP is not an ethical code, but a procedural regulatory manual based on the regulatory frameworks of the US, Japan, and Europe. Thus, it is a description of existing procedures, not an aspirational document. It is not the procedural nuances that are at stake, but rather the moral reasoning that forms the basis of a culture of ethically responsible research."[112] Others might differ with Goodyear on this point because the standardization of these procedures does provide a better infrastructure for human research protections. Is this not then an ethical code?

Some defend the change, saying that the ICH guidelines are more concrete and less subject to interpretation, thus ensuring better data.[113] They also provide a basis for human subjects protection by requiring that an IRB oversee trials. Others are less charitable, saying that the United States is demonstrating unilateralism, as it has with other global agreements in the last few years.

So in some cases, such as certain multiple sclerosis trials, the FDA can now demand placebo-controlled trials when such trials would be considered illegal and unethical overseas. Ironically, much of the opposition to placebos stemmed from African trials in which the FDA accepted AZT trials against placebos, at the same time insisting that similar trials in the United States be conducted as a comparison against proven effective treatment rather than placebos.

Concerns about the United States' unilateral decision to withdraw the Helsinki requirement have been depicted as

- Entrenching different standards for different parts of the world (ethical pluralism)
- Establishing the United States' right to unique policies (exceptionalism)
- Imposing one country's standards on others (moral imperialism).[114]

The 2008 revision of the Declaration of Helsinki also places stronger emphasis on protections for vulnerable populations and potential benefits to communities. Despite these lofty goals, the reality is far different. As Indian journalist (and executive editor of the *Indian Journal of Medical Ethics*) Sandhya Srinivasan reports in an in-depth analysis of four clinical trials in India, "they were conducted on vulnerable groups, and they were conducted primarily or exclusively in countries where concerns have been raised about the quality of regulation of such trials. In addition, in the case of lapatinib, the drug is very expensive and therefore unaffordable for most people who would need it." While these specific studies—Glaxo's phase 2 trial of lapatinib for advanced breast cancer, two placebo-controlled trials of Astra Zeneca's antipsychotic drug quetiapine fumarate extended release, and Johnson & Johnson's placebo-controlled trial of the antipsychotic drug risperidone—were conducted prior to 2008, the pattern of violation of the Helsinki guidelines persists.[115] Some problems are actually worsening as more trials are being shifted to India and other developing countries.

In India, for example, the Drugs and Cosmetics Rules were amended in 2009 to allow clinical trials (phase 2 trials) to be done in that country at the same time as in other countries, rather than lagging behind to await trial results that might detect problems. Since then, the number of new trials in India rose from 100 in 2005, when the new rules took effect, to about 500 in 2008.[116] (Phase 1 trials are allowed only for Indian discoveries or for foreign drugs if they are of special relevance to Indian health.)[117, 118]

Earlier-phase trials further take advantage of the extreme poverty and vulnerabilities of patients, with little likelihood that either the subjects or the broader community will truly benefit. As the FDA demands more placebo-controlled trials, an available and willing population is found in India (and elsewhere), and the Drug Controller General of India (the FDA equivalent) is willing to turn a blind eye to the resultant problems, "permitting a number of unethical trials . . . [suggesting that the office] places greater value on the potential financial returns of clinical trial outsourcing than on protecting the people who take part in drug trials in India."[119]

Concerns regarding access to care are not limited to less developed countries. A related ethical dilemma in this country involves the financial incentive for uninsured patients to participate in trials. Such patients often are motivated by the greater access to free medical care provided on a trial. With some medications, particularly those for HIV and the newer classes of drugs, such as for rheumatoid arthritis, participation in a trial may gain patients long-term access to care they would otherwise be unable to afford.

It is less clear whether there are ethical problems in the implementation of overseas trials as well as in the design. Maybe this is, in large part, cultural as American subjects are perhaps more likely to question information than are many of their counterparts elsewhere. However, universal concerns about coercion and who should participate, as well as about the ability of subjects to understand what participation means or what, if any, alternatives they might have to participation in a clinical trial, are universal.

Another ethical debate regarding research trials in developing countries concerns the issues of race and gender as they relate to illnesses such as AIDS. For example, the AIDS epidemic is devastating sub-Saharan Africa, where up to one in four people is HIV infected.[120] In one survey of AIDS patients in South Africa, 88 percent of the women said they felt they had to participate in a trial, almost a third thought there would be repercussions if they did not participate, and almost all did not believe they were allowed to withdraw from a trial. One might argue that it is inherently too coercive to conduct trials in a country lacking basic healthcare, where participation might appear to provide the only access to care.[121] Others might counter that access to some care is better than none and that the trial findings will benefit the entire population, rather than just one person, and are therefore justified.

Unfortunately, there are still further problems with studies conducted overseas. For example, the FDA has little ability (or personnel) to monitor trials outside the United States. Pharmaceutical companies are rapidly shifting trials overseas because of the lower cost, the abundance of patients who are willing to be subjects, and the fact that some illnesses are simply more common in other countries.[122] Another temptation is that regulatory agencies may not be as strict in some countries as they are in the United States.[123] Consent may be easier to obtain in countries that are more authoritarian or where treatment options may be fewer. Or, as a Hungarian researcher phrased it, "Patients in Western countries—and in the United States especially—have an overdeveloped sense of their rights and a fear of being harmed."[124]

On one hand, one might ask if different standards for studies in different countries are justified by the local economic conditions and profound poverty. Are different standards justified by the degree of devastation wrought by a disease? Are they justified when no viable alternative treatments are available, so the subjects are no worse off than if they were not participating in the study?[125] On the other hand, studies with different standards do not meet the principle of distributive justice because the local study populations will not significantly benefit from the research if the new therapies will not be affordable to them, although they are taking a higher proportion of the risk. Some view research on people of color in developing countries as profoundly racist if the studies are held to different and lower standards than would now be allowed in the United States. Should ethical standards be absolute, or should they be allowed to vary depending on local or regional conditions?

Justice and Societal Needs

An extension of the debate regarding research in developing countries is the debate surrounding allocation of resources even in the more prosperous ones, such as the United States. A thorough discussion is available through Public Agenda, a broad-based opinion research organization that provides extensive background information on its Web site.[126] The issue is categorized here as how to allocate limited resources, and it raises three questions:

1. Should public funding for practical or applied research be increased from the current 1 percent of the federal government's budget to direct resources toward improving quality of life, particularly for people with common diseases, such as diabetes?
2. Should these same public funds instead be directed toward basic science research, such as research on the mechanisms of disease, since this area has the broadest potential, even though it provides little or no immediate

financial or therapeutic return? This would leave the drug industry to fund research on clinical applications.

3. Instead of spending public monies on research for the future or on "designer" drugs that may benefit only a small segment of the population, shouldn't we instead be spending tax revenue on promoting and ensuring basic healthcare for all?

The focus of research endeavors has been described as another example of the failure of distributive justice. In this case, the balance is tilted toward the affluent members of society because most clinical research is profit driven. Research on AIDS, particularly for affordable therapies useful in developing countries, lags well behind more expensive and more profitable higher tech solutions. Similarly, relatively little research has been done on lupus, an illness that disproportionately affects black women.

Social Justice and Drug Development

Over the past 5 years I've become much more aware of and concerned about social justice issues as they relate to drug development. I'll review here a few examples of issues that have particularly caught my attention and raised my sense of indignation. I invite readers to engage in a dialogue about these issues via my Web site and blog.

Perhaps my greatest sense of outrage comes from our society's priorities, which I find misguided in many ways, particularly given the state of the global economy, unemployment, and the healthcare crisis in the United States wrought by insurers and their lobbyists. I looked briefly at NIH funding changes between 2005 and 2008 and was curious about some of the priorities. For example, despite the growing menace of antibiotic-resistant

View from the Trenches

Having briefly worked in impoverished areas of India and Peru, I strongly believe that consideration of the local conditions and the ability to provide the hope of improvement over the baseline care available define both the moral high ground and the only practical route. Further, I would hope for a shift back toward developing treatments that will help most of the global population, such as treatments for infections and malnourishment, rather than developing drugs—especially "lifestyle" drugs—that are inaccessible except to the affluent few.

bacteria, the latter ranked 86th in funding. Pharmaceutical companies are no longer making significant investments in this area either, the drugs are being excessively used, and various chain stores have questionable programs touting "free" antibiotics. While such a program has some value to patients who can ill-afford the medications, it also encourages overprescribing them as does their over-the-counter availability in many countries.[127]

Similarly, funding for injuries to the head and spine has dropped significantly. Teen pregnancy ranked 163rd, and funding has dropped. Who needs to study this public health and societal problem when abstinence is the answer, anyway?

Lifestyle Drugs

Television programs are littered with direct-to-consumer (DTC) advertising, particularly for drugs for erectile dysfunction—which can cost as much as $15 a pop. These drugs, as well as those for baldness and other cosmetic concerns, were actually covered under Medicare drug benefit legislation in 2003, although many other classes of drugs were excluded. And this, despite the fact that the price of Viagra has shot up 108 percent in the past 10 years.[128]

The reason for the barrage of DTC advertising is probably because it is so effective. Patients see the ads and then pressure their physicians for a prescription. It is easier and faster for doctors to acquiesce and write the prescription than to enter into lengthy discussions with patients and risk losing them to a competitor's practice.

Dr. Marcia Angell, former editor in chief of the *New England Journal of Medicine*, says that DTC ads actually promote "illnesses" through the power of suggestion: "Once upon a time, drug companies promoted drugs to treat diseases. Now it is often the opposite. They promote diseases to fit their drugs."[129]

A new drug is on the horizon for men. Ed Silverman reports in "Come Again? A Spray for Premature Ejaculation" that this new spray anesthetic delayed premature ejaculation an average of a whopping 108 seconds. Silverman wryly asks, "How long do you think it will take before PE and ED combo therapies are tested?"[130]

An op-ed shares my dismay over public funding for lifestyle drugs (those used generally for cosmetic purposes or "to perform an activity 'on demand' or without consequences, ameliorate an imprudent binge, or modify effects of aging"):[131]

"As we consider our goals for the New Year, what is more important to American taxpayers: free Viagra or providing essential food, health care and education for our neediest families? According to our congressional leaders, free Viagra is the priority."[132]

Many would argue that funding of drugs for impotence or baldness is also unjustly favoring men, as contraceptives and drugs for women's illnesses are often excluded from coverage.

In 2008, the FDA gave a Christmas gift to the pharmaceutical industry, announcing approval of Allergan's Latisse. This "New Prescription Product Increases Length, Thickness and Darkness of Eyelashes." You can read the nauseating details in Allergan's shareholder news flash.[133] While this drug, like Rogaine for baldness, was discovered as a "side effect" observed during trials for a legitimate medical indication—glaucoma with bimatoprost ophthalmic drops (Latisse) and blood pressure with minoxidil (Rogaine)—one has to ask, "Doesn't the FDA have anything better to do?" This will surely become one of those drugs destined to create a disease—the tragedy of hypotrichosis of the eyelashes.

Profiting from Orphan Diseases

Recently Genzyme, as the sole provider of treatment for Gaucher's disease, demonstrated a new model for the pharmaceutical industry for pricing and marketing drugs for orphan diseases. As Stephen Heuser explained, "Genzyme's solution, elegant in its way, was to set a price high enough to earn a substantial profit no matter how small its pool of patients. Then the company . . . show[ed] that American health insurers could be persuaded to pay the six-figure price tag. And with the only effective treatment for Gaucher disease, Genzyme never needed to lower the price, even as production efficiencies raised profit margins on the drug to as much as 90 percent." The price? Only $160,000 per year per patient. When it had saturated the U.S. market, "Genzyme created divisions within the company to find overseas patients; it hired experts to cajole balky governments into paying for the patients' Cerezyme doses."[134]

Neglected Tropical Diseases: Putting Drug Development in Context

Neglected tropical diseases (NTDs) are the diseases of "the bottom billion." They primarily affect people subsisting on less than $2 per day, 2.7 billion people[135] (almost half the world's population), of whom over 1.4 billion lived on less than $1.25 per day in 2008.[136] NTDs are typically "Biblical diseases"—afflictions that have burdened humanity for centuries. Many of these diseases are disabling and very deforming, causing great stigma and social isolation as well as physical scarring. NTDs have received relatively little attention because they affect the voiceless, the most vulnerable, impoverished, and marginalized populations in society, often living out of sight in rural areas of low-income countries and densely crowded urban slums. NTDs also promote further cycles of poverty by impairing child development, pregnancy, and worker productivity. There are no commercial markets for products that target these diseases.[137, 138, 139] Yet as leaders note, "interventions, when applied, have a history of success."[140]

A DALY (disability-adjusted life year) is a metric that the World Health Organization uses to standardize the description of the impact of diseases. The DALY reflects the total amount of healthy life lost, to all causes, whether from premature mortality or from some degree of disability during a period of time. The DALY ranking of communicable diseases showed a burden (in millions) for HIV/AIDS of 84.5; NTDs, 56.6; malaria, 46.5; and tuberculosis, 34.7.[141] In contrast, the impact of coronary artery disease is 58.6 DALYs, which is about the same as for all the NTDs combined, but spending is 100 times more than for NTDs, which is only 62 cents per DALY.[142]

The biggest problems with regard to NTDs include infections caused by helminths, especially soil-transmitted worms, which are the NTDs with the largest global burden, with a 3 million DALY impact. These include Ascaris (roundworm), which infects almost all children in developing countries, resulting in malnutrition and stunted growth and development; trichuris (whipworm), which infects 800 million people; and hookworm, which infects 600 million people. Yet for 2 cents per person annually, soil-transmitted helminth infections can be readily treated with albendazole or mebendazole, restoring the victims' ability to learn and earn and breaking the cycle of poverty.[143]

Schistosomiasis is acquired by swimming or working in fresh water, whereby the larvae enter through the skin. It infects 200 million people and has an impact of 1.7 million DALYs.[144]

Fascinating work suggests that infection with schistosomiasis, which often causes bladder and genital lesions and bleeding, may increase susceptibility to HIV. Want to reduce AIDs infections? What's the return on investment of 25 cents for a single dose of praziquantel if you can reduce AIDS?

Mosquito-borne lymphatic filariasis (elephantiasis) affects 120 million people, mostly in India and Africa, with a loss of 5.8 million DALYs. LF has a disproportionate effect on men as it is the major cause of hydrocele. While LF costs $2 billion in lost productivity, it could be readily treated with only one annual treatment of albendazole plus either diethylcarbamazine (DEC) or ivermectin.[145]

Onchocerciasis (river blindness) control is one of the great success stories, both of society's ability to do good and of pharmaceutical philanthropy. The filarial worm is transmitted by bites from black flies. While its DALY is only .5 million, infecting 18 million people, it causes severe rash and blindness—up to 50 percent of adult men may be blinded in some areas. Merck has been a model of philanthropy, donating 60 million doses per year of ivermectin, which also eradicates filariasis. (Merck's philanthropy is especially notable because, like Genzyme, it was the sole manufacturer of an important drug. Unlike Genzyme, Merck chose not to exploit that advantage.)[146]

Other NTDs include Guinea worm, protozoan NTDs (Chagas and leishmania), and bacterial infections (leprosy, Buruli ulcer, and trachoma).

Why Care?

For perspective on priorities in drug development, note that by 2020 the population of the United States will decline to 4 percent of the world total while that of developing countries will climb to 84 percent. Out of $2 trillion in annual healthcare expenditures, 90 percent goes to the top countries and regions (United States, Japan, Europe, Canada, Australia, Hong Kong, Singapore, and Israel). Only 10 percent of resources go to the people who bear 90 percent of the disease burden.[147]

Other studies show that as funding for the military goes up, public health and education are shortchanged.[148] While U.S. spending is low on the basis of gross domestic product, the country spent $420.7 billion on the military (2005), which was 43–47 percent of global military spending. China and Russia, our closest competitors on the military front, each came in at $62 billion, or 6 percent of global military spending.[149]

In a provocative essay, University of Virginia professor Dr. Richard Guerrant discusses the disparities between economies and notes that while the high income countries and regions account for 18 percent of the global population, they consume more than 60 percent of global resources. He goes on to examine the destabilizing influence such vast disparities create. Malnutrition and infections are the largest causes of mortality around the world, yet relatively few resources are directed toward these problems. Guerrant ends hopefully, noting that, if not for the most noble reasons, "perhaps for the first time in human evolution, we can begin to perceive the *survival advantage of caring about the other person*, the poor in the tropics."[150]

More recently, Dr. Peter Hotez* echoes the foreign policy advantage of addressing these diseases, noting that more than half of those infected come from Yemen, Somalia, Sudan, and Afghanistan, with other pockets occurring in countries with nuclear arms capabilities, including India, Pakistan, China, Iran, and North Korea. Dr. Hotez makes a strong argument for the cost-effectiveness of using medical diplomacy as a tool to gain global security.[151]

As we've seen, the NTDs as a group create an enormous burden—and this is not including the impact of deaths from pneumonia, malaria, TB, HIV/AIDS, and even childhood diarrhea, all of which have a disproportionate toll on the world's poor. Treating the NTDs alone would be relatively easy. A "Rapid Impact" package of only four drugs—albendazole or mebendazole, DEC or ivermectin, praziquantel, and azithromycin—will treat seven major NTDs (three helminth infections, schistosomiasis, filariasis, river blindness, and trachoma). The cost of this Rapid Impact package? Just 50 cents—including drugs, delivery, equipment, distribution, education materials, and training, monitoring, and evaluation—or only $200 million per year, to treat 500 million people. It's such a bargain compared to most everything else we do.[152] The collateral benefits are numerous as well, including less anemia and malnutrition, resulting in improved growth, educational performance, and later earning capacity. Why haven't we done this?

What Have We Chosen as Priorities Instead?

While few drugs have been available for sleeping sickness in the past (suramin, pentamidine, and melarsoprol, an arsenic derivative), Sanofi-Aventis developed a new drug, eflornithine. Unfortunately, it stopped production of IV eflornithine in 1999 due to lack of profit. After protests and arm-twisting from

---

* Peter J. Hotez is distinguished research professor and chair of the Department of Microbiology, Immunology and Tropical Medicine at George Washington University. He is also president of the Sabin Vaccine Institute.

Doctors Without Borders (aka Médecins Sans Frontières, MSF) and WHO, it resumed production in 2001. During this period, however, it continued to make topical eflornithine. Why? For unwanted facial hair! The company's ad for Vaniqa said, "What a burden that has been lifted from my life! I feel so free now to be who I really am. I'm not at all self-conscious with people."[153] Vaniqa cost $1–$2 per day.

Disparities: Did you know that several years ago, the amount you'd pay for one "little blue pill" (Viagra) or one latte was enough to feed three people for one day or could treat a number of people to eradicate the seven major NTDs?[154] Or that consumer expenditures for cosmetics are estimated to exceed $35 billion annually in the United States, or more than $100 per person?[155] There is a rapidly widening gap between the haves and the have-nots. This is inequitable and is a major force in the growth of world instability. If for nothing more than self-interest, as the late Harvard economics professor John Kenneth Galbraith cogently warned, "It is time for privileged people to move beyond self satisfied complacency."[156]

It should be noted that pharmaceuticals do make significant charitable donations—just ask them. PhRMA (the industry group) reports that its members account for 34 percent of corporate donations, far more than the next largest contributing industry, and have provided billions of dollars in donations.[157]

A recent study analyzed investments for NTD research and development in 2007. Nearly 80 percent of the $2.5 billion (public and private) in funding was for the "big three": HIV/AIDS, TB, and malaria. Significant progress has been made particularly with HIV/AIDS as it has assumed a higher governmental priority.

In 2003, the U.S. government committed $15 billion for the President's Emergency Plan for AIDS Relief (PEPFAR) to provide antiretroviral therapy and efforts to reduce infection. And with generics, the cost for first-generation antiretroviral drugs has decreased from $10,000 to less than $100 per patient per year—a vast improvement but still extraordinarily expensive for many developing countries. Fortunately, international donation and granting facilities exist to compensate for local governments' inability to provide for their populations. What do local governments do with their assets? Perhaps this is another case of misplaced priorities. In 2006, a number of countries created UNITAID, a drug purchase facility financed with a tax on airplane tickets for sustainable funding. Now in partnership with the Gates Foundation, UNITAID, like the Global Fund, focuses on decreasing the price of priority medicines, thereby improving access. The World Health Assembly also proposed a patent pool administered by UNITAID to spur drug discovery and development.

Doctors Without Borders cleverly employed YouTube videos to educate people about the benefits of patent pools, resulting in a campaign that successfully encouraged the UNITAID decision in December 2009 to set up and fund the licensing agency to implement this project.[158] The downsides include the valuation of contributions, concerns about intellectual property ownership, and the cherry-picking of countries that might benefit from the pool.[159]

One other exciting R&D innovation is the new approach that Pfizer and Glaxo are taking. Instead of eliminating major competition through mergers or competing with relatively small staffs, in November 2009, the two huge corporations spun off their HIV/AIDS units into a joint research alliance, ViiV Healthcare, solely devoted to this issue.

While malaria, TB, and HIV/AIDS have been benefiting from increasing attention, "other equally high-burden diseases as measured by DALYs . . . ,

"Open Labs, Open Minds"[160]

In a surprising speech to the Council on Foreign Relations on January 20, 2010, GlaxoSmithKline's CEO, Andrew Witty, announced an innovative new program to combat malaria and NTDs with three major components. The first is opening a knowledge pool, containing 800 of the company's patents and related information, to researchers in these areas, with administration by the nonprofit BIO Ventures for Global Health. The second is creating the "Open Lab" center, where up to 60 independent researchers can go to work on their own projects, using Glaxo's infrastructure and the expertise of its teams. The third element is opening selected data to researchers—in this case, making freely available to others 13,500 compounds potentially useful as antimalarials.

Glaxo has the leading candidate for a malaria vaccine and hopes to seek approval in 2012. One of the most welcome announcements because of its more immediate impact, is the decision to market the vaccine at an astonishingly reasonable price of manufacturing cost plus 5 percent profit—and then to plow the profits right back into research for NTDs.

Some people question GSK's motives and note that only a very small percentage of the company's profits come from the poorest countries. But whatever the motives—and rarely is something all good or all bad—this looks like a winning plan for all and one that will hopefully be copied by others.

such as pneumonia and the diarrhoeal illnesses, collectively received less the 6% of total funding." Pharmaceutical companies provided about 9 percent of the funding; the Gates Foundation, 18 percent; the NIH, 42 percent.[161]

The outlook for NTD research has significantly improved in recent years. Between 1975 and 1999, there were only 13 new drugs for NTDs. Since 2000, three dedicated institutes have been set up by pharmaceutical companies, as well as four public-private partnerships, with large funding by philanthropies. In the partnership model, the multinational corporations can "significantly reduce R&D costs by re-focusing in-house activity from late-stage clinical development to early-pipeline R&D, which requires a significantly smaller investment. It is notable that 80 per cent of current multinational neglected disease projects are now early-pipeline R&D." The private groups then take over the conduct of the clinical trials, the more expensive part of the development.

These partnerships have been achieving a good measure of success. However, much of the progress has focused on malaria and TB—all but 8 of 63 drugs being evaluated—rather than the more neglected diseases.[162]

Not long ago we were told that banks were "too big to fail." Next we were told that pharmaceutical companies, despite repeated misuse of their position, were too important to punish meaningfully. Besides their promotion of off-label uses of certain drugs that caused unnecessary expense and risks for individuals, the current business climate with pharmaceutical companies allows behaviors that are putting us all at risk. For example, while little attention is being paid to the critical need to develop new antibiotics for multidrug-resistant organisms because the profits pale in comparison to those for drugs for chronic diseases or entertainment, Pfizer and others are squandering our limited antibiotic arsenal by promoting the use of important drugs (like linezolid irresponsibly). And instead of focusing on urgent health needs, they continue to add new lifestyle drugs and drugs in search of diseases, like Latisse, for the important indication of "inadequate" eyelashes.

This focus, while understandable from an economic perspective for the drug company and its stockholders, results in the health needs of the poor being neglected and widens the wealth and power gap, leaving the poor even more marginalized.[163] Should we use the influence of our government to change incentives toward benefiting the broadest base of the population?

Should we perhaps seek to have WHO contract with the pharmaceutical industry on a "work for hire" basis to develop drugs for NTDs? Funding could come through the UN and through foundations. The IPs for these drugs would be owned by WHO and could be licensed for a nominal fee to plants located in the affected regions, thus providing economic benefits from the manufacturing of the drugs as well as reduced morbidity and mortality in the afflicted populations.

Other elements of enlightened self-interest exist as well. With globalization, a number of emerging infections are now affecting the most developed countries as well as the poorer ones, including cholera, diphtheria, measles, cyclospora, TB and multidrug resistant TB, and other bacterial infections.[164] Most recently, we've seen SARS (severe acute respiratory syndrome), avian influenza, and now Influenza A H1N1. SARS was stopped, in large part, by unparalleled global cooperation and sharing of scientific discoveries and resources. It is less certain that this will happen with the H1N1 flu.

The outlook for NTDs is improving, however, with important recent partnerships in addition to donations. For example, Sanofi-Aventis worked out a partnership with the Drugs for Neglected Diseases Initiative (DNDi) to develop fexinidazole, the only new drug in development for sleeping sickness, in addition to continuing to help WHO by supplying eflornithine. Doctors Without Borders provides kits to administer the IV medication. In 2008, the Nifurtimox-Eflornithine Combination Trial was completed successfully, with Bayer joining the partnership by donating the nifurtimox. The combo markedly shortens the need for IV therapy.[165]

Sanofi-Aventis further redeemed itself by selling its important antimalarial combination drug, artemisinin plus amodiaquine (ASAQ), to WHO at cost, less than $1 per treatment course.[166]

Merck is perhaps the best known for its very generous support of attempts to eradicate NTDs with ivermectin, for onchocerciasis and filariasis.

Other notable public-private partnerships in this area include the following:

- GlaxoSmithKline's research of new therapies for the big three of WHO's priority infectious diseases (malaria, TB, and HIV/AIDS) and donations of albendazole for lymphatic filariasis
- Merck and DND's focus on visceral leishmaniasis and Chagas disease (in addition to Merck's very generous donations)

- Merck KGaA, WHO, and MedPharm's Schistosomiasis Control Initiative, including praziquantel donations
- Pfizer's International Trachoma Initiative; Diflucan Donation Program for candidal esophagitis in AIDS (Africa); sharing of large chemical libraries with Medicine for Malaria Venture and DNDi for screening—searching for new chemical matter for malaria and kinetoplastid disease, respectively; WHO partnership whereby young scientists receive fellowships to work in research labs alongside experienced scientists and then return to their countries and set up their own labs and research; and WHO fellowship that allows developing world clinicians to join a development program and learn the art and science of clinical development—then return to their countries and educate others
- Sanofi-Aventis, Doctors Without Borders, and DNDi's partnership to develop ASAQ for malaria
- Johnson & Johnson's Children without Worms mebendazole donations for soil-transmitted helminth diseases
- Novartis's Institute for Tropical Diseases partnership with the Singapore Economic Development Board, researching dengue, TB, and malaria, and the Novartis Vaccines Institute for Global Health, focusing on diarrheal illnesses

It is heartening to see the changes that are gradually occurring.

It seems that a great deal of suffering could be alleviated and a substantial economic gain realized at a very reasonable cost if we were to find ways to enhance the development and distribution of drugs targeting NTDs, which affect 2.7 billion people, the poorest of the poor. In combination with policies targeting the health impacts of increased globalization noted above, a very real and important impact could be made in the lives of many, many people for a very small investment. In 2002, Kofi Anan reflected on the UN Millennium Development Goals, which include increasing access to food and safe drinking water and halting the incidence of HIV/AIDS and other infections. Noting the inextricable link between poverty, disease, and security, he said, paraphrasing Martin Luther King Jr., "Let us recognize that extreme poverty anywhere is a threat to human security everywhere. Let us recall that poverty is a denial of human rights. For the first time in history, in this age of unprecedented wealth and technical prowess, we have the power to save humanity from this shameful scourge. Let us summon the will to do it."[167]

Conclusion

It appears likely that ethical issues will remain a major topic of concern for the research clinician. The development, adoption, and diffusion of new technologies will generate new topics of debate. Issues affecting women, the use of fetal tissue, end of life concerns, the conduct of research in developing countries, poverty, and a myriad of other societal concerns will continue to demand increasing attention. Unfortunately, it appears that our society is becoming increasingly polarized around these issues. Given further scientific and medical advances, ethics will be a major topic to be carefully considered in the future, and it is an area of study worthy of being explored by all clinical investigators. (Suggestions for further reading and exploration are given in appendix B.) Our debates can and should be thoughtful and considered, opposing groups must truly listen to each other's concerns, and we must somehow find common ground.

CHAPTER 10

Opportunities and Training in Clinical Research

> Careers, like rockets, don't always take off on time.
> The trick is to always keep the engine running.
> —GARY SINISE

This chapter outlines an array of clinical research career options for physicians, coordinators, and people in related occupations.

While some reports about the outlook for the drug development industry in the United States have been rather gloomy, focusing on the significant shift overseas, others are quite optimistic. The Bureau of Labor Statistics' 2010–11 *Career Guide to Industries* attributes its encouraging perspective to the growth in the biotechnology industry; the aging population, who consume higher amounts of healthcare services; the increasing popularity of lifestyle drugs; and "the rising health consciousness and expectations of the general public." The news is particularly good for medical scientists: the BLS projects growth of 22–50 percent between 2008 and 2018.[1]

The outlook for coordinators and CRAs is also good over the next decade, with the BLS projecting an increase of approximately 20 percent, compared to a projected 11 percent increase for all industries combined. Yet surveys show that 75 percent of CRCs received no formal training in coordination on the job and that training needs to be standardized.[2]

Since the first edition, the number and variety of formal training options for coordinators and CRAs and those in the regulatory affairs and medical device related fields have increased greatly. Courses include those leading to associate's and bachelor's degrees, dual degree programs, and medical scientist training and are taught in both academic and clinical settings. The final section of this chapter, expanded in appendix C, lists specific professional training resources for physicians, for coordinators, and for other health professionals. A detailed list of programs, categorized by career goal, is available on my Web site (http://conductingclinicalresearch.com).

Enhancing Your Practice

Clinical research is a very effective way to augment and expand your practice. For example, as an active practitioner, you can use your experience with clinical trials to enhance your image as a local expert in your field. In addition to patient care, you can accept public speaking engagements about your trial experience, which can further serve as advertisement for your practice.

Medical practices are having increasing difficulty recruiting and retaining practitioners, particularly in rural and lower income areas. At the same time that this need is increasing, counterpressures are discouraging doctors from continuing in practice. Income has plateaued or diminished at the same time that overhead has skyrocketed. Much of this is due to personnel costs—increases in both salaries and benefits and an increase in the number of staff required for handling insurance authorizations, billing and coding, complying with HIPAA regulations, and meeting other clerical requirements. Staff benefits and malpractice insurance costs are skyrocketing while managed care is restricting visits and reimbursement.

Conducting clinical research can provide a welcome relief from the growing financial burden of practice management. It can subsidize the care of uninsured patients as well as provide a comfortable cushion of income that helps offset the losses from these other, increasingly expensive, areas of overhead.

The added income from clinical trials research can comfortably supplement your regular patient care income. However, substantial costs are involved, both financially and in terms of time invested. A 2002 CenterWatch survey of clinical trial study sites revealed the allocation of operating income as shown in figure 9.1.[3]

In terms of net profit, CenterWatch data suggest that a typical phase 3 trial receives a grant of $30,000: $3,000 per patient for 10 patients. Ten to 20 percent of this might be expected profit, if all goes well, or $3,000–$6,000 per study per year. Phase 2 trials, which involve dose finding, pharmacokinetics, and safety evaluations, are often more complicated; they are also better compensated.

Cullen Vogelson, experienced as a clinical research coordinator, monitor, and study manager, and a former assistant editor of *Modern Drug Discovery*, has written an excellent series of articles explaining clinical research.[4] He is more balanced and charitable in his assessment of physician motivation than is most of the news media. He observes, "Clinical research allows physicians to aid patients who cannot be helped by available treatments. It allows them to provide not just high quality, but often expensive, cutting-edge healthcare to those who lack even the most basic form of insurance. Finally, it provides a way for physicians to not only treat patients but also participate in the advancement of scientific knowledge and understanding that may lead to vast improvements in medicine for all."[5]

Brief Training Options

Research training opportunities in the medical school curriculum are still quite limited. Much research training is acquired informally, on the job.

1
THIS IS NOT LEGAL TENDER
AND SHALL NOT BE USED FOR SUCH
F285937448B
WASHINGTON
Salaries 58%
Patient recruitment 6%
Marketing and sales 4%
Training 3%
Overhead 17%
Operating profit 12%

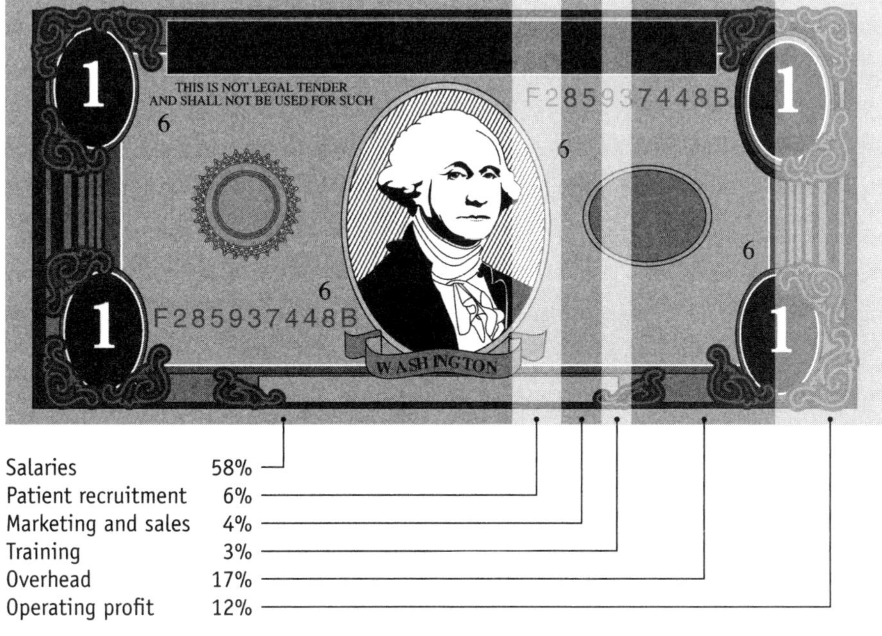

Figure 9.1 Where does the grant money go?

View from the Trenches

Living in an economically depressed rural community, I see many patients who avoid getting medical care or taking medicine because of the expense. Clinical trials provide free quality care to those who could not otherwise afford any care. The quality of my care has also certainly been enhanced by the education I receive, often from experts in their field, at investigator's meetings and conferences.

You can learn a great deal of useful information by attending investigator's meetings. I would highly recommend attending the meetings, especially if you are relatively new to clinical research or if you have little experience with a newer agent or a particular class of drug. Investigator's meetings are educational and are also a great way to meet interesting people and to network, often leading you to other study opportunities.

The investigator's meeting provides a crash course in all aspects of an investigational drug. It usually includes a scientific background presentation by a bench (research) scientist. Then the medical monitor reviews clinical data from earlier trials, if available. Pharmacokinetics of the drug are reviewed. The MRA or CRA will cover other topics relating to protocol implementation, gathering of pharmacoeconomic data, review of CRFs, and so on. Investigator's meetings are also likely to include presentations from laboratory personnel and regulatory folk. Most of the actual protocol conduct can be readily acquired from the CRA and the review of the protocol. Often, you will hear considerable discussion of pathophysiology and preclinical or early clinical testing that is quite useful and not as readily acquired elsewhere. Protocol design issues can generate intense arguments that are both educational and interesting. Sometimes the discussion revolves around the balance between what is intellectually the soundest way of analyzing a problem versus what is clinically practical. Often, discussion involves what the comparators should be or for how long treatment should be given or how much lab work is necessary. Heated discussions may occur over inclusion and exclusion criteria for selecting patients and whether investigators think that the trial will produce useful data. It is unlikely, however, that the sponsor will make substantive changes to the protocol at this stage unless very serious concerns are expressed.

Personally meeting and developing a relationship with the sponsor's team is also helpful. You can get a sense of what dealing with various individuals will be like that you simply can't acquire without the face-to-face contact. Additionally, the investigator's meeting is a useful place to network and meet others you might be able to work with in the future or share information with about upcoming trials. An added bonus of going to these meetings is that they are generally set in very nice locations as an incentive to boost attendance.

An effort is currently underway to better standardize physician training in research. Web-based training is available for ethics and good clinical practices at several sites. One particularly helpful site is that of the NIH (http://cme.cancer.gov/clinicaltrials/learning/humanparticipant-protections.asp).[6] Similar topics are covered at several universities' Web sites, such as those of the Washington University School of Medicine, the University of Iowa, and others listed in appendix C. Brief formal courses are available through groups such as the Drug Information Association (DIA), the Association of Clinical Research Professionals (ACRP), and the American Academy of Pharmaceutical Physicians. Certification, if you wish to pursue that, is available through the Certified Physician Investigator examination, offered by the American Academy of Pharmaceutical Physicians. "Introduction to the Principles and Practice of Clinical Research" is an innovative on-line video course developed by the NIH and available at http://www.nihtraining.com.[7]

I would also highly recommend initially working as a subinvestigator on a trial and getting on-the-job training in that manner. There is no better way of learning than by trying new things in gradual increments. Remember the medical school adage, "See one, do one, teach one"?

Formal Training Programs

Clinical research physicians are considered a rare and prized commodity. In 1966, more than half the NIH research grant recipients had medical degrees; in 1977 it was only one-third.[8] Between 1984 and 1999, the percentage of U.S. physician-scientists declined from 4.2 to 1.8 percent—and only a portion of these conduct patient-oriented research.[9] In 2000, Dr. David G. Kaufman, president of the Federation of American Societies for Experimental Biology (FASEB), testified before Congress regarding the critical shortfall in the number of physician-scientists, further noting that the proportion of physician researchers under the age of 45 was at an all-time low. He expressed that this was particularly troublesome as "young investigators

View from the Trenches

I had some on-the-job training during my fellowship, during which I designed and conducted a vaccine trial studying mucosal immunity in response to an oral vaccine. I received good mentoring on that project. But that brief clinical foray, and the subsequent months filtering spit and nasal secretions, then assaying antibody response by tissue culture and by an enzyme-linked assay (ELISA), was a far cry from conducting trials as a PI for commercial sponsors. Given my isolated practice setting, I had to learn about the industry's trials on my own, from my monitors, at investigator's meetings, and primarily from my variety of experiences.

I have since arranged training on my studies for some of my colleagues. They got a "no risk" opportunity to see what was involved in conducting a trial as well as some additional income. Their time involvement was limited, being scheduled for no more than 3 hours of study patient visits per week (for these particular trials), and generally less. I enjoyed the camaraderie and benefited by having access to additional patients as well as backup coverage for weekends and vacations. I urge you to explore this apprenticeship option.

have frequently been the source of the novel insights that have led to major scientific breakthroughs."[10]

The reasons for the shortfall are many. Medical training is woefully inadequate in preparing students to design and implement research protocols, and it is also lacking in preparation for the technical aspects of conducting research. Also, the increasingly heavy debt faced by graduating physicians is often molding career decisions. Young physicians, who are ill prepared for the business aspects of practice, are under severe constraints. As they are already struggling to balance managing debt, launching a career, and starting a family, many of them simply cannot fathom further continuing their education.[11]

The Association of American Medical Colleges' conference (see "Breaking the Scientific Bottleneck" in chapter 7) and the Institute of Medicine's Committee on Addressing Career Paths for Clinical Research brought recognition that there were few training opportunities for clinical investigators. The need for experts in "translational research"—those who can bridge the gap between pure bench research in molecular biology, cell biology and genetics, and clinical care—received particular recognition. Thus, physicians who can understand the implications and application of basic research for patient care are at a premium.[12]

Subsequently, programs to train such physicians have been developed across the country. These programs receive NIH grants to provide the infrastructure for training in clinical research careers, especially targeting those doctors with an academic bent. They fall under the umbrella of the NIH Roadmap initiative, administered via the NIH's National Center for Research Resources. In 2006, Clinical and Translational Science Awards (CTSAs) were granted to 12 academic centers to encourage clinical and translational research. By 2012, 60 academic health centers and their related institutions are expected to be part of the CTSA consortium.[13]

A common thread to these programs is a somewhat standardized curriculum designed to give clinical researchers from disparate disciplines a common language. Typical formal coursework includes the following:

- Epidemiology: for example, clinical trial design, observational study design, issues in bias, and methods of clinical measurement, including quality of life
- Biostatistics: basic biostatistics and computer-based training for data management and analysis
- Decision analysis: cost-effectiveness and meta-analysis
- Ethics: issues including informed consent and conflict of interest
- Legal and regulatory issues related to clinical research
- Skills: instruction in developing hypotheses, designing clinical research projects, writing grants, writing scientific papers, and making oral presentations

These programs are generally 2 years long, occasionally 3. They are a best buy and a remarkably good deal. For doctoral degree students, grants are available. The NIH explains the generosity of its grant, noting that the Clinical Research Loan Repayment Program is vital "to efforts to attract health professionals to careers in clinical research. In exchange for a 2-year commitment to clinical research, NIH will repay up to $35,000 per year of educational debt, pay an additional 39 percent of the repayments to cover your Federal taxes, and may reimburse state taxes resulting from these payments."[14] The 2-year commitment is for 20 or more hours per week. In 2003, 1,200 students applied and 730 received awards. A partial listing of career development awards training programs is presented in appendix C.

Conclusion

This chapter surveyed the major resources available to provide formal training in clinical research in both academic and clinical settings. The information regarding training programs is expanded in appendix C, where you will find specific resources for professional training for many research-related healthcare careers. You've also seen how you might enhance your own career, personally and financially, by taking professional training in clinical research.

Epilogue

> The future is not a gift: it is an achievement.
> Every generation helps make its own future.
> This is the essential challenge of the present.
> —ROBERT F. KENNEDY

You are now well equipped to venture out and join the exciting area of clinical research. You have in this book many of the resources that you will need, culled from more than 20 years of experience successfully conducting clinical trials in a solo practice. Your path should be infinitely easier. You just need to decide if this is what you really want to do—if it is, take the plunge.

I have tried to provide you with an exhaustive account of what is involved—from the tiniest mundane details to the emotionally gratifying aspects to the difficult and oftentimes ugly controversies you may encounter. While you will face tedious details and difficulties, I hope that you will experience the same sense of fulfillment that I do from working on developing new treatments for diseases and helping future generations and that you will allow the difficult issues you encounter to broaden your perspective and further your growth.

Before you move on to the appendices, I thought I'd elaborate on the personality characteristics of infectious disease doctors, as humorously (and insightfully) described by Julia Bess Frank in the *New England Journal of Medicine.*[1]

Laments of a Clinical Clerk

Of all my consultants, most easy to please
Is the fellow who comes from infectious disease.
His wants are so simple! His needs are so few!
Just gather some sputum, blood cultures times two,
X-ray the patient from guggle to zatch,
Examine the urine, both cath and clean catch;
It takes but a moment to do an L.P.,
Swab wound, throat and cervix, yank out the I.V.

When all of the data at last are collected,
The last culture plated, the last slide inspected,
The attending arrives to review and recap
(While intern and student enjoy a brief nap):
He broods with the air of a scribe with papyrus
And gives his opinion: "Most likely a virus.
Don't bother to fix it; can't treat it, can't cure it,
Though superinfection may later obscure it.
Should there be recurrence of fever or pain
Go back to square one and start over again!"

Appendices

APPENDIX A

Background Resource Information

Contents

Time Line of Drug Development and Drug Law Milestones 350

Trials Gone Wrong 356

Lessons Learned from the TeGenero Trial 359

World Medical Association Declaration of Helsinki 367

The Belmont Report: *Ethical Principles and Guidelines for the Protection of Human Subjects of Research* 373

Nuremberg Code Regulations 385

Time Line of Drug Development and Drug Law Milestones

This table provides more details to complement the historical highlights given in chapter 1.[1]

Year	Milestone	Status	Description
1813	Vaccine Act	U.S. law	Response to contaminated smallpox vaccines.
1848	Import Drugs Act	U.S. law	Response to counterfeit, contaminated, or adulterated drugs.
1880	Peter Collier, chief chemist, U.S. Department of Agriculture	Failed	First major attempt at passage of a national food and drug law—failed.
1902	Biologics Control Act	U.S. law	To ensure purity and safety of serums and vaccines.
1906	Food and Drugs Act	U.S. law	Required "only that drugs meet standards of strength and purity. The burden of proof was on FDA to show that a drug's labeling was false and fraudulent before it could be taken off the market."[2]
1911	U.S. v. Johnson	Supreme Court ruling	Found that the 1906 Food and Drugs Act does not prohibit false claims of efficacy—but does prohibit false or misleading statements about the ingredients or identity of a drug.
1938	Food, Drug, and Cosmetic (FD&C) Act of 1938	U.S. law in response to "Elixir Sulfanilamide," which led to 107 deaths	"For the first time, required a manufacturer to prove the safety of a drug before it could be marketed."[3] Established the need for human trials before approval and marketing.
1939	Food and Drug Administration	Established first standards for processed food.	
1945	Penicillin Amendment	Amendment to the 1938 FD&C Act	Required FDA certification of all penicillin for safety and efficacy; later extended to all antibiotics. Abolished in 1983.
1947	Nuremberg Code[4]	International code of ethics in response to World War II war crimes	Informed consent required for experiments. Benefit to science must be weighed against risks and suffering of experimental subjects. See chapter 7, "Ethical Issues in Human Subjects Research."

Year	Milestone	Status	Description
1949	International Code of Medical Ethics of the World Medical Association, including the Declaration of Geneva[5]	International code of professional ethics	A physician shall act only in the patient's interest when providing medical care. See chapter 7.
1951	Durham-Humphrey Amendment	U.S. law "Caution: Federal law prohibits . . ."	Required "that any drug be labeled for sale by prescription only." Defined prescription drugs as those "unsafe for self-medication."[6]
1958	Food Additives Amendment Delaney Proviso	Amendment to the FD&C Act	Required food additive manufacturers to demonstrate safety. Prohibited food additives shown to be carcinogenic in animals or people.
1962	Kefauver-Harris Amendments to the 1938 FD&C Act Public Law 87-781; 76 Stat. 788-89	First U.S. law requiring informed consent[7] A direct response to the thalidomide disaster in 1961, in which the use of that drug during pregnancy was found to be associated with severe congenital anomalies, called fetal amelia and phocomelia, in which arms and legs develop only as small, weblike limbs8	Empowered the FDA to ban drug experiments in humans pending animal trials for safety. Mandated informed consent from patients receiving nonapproved drugs. Required firms to prove efficacy as well as safety of their drugs; applied retroactively to 1938.Required reporting of adverse events to the FDA. Required drug advertising to report risks as well as benefits.
1963	FDA regulations 21 CFR 130.3, later incorporated in 45 CFR 46 (see below)	U.S. regulations	Clinical investigators required to certify that informed consent was properly obtained.
1964	Declaration of Helsinki signed by United States (revised in 1975, 1983, 1989)	International ethical guidelines	Expanded ethical and informed consent requirements, especially for minors and consent by surrogates. See "Historical Context" in chapter 7.
1965	HR 2, Drug Abuse Control Amendments of 1965	U.S. regulations in response to Bay of Pigs invasion	Counterfeit drug ban.[9]

Year	Milestone	Status	Description
1966	U.S. Surgeon General policy statement to the Heads of the Institutions Conducting Research with Public Health Service Grants	U.S. policy	Origin of Institutional Review Boards (IRBs). Required that all human subject research undergo independent review prior to implementation.
1966	FDA Regulations 21 CFR 130.37, later incorporated in 45 CFR 46 (see below)	U.S. regulations	Defined specific elements and requirements of informed consent.
1966	Guidelines for Reproductive Studies for Safety Evaluation of Drugs for Human Use	U.S. regulations	Refined requirements for developmental testing and assessing teratogenic effects.[10]
1974–1978	Regulations for the Protection of Human Subjects of Biomedical and Behavioral Research[11] 45 CFR 46	U.S. regulations Subpart B Subpart C	Established IRB procedures. Provided special protections for pregnant women and fetuses. Provided special protections for prisoners.
1979	Belmont Report issued by the National Commission for the Protection of Human Subjects of Biomedical and Behavioral Research[12]	U.S. ethical guidelines	Set out principles of respect, beneficence, and justice. See "Historical Context" in chapter 7.
1980–1983	President's Commission for the Study of Ethical Problems in Medicine and Biomedical and Behavioral Research (President's Commission)	Recommendations became basis of 10 CFR 745 ("Common Rule"), below	Recommended that all federal agencies adopt the human subject regulations of the Department of Health and Human Services (DHHS, formerly DHEW).
1981	FDA regulations revised regarding informed consent (21 CFR 50) and IRBs (21 CFR 56)	U.S. regulations	Revised to correspond to DHHS regulations.
1983	Anti-Tampering Act	U.S. law	Required tamper-resistant packaging; made tampering a crime.

Year	Milestone	Status	Description
1983	45 CFR 46 Subpart D	U.S. regulations	Special protections for children.
1983	Orphan Drug Act	U.S. regulations	Provided incentives for developing drugs for rare diseases, including major tax deductions and exclusive marketing rights.
1984	Drug Price Competition and Patent Term Restoration Act, aka "Hatch-Waxman Amendments"; 180-day generic drug exclusivity http://www.fda.gov.cder	U.S. regulations	Extended patent life by up to 5 years to compensate patent holders for marketing time lost during development and approval. Established the Abbreviated New Drug Application (ANDA) approval process, permitting generic versions of approved drugs to be approved without a full New Drug Application. Granted market exclusivity incentive to the first generic applicant.
1991	Common Federal Policy for the Protection of Human Subjects ("Common Rule") 10 CFR 745	U.S. regulations	Sixteen agencies adopted the regulations of 45 CFR 46 subpart A. Many adopted subparts B, C, D.
1988–1992	FDA Expanded Access and Expedited Approval of New Therapies Related to HIV/AIDS—Interim	U.S. regulations prompted by AIDS activism	Provided expedited approval of drugs for serious and life-threatening diseases (AIDS).
	Final rule[13]		Allowed that phase 2 studies may provide adequate data to support approval.
		Surrogate end points	Allowed approval of drugs based on surrogate end points that reasonably predict that a drug provides clinical benefit.
1992	Prescription Drug User Fee Act (PDUFA)	U.S. law	Requires pharmaceutical industry to pay application fees, which are used to hire more reviewers to speed the approval process.
1995	Final report of Advisory Committee on Human Radiation Experiments (created in 1994)[14]	Report	Addressed issues for when research must be kept secret.
1995–2001	National Bioethics Advisory Commission (NBAC)[15]	Report	Series of ethical and policy reports.

Year	Milestone	Status	Description
1996	FDA regulations revised 21 CFR 50.24	U.S. regulations	Allowed exceptions from informed consent for research studies involving emergency research.
1996	International Conference on Harmonisation, Guideline E6: Good Clinical Practice, Consolidated Guidance	International guidelines	Established good clinical practices guidelines as an international standard that provides public assurance that trial subjects are protected. United States, European Union, and Japan are all signatories.
2000	World Health Organization Operational Guidelines for Ethics Committees That Review Biomedical Research[16]	International guidelines	Guidance with roles and requirements for ethics committees around the world.
2001	Best Pharmaceuticals for Children Act[17] Suspension of Rule requiring pediatric studies of medicines for children[18]	U.S. law	Encouraged studies of drugs in children. Provided incentives for manufacturers to conduct pediatric trials.
2002	FDA Rule on Products to Treat Exposure to Toxic Substances[19]	U.S. regulations	Response to terrorism; emergency preparedness.
2002[19]	Medical Device User Fee and Modernization Act	U.S. law	Like PDUFA, requires device manufacturers to fund inspections.
2003	Pediatric Research Equity Act	U.S. law	Requires research into pediatric applications for new drugs and biological products.
2004	Project BioShield	U.S. law	Authorizes FDA to expedite its review procedures for counterterrorism.
2004	Critical Path Initiative (CPI)	FDA	New strategy "to tackle the steep decline in the number of innovative medical products being submitted for approval—and getting to patients—despite the enormous breakthroughs being made in biomedical science."[20]
2007	Food and Drug Administration Amendments Act (FDAAA)	U.S. law	Requires a plan for pediatric testing before adult studies are complete.
2007	Sentinel Initiative	Part of FDAAA	Requires "active surveillance" for risks postmarketing.

Year	Milestone	Status	Description
2007	Clinical Trials Registry	Part of FDAAA	Expands the types of clinical trials that must be registered at ClinicalTrials.gov and the type of data that must be submitted. Will prevent negative outcomes in trials from being hidden.
2008	FDA Clinical Trials Transformation Initiative (CTTI)	Part of FDAAA	Formed a public-private task force to improve monitoring and reporting of AEs.
2008	Genetic Information Nondiscrimination Act (GINA)	U.S. law	Protects genetic information from being used against individuals in employment or health insurability.
2008	Acceptance of Foreign Clinical Trial Data	FDA	No longer requires non-U.S. trials to be conducted under the Declaration of Helsinki standards. Also addresses multiregional trials.
2008	*Riegel v. Medtronic*	Supreme Court ruling[21]	"Preemption": device manufacturers cannot be sued under state law if the device received marketing approval from the FDA.
2009	American Recovery and Reinvestment Act (ARRA)	U.S. law	Provides $10 billion for "scientific research and facilities" through 2010.
2009	Health Information Technology for Economic and Clinical Health Act (HITECH Act)	Part of ARRA	Requirements for electronic medical records.
2009	Executive Order 13505: "Removing Barriers to Responsible Scientific Research involving Human Stem Cells"		Rescinded some restrictions on federal funding for human embryonic stem cell research.
2009	IRB registry	Code of Federal Regulations (45 CFR 46)	Required if the research is conducted or supported by DHHS.
2009	Wyeth v. Levine	Supreme Court ruling[22]	No preemption for drug manufacturers

Trials Gone Wrong

This table provides more details on the rationale and need for strict safety measures in clinical trials, as discussed in chapter 4.

Case	Problem	Issue	Charge	Outcome	Lessons learned
Kathryn Hamilton v. Hutchinson Cancer Research Center	Consent	Lack of informed consent; financial conflict of interest	Patient not informed of risks and ineffectiveness of drugs nor of significant financial conflict of interest.	Patient died	Oversight and financial disclosures are needed.
Cheryl Mathias, whistleblower against University of Oklahoma melanoma trial		Lack of informed consent	PI lied to patients about risks.		
***Nicole Wan v. University of Rochester* (continued on next page)**	Study conduct	Experience of investigator	Intern allowed to do a bronchoscopy.	19-year-old healthy volunteer died of lidocaine (an approved and widely used drug) toxicity.	Safety net must include adequate training and supervision of investigator.
	Protocol	Inadequate safeguard	Failure to establish maximum dose of lidocaine for healthy subjects		Have safety net: limit amount of lidocaine on procedure tray.
	Protocol	Inadequate safeguard	No statement in protocol that procedure was to be terminated if lidocaine exceeded specified amount		Specify safeguards.
	Data/ regulation	Lack of documentation	No log of amount of lidocaine and timing of administration	Required better documentation.	Call off procedure if documentation is inadequate.

Case	Problem	Issue	Charge	Outcome	Lessons learned
***Nicole Wan v. University of Rochester*, continued**	Study conduct	Lack of monitoring	Patient was discharged despite reporting feeling poorly.	NY required research procedures on healthy volunteers to offer all safety precautions as provided to clinical patients.	Better monitoring and procedures for follow-up
Jesse Gelsinger	Preclinical safety	Lack of consent	Final consent omitted information that monkeys had died from prescriptions.	18-year-old volunteer died.	
	Protocol (dose escalation)	Safety reporting of AEs ignored	PI failed to report adverse events in earlier subjects to FDA.	PI disbarred; civil suit filed.	
	Recruitment/ consent	Coercion in recruiting	Description included "very low doses" and "promising results."		
	IRB	Financial conflict of interest	University of Pennsylvania researchers held patents and stock holdings, not disclosed.		Financial conflict of interest reporting requirements were tightened.
	Study conduct	Gross protocol violation	Two prior subjects developed liver toxicity that should have stopped the trial.		Better oversight is needed—monitoring and IRB.
	Study conduct	Major protocol violation	Gelsinger's ammonia level exceeded allowable inclusion criteria.		Entry criteria should not be altered by PI.

Case	Problem	Issue	Charge	Outcome	Lessons learned
Ellen Roche v. Johns	Protocol	Lack of adequate background research	Prior reports of hexamethonium toxicity and withdrawal were not heeded.	Healthy 24-year-old volunteer in asthma study died.	Thorough literature search prior to research is required.
	IRB	Inadequate IRB review and oversight	One IRB, meeting every 2 weeks, responsible for 800 new proposals and annual reviews.		More IRBs were established.
			Culture viewed oversight process as a barrier to research rather than a safeguard.		
	Recruit-ment	Possible coercion	Roche worked in Hopkins asthma center.		Avoid enrolling friends, family, employees.
	Study conduct	Inhalation medication not properly prepared			
	Regula-tory, IRB	IND was not sought or required by IRB			
	Regulatory		PI failed to report prior AEs.		
	Consent	Volunteer not told of hexamonium risks			
Suzanne Davenport	Consent, subject injury	Who pays for subject injury unclear			
TeGenero	Consent				

Lessons Learned from the TeGenero Trial

This table is a summary of some of the major criticisms of the TeGenero trial (discussed in chapter 8) gleaned from literature and experts, as well as their suggestions for how to prevent such a disaster from ever recurring.

Element of trial	Criticism/violation	Lessons learned
STUDY DESIGN		
Dosing is typically given to subjects at staggered intervals, allowing for detection of adverse events before proceeding with other subjects. In some studies, an additional safety measure is taken by administering a tiny "test dose" before the regular dose.	"TGN1412 study personnel administered the study drug in quick order without test doses, at about ten-minute intervals. As it turned out, obvious negative reactions to the drug appeared in the first subjects before the study drug was administered to the last subjects. The question is thus why administration continued despite the initial negative reactions."[23]	Minimum dosing intervals between subjects should be specified, especially for early phase studies.
While referring to dose escalation between groups, the informed consent form (ICF) states, "the next scheduled dose will be confirmed only after the review of all relevant safety data of the preceding group. Therefore . . . may be subject to change based on this safety data."[24]	The subjects, all in group 1, received the investigational drug at about 10-minute intervals.	This type of dosing is irresponsible for a first-in-human trial, especially of an immune-affecting drug.
Initial dosing is often established as 1/10 of the "No observable adverse effect level" (NOAEL). For this study, "human equivalent dose" and safety margins led to a starting dose of 0.1 milligrams per kilogram (mg/kg), or 100 micrograms per kilogram (μ/kg) or a 160-fold safety margin.	Using Minimal Anticipated Biological Effect Level (MABEL) and the Committee for Medicinal Products for Human Use's "Position Paper on Non-Clinical Safety Studies to Support Clinical Trials with a Single Microdose" would have resulted in a starting dose of 5 μ/kg.[25]	Dosing should perhaps be based on the Minimal Anticipated Biological Effect Level.

Element of trial	Criticism/violation	Lessons learned
In animal studies, "moderate elevations of IL-2, IL-5 and IL-6 serum levels were observed upon TGN1412 treatment in individual animals, however, no clinical signs of a first-dose cytokine release syndrome (CRS) were observed."[26]	Investigators knew the dose given to monkeys was pharmacologically active at 5 mg/kg.	
An IV bolus of the study drug was administered.		Slow IV infusion over hours is more appropriate, allowing stopping if AEs develop.
Healthy volunteers were used as test subjects.		First-in-human tests should be considered in patients rather than in healthy volunteers (especially for oncology drugs).
Limited backup coverage was in place. "Since only a weak increase in cytokine levels were observed at 5 mg/kg TGN1412 in cynomolgus monkeys, no CRS is expected . . . subjects will be closely monitored for first-dose CRS."[27]	Limited 24-hour coverage was in place, and not at level of expertise to support this magnitude of SAE. No specific provisions for monitoring were included in the protocol.[28]	Better contingency plans must be in place, or such initial studies should be done in an ICU. Consider specialized Phase 1 units.[29]
IRB APPROVAL		
The IRB approved the study.	How much expertise was on the panel that approved this study? Did the panel include immunologists? How much did the panelists rely on information from the investigator and sponsor?	Experts should participate in an independent literature review as part of the IRB review.
ADHERENCE TO PROTOCOL/GCP		
Investigator training and experience should adhere to GCP.	"MHRA Inspectors were not satisfied that the individual (physician) had adequate training and experience for their role."[30]	Better oversight is needed by the sponsor and CRO, as well as the IRB, of the level of experience required to conduct a trial safely.

Element of trial	Criticism/violation	Lessons learned
Blinding procedures should adhere to GCP.	"The placebo volunteers were permitted to leave the trial before appropriate checks were undertaken to confirm that they were the two subjects that had received the placebo."[31]	Careful unblinding checks and SOPs are needed.
READABILITY OF CONSENT		
Consent forms are required to be "understandable" and are typically pitched at no higher than eighth grade level.	"The TGN1412 ICF is written at the 14th-grade (2nd-year of college) level. 29 percent of the sentences are written at a graduate school level."[32]	See "Health Literacy and Informed Consent" in chapter 5. Consents should be reviewed for readability.
BIASED LANGUAGE		
"Expert advice from immunologists has been sought in designing the protocol to minimise your risks, including a robust screening process that takes into account your immune status, and repeated *thorough* assessments of immune function," " . . . the following unintended effects may *theoretically* be encountered during any trial with a monoclonal antibody drug . . . ," "At the end of the study (on Day 43) you will be asked to return to the Unit to give blood and urine samples for *routine analysis*," and "This study has been *carefully* reviewed and approved by an Independent Research Ethics Committee. One of the obligations of the Committee is to safeguard the interests of volunteers."[33] "[T]hose for whom the trial would not be safe are literally 'screened out.'"[34]		Words that tend to downplay risks—"robust screening," "thorough assessments," "theoretically" a problem, "carefully reviewed and approved"—should be avoided.

Element of trial	Criticism/violation	Lessons learned
RECRUITMENT		
Recruitment should not employ excessive inducement.	"The TGN1412 study's subject recruitment posting at www.drugtrial.co.uk stated, 'You'll have plenty of time to read or study or just relax—with digital TV, pool table, videogames, DVD player and now FREE Internet access! You can even just catch up on some sleep!'"[35] "For your time, and to compensate for any inconvenience, a payment of £2000 will be made on completion of the study."[36]	A vacation and £2000 for 3 nights and a few follow-ups sounds pretty good. How did the IRB approve this?
INSURANCE COVERAGE		
The sponsor needs adequate insurance.	Insurance coverage was not confirmed.	The investigator has a duty to be sure the sponsor has adequate insurance to cover for catastrophes and that the clinical trial agreement provides subject injury protections.
HELSINKI REQUIREMENTS		
"Medical research involving human subjects must . . . be based on a thorough knowledge of the scientific literature . . . and on adequate laboratory and, where appropriate, animal experimentation" (principle 11).	Among other articles, "a 2002 article in the Journal of Clinical Immunology warned that 'caution should be taken in the development of immunotherapies targeting [T cell] costimulatory pathways' such as the CD28 receptor."[37]	Experts should participate in an independent literature review as part of the IRB review.

Element of trial	Criticism/violation	Lessons learned
"Every medical research project involving human subjects should be preceded by careful assessment of predictable risks and burdens in comparison with foreseeable benefits to the subject or to others" (principle 16).	Risks are buried on page 6. "The study protocol states that, after administration of TGN1412, a 'cytokine storm,' defined as a 'massive cytokine release,' 'may theoretically be encountered.' In the ICF, the 'cytokine storm' is downgraded to a 'cytokine release,' a much less intimidating term. The ICF states that '. . . unintended effects may theoretically' include '. . . cytokine release (causing a hives-like allergic reaction) . . . .'"[38]	See "Health Literacy and Informed Consent," in chapter 5, which recommends putting risks on the first page.
"The subjects must be volunteers and informed participants in the research project" (principle 20).	"Statements such as 'Risk of anaphylaxis applies to all studies at PAREXEL, with drugs at every stage of development [and the staff are well trained in anticipation of this (unlikely) possibility. Anaphylaxis could occur any time you encounter any new drug, cosmetic or even foodstuff in a restaurant (peanuts and shellfish are famous for causing it)]' and 'any drug can cause a serious allergic reaction in susceptible individuals. For example, penicillin and even aspirin can be life-threatening to some people,' may be factually correct but tend to downplay these risks."[39]	The consent greatly minimized risks, particularly given the nature of the study. The IRB should have caught this. (On the other hand, sometimes we all make such analogies to try to simplify the consent and make it more understandable and relevant to subjects' prior experiences.)

Element of trial	Criticism/violation	Lessons learned
ELEMENTS IN THE INFORMED CONSENT		
"The trial treatment(s) and the probability for random assignment to each treatment." . . . [ICH]	"ICH requires a statement of the randomization probabilities, which is missing. Instead, the statement ' . . . volunteers will be "randomized" to receive either a single dose of the study drug or a placebo' implies a 50:50 randomization ratio. The actual ratio was 3:1 study drug to placebo."[40]	Informed consents must be accurate and explicit in informed consent.
"The anticipated prorated payment, if any, to the subject for participating in the trial. [ICH]"	"The calculation of the prorated payment is not disclosed in the statement 'If you withdraw from the study prior to completion, you will be paid on a proportional basis.'[41] The ICF states, "I understand that my rights to compensation may be affected . . . if I fail to adhere to the requirements of the study." No further detail is given. [42]	Payment should be prorated on a scale so as to be clear and noncoercive—for example, payment per visit or event—rather than requiring completion.
"The anticipated expenses, if any, to the subject for participating in the trial. [ICH] Any additional costs to the subject that may result from participation in the research. [CFR]" (Twelve visits were required after the initial overnight stays, over a period of 10 weeks.)	"The ICF says the stipend is to 'compensate for any inconvenience,' without mentioning transportation and other costs related to regular and extra visits, which, however, should be obvious to the subject. As of April 9, 2006, one of the injured Subjects, Rob O., has been paying his own, 50 cab fares for follow-up medical care visits without reimbursement."[43]	Informed consents need to be specific as to what is covered by the sponsor.

Element of trial	Criticism/violation	Lessons learned
"The compensation and/or treatment available to the subject in the event of trial-related injury. [ICH] For research involving more than minimal risk, an explanation as to whether any compensation and an explanation as to whether any medical treatments are available if injury occurs and, if so, what they consist of, or where further information may be obtained. [CFR]"	"According to guidelines laid down by the Association of the British Pharmaceutical Industry, Sponsor compensates 'for any significant deterioration in health or well-being caused directly by your participation in the study.' The National Health Service presumably provides free treatment for minor medical care and injuries that are indirectly caused by the study. Foreign nationals (who, according the protocol, are not excluded from participating) may not be covered by the National Health Service and therefore may not have coverage for minor medical care."[44]	Volunteers must be protected. The investigators should be sure insurance coverage is available and that compensation is spelled out in the CTA and informed consent.
"A contact point where [the subject] may obtain further information about the trial. [MHU] The person(s) to contact for further information regarding the trial and the rights of trial subjects, and whom to contact in the event of trial-related injury. [ICH] An explanation of whom to contact for answers to pertinent questions about the research and research subjects' rights, and whom to contact in the event of a research-related injury to the subject. [CFR]"	"The statement 'If you have any point of concern, before during or after the study, you can discuss this with the Principal Investigator or Unit Medical Director, *then* you may approach the Ethics Committee . . . ' [Italics added] potentially puts the subject in a very awkward situation if he/she wants to contact the Ethics Committee, which is unidentified in the ICF."[45]	Subjects must be provided with freely available IRB or ethics committee contacts.

Element of trial	Criticism/violation	Lessons learned
"The subject [may] withdraw from the trial at any time. [MHU] The subject's participation in the trial is voluntary and the subject may refuse to participate or withdraw from the trial, at any time, without penalty or loss of benefits to which the subject is otherwise entitled. [ICH] Participation is voluntary, refusal to participate will involve no penalty or loss of benefits to which the subject is otherwise entitled, and the subject may discontinue participation at any time without penalty or loss of benefits to which the subject is otherwise entitled. The consequences of a subject's decision to withdraw from the research and procedures for orderly termination of participation by the subject. [CFR]"	"The statement 'If you leave the study and exercise your right not to give a reason, . . . no payment need be made to you' is a significant penalty for subjects who are participating for financial compensation. Of course, the Subject can provide a false reason. Paying the stipend at completion of the study may coerce the Subject to stay to the end of a study that may have a duration as long as 'approximately 10 weeks.'"[46]	Coercion must be avoided.

World Medical Association Declaration of Helsinki

Ethical Principles for Medical Research Involving Human Subjects

Adopted by the 18th WMA General Assembly, Helsinki, Finland, June 1964, and amended by the:

- 29th WMA General Assembly, Tokyo, Japan, October 1975
- 35th WMA General Assembly, Venice, Italy, October 1983
- 41st WMA General Assembly, Hong Kong, September 1989
- 48th WMA General Assembly, Somerset West, Republic of South Africa, October 1996
- 52nd WMA General Assembly, Edinburgh, Scotland, October 2000
- 53rd WMA General Assembly, Washington 2002 (Note of Clarification on paragraph 29 added)
- 55th WMA General Assembly, Tokyo 2004 (Note of Clarification on Paragraph 30 added)
- 59th WMA General Assembly, Seoul, October 2008

A. INTRODUCTION

1. The World Medical Association (WMA) has developed the Declaration of Helsinki as a statement of ethical principles for medical research involving human subjects, including research on identifiable human material and data. The Declaration is intended to be read as a whole and each of its constituent paragraphs should not be applied without consideration of all other relevant paragraphs.
2. Although the Declaration is addressed primarily to physicians, the WMA encourages other participants in medical research involving human subjects to adopt these principles.
3. It is the duty of the physician to promote and safeguard the health of patients, including those who are involved in medical research. The physician's knowledge and conscience are dedicated to the fulfilment of this duty.
4. The Declaration of Geneva of the WMA binds the physician with the words, "The health of my patient will be my first consideration," and the International Code of Medical Ethics declares that, "A physician shall act in the patient's best interest when providing medical care."
5. Medical progress is based on research that ultimately must include studies involving human subjects. Populations that are underrepresented in medical research should be provided appropriate access to participation in research.

6. In medical research involving human subjects, the well-being of the individual research subject must take precedence over all other interests.

7. The primary purpose of medical research involving human subjects is to understand the causes, development and effects of diseases and improve preventive, diagnostic and therapeutic interventions (methods, procedures and treatments). Even the best current interventions must be evaluated continually through research for their safety, effectiveness, efficiency, accessibility and quality.

8. In medical practice and in medical research, most interventions involve risks and burdens.

9. Medical research is subject to ethical standards that promote respect for all human subjects and protect their health and rights. Some research populations are particularly vulnerable and need special protection. These include those who cannot give or refuse consent for themselves and those who may be vulnerable to coercion or undue influence.

10. Physicians should consider the ethical, legal and regulatory norms and standards for research involving human subjects in their own countries as well as applicable international norms and standards. No national or international ethical, legal or regulatory requirement should reduce or eliminate any of the protections for research subjects set forth in this Declaration.

B. PRINCIPLES FOR ALL MEDICAL RESEARCH

11. It is the duty of physicians who participate in medical research to protect the life, health, dignity, integrity, right to self-determination, privacy, and confidentiality of personal information of research subjects.

12. Medical research involving human subjects must conform to generally accepted scientific principles, be based on a thorough knowledge of the scientific literature, other relevant sources of information, and adequate laboratory and, as appropriate, animal experimentation. The welfare of animals used for research must be respected.

13. Appropriate caution must be exercised in the conduct of medical research that may harm the environment.

14. The design and performance of each research study involving human subjects must be clearly described in a research protocol. The protocol should contain a statement of the ethical considerations involved and should indicate how the principles in this Declaration have been addressed. The protocol should include information regarding funding, sponsors, institutional affiliations, other potential conflicts of interest, incentives for subjects and provisions for treating and/or compensating subjects who are harmed as a consequence of participation in the research study. The protocol should describe arrangements

for post-study access by study subjects to interventions identified as beneficial in the study or access to other appropriate care or benefits.

15. The research protocol must be submitted for consideration, comment, guidance and approval to a research ethics committee before the study begins. This committee must be independent of the researcher, the sponsor and any other undue influence. It must take into consideration the laws and regulations of the country or countries in which the research is to be performed as well as applicable international norms and standards but these must not be allowed to reduce or eliminate any of the protections for research subjects set forth in this Declaration. The committee must have the right to monitor ongoing studies. The researcher must provide monitoring information to the committee, especially information about any serious adverse events. No change to the protocol may be made without consideration and approval by the committee.
16. Medical research involving human subjects must be conducted only by individuals with the appropriate scientific training and qualifications. Research on patients or healthy volunteers requires the supervision of a competent and appropriately qualified physician or other health care professional. The responsibility for the protection of research subjects must always rest with the physician or other health care professional and never the research subjects, even though they have given consent.
17. Medical research involving a disadvantaged or vulnerable population or community is only justified if the research is responsive to the health needs and priorities of this population or community and if there is a reasonable likelihood that this population or community stands to benefit from the results of the research.
18. Every medical research study involving human subjects must be preceded by careful assessment of predictable risks and burdens to the individuals and communities involved in the research in comparison with foreseeable benefits to them and to other individuals or communities affected by the condition under investigation.
19. Every clinical trial must be registered in a publicly accessible database before recruitment of the first subject.
20. Physicians may not participate in a research study involving human subjects unless they are confident that the risks involved have been adequately assessed and can be satisfactorily managed. Physicians must immediately stop a study when the risks are found to outweigh the potential benefits or when there is conclusive proof of positive and beneficial results.
21. Medical research involving human subjects may only be conducted if the importance of the objective outweighs the inherent risks and burdens to the research subjects.

22. Participation by competent individuals as subjects in medical research must be voluntary. Although it may be appropriate to consult family members or community leaders, no competent individual may be enrolled in a research study unless he or she freely agrees.

23. Every precaution must be taken to protect the privacy of research subjects and the confidentiality of their personal information and to minimize the impact of the study on their physical, mental and social integrity.

24. In medical research involving competent human subjects, each potential subject must be adequately informed of the aims, methods, sources of funding, any possible conflicts of interest, institutional affiliations of the researcher, the anticipated benefits and potential risks of the study and the discomfort it may entail, and any other relevant aspects of the study. The potential subject must be informed of the right to refuse to participate in the study or to withdraw consent to participate at any time without reprisal. Special attention should be given to the specific information needs of individual potential subjects as well as to the methods used to deliver the information. After ensuring that the potential subject has understood the information, the physician or another appropriately qualified individual must then seek the potential subject's freely-given informed consent, preferably in writing. If the consent cannot be expressed in writing, the non-written consent must be formally documented and witnessed.

25. For medical research using identifiable human material or data, physicians must normally seek consent for the collection, analysis, storage and/or reuse. There may be situations where consent would be impossible or impractical to obtain for such research or would pose a threat to the validity of the research. In such situations the research may be done only after consideration and approval of a research ethics committee.

26. When seeking informed consent for participation in a research study the physician should be particularly cautious if the potential subject is in a dependent relationship with the physician or may consent under duress. In such situations the informed consent should be sought by an appropriately qualified individual who is completely independent of this relationship.

27. For a potential research subject who is incompetent, the physician must seek informed consent from the legally authorized representative. These individuals must not be included in a research study that has no likelihood of benefit for them unless it is intended to promote the health of the population represented by the potential subject, the research cannot instead be performed with competent persons, and the research entails only minimal risk and minimal burden.

28. When a potential research subject who is deemed incompetent is able to give assent to decisions about participation in research, the physician must seek that assent in addition to the consent of the legally authorized representative. The potential subject's dissent should be respected.

29. Research involving subjects who are physically or mentally incapable of giving consent, for example, unconscious patients, may be done only if the physical or mental condition that prevents giving informed consent is a necessary characteristic of the research population. In such circumstances the physician should seek informed consent from the legally authorized representative. If no such representative is available and if the research cannot be delayed, the study may proceed without informed consent provided that the specific reasons for involving subjects with a condition that renders them unable to give informed consent have been stated in the research protocol and the study has been approved by a research ethics committee. Consent to remain in the research should be obtained as soon as possible from the subject or a legally authorized representative.

30. Authors, editors and publishers all have ethical obligations with regard to the publication of the results of research. Authors have a duty to make publicly available the results of their research on human subjects and are accountable for the completeness and accuracy of their reports. They should adhere to accepted guidelines for ethical reporting. Negative and inconclusive as well as positive results should be published or otherwise made publicly available. Sources of funding, institutional affiliations and conflicts of interest should be declared in the publication. Reports of research not in accordance with the principles of this Declaration should not be accepted for publication.

C. ADDITIONAL PRINCIPLES FOR MEDICAL RESEARCH COMBINED WITH MEDICAL CARE

31. The physician may combine medical research with medical care only to the extent that the research is justified by its potential preventive, diagnostic or therapeutic value and if the physician has good reason to believe that participation in the research study will not adversely affect the health of the patients who serve as research subjects.

32. The benefits, risks, burdens and effectiveness of a new intervention must be tested against those of the best current proven intervention, except in the following circumstances:

    - The use of placebo, or no treatment, is acceptable in studies where no current proven intervention exists; or
    - Where for compelling and scientifically sound methodological reasons the use of placebo is necessary to determine the efficacy or safety of an intervention and the patients who receive placebo or no treatment will not be subject to any risk of serious or irreversible harm. Extreme care must be taken to avoid abuse of this option.

33. At the conclusion of the study, patients entered into the study are entitled to be informed about the outcome of the study and to share any benefits that result from it, for example, access to interventions identified as beneficial in the study or to other appropriate care or benefits.

34. The physician must fully inform the patient which aspects of the care are related to the research. The refusal of a patient to participate in a study or the patient's decision to withdraw from the study must never interfere with the patient-physician relationship.

35. In the treatment of a patient, where proven interventions do not exist or have been ineffective, the physician, after seeking expert advice, with informed consent from the patient or a legally authorized representative, may use an unproven intervention if in the physician's judgement it offers hope of saving life, re-establishing health or alleviating suffering. Where possible, this intervention should be made the object of research, designed to evaluate its safety and efficacy. In all cases, new information should be recorded and, where appropriate, made publicly available.

The Belmont Report: *Ethical Principles and Guidelines for the Protection of Human Subjects of Research*

The National Commission for the Protection of Human Subjects of Biomedical and Behavioral Research

April 18, 1979

AGENCY: Department of Health, Education, and Welfare.

ACTION: Notice of Report for Public Comment.

SUMMARY: On July 12, 1974, the National Research Act (Pub. L. 93-348) was signed into law, there-by creating the National Commission for the Protection of Human Subjects of Biomedical and Behavioral Research. One of the charges to the Commission was to identify the basic ethical principles that should underlie the conduct of biomedical and behavioral research involving human subjects and to develop guidelines which should be followed to assure that such research is conducted in accordance with those principles. In carrying out the above, the Commission was directed to consider: (i) the boundaries between biomedical and behavioral research and the accepted and routine practice of medicine, (ii) the role of assessment of risk-benefit criteria in the determination of the appropriateness of research involving human subjects, (iii) appropriate guidelines for the selection of human subjects for participation in such research and (iv) the nature and definition of informed consent in various research settings.

The Belmont Report attempts to summarize the basic ethical principles identified by the Commission in the course of its deliberations. It is the outgrowth of an intensive four-day period of discussions that were held in February 1976 at the Smithsonian Institution's Belmont Conference Center supplemented by the monthly deliberations of the Commission that were held over a period of nearly four years. It is a statement of basic ethical principles and guidelines that should assist in resolving the ethical problems that surround the conduct of research with human subjects. By publishing the Report in the Federal Register, and providing reprints upon request, the Secretary intends that it may be made readily available to scientists, members of Institutional Review Boards, and Federal employees. The two-volume Appendix, containing the lengthy reports of experts and specialists who assisted the Commission in fulfilling this part of its charge, is available as DHEW Publication No. (OS) 78-0013 and No. (OS) 78-0014, for sale by the Superintendent of Documents, U.S. Government Printing Office, Washington, D.C. 20402.

Unlike most other reports of the Commission, the Belmont Report does not make specific recommendations for administrative action by the Secretary of Health, Education, and Welfare. Rather, the Commission recommended that the Belmont Report be adopted in its entirety, as a statement of the Department's policy. The Department requests public comment on this recommendation.

Members of the Commission of Biomedical and Behavioral Research

Kenneth John Ryan, M.D., Chairman, Chief of Staff, Boston Hospital for Women.

Joseph V. Brady, Ph.D., Professor of Behavioral Biology, Johns Hopkins University.

Robert E. Cooke, M.D., President, Medical College of Pennsylvania.

Dorothy I. Height, President, National Council of Negro Women, Inc.

Albert R. Jonsen, Ph.D., Associate Professor of Bioethics, University of California at San Francisco.

Patricia King, J.D., Associate Professor of Law, Georgetown University Law Center.

Karen Lebacqz, Ph.D., Associate Professor of Chouristian Ethics, Pacific School of Religion.

*** David W. Louisell, J.D., Professor of Law, University of California at Berkeley.

Donald W. Seldin, M.D., Professor and Chairman, Department of Internal Medicine, University of Texas at Dallas.

Eliot Stellar, Ph.D., Provost of the University and Professor of Physiological Psychology, University of Pennsylvania.

*** Robert H. Turtle, LL.B., Attorney, VomBaur, Coburn, Simmons & Turtle, Washington, D.C.

Table of Contents

Ethical Principles and Guidelines for Research Involving Human Subjects

A. Boundaries Between Practice and Research

B. Basic Ethical Principles

1. Respect for Persons
2. Beneficence
3. Justice

C. Applications

1. Informed Consent
2. Assessment of Risk and Benefits
3. Selection of Subjects

*** Deceased.

Ethical Principles & Guidelines for Research Involving Human Subjects

Scientific research has produced substantial social benefits. It has also posed some troubling ethical questions. Public attention was drawn to these questions by reported abuses of human subjects in biomedical experiments, especially during the Second World War. During the Nuremberg War Crime Trials, the Nuremberg code was drafted as a set of standards for judging physicians and scientists who had conducted biomedical experiments on concentration camp prisoners. This code became the prototype of many later codes* intended to assure that research involving human subjects would be carried out in an ethical manner.

The codes consist of rules, some general, others specific, that guide the investigators or the reviewers of research in their work. Such rules often are inadequate to cover complex situations; at times they come into conflict, and they are frequently difficult to interpret or apply. Broader ethical principles will provide a basis on which specific rules may be formulated, criticized and interpreted.

Three principles, or general prescriptive judgments, that are relevant to research involving human subjects are identified in this statement. Other principles may also be relevant. These three are comprehensive, however, and are stated at a level of generalization that should assist scientists, subjects, reviewers and interested citizens to understand the ethical issues inherent in research involving human subjects. These principles cannot always be applied so as to resolve beyond dispute particular ethical problems. The objective is to provide an analytical framework that will guide the resolution of ethical problems arising from research involving human subjects.

This statement consists of a distinction between research and practice, a discussion of the three basic ethical principles, and remarks about the application of these principles.

A. Boundaries Between Practice and Research

It is important to distinguish between biomedical and behavioral research, on the one hand, and the practice of accepted therapy on the other, in order to know what activities ought to undergo review for the protection of human subjects of research. The distinction between research and practice is blurred partly because both often occur together (as in research designed to evaluate a therapy) and partly because notable departures from standard practice are often called "experimental" when the terms "experimental" and "research" are not carefully defined.

---

* Since 1945, various codes for the proper and responsible conduct of human experimentation in medical research have been adopted by different organizations. The best known of these codes are the Nuremberg Code of 1947, the Helsinki Declaration of 1964 (revised in 1975), and the 1971 Guidelines (codified into Federal Regulations in 1974) issued by the U.S. Department of Health, Education, and Welfare Codes for the conduct of social and behavioral research have also been adopted, the best known being that of the American Psychological Association, published in 1973.

For the most part, the term "practice" refers to interventions that are designed solely to enhance the well-being of an individual patient or client and that have a reasonable expectation of success. The purpose of medical or behavioral practice is to provide diagnosis, preventive treatment or therapy to particular individuals.* By contrast, the term "research' designates an activity designed to test an hypothesis, permit conclusions to be drawn, and thereby to develop or contribute to generalizable knowledge (expressed, for example, in theories, principles, and statements of relationships). Research is usually described in a formal protocol that sets forth an objective and a set of procedures designed to reach that objective.

When a clinician departs in a significant way from standard or accepted practice, the innovation does not, in and of itself, constitute research. The fact that a procedure is "experimental," in the sense of new, untested or different, does not automatically place it in the category of research. Radically new procedures of this description should, however, be made the object of formal research at an early stage in order to determine whether they are safe and effective. Thus, it is the responsibility of medical practice committees, for example, to insist that a major innovation be incorporated into a formal research project.**

Research and practice may be carried on together when research is designed to evaluate the safety and efficacy of a therapy. This need not cause any confusion regarding whether or not the activity requires review; the general rule is that if there is any element of research in an activity, that activity should undergo review for the protection of human subjects.

B. Basic Ethical Principles

The expression "basic ethical principles" refers to those general judgments that serve as a basic justification for the many particular ethical prescriptions and evaluations of human actions. Three basic principles, among those generally accepted in our cultural tradition, are particularly relevant to the ethics of research

---

* Although practice usually involves interventions designed solely to enhance the well-being of a particular individual, interventions are sometimes applied to one individual for the enhancement of the well-being of another (e.g., blood donation, skin grafts, organ transplants) or an intervention may have the dual purpose of enhancing the well-being of a particular individual, and, at the same time, providing some benefit to others (e.g., vaccination, which protects both the person who is vaccinated and society generally). The fact that some forms of practice have elements other than immediate benefit to the individual receiving an intervention, however, should not confuse the general distinction between research and practice. Even when a procedure applied in practice may benefit some other person, it remains an intervention designed to enhance the well-being of a particular individual or groups of individuals; thus, it is practice and need not be reviewed as research.

** Because the problems related to social experimentation may differ substantially from those of biomedical and behavioral research, the Commission specifically declines to make any policy determination regarding such research at this time. Rather, the Commission believes that the problem ought to be addressed by one of its successor bodies.

involving human subjects: the principles of respect of persons, beneficence and justice.

1. **Respect for Persons**—Respect for persons incorporates at least two ethical convictions: first, that individuals should be treated as autonomous agents, and second, that persons with diminished autonomy are entitled to protection. The principle of respect for persons thus divides into two separate moral requirements: the requirement to acknowledge autonomy and the requirement to protect those with diminished autonomy.

   An autonomous person is an individual capable of deliberation about personal goals and of acting under the direction of such deliberation. To respect autonomy is to give weight to autonomous persons' considered opinions and choices while refraining from obstructing their actions unless they are clearly detrimental to others. To show lack of respect for an autonomous agent is to repudiate that person's considered judgments, to deny an individual the freedom to act on those considered judgments, or to withhold information necessary to make a considered judgment, when there are no compelling reasons to do so.

   However, not every human being is capable of self-determination. The capacity for self-determination matures during an individual's life, and some individuals lose this capacity wholly or in part because of illness, mental disability, or circumstances that severely restrict liberty. Respect for the immature and the incapacitated may require protecting them as they mature or while they are incapacitated.

   Some persons are in need of extensive protection, even to the point of excluding them from activities which may harm them; other persons require little protection beyond making sure they undertake activities freely and with awareness of possible adverse consequence. The extent of protection afforded should depend upon the risk of harm and the likelihood of benefit. The judgment that any individual lacks autonomy should be periodically reevaluated and will vary in different situations.

   In most cases of research involving human subjects, respect for persons demands that subjects enter into the research voluntarily and with adequate information. In some situations, however, application of the principle is not obvious. The involvement of prisoners as subjects of research provides an instructive example. On the one hand, it would seem that the principle of respect for persons requires that prisoners not be deprived of the opportunity to volunteer for research. On the other hand, under prison conditions they may be subtly coerced or unduly influenced to engage in research activities for which they would not otherwise volunteer. Respect for persons would then dictate that prisoners be protected. Whether to allow prisoners to "volunteer" or to "protect" them presents a dilemma. Respecting persons, in most hard cases, is often a matter of balancing competing claims urged by the principle of respect itself.

2. **Beneficence**—Persons are treated in an ethical manner not only by respecting their decisions and protecting them from harm, but also by making efforts to

secure their well-being. Such treatment falls under the principle of beneficence. The term "beneficence" is often understood to cover acts of kindness or charity that go beyond strict obligation. In this document, beneficence is understood in a stronger sense, as an obligation. Two general rules have been formulated as complementary expressions of beneficent actions in this sense: (1) do not harm and (2) maximize possible benefits and minimize possible harms.

The Hippocratic maxim "do no harm" has long been a fundamental principle of medical ethics. Claude Bernard extended it to the realm of research, saying that one should not injure one person regardless of the benefits that might come to others. However, even avoiding harm requires learning what is harmful; and, in the process of obtaining this information, persons may be exposed to risk of harm. Further, the Hippocratic Oath requires physicians to benefit their patients "according to their best judgment." Learning what will in fact benefit may require exposing persons to risk. The problem posed by these imperatives is to decide when it is justifiable to seek certain benefits despite the risks involved, and when the benefits should be foregone because of the risks.

The obligations of beneficence affect both individual investigators and society at large, because they extend both to particular research projects and to the entire enterprise of research. In the case of particular projects, investigators and members of their institutions are obliged to give forethought to the maximization of benefits and the reduction of risk that might occur from the research investigation. In the case of scientific research in general, members of the larger society are obliged to recognize the longer term benefits and risks that may result from the improvement of knowledge and from the development of novel medical, psychotherapeutic, and social procedures.

The principle of beneficence often occupies a well-defined justifying role in many areas of research involving human subjects. An example is found in research involving children. Effective ways of treating childhood diseases and fostering healthy development are benefits that serve to justify research involving children—even when individual research subjects are not direct beneficiaries. Research also makes it possible to avoid the harm that may result from the application of previously accepted routine practices that on closer investigation turn out to be dangerous. But the role of the principle of beneficence is not always so unambiguous. A difficult ethical problem remains, for example, about research that presents more than minimal risk without immediate prospect of direct benefit to the children involved. Some have argued that such research is inadmissible, while others have pointed out that this limit would rule out much research promising great benefit to children in the future. Here again, as with all hard cases, the different claims covered by the principle of beneficence may come into conflict and force difficult choices.

3. **Justice**—Who ought to receive the benefits of research and bear its burdens? This is a question of justice, in the sense of "fairness in distribution" or "what is deserved." An injustice occurs when some benefit to which a person

is entitled is denied without good reason or when some burden is imposed unduly. Another way of conceiving the principle of justice is that equals ought to be treated equally. However, this statement requires explication. Who is equal and who is unequal? What considerations justify departure from equal distribution? Almost all commentators allow that distinctions based on experience, age, deprivation, competence, merit and position do sometimes constitute criteria justifying differential treatment for certain purposes. It is necessary, then, to explain in what respects people should be treated equally. There are several widely accepted formulations of just ways to distribute burdens and benefits. Each formulation mentions some relevant property on the basis of which burdens and benefits should be distributed. These formulations are (1) to each person an equal share, (2) to each person according to individual need, (3) to each person according to individual effort, (4) to each person according to societal contribution, and (5) to each person according to merit.

Questions of justice have long been associated with social practices such as punishment, taxation and political representation. Until recently these questions have not generally been associated with scientific research. However, they are foreshadowed even in the earliest reflections on the ethics of research involving human subjects. For example, during the 19th and early 20th centuries the burdens of serving as research subjects fell largely upon poor ward patients, while the benefits of improved medical care flowed primarily to private patients. Subsequently, the exploitation of unwilling prisoners as research subjects in Nazi concentration camps was condemned as a particularly flagrant injustice. In this country, in the 1940's, the Tuskegee syphilis study used disadvantaged, rural black men to study the untreated course of a disease that is by no means confined to that population. These subjects were deprived of demonstrably effective treatment in order not to interrupt the project, long after such treatment became generally available.

Against this historical background, it can be seen how conceptions of justice are relevant to research involving human subjects. For example, the selection of research subjects needs to be scrutinized in order to determine whether some classes (e.g., welfare patients, particular racial and ethnic minorities, or persons confined to institutions) are being systematically selected simply because of their easy availability, their compromised position, or their manipulability, rather than for reasons directly related to the problem being studied. Finally, whenever research supported by public funds leads to the development of therapeutic devices and procedures, justice demands both that these not provide advantages only to those who can afford them and that such research should not unduly involve persons from groups unlikely to be among the beneficiaries of subsequent applications of the research.

C. Applications

Applications of the general principles to the conduct of research leads to consideration of the following requirements: informed consent, risk/benefit assessment, and the selection of subjects of research.

1. **Informed Consent**—Respect for persons requires that subjects, to the degree that they are capable, be given the opportunity to choose what shall or shall not happen to them. This opportunity is provided when adequate standards for informed consent are satisfied.

   While the importance of informed consent is unquestioned, controversy prevails over the nature and possibility of an informed consent. Nonetheless, there is widespread agreement that the consent process can be analyzed as containing three elements: information, comprehension and voluntariness.

   Information. Most codes of research establish specific items for disclosure intended to assure that subjects are given sufficient information. These items generally include: the research procedure, their purposes, risks and anticipated benefits, alternative procedures (where therapy is involved), and a statement offering the subject the opportunity to ask questions and to withdraw at any time from the research. Additional items have been proposed, including how subjects are selected, the person responsible for the research, etc.

   However, a simple listing of items does not answer the question of what the standard should be for judging how much and what sort of information should be provided. One standard frequently invoked in medical practice, namely the information commonly provided by practitioners in the field or in the locale, is inadequate since research takes place precisely when a common understanding does not exist. Another standard, currently popular in malpractice law, requires the practitioner to reveal the information that reasonable persons would wish to know in order to make a decision regarding their care. This, too, seems insufficient since the research subject, being in essence a volunteer, may wish to know considerably more about risks gratuitously undertaken than do patients who deliver themselves into the hand of a clinician for needed care. It may be that a standard of "the reasonable volunteer" should be proposed: the extent and nature of information should be such that persons, knowing that the procedure is neither necessary for their care nor perhaps fully understood, can decide whether they wish to participate in the furthering of knowledge. Even when some direct benefit to them is anticipated, the subjects should understand clearly the range of risk and the voluntary nature of participation.

   A special problem of consent arises where informing subjects of some pertinent aspect of the research is likely to impair the validity of the research. In many cases, it is sufficient to indicate to subjects that they are being invited to participate in research of which some features will not be revealed until the research is concluded. In all cases of research involving incomplete disclosure, such research is justified only if it is clear that (1) incomplete disclosure is truly necessary to accomplish the goals of the research, (2) there are no undisclosed risks to subjects that are more than minimal, and (3) there is an adequate plan for debriefing subjects, when appropriate, and for dissemination of research results to them. Information about risks should never be withheld for the purpose of eliciting the cooperation of subjects, and truthful answers should always be given to direct questions about the research. Care should be taken to distinguish cases in which disclosure would destroy or invalidate the research from cases in which disclosure would simply inconvenience the investigator.

Comprehension. The manner and context in which information is conveyed is as important as the information itself. For example, presenting information in a disorganized and rapid fashion, allowing too little time for consideration or curtailing opportunities for questioning, all may adversely affect a subject's ability to make an informed choice.

Because the subject's ability to understand is a function of intelligence, rationality, maturity and language, it is necessary to adapt the presentation of the information to the subject's capacities. Investigators are responsible for ascertaining that the subject has comprehended the information. While there is always an obligation to ascertain that the information about risk to subjects is complete and adequately comprehended, when the risks are more serious, that obligation increases. On occasion, it may be suitable to give some oral or written tests of comprehension.

Special provision may need to be made when comprehension is severely limited—for example, by conditions of immaturity or mental disability. Each class of subjects that one might consider as incompetent (e.g., infants and young children, mentally disable patients, the terminally ill and the comatose) should be considered on its own terms. Even for these persons, however, respect requires giving them the opportunity to choose to the extent they are able, whether or not to participate in research. The objections of these subjects to involvement should be honored, unless the research entails providing them a therapy unavailable elsewhere. Respect for persons also requires seeking the permission of other parties in order to protect the subjects from harm. Such persons are thus respected both by acknowledging their own wishes and by the use of third parties to protect them from harm.

The third parties chosen should be those who are most likely to understand the incompetent subject's situation and to act in that person's best interest. The person authorized to act on behalf of the subject should be given an opportunity to observe the research as it proceeds in order to be able to withdraw the subject from the research, if such action appears in the subject's best interest.

Voluntariness. An agreement to participate in research constitutes a valid consent only if voluntarily given. This element of informed consent requires conditions free of coercion and undue influence. Coercion occurs when an overt threat of harm is intentionally presented by one person to another in order to obtain compliance. Undue influence, by contrast, occurs through an offer of an excessive, unwarranted, inappropriate or improper reward or other overture in order to obtain compliance. Also, inducements that would ordinarily be acceptable may become undue influences if the subject is especially vulnerable.

Unjustifiable pressures usually occur when persons in positions of authority or commanding influence—especially where possible sanctions are involved—urge a course of action for a subject. A continuum of such influencing factors exists, however, and it is impossible to state precisely where justifiable persuasion ends and undue influence begins. But undue influence would include actions such as manipulating a person's choice through the controlling influence of a close relative and threatening to withdraw health services to which an individual would otherwise be entitle.

2. **Assessment of Risks and Benefits**—The assessment of risks and benefits requires a careful arrayal of relevant data, including, in some cases, alternative ways of obtaining the benefits sought in the research. Thus, the assessment presents both an opportunity and a responsibility to gather systematic and comprehensive information about proposed research. For the investigator, it is a means to examine whether the proposed research is properly designed. For a review committee, it is a method for determining whether the risks that will be presented to subjects are justified. For prospective subjects, the assessment will assist the determination whether or not to participate.

The Nature and Scope of Risks and Benefits. The requirement that research be justified on the basis of a favorable risk/benefit assessment bears a close relation to the principle of beneficence, just as the moral requirement that informed consent be obtained is derived primarily from the principle of respect for persons. The term "risk" refers to a possibility that harm may occur. However, when expressions such as "small risk" or "high risk" are used, they usually refer (often ambiguously) both to the chance (probability) of experiencing a harm and the severity (magnitude) of the envisioned harm.

The term "benefit" is used in the research context to refer to something of positive value related to health or welfare. Unlike, "risk," "benefit" is not a term that expresses probabilities. Risk is properly contrasted to probability of benefits, and benefits are properly contrasted with harms rather than risks of harm. Accordingly, so-called risk/benefit assessments are concerned with the probabilities and magnitudes of possible harm and anticipated benefits. Many kinds of possible harms and benefits need to be taken into account. There are, for example, risks of psychological harm, physical harm, legal harm, social harm and economic harm and the corresponding benefits. While the most likely types of harms to research subjects are those of psychological or physical pain or injury, other possible kinds should not be overlooked.

Risks and benefits of research may affect the individual subjects, the families of the individual subjects, and society at large (or special groups of subjects in society). Previous codes and Federal regulations have required that risks to subjects be outweighed by the sum of both the anticipated benefit to the subject, if any, and the anticipated benefit to society in the form of knowledge to be gained from the research. In balancing these different elements, the risks and benefits affecting the immediate research subject will normally carry special weight. On the other hand, interests other than those of the subject may on some occasions be sufficient by themselves to justify the risks involved in the research, so long as the subjects' rights have been protected. Beneficence thus requires that we protect against risk of harm to subjects and also that we be concerned about the loss of the substantial benefits that might be gained from research.

The Systematic Assessment of Risks and Benefits. It is commonly said that benefits and risks must be "balanced" and shown to be "in a favorable ratio." The metaphorical character of these terms draws attention to the difficulty of making precise judgments. Only on rare occasions will quantitative techniques be available for the scrutiny of research protocols. However, the idea of systematic, nonarbitrary analysis of risks and benefits should be emulated insofar as possible. This ideal requires those making decisions about the justifiability of research to be thorough in the accumulation and assessment of information about all aspects of the research, and to consider alternatives systematically. This procedure renders the assessment of research more rigorous and precise, while making communication between review board members and investigators less subject to misinterpretation, misinformation and conflicting judgments. Thus, there should first be a determination of the validity of the presuppositions of the research; then the nature, probability and magnitude of risk should be distinguished with as much clarity as possible. The method of ascertaining risks should be explicit, especially where there is no alternative to the use of such vague categories as small or slight risk. It should also be determined whether an investigator's estimates of the probability of harm or benefits are reasonable, as judged by known facts or other available studies.

Finally, assessment of the justifiability of research should reflect at least the following considerations: (i) Brutal or inhumane treatment of human subjects is never morally justified. (ii) Risks should be reduced to those necessary to achieve the research objective. It should be determined whether it is in fact necessary to use human subjects at all. Risk can perhaps never be entirely eliminated, but it can often be reduced by careful attention to alternative procedures. (iii) When research involves significant risk of serious impairment, review committees should be extraordinarily insistent on the justification of the risk (looking usually to the likelihood of benefit to the subject—or, in some rare cases, to the manifest voluntariness of the participation). (iv) When vulnerable populations are involved in research, the appropriateness of involving them should itself be demonstrated. A number of variables go into such judgments, including the nature and degree of risk, the condition of the particular population involved, and the nature and level of the anticipated benefits. (v) Relevant risks and benefits must be thoroughly arrayed in documents and procedures used in the informed consent process.

3. **Selection of Subjects**—Just as the principle of respect for persons finds expression in the requirements for consent, and the principle of beneficence in risk/benefit assessment, the principle of justice gives rise to moral requirements that there be fair procedures and outcomes in the selection of research subjects.

   Justice is relevant to the selection of subjects of research at two levels: the social and the individual. Individual justice in the selection of subjects would require that researchers exhibit fairness: thus, they should not offer potentially beneficial research only to some patients who are in their favor or select only "undesirable" persons for risky research. Social justice requires that distinction be drawn between classes of subjects that ought, and ought not, to participate in any particular kind of research, based on the ability of members of that class to bear burdens and on the appropriateness of placing further burdens on already burdened persons. Thus, it can be considered a matter of social justice that there is an order of preference in the selection of classes of subjects (e.g., adults before children) and that some classes of potential subjects (e.g., the institutionalized mentally infirm or prisoners) may be involved as research subjects, if at all, only on certain conditions.

   Injustice may appear in the selection of subjects, even if individual subjects are selected fairly by investigators and treated fairly in the course of research. Thus injustice arises from social, racial, sexual and cultural biases institutionalized in society. Thus, even if individual researchers are treating their research subjects fairly, and even if IRBs are taking care to assure that subjects are selected fairly within a particular institution, unjust social patterns may nevertheless appear in the overall distribution of the burdens and benefits of research. Although individual institutions or investigators may not be able to resolve a problem that is pervasive in their social setting, they can consider distributive justice in selecting research subjects.

   Some populations, especially institutionalized ones, are already burdened in many ways by their infirmities and environments. When research is proposed that involves risks and does not include a therapeutic component, other less burdened classes of persons should be called upon first to accept these risks of research, except where the research is directly related to the specific conditions of the class involved. Also, even though public funds for research may often flow in the same directions as public funds for healthcare, it seems unfair that populations dependent on public healthcare constitute a pool of preferred research subjects if more advantaged populations are likely to be the recipients of the benefits.

   One special instance of injustice results from the involvement of vulnerable subjects. Certain groups, such as racial minorities, the economically disadvantaged, the very sick, and the institutionalized may continually be sought as research subjects, owing to their ready availability in settings where research is conducted. Given their dependent status and their frequently compromised capacity for free consent, they should be protected against the danger of being involved in research solely for administrative convenience, or because they are easy to manipulate as a result of their illness or socioeconomic condition.[47]

Nuremberg Code Regulations

1. The voluntary consent of the human subject is absolutely essential. This means that the person involved should have legal capacity to give consent; should be so situated as to be able to exercise free power of choice, without the intervention of any element of force, fraud, deceit, duress, overreaching, or other ulterior form of constraint or coercion; and should have sufficient knowledge and comprehension of the elements of the subject matter involved as to enable him to make an understanding and enlightened decision. This latter element requires that before the acceptance of an affirmative decision by the experimental subject there should be made known to him the nature, duration, and purpose of the experiment; the method and means by which it is to be conducted; all inconveniences and hazards reasonable to be expected; and the effects upon his health or person which may possibly come from his participation in the experiment. The duty and responsibility for ascertaining the quality of the consent rests upon each individual who initiates, directs or engages in the experiment. It is a personal duty and responsibility which may not be delegated to another with impunity.
2. The experiment should be such as to yield fruitful results for the good of society, unprocurable by other methods or means of study, and not random and unnecessary in nature.
3. The experiment should be so designed and based on the results of animal experimentation and a knowledge of the natural history of the disease or other problem under study that the anticipated results will justify the performance of the experiment.
4. The experiment should be so conducted as to avoid all unnecessary physical and mental suffering and injury.
5. No experiment should be conducted where there is an a priori reason to believe that death or disabling injury will occur; except, perhaps, in those experiments where the experimental physicians also serve as subjects.
6. The degree of risk to be taken should never exceed that determined by the humanitarian importance of the problem to be solved by the experiment.
7. Proper preparations should be made and adequate facilities provided to protect the experimental subject against even remote possibilities of injury, disability, or death.
8. The experiment should be conducted only by scientifically qualified persons. The highest degree of skill and care should be required through all stages of the experiment of those who conduct or engage in the experiment.
9. During the course of the experiment the human subject should be at liberty to bring the experiment to an end if he has reached the physical or mental state where continuation of the experiment seems to him to be impossible.

10. During the course of the experiment the scientist in charge must be prepared to terminate the experiment at any stage, if he has probable cause to believe, in the exercise of the good faith, superior skill and careful judgment required of him that a continuation of the experiment is likely to result in injury, disability, or death to the experimental subject.[48]

APPENDIX B

Suggested Resources

Contents

General Information	388
Organizations	389
Journals	389
Food and Drug Administration	390
Non-FDA Regulatory Information	393
Human Research Protection	393
Miscellaneous Resources	396
Career Information	397
Major Pharmaceutical Sponsors	398
Major Contract Research Organizations	400

General Information

The Web sites listed here are all sites that you will want to explore and become familiar with.

CenterWatch
http://www.centerwatch.com

A for-profit company that matches investigators with pharmaceutical companies. The site includes extensive sections on various topics regarding clinical research.

Clinical Trials Networks Best Practices (Duke Clinical Research Institute)
https://www.ctnbestpractices.org/

Superb resource center with training modules, sample forms, and educational and reference tools.

FDA Center for Drug Evaluation and Research
http://www.fda.gov.cder

Information and regulations.

Institute of Medicine of the National Academy of Sciences
http://www.iom.edu

Extensive information about ethics and research protection.

National Institutes of Health
http://www.nih.gov
http://www.clinicaltrials.gov

The primary government biomedical research agency. This excellent site provides education about ethics, patient protections, regulations, and training, among other things.

Dictionary

MediLexicon
http://www.medilexicon.com

A dictionary of terms related to medicine and pharmaceutical companies.

Regulations

RegSource
http://www.regsource.com

An excellent resource providing complete U.S., European, and other global regulatory information on drugs, biotechnology, and medical devices.

Organizations

American Academy of Pharmaceutical Physicians and Investigators
http://www.appinet.org

Association of Clinical Research Professionals (ACRP)
http://www.acrpnet.org

Extensive resources for continuing education and professional development.

Drug Information Association (DIA)
http://www.diahome.org

Information about conferences and training.

Regulatory Affairs Professionals Society (RAPS)
http://www.raps.org

Society for Clinical Data Management
http://www.scdm.org

A professional society founded to advance clinical data management as a discipline.

Society for Clinical Research Associates (SoCRA)
http://www.socra.org

A source for education and training.

Journals

Applied Clinical Trials
http://www.actmagazine.com

A monthly journal providing a wealth of information of use to research clinicians. Subscription is free.

Drug Information Journal

A monthly journal for DIA members.

The Monitor

A quarterly newsletter for members of the ACRP.

Modern Drug Discovery
http://pubs.acs.org/journals/mdd/back.html

A very interesting, though often more technical, journal from the American Chemical Society. The journal stopped publishing in December 2004. Back issues are worth browsing.

Clinical Trials Advisor
http://www.clinicaltrialsadvisor.com

One of many business-oriented subscription newsletters produced by FDANews.

Regulatory Affairs Focus

A monthly journal for members of the RAPS.

Food and Drug Administration

Food and Drug Administration home page
http://www.fda.gov

The FDA Web site is complex. Following is a list of specific sites under the umbrella of the FDA that are likely to be of use.

Bioresearch Monitoring Information System File
http://www.fda.gov/cder/foi/special/bmis/index.htm

Clinical investigators, CROs, and IRBs abstracted from Forms FDA 1571 and 1572.

CBER (Center for Biologics Evaluation and Research)
http://www.fda.gov/cber

CBER Guidelines
http://www.fda.gov/cber/guidelines.htm

CDER (Center for Drug Evaluation and Research)
http://www.fda.gov.cder

CDER Guidance Documents
http://www.fda.gov/Drugs/GuidanceComplianceRegulatoryInformation/Guidances/default.htm

CDRH (Center for Devices and Radiological Health)
http://www.fda.gov/cdrh

CDRH Bioresearch Monitoring
http://www.fda.gov/cdrh/comp/bimo.html

CDRH Device Advice
http://www.fda.gov/cdrh/devadvice/

CDRH Guidance (Medical Devices)
http://www.fda.gov/medicaldevices/deviceregulationandguidance/guidancedocuments/default.htm

Center for Biologics Evaluation and Research (see CBER)

Center for Devices and Radiological Health (see CDRH)

Center for Drug Evaluation and Research (see CDER)

Clinical Investigator Disqualifications Proceedings
http://www.fda.gov/RegulatoryInformation/FOI/ElectronicReadingRoom/ucm143242.htm

Computerized Systems Used in Clinical Trials
http://www.fda.gov/ICECI/EnforcementActions/BioresearchMonitoring/ucm135196.htm

Debarred Persons List
http://www.fda.gov/ora/compliance_ref/debar/

Disqualified/Restricted/Assurances Lists for Clinical Investigators
http://www.fda.gov/ora/compliance_ref/bimo/dis_res_assur.htm

Drug Approvals List
http://www.fda.gov/Drugs/InformationOnDrugs/default.htm

Electronic Regulatory Submissions and Review
http://www.fda.gov/cder/regulatory/ersr/

Expedited Safety Reporting Requirements
http://www.fda.gov/Safety/MedWatch/HowToReport/ucm085692.htm

FDA Organizational Chart
http://www.fda.gov/AboutFDA/CentersOffices/OrganizationCharts/default.htm

Freedom of Information Reading Room
http://www.fda.gov/foi/

Information for Health Professionals
http://www.fda.gov/oc/oha/

International Conference on Harmonisation (ICH) Guidances
http://www.fda.gov/cber/ich/ichguid.htm

Investigational Device Exemptions (IDE) Policies and Procedures
http://www.fda.gov/MedicalDevices/DeviceRegulationandGuidance/HowtoMarketYourDevice/InvestigationalDeviceExemptionIDE/default.htm

IRB Operations and Clinical Investigation Requirements
http://www.fda.gov/downloads/RegulatoryInformation/Guidances/ucm127630
.pdf

Laws Enforced by FDA
http://www.fda.gov/opacom/laws/lawtoc.htm

Laws, Food, Drug, and Cosmetic Act
http://www.fda.gov/opacom/laws/fdcact/fdctoc.htm

Letters Providing Clinical Investigators with Notice of Initiation of Disqualification Proceedings and Opportunity to Explain
http://www.fda.gov/foi/nidpoe/default.html

MedWatch
http://www.fda.gov/medwatch/

Modernization Act of 1997, CDER-Related Documents
http://www.fda.gov/RegulatoryInformation/Legislation/FederalFoodDrugandCosmeticActFDCAct/SignificantAmendmentstotheFDCAct/FDAMA/default.htm

National Drug Code (NDC) directory
http://www.fda.gov/cder/ndc/

Orange Book (Approved Drugs)
http://www.fda.gov/Drugs/InformationOnDrugs/ucm129662.htm

Pediatric Medicine Page
http://www.fda.gov/cder/pediatric/

Pharmacy Compounding
http://www.fda.gov/Drugs/GuidanceComplianceRegulatoryInformation/PharmacyCompounding/default.htm

Warning Letters
http://www.fda.gov/foi/warning.htm

Non-FDA Regulatory Information

Clinical Trials Registry
http://www.clinicaltrials.gov

Government Printing Office
http://www.gpoaccess.gov/index.html

Federal Register, Code of Federal Regulations, *and* Congressional Record.

International Conference on Harmonisation of Technical Requirements for Registration of Pharmaceuticals for Human Use (ICH)
http://www.ich.org

RegSource
http://www.regsource.com

An extensive source of information about regulatory affairs, the FDA, Federal Register, and clinical trials.

Human Research Protection

Applied Research Ethics National Association (ARENA)
http://www.arena.org

Association for the Accreditation of Human Research Protection Programs (AAHRPP)
http://www.aahrpp.org

Bioethics Resources on the Web, National Institutes of Health
http://www.nih.gov/sigs/bioethics

Resources including instruction.

Code of Federal Regulations
http://www.gpoaccess.gov/index.html

Council for Certification of IRB Professionals (CCIP)
http://www.ptcny.com/clients/CCIP/

An affiliate of ARENA.

Department of Energy: Protection of Human Subjects Page
http://humansubjects.energy.gov/

Institute of Medicine, a component of the National Academy of Sciences (NAS)
http://www.iom.edu

Instruction in Responsible Conduct of Research.

International Conference on Harmonisation of Technical Requirements for Registration of Pharmaceuticals for Human Use (ICH)
http://www.ich.org

Office of Human Research Protection (OHRP), Department of Health and Human Services
http://www.hhs.gov/ohrp/

Public Responsibility in Medicine and Research
http://www.primr.org

University of Iowa:
Clinical Trials Office
http://research.uiowa.edu/dsp/main/?get=clintrial
Human Subjects Office
http://research.uiowa.edu/hso/

University of Michigan IRB
http://www.med.umich.edu/irbmed/

University of Southern California IRB
http://ccnt.hsc.usc.edu/irb/docs/instruction.htm

University of Washington
https://www.washington.edu/research/hsd/

Further Reading: Human Research Protection

***Ethical and Policy Issues in Research Involving Human Participants.* National Bioethics Advisory Commission.**
http://bioethics.georgetown.edu/nbac/pubs.html

***Future of Drug Safety: Promoting and Protecting the Health of the Public.* Institute of Medicine. Washington, DC: National Academy Press, 2007.**
http://www.nap.edu/catalog.php?record_id=11750

Institute of Medicine of the National Academy of Sciences
http://www.iom.edu/IOM/IOMHome.nsf/Pages/human+research+protections

One of my favorite resources, providing extensive on-line resources and free, full-text on-line copies of its library, with books and reports written by experts in their fields.

***Institutional Review Boards: A Time for Reform.* OEI-01-97-00193. Washington, DC: DHHS, 1998.**
http://www.oig.hhs.gov/oei/reports/oei-01-97-00193.pdf

***IRB Guidebook*, Office for Human Research Protections.**
http://www.ohrp.osophs.dhhs.gov/irb/irb_guidebook.htm

National Bioethics Advisory Committee
http://bioethics.georgetown.edu/nbac/ (archive)

National Human Research Protections Advisory Committee
http://www.hhs.gov/ohrp/nhrpac/nhrpac.htm

Office for Human Research Protections
http://www.hhs.gov/ohrp/

Oversight of Clinical Investigators. DHHS Office of Inspector General. FDA OEI-05-99-00350. Washington, DC: DHHS, 2000.
http://www.oig.hhs.gov/oei/reports/oei-05-99-00350.pdf

Prescription for Harm: The Decline in FDA Enforcement Activity. Committee on Oversight and Government Reform, United States House of Representatives, 2006.
http://oversight.house.gov/index.php?option=com_content&view=article&id=2558&catid=44:legislation

Preserving Public Trust: Accreditation and Human Research Participant Programs. Institute of Medicine. Washington, DC: National Academy Press, 2001.
http://www.nap.edu/openbook/0309073286/html/

Protecting Subjects, Preserving Trust, Promoting Progress—Policy and Guidelines for the Oversight of Individual Financial Interests in Human Subjects Research. Association of American Medical Colleges Task Force on Financial Conflicts of Interest in Clinical Research. Protecting Subjects; Washington, DC: AAMC, 2001.
http://www.aamc.org/research/coi/start.htm

Protecting Human Research Subjects: Status of Recommendations, OEI-01-97-00197. Washington, DC: DHHS, 2000.
http://www.oig.hhs.gov/oei/reports/oei-01-97-00197.pdf

Recruiting Human Subjects: Pressures in Industry-Sponsored Clinical Research. DHHS Office of Inspector General. OEI-01-97-00195. Washington, DC: DHHS, 2000.
http://www.oig.hhs.gov/oei/reports/oei-01-97-00195.pdf

Recruiting Human Subjects: Sample Guidelines for Practice. DHHS Office of Inspector General OEI-01-97-00196. Washington, DC: DHHS, 2000.
http://www.oig.hhs.gov/oei/reports/oei-01-97-00196.pdf

Report on Individual and Institutional Financial Conflict of Interest. Task Force on Research Accountability. Association of American Universities Washington, DC: AAU, 2001.
http://www.aau.edu/research/COI.01.pdf

Report on University Protections of Human Beings Who Are the Subjects of Research. Association of American Universities Task Force on Research Accountability. Washington, DC: AAU, 2000.
http://www.aau.edu/reports/HumSubRpt06.28.00.pdf

Responsible Conduct of Research Education Resources
http://rcrec.org/

***Responsible Research: A Systems Approach to Protecting Research Participants*, IOM**
http://www.iom.edu/Reports/2002/Responsible-Research-A-Systems-Approach-to-Protecting-Research-Participants.aspx

***Scientific Research: Continued Vigilance Critical to Protecting Human Subjects.* General Accounting Office. GAO/HEHS-96-72. Washington, DC: GAO (1996).**
http://www.gao.gov/cgi-bin/getrpt?GAO/HEHS-96-72

Veterans' Administration Office of Research Compliance and Assurance (ORCA)
http://www1.va.gov/oro/

Miscellaneous Resources

caBIG Cancer Biomedical Informatics Grid
https://cabig.nci.nih.gov/

Clinical Research Study Investigator's Toolbox
http://www.nia.nih.gov/ResearchInformation/CTtoolbox/

Includes a number of templates ranging from writing the protocol to obtaining consent to reporting adverse events.

FDC "Pink Sheet"
http://www.thepinksheet.com/FDC/Weekly/pink/Prev1Toc.htm

An electronic news source regarding new prescription drugs.

FDC "Tan Sheet"
http://www.thetansheet.com/FDC/Weekly/Tan/TOC.htm

An electronic news source regarding new nonprescription drugs.

Federal Investigator Registry of Biomedical Informatics Research Data (FIREBIRD)
https://firebird.nci.nih.gov/Firebird/

Enables investigators to complete electronic submission of clinical trial documentation to trial sponsors and regulatory bodies. A profile and related regulatory documents are all kept in one handy repository. Unlike the major electronic data capture vendors, such as PhaseForward and Medidata, OpenClinica, a small player, is worthy of mention because it is a freely available, open source Web-based software with a number of modules that can be modified for specific sites or trials.

Guidance Documents
http://www.fda.gov/AboutFDA/ContactFDA/StayInformed/GetEmailUpdates/default.htm

List of Investigators Subject to Administrative Action, PHS
http://www.silk.nih.gov/public/cbz1bje.@www.orilist.html

Career Information

Association of Clinical Research Professionals (ACRP) Career Center
http://www.acrpnet.org

JobWatch
http://www.centerwatch.com/careers/jwads.html

Research careers
http://www.centerwatch.com/careers/careers.html

Science Careers from American Association for the Advancement of Science (AAAS) Science Magazine
http://sciencecareers.sciencemag.org/

Society for Clinical Data Management
http://www.scdm.org

Major Pharmaceutical Sponsors

Abbott
http://www.abbott.com

Amgen
http://www.amgen.com

Arpida
http://www.evolva.com/
Merged with Evolva in 2009.

AstraZeneca
http://www.astrazeneca.com

Aventis Pharmaceuticals
http://en.sanofi-aventis.com/
Now a part of Sanofi-Aventis.

Bayer
http://www.pharma.bayer.com/scripts/pages/en/index.php

Boehringer Ingelheim
http://www.boehringer-ingelheim.com

Bristol-Myers Squibb
http://www.bms.com

Chiron
http://www.novartis.com/
Chiron acquired by Novartis in 2006.

Eli Lilly and Company
http://www.lilly.com

GlaxoSmithKline
http://www.gsk.com
Was Glaxo-Wellcome and SmithKline Beecham.

Hoechst
Now part of Sanofi-Aventis.

Hoffman-LaRoche
http://www.roche.com

Janssen
http://www.janssen-cilag.com

Johnson & Johnson
http://www.jnj.com

Merck
http://www.merck.com

Novartis
http://www.novartis.com

Ortho-McNeil
http://www.ortho-mcneil.com/ortho-mcneil/company.html
Now part of ORTHO-MCNEIL-JANSSEN group of J&J.

Parke-Davis
http://www.pfizer.com
Was Warner Lambert; now Pfizer.

Pharmacia
http://www.pfizer.com
Was Upjohn Pharmacia; now Pfizer.

Procter & Gamble
http://www.pg.com

Rhone-Poulenc Rorer
http://en.sanofi-aventis.com/
Now part of Sanofi-Aventis Pasteur.

Sandoz
http://www.novartis.com
Now Novartis.

Sanofi-Aventis Pasteur
http://www.sanofipasteur.com

Schering-Plough
http://www.merck.com/

SmithKline Beecham
http://www.gsk.com
Now GlaxoSmithKline.

Wyeth
http://www.pfizer.com/welcome/

Major Contract Research Organizations

Acurian
http://www.acurian.com

Cato Research Ltd.
http://www.cato.com

Celerion
http://www.celerion.com

Charles River Laboratories
http://www.criver.com

Covance
http://www.covance.com

ICON
http://www.iconus.com

Kendle
http://www.kendle.com

MDS Pharma Services
Now Celerion.

Omnicare
http://www.omnicarecr.com

Parexel
http://www.parexel.com

Pharmanet
http://www.pharmanet.com

PPD (Pharmaceutical Product Development)
http://www.ppdi.com

PRA International
http://www.prainternational.com

Quintiles
http://www.quintiles.com

APPENDIX C

Career Information and Training Programs

Contents

Career Information and Resources	402
Selected Overview Courses in Clinical Research	403
Certificate Programs	404
Distance Learning Courses and Self-Study Aids	405
Academic Programs	407
International Programs	438

The contents of the following lists are not exhaustive but represent the resources that appeared to be helpful for readers of this book. Please note that Web sites and URLs change faster than any normal person can keep up with; they were accurate at the time of writing. If a Web site is no longer in existence, you might try the Way Back Machine, http://web.archive.org/collections/web.html, unless, of course, it has disappeared now, too. Please send any corrections or changes to info@conductingclinicalresearch.com.

Career Information and Resources

Academy of Pharmaceutical Physicians and Investigators (APPI)
http://www.appinet.org/

American Association of Medical Colleges (AAMC)
http://www.aamc.org/research/clinicalresearch/start.htm

- *Clinical Research*

http://www.aamc.org/research/start.htm

- *Medical Research*

Association of Clinical Research Professionals (ACRP)
http://www.acrpnet.org

Drug Information Association
http://www.diahome.org

Regulatory Affairs Professionals Society (RAPS)
http://www.raps.org

Society of Clinical Research Associates (SOCRA)
http://socra.org/

Careers in Specific Areas

Biochemistry or biological sciences

Federation of American Societies for Experimental Biology, 9650 Rockville Pike, Bethesda, MD 20814
http://www.faseb.org

Biological sciences

American Institute of Biological Sciences, Suite 200, 1444 I St. NW, Washington, DC 20005
http://www.aibs.org

Education for scientific and technical careers

Alfred P. Sloan Foundation
http://www.sloan.org/programs/edu_careers.shtml

Fields of study leading to master's degree

Professional Science Master's
http://www.sciencemasters.com/

Microbiology

American Society for Microbiology, Office of Education and Training-Career Information, 1325 Massachusetts Ave. NW, Washington, DC 20005
http://www.asm.org

Pharmaceutical sciences (brochure)

American Association of Pharmaceutical Scientists (AAPS), 2107 Wilson Blvd., Suite #700, Arlington, VA 22201
http://www.aaps.org/sciaffairs/careerinps.htm

Physiology

American Physiological Society, Education Office, 9650 Rockville Pike, Bethesda, MD 20814
http://www.the-aps.org

Regulatory affairs

San Diego State University
Center for Bio/Pharmaceutical and Biodevice Development
http://interwork.sdsu.edu/cbbd/regaffairs/regaffairs.htm

- *Master of Science in Regulatory Affairs and Certificate Program (distance learning)*

Selected Overview Courses in Clinical Research

Clinical Research Training Online (at NIH)
http://www.cc.nih.gov/training/training/crt/info.html

Introduction to the Principles and Practice of Clinical Research (IPPCR)
http://ippcr.nihtraining.com/ (online)

Protecting Human Research Participants (at NIH)
http://phrp.nihtraining.com/users/login.php

Principles of Clinical Pharmacology (at NIH)
http://www.cc.nih.gov/training/training/principles.html

- *NIH free course!*

Public Responsibility in Medicine and Research (PRIM&R)
http://www.primr.org/Education.aspx?id=58

- Investigator 101 *CD-ROM*

See also ACRP and DIA courses below.

Certificate Programs

Association of Clinical Research Professionals (ACRP)
http://www.acrpnet.org

- *Courses (classroom and online) and certification of clinical research coordinators, clinical research associates, and investigators*

Academy of Pharmaceutical Physicians and Investigators (APPI)
http://www.appinet.org

- *Certified physician investigator course*

Drug Information Association (DIA)
http://www.diahome.org

- *Certificate programs in project management, clinical research, or clinical safety and pharmacovigilance*

Regulatory Affairs Professionals Society (RAPS)
http://www.raps.org

- *Regulatory affairs certificate programs in medical devices or pharmaceuticals*

Society of Clinical Research Associates (SOCRA)
http://socra.org

- *Certificate Program for Clinical Research Professionals*

Many of these courses may be taken individually or as part of a complete degree program.

Many of the master's degree programs listed below also have courses that can be taken individually or toward a certificate. See also the *Applied Clinical Trials* annual December issue, which focuses on educational resources.

Please also see http://conductingclinicalresearch.com for more specific URLs and updates.

Distance Learning Courses and Self-Study Aids

See also Selected Overview Courses in Clinical Research and certificate programs above.

Arizona State University College of Nursing and Health Innovation
http://nursingandhealth.asu.edu/programs/nursing/

- *Master of Science degree in Clinical Research Management (MSCRM)*
- *Graduate Certificate, Clinical Research Management*

Boston University
http://www.bu.edu/online/online_programs/certificate_programs/clinical_investigation.html

- *Graduate Certificate in Clinical Investigation*

Collaborative Institutional Training Initiative (CITI)
https://www.citiprogram.org
A collaboration between the University of Miami and the Fred Hutchinson Cancer Research Center for a Web-based training program in human research subjects protections.

- *Basic courses in the protection of human research subjects—biomedical focus, social and behavioral focus, and refresher courses*
- *Good clinical practice course*
- *Health Information Privacy and Security course (HIPS)*
- *Laboratory animal welfare courses for investigators and IACUC members*
- *Responsible Conduct of Research (RCR)*

Drexel University
http://www.drexel.com/online-degrees

- *Certificate in the Study of Clinical Research*
- *Master of Science in Nursing in Clinical Trials Research*
- *Master of Science in Clinical Research Organization and Management*

Duke University, Graduate School of Nursing
Clinical Research Management Specialty
http://nursing.duke.edu/modules/son_academic/index.php?id=94

- *Master of Science in Nursing (MSN) in Clinical Research Management*
- *Nondegree certificate*
  http://nursing.duke.edu/modules/son_academic/index.php?id=7

Gwinnett Technical College
http://www.gwinnetttech.edu

- *Clinical Research Professional (CRP) Certificate (online)*
- *Certificate in Clinical Research*

London School of Hygiene and Tropical Medicine
http://www.lshtm.ac.uk/prospectus/masters/dmsct.html

- *Postgraduate Diploma and Master of Science in Clinical Trials (online)*

Michigan State University
http://nursing.msu.edu/cracrc.aspx

- *Clinical Research Monitoring and Coordination Certificate course (online)*

National Council of University Research Administrators (NCURA)
http://www.ncura.edu/content/educational_programs/online/clinical_trials/

- *A Primer on Clinical Trials (online tutorial on clinical trials management)*

Thomas Edison State College
http://www.tesc.edu/2248.php

- *Graduate Certificate in Clinical Trials Management*

University of California, Berkeley, Extension
http://extension.berkeley.edu/cert/clinical.html

- *Professional Certificate in Clinical Research Conduct and Management*

University of California, Irvine
http://ocw.uci.edu/courses/course.aspx?id=24

- *Fundamentals of Clinical Trials*

University of Canberra
http://www.canberra.edu.au/courses/index.cfm?action=detail&courseid=463AA

- *Graduate Certificate in Clinical Trials Management (online)*

University of Illinois at Chicago
http://www.uic.edu/sph/clinicalresearch/

- *Clinical Research Methods Online Certificate Program*

University of Liverpool
http://www.liv.ac.uk/study/online/

- *Master of Science in Clinical Research Administration (MSCRA) (online)*

University of Medicine and Dentistry of New Jersey, School of Health Related Professions, Biopharma Educational Initiative
http://shrp.umdnj.edu/programs/biopharma/index.html

- *Certificates (postbaccalaureate) in Regulatory Affairs, Clinical Recruitment Sciences, and Clinical Trials Informatics*
- *Master of Science in Clinical Trial Sciences, Clinical Trials Management and Recruitment Sciences, Clinical Trials Informatics, and Regulatory Affairs*

Vanderbilt University
http://www.nursing.vanderbilt.edu

- *Master of Science in Nursing in Clinical Research Management (distance learning)*

Note: The CNS and CNL (Clinical Management) specialty program has been discontinued because of low enrollment numbers. Vanderbilt will continue to offer clinical management courses to students currently enrolled in the program.

Walden University
http://www.waldenu.edu/Degree-Programs/Masters.htm

- *Master of Science in Clinical Research Administration*

Academic Programs

Many of these programs are for postdoctoral students in medicine, nursing, or pharmacology. Some of the nondegree programs can be taken by others. Many courses now target clinical research coordinators and associates. These can be found on pages 425–429.

A notation of NIH, NCCR, CTSA, or CTSI next to an entry indicates that the program has federal funding and is intended for those seeking a career in academic medicine. These institutions tend to offer advanced degrees in many disciplines. This listing is not comprehensive and will change as more Clinical and Translational Science Awards (CTSA) grants are awarded. See http://www.ctsaweb.org/.

A notation of K, T, or F (for example, "K30") indicates that Career Development Awards are available. These are found particularly at research centers that are part of the CTSA consortium. For further information on these postgraduate grants, see http://grants.nih.gov/grants/funding/funding_program.htm and http://funding.niaid.nih.gov/ncn/training/default_career.htm.

A list of CTSA awardees and members of each institution's consortium is available at the NIH's National Center for Research Resources (NCRR) page, as well as links to career development awards funding. See http://www.ncrr.nih.gov/clinical_research_resources/clinical_and_translational_science_awards/consortium_directory/.

Biostatistics

Columbia University
http://www.mailman.columbia.edu/academics/degree-offerings/biostatistics

- *Master's in Biostatistics*
- *Patient-oriented research track*
- *Clinical research methods track*

The Dartmouth Institute
http://tdi.dartmouth.edu/centers/education/degrees/ms/

- *Master of Science in Clinical/Health Service Research (Biostatistics and Epidemiology)*
- *Master of Public Health*

Michigan State University
http://www.epi.msu.edu/

- *Training Clinical Researchers in Community Settings (TRECOS)*
- *Certificate in Biostatistics or Clinical Nursing Research*

North Carolina State University
http://www.stat.ncsu.edu

- *Master's and PhD in biomedical statistics*

University of Iowa
http://www.public-health.uiowa.edu/biostat/

- *Graduate training program in clinical investigation*
- *Master's in Clinical Investigation, Epidemiology, or Biostatistics*
- *PhD in Biostatistics*
- *Certificate in Clinical Investigation*

University of Michigan
http://www.sph.umich.edu/biostat/programs/clinical-stat/index.html

- *Training program in clinical research*
- *Master of Science Degree in Clinical Research Design and Statistical Analysis*
- *Nondegree certificate program*
- *PhD in Biostatistics*

University of North Texas Health Science Center
http://www.hsc.unt.edu/education/sph/biostats.cfm

- *Master of Public Health in Biostatistics with Clinical Research emphasis*

University of Pennsylvania, Center for Clinical Epidemiology and Biostatistics
http://www.cceb.med.upenn.edu/education

- *Master of Science in Clinical Epidemiology or Biostatistics*
- *PhD or MD/PhD in Epidemiology*

University of Wisconsin
http://www.biostat.wisc.edu/Educational_Resources/trainstudcapstoneclintrials.htm

- *Biostatistics and Medical InformaticsClinical Trials Program*
- *Certificate Program in Clinical Research Methodology and Statistical Analysis*

Virginia Commonwealth University
http://www.biostatistics.vcu.edu/programs/clinical/msClinical.html

- *Master of Science in Biostatistics, Clinical Research and Biostatistics concentration*

Clinical Research or Investigation

Albert Einstein College of Medicine
Albert Einstein-Montefiore Institute for Clinical and Translational Research (CTSA)
http://www.einstein.yu.edu/ictr/pci.aspx?id=21455

- *Clinical Research Training Program*
- *Master of Science Degree in Clinical Research Methods*

American University of Health Sciences
http://www.auhs.edu/about.html

- *Master's in Clinical Research*
- *Certificate in Clinical Research (for CRA/CRC)*

Atlanta Clinical and Translational Science Institute
http://www.actsi.org/ (see Emory University)

Baylor College of Medicine
http://www.bcm.edu/cstp

- *Clinical Scientist Training Program (K30)*
- *Master's or PhD Degree in Clinical Investigation*
- *Nondegree certificate*

Boston University School of Medicine
http://www.bu.edu/maci/

- *Master's in Clinical Investigation*

Boston University Metropolitan College
http://www.bu.edu/met/adult_college_programs/index.html

- *Certificate in Clinical Research (undergraduate)*
- *Bachelor of Science (BS) in Biomedical Laboratory and Clinical Sciences*

Campbell University School of Pharmacy
http://campbellpharmacy.net/academics/index.html

- *Bachelor's in Clinical Research (BSCR)*
- *Master's in Clinical Research (MSCR)*
- *Doctor of Pharmacy/Master of Science in Pharmaceutical Sciences (PharmD/MSPS)*
- *Doctor of Pharmacy/Master of Science in Clinical Research (PharmD/MSCR)*

Case Western Reserve
http://mediswww.cwru.edu/CRSP/courses.cfm

- *Clinical Research Scholars Program*
- *Master of Science in Clinical Research*

Charles Drew University
http://www.cdrewu.edu/page/1086

- *Master's in Clinical Research (MSCR)*

Clinical and Translational Science Institute (Boston University)
http://ctsi.bu.edu/

Columbia University
http://irvinginstitute.columbia.edu/education/irving_scholars.html

Irving Institute for Clinical and Translational Research (CTSA)

- *Master of Science Degree in Biostatistics/Patient Oriented Research and career development awards*

Colorado Clinical and Translational Sciences Institute
http://cctsi.ucdenver.edu

- *Master of Science or PhD in Clinical Science (MSCS)*

Duke University School of Medicine
http://crtp.mc.duke.edu

- *Master of Health Sciences in Clinical Research*
- *Nondegree option*

Duke-NIH Training Program in Clinical Research
http://www.cc.nih.gov/training/duke.html

- *Master of Health Sciences in Clinical Research*
- *Nondegree option*

Duke Translational Medicine Institute (CTSA)
http://www.dtmi.duke.edu/

Emory University Laney Graduate School
http://www.gs.emory.edu/academics/index.php?entity_id=96

- *Master's in Clinical Research*

Emory University Rollins School of Public Health
www.sph.emory.edu/CRCA/

- *Master's in Clinical Research*

Emory University Woodruff Health Sciences Center
http://whsc.emory.edu/home/about/index.html

- *Master's in Clinical Research*

http://www.actsi.org/areas/retcd/kl2/index.html

- *Medical Scientist Training Program (TL1 dual-degree program)*
- *Mentored Clinical and Translational Research Scholars Program supports career development for junior faculty (KL2: MD, PhD, or MD/PhD)*
- *Short-term training*
  http://www.actsi.org/areas/reted/short_term/index.html

Harvard Catalyst (The Harvard Clinical and Translational Science Center) Clinical and Translational Science Center consortium (NIH)
http://catalyst.harvard.edu/home.html

Harvard Medical School
http://www.hms.harvard.edu/gradprograms/scsp/

- *Scholars in Clinical Science Program (CTSA program)*
- *Master of Medical Science*

http://www.jbcc.harvard.edu/trainings.htm (postdoctoral candidates)

- *The Stuart T. Hauser Research Training Program in Biological and Social Psychiatry*

Harvard School of Public Health
http://www.hsph.harvard.edu/academics/clinical-effectiveness

Summer Program in Clinical Effectiveness

Indiana University Regenstrief Institute for Health Care
http://www.regenstrief.org/training/#cite

- *Clinical Investigator and Translational Education (CITE)*
- *Master of Science in Clinical Research (postdoctoral)*

Johns Hopkins University Schools of Medicine and Public Health
http://www.jhsph.edu/gtpci/

- *Graduate Training Program in Clinical Investigation*
- *PhD or Master of Health Sciences (MHS) Degree in Clinical Investigation*

http://www.jhsph.edu/gtpci/continuing_ed/clinical_research.html

- *Summer Intensive Course in Clinical Research Methods (for postdoctoral, junior faculty)*

Johns Hopkins Institute for Clinical and Translational Research (NIH CTSA)
http://ictr.johnshopkins.edu/

Loyola University Chicago
http://www.stritch.luc.edu/depts/prevmed/Main/CRM/CRM.htm

- *Master's in Clinical Research Methods*

Mayo Center for Translational Science Activities
http://ctsa.mayo.edu/education/masters-degree.html

- *Mentored Career Development Program, KL2 postdoctoral*
- *Master's Degree in Clinical Research (CTSA)*
- *Master's Degree in Clinical and Translational Science*

Mayo Clinic
http://www.mayo.edu

- *Medical Scientist Training Program (MSTP)*
- *MD/PhD*
- *Clinical and Translational Science (CTS) PhD Program*
- *Clinical Research Training Program (CRTP)*
- *Master's in Clinical Research*
- *Postbaccalaureate Research Education Program*

Medical College of Wisconsin
http://www.mcw.edu/scholars

- *Clinical Research Scholars Program*
- *Certificate Program in Research Ethics*
- *Master of Arts Degree in Bioethics*
- *PhD in Biostatistics*

See also Clinical and Translational Science Institute (CTSI) of Southeast Wisconsin

http://ctsi.mcw.edu/index.php

- *Master of Science in Clinical and Translational Science*
- *Basic and Translational Science PhD*

Medical University of South Carolina Clinical and Translational Research (SCTR) Institute (CTSA)

http://www.sctrinstitute.org/education/MSCR.html

- *Master's in Clinical Research*

Michigan State University Clinical and Translational Sciences Institute (MSU-CTSI)

https://ctsi.msu.edu/

- *Master's or MD/PhD (K12 and T32) in clinical research*

Morehouse School of Medicine

http://www.msm.edu/Academics/

- *Master's in Clinical Research*

(see Emory University and Atlanta Clinical and Translational Science Institute)

The Morehouse School of Medicine (MSM) Community Practitioner's Network is particularly interested in encouraging minority participation in clinical research.

Mount Sinai School of Medicine, Institutes for Clinical and Translational Sciences

http://www.mssm.edu/research/institutes

- *Master's in Biomedical Science and other MD/PhD*

Mount Sinai School of Medicine Clinical Research Training Program

http://www.mssm.edu/about-us/diversity/initiatives/clinical-training-program

- *Master's in Clinical Research (postdoctoral)*

Mount Sinai School of Medicine, Union Graduate College

http://www.bioethics.uniongraduatecollege.edu/

- *Master of Science or Certificate Degree in Bioethics*

New York University-HHC Clinical and Translational Science Institute (CTSA)

http://ctsi.med.nyu.edu/

NIH Center for Cancer Research (CCR)

http://ccr.cancer.gov/careers/clinical_programs_invest.asp

- *Clinical Investigator Development Program*
- *Fellowship training for MDs interested in oncologic research*

NIH Clinical Center Sabbatical in Clinical Research Management

http://www.cc.nih.gov/training/sabbatical/

Northwestern University Center for Biotechnology
http://www.mbp.northwestern.edu

- *Master's in Biotechnology*
- *Nondegree programs*

Northwestern University Clinical and Translational Sciences (NUCATS) Institute (CTSA)
http://www.nucats.northwestern.edu/education/MSCI/

- *Master's in Clinical Investigation*

Northwestern University Feinberg School of Medicine
http://www.feinberg.northwestern.edu/research/graduate-programs.html

Ohio State University Center for Clinical and Translational Science (CTSA)
http://medicalcenter.osu.edu/research/translational_research/ccts/Pages/index.aspx

Ohio State University College of Medicine
http://medicine.osu.edu

- *Master of Science in Medical Science*
- *Master of Public Health in Clinical Investigation*

Ohio State University College of Optometry
http://optometry.osu.edu/graduate

- *Graduate Program in Vision Science*
- *Master's and PhD in Vision Science*

Oregon Health and Science University Clinical and Translational Research Institute (OCTRI) (CTSA)
http://www.ohsu.edu/xd/education/schools/school-of-medicine/academic-programs/hip/program

- *Human Investigations Program (HIP)*
- *Master's and Certificate of Training in Human Investigations, or nondegree courses for postdoctoral*
- *Master of Clinical Research (MCR)*

Penn State Clinical and Translational Science Institute
http://pennstatehershey.org/sites/ctsi

Penn State General Clinical Research Training Center
http://www.pennstatehershey.org/web/gcrc/home

- *Master of Science Degree in Health Evaluation Sciences*

Regis College
http://www.regiscollege.edu/academics/details.aspx?id=6450

- *Graduate Certificate in Health Product Regulation or Clinical Research*

Rockefeller University Center for Clinical and Translational Science (CTSA)
http://www.rockefeller.edu/ccts

- *Certificate in Clinical and Translational Science Program*

Rush University
http://www.rushu.rush.edu

- *Master's in Clinical Research*
- *K23 research grant for physicians*

Scripps Translational Science Institute
http://www.stsiweb.org/index.php/education_training/

- *Master's in Clinical Investigation (CTSA)*

Stanford University
Spectrum, the Stanford Center for Clinical and Translational Education and Research (CTSA)
http://sccter.stanford.edu/

State University of New York Upstate Medical University
http://www.upstate.edu/grad/programs/pharmacology.php

- *Master's, PhD, or MD/PhD*

Thomas Jefferson University
http://www.jefferson.edu/JCGS

- *Certificate Program in Clinical Research (graduate)*
- *Master of Science Program in Pharmacology*
- *Clinical research scientist specialization track*
- *Human investigation (K30)*
- *Clinical research scientist*

Tufts Clinical and Translational Science Institute
http://www.tuftsctsi.org/

- *Certificate, Master of Science, or PhD in Clinical Research (CTSA)*

Tufts Medical Center, Sackler School Clinical Research Graduate Program
http://www.nemc.org/dccr/clinical_research_information.htm

- *Master of Science/PhD programs in clinical research*

Tufts University Institute for Clinical Research and Health Policy Studies
http://160.109.101.132/icrhps/gradprog/default.asp

- *Master's and PhD degrees in Clinical Research*

University of Alabama, Birmingham
Center for Clinical and Translational Science (CTSA)
www.ccts.uab

- *Certificate and graduate programs*

University of Arkansas
Arkansas Center for Clinical and Translational Research (CTSA)
http://www.uams.edu/cctr/

- *Certificate, Master's and PhD in Clinical and Translational Sciences*

University of Arizona
http://www.publichealth.arizona.edu/azcrtp/

- *Arizona Clinical Research Training Program (AzCRTP), a graduate certificate (postdoctoral)*

University of California, Davis Clinical and Translational Science Center
http://www.ucdmc.ucdavis.edu/ctsc/ (CTSA)

- *Multiple degree and career programs*

University of California, Los Angeles
http://dgsom.healthsciences.ucla.edu/education/mscr/

- *Master's degree in Clinical Research (Biomathematics)*

http://149.142.238.229/k30/curriculum.asp

- *K30@UCLA Graduate Training Program in Translational Investigation*
- *Master's in Clinical Research or certificate program (CTSA)*

University of California, San Diego (CTSA)
http://crest.ucsd.edu/

- *Clinical Research Enhancement through Supplemental Training (CREST)*

http://meded.ucsd.edu/ugme/goddp/index.cfm

- *Master of Advanced Studies in Clinical Research*

University of California, San Francisco
http://www.epibiostat.ucsf.edu/courses/overview.html

- *Training in Clinical Research (TICR) Program*
- *Summer clinical research workshop*
- *Advanced Training in Clinical Research (ATCR) Certificate*
- *Master's Degree Program in Clinical Research*

University of California, San Francisco Clinical and Translational Science Institute
http://ctsi.ucsf.edu/ (CTSA)

- *Multiple degree and career programs*

University of Chicago
http://health.bsd.uchicago.edu/Education/CRTP

- *Clinical Research Training Program*
- *Master of Science in Health Studies*
- *Nondegree certificate program*

University of Chicago Institute for Translational Medicine (CTSA)
http://itm.uchicago.edu/

- *Master of Science in Health Studies*
- *PhD in Health Studies*

University of Cincinnati
http://www.eh.uc.edu/clinicalresearch/

- *Master of Science Degree Program in Clinical and Translational Research (CTSA)*
- *Certificate in Clinical and Translational Research*
- *Certificate in Clinical Research*
- *Clinical Research Certificate Program (postbaccalaureate)*

University of Colorado Health Science
http://www.uchsc.edu/clinicalscience/

- *Clinical Science PhD Program (CTSA)*

University of Florida
http://www.medicine.ufl.edu/appci/

- *Advanced Postgraduate Program in Clinical Investigation (APPCI)*
- *Certificate Program or a Master's Degree in Clinical and Translational Science (MS-CTS), Public Health (MPH), or Epidemiology (MS-Epi)*
- *Nondegree programs for predoctoral trainees and research coordinators*

http://pharmreg.dce.ufl.edu/ethics.html

- *Master of Science in Pharmacy with Major in Clinical Research Regulation and Ethics*

University of Florida Clinical and Translational Science Institute

https://www.ctsi.ufl.edu/

- *Master's or PhD in Clinical Trial Science*

University of Hawaii, Manoa

http://www2.hawaii.edu/~mscr/

- *Master of Science in Clinical Research (CTSA)*
- *PhD in Clinical Research*

University of Illinois at Chicago, Center for Clinical and Translational Science

http://cores33webs.mede.uic.edu/crtp/home.htm

- *Clinical Research Training Program (CRTP) (NCCR)*
- *Master of Science in Clinical and Translational Science*

University of Iowa

http://research.uiowa.edu/

- *Graduate training program in clinical investigation*
- *Master's in Clinical Investigation, Epidemiology, or Biostatistics*
- *Certificate in Clinical Investigation*

University of Iowa Institute for Clinical and Translational Science

http://icts.uiowa.edu/content/training-and-education

- *Master's and PhD Degrees in Translational Biomedicine*
- *Master of Science and PhD degree programs in Clinical and Translational Research, a year-long certificate program*

University of Kentucky

http://www.research.uky.edu/gs/gradprogs.html

- *Master's in Clinical Research Design*

University of Kentucky Center for Clinical and Translational Science

http://www.ccts.uky.edu

- *Graduate Certificate in Clinical Research Skills*

University of Maryland School of Medicine

http://medschool.umaryland.edu

- *Master's or nondegree certificate in Clinical Research*
- *Master's Degree in Clinical Research (Department of Epidemiology and Preventive Medicine)*

University of Massachusetts Medical School

http://www.umassmed.edu/cphr/index.aspx

- *Clinical and Population Health Research Doctoral Program*

University of Michigan
http://www.michr.umich.edu

- *Multidisciplinary Clinical Researchers in Training Program (MCRiT)*
  - *Master of Science in Clinical Research degree*

http://www.psc.isr.umich.edu/research/project-detail/34473

University of Michigan Institute for Clinical and Health Research (NIH, CTSA, KL2)

  - *Mentored Clinical Scholars Program*
  - *Master of Science Degree in Clinical Research Design and Statistical Analysis (CTSA now)*
- *Robert Wood Johnson Clinical Scholars Program*

University of Minnesota
http://www.catalogs.umn.edu/grad/programs/g034.html

- *Master of Science or PhD in Clinical Research*

University of Minnesota School of Public Health
http://www.sph.umn.edu/programs/cr/competencies.asp

- *Master of Science or Master of Public Health in Clinical Research*

University of North Carolina School of Medicine
http://www.med.unc.edu/

- *K30 clinical research curriculum*
- *Robert Wood Johnson Clinical Scholars Program*
- *Master of Science in Clinical Research (MSCR)*

University of North Carolina School of Nursing–Wilmington
http://www.uncw.edu/son/academic-ClinicalResearch.htm

- *Bachelor of Science in Clinical Research Program*

University of North Carolina–North Carolina Translational and Clinical Sciences (TraCS) Institute (CTSA)
http://tracs.unc.edu/

- *Clinical Research Curriculum*
- *Master of Public Health and others*

University of Pennsylvania Institute for Translational Medicine and Therapeutics (CTSA consortium)
http://www.itmat.upenn.edu/

- *Master's in Translational Research and other programs*
- *Robert Wood Johnson Clinical Scholars Program*

University of Pittsburgh Institute for Clinical Research Education
http://www.icre.pitt.edu/

- *Master's or nondegree certificate in Clinical Research*
- *PhD in Clinical and Translational Science*

University of Pittsburgh Clinical and Translational Science Institute (CTSA)
http://www.ctsi.pitt.edu

- *Multiple programs*

University of Rochester Medical Center
http://www.urmc.rochester.edu/

- *Clinical Research Training Program*
- *Office of Human Subject Protection*
- *Cancer Control Research Training Program*
- *Master of Public Health in Clinical Investigation or Master of Science in Medical Statistics*

University of Rochester Clinical and Translational Science Institute
http://www.urmc.rochester.edu/ctsi/

- *Master of Science in Clinical Investigation (MSCI)*
- *Master of Science in Translational Research (MSTR)*
- *Master's Degree in Public Health (MPH)*
- *PhD in a health-related discipline (including translational biomedical research)*
- *PhD program in Translational Biomedical Science*
- *Medical Scientist Training Program (MD/PhD)*

University of Tennessee
http://www.uthsc.edu/prevmed/pm/k30certificateprogram.html

- *Certificate in Clinical Research (postdoctoral)*

University of Texas Medical Branch
http://www.utmb.edu/gcrc/education/Ed_CREO.htm

- *Master's or PhD in Clinical Science or Biomedical Science*

University of Texas Medical Branch, Institute for Translational Sciences
http://www.its.utmb.edu/ (CTSA)

- *Multiple degrees*

University of Texas Health Science Center at San Antonio Institute for the Integration of Medicine and Science/Clinical-Translational Research
http://iims.uthscsa.edu/ed_welcome.html

- *Master of Science in Clinical Investigation (MSCI)*
- *Doctoral Degree in Translational Science*
- *Certificate Program in Translational Science*

University of Texas Medical School at Houston Center for Clinical Research and Evidence-Based Medicine
http://ped1.med.uth.tmc.edu/neo/center/programs/index_002.html

- *Master's in Clinical Research*

University of Texas Health Science Center at Houston, Center for Clinical and Translational Sciences
http://ccts.uth.tmc.edu/ (Consortium) (CTSA)

- *Multiple degrees*

University of Texas Southwestern Medical Center at Dallas
http://www3.utsouthwestern.edu/clinicalresearch/

- *Proficiency Certificate in Clinical Investigation (PCCI)*
- *Master of Public Health (MPH)*

University of Texas Southwestern Medical Center, Texas Clinical and Translational Science Initiative
http://www.utsouthwestern.edu/utsw/home/home/research/ctsa

- *Consortium (CTSA) including Southwestern Medical Center*
- *Certificate, Master's, and PhD programs*

University of Utah Center for Clinical and Translational Science
http://www.ccts.utah.edu/

- *Master's in Clinical Investigation (postdoctoral) (CTSA)*

University of Virginia School of Medicine
http://www.healthsystem.virginia.edu/internet/phs/ms/mshome.cfm

- *Master's Degree in Health Evaluation Sciences (now MSCR)*
- *Master of Science Degree in Clinical Research*

University of Washington
http://pce.uw.edu/finder.aspx

- *Certificate in Clinical Trials*
- *Master's Degree (Master of Public Health or Master of Science in epidemiology), clinical research track*

University of Washington Institute of Translational Health Sciences
http://www.iths.org

- *ITHS KL2 Multidisciplinary Clinical Research Career Development Program (CTSA)*

University of Wisconsin School of Medicine and Public Health
http://www.pophealth.wisc.edu/Research

- *Master of Public Health*
- *Master of Science in Population Health*
- *PhD in Population Health*

University of Wisconsin, Madison General Clinical Research Center
http://www.medsch.wisc.edu/UWGCRC/cipp.htm

- *Clinical Investigator Preparatory Program*

University of Wisconsin–Madison Institute for Clinical and Translational Research (CTSA consortium)
https://ictr.wisc.edu

Vanderbilt Institute for Clinical and Translational Research
http://www.mc.vanderbilt.edu/victr/pub/

- *Multiple programs, including medical students, Master's in Clinical Investigation, Master of Public Health, and career development (CTSA)*

Villanova University School of Nursing
http://www.villanova.edu/nursing

- *Introduction to Clinical Research*

Wake Forest University
http://ctsfh.wfu.edu/education-core

- *Clinical and population translational sciences*
- *Master's (MS) or MD/MA in Clinical and Population Translational Sciences (CTSA) or Molecular Medicine and Translational Science*
- *MD/PhD or PhD in Molecular Medicine*
- *Graduate Certificate in Bioethics*
- *Master's Degree in Bioethics*

Washington University in St. Louis Institute of Clinical and Translational Sciences Clinical Research Training Center (CRTC)
http://icts.wustl.edu/cores/crtc.aspx

- *Certificate or Master's Degree in Clinical Investigation*

Wayne State University
http://www.med.wayne.edu/em/research/clinical.asp

- *Emergency Medicine Clinical Research Fellowship*

Wayne State University and Perinatology Research Branch
http://www.med.wayne.edu/prb/home.htm

- *Maternal-Fetal Medicine Fellowship*

Weill Cornell Medical College (CTSA consortium)
http://www.med.cornell.edu/ctsc/training_and_education/

- *Clinical and Translational Education Program (CTEP)*
- *Certificate in Clinical Investigation*
- *Master's in Clinical Investigation*
- *Career scholars program (KL2, TL1)*

West Virginia University
http://www.hsc.wvu.edu/ResOff/PhDPrograms/BioMedSci.aspx

- *Graduate training in the biomedical sciences*
- *Schools of Medicine and Pharmacy*
- *Master's, PhD, and dual degree programs*

Yale University School of Medicine
http://info.med.yale.edu/invmed/

- *PhD in Investigative Medicine*
- *Robert Wood Johnson Clinical Scholars Program*

Clinical Pharmacology

Clinical Pharmacology Study Group (CPSG)
http://www.mcphs.edu/academics/programs/residencies_and_fellowships/clinical_pharmacology/

- *Postdoctoral program for doctors of pharmacy (Pharm Ds) leading to certificate as investigational pharmacist*

Massachusetts College of Pharmacy
http://www.mcphs.edu/academics/masters_and_doctoral_programs/

- *Master's or PhD in Pharmacology*
- *Master's in Drug Discovery and Development*
- *Master's in Pharmaceutics*

NIH Clinical Center
http://www.cc.nih.gov/researchers/training.shtml

Ohio State University College of Medicine Division of Clinical Trials
http://clinpharm.osu.edu/mastersprogram/index.cfm

- *Master's Program in Pharmacology*
- *Master's Degree in Clinical trials*
- *Fellowship certification in clinical research*

Thomas Jefferson University, Jefferson Medical College
http://www.jefferson.edu/clinpharm/

- *Master's in Pharmacology (K30), clinical research scientist tract*
- *Human investigation specialization track*

University of Minnesota College of Pharmacy
http://www.catalogs.umn.edu/grad/programs/g156.html

- *Master's or PhD in Experimental and Clinical Pharmacology (ECP)*

Virginia Commonwealth University
http://www.pharmacy.vcu.edu/pharmacy/page.aspx?id=58

- *Master's and PhD in Pharmacy Administration*

Clinical Research Administration

Drexel (online)
http://www.drexel.com/online-degrees/biomedical-degrees/index.aspx

- *Master of Science in Clinical Research Organization and Management*
- *Nondegree certificate*

Eastern Michigan University
http://www.emich.edu/hs/cra/

- *Nondegree certificate program (postbaccalureate)*
- *Master of Science in Clinical Research Administration (CRAD)*

George Washington University
http://www.gwumc.edu

- *Bachelor of Science or Master's in Clinical Research Administration*
- *BS/MS in Clinical Research Administration (dual degree program)*

Northwestern University
http://www.scs.northwestern.edu/grad/crra/professional_graduate.cfm

- *Master of Science in Clinical Research and Regulatory Administration*
- *Graduate Certificate in Clinical Research and Regulatory Administration*

Rochester Institute of Technology Center for Bioscience Education and Technology (CBET)
http://www.rit.edu/~w-cbet/cr/

- *Bachelor's in Clinical Research Management*
- *Master of Science in Clinical Research Management*

Temple University School of Pharmacy
http://www.temple.edu/pharmacy_qara/pdf/brochure_certificateinclinicaltrialmanagement.pdf

- *Clinical Trial Management Certificate and Postmaster's Certificate*

Touro University International (now TUI University)
http://www.tuiu.edu/description.asp?main_cou_id=641

- *Graduate Certificate in Clinical Research Administration (postbaccaclureate, online)*

University of California, San Diego, Extension
http://extension.ucsd.edu/programs/index.cfm?vAction=certDetail&vCertificateID=140

- *Specialized Certificate in Clinical Trials Administration*

University of Liverpool
http://www.liv.ac.uk

- *Master of Science in Clinical Research Administration*

University of Southern California
http://regulatory.usc.edu/

- *Certificate in Regulatory and Clinical Affairs*
- *Master of Regulatory Science*
- *Doctor of Regulatory Science (DRSc)*

Clinical Research Coordinator/Associates Courses

American University of Health Sciences
http://www.auhs.edu/about.html

- *Certificate in Clinical Research*

Anoka Ramsey Community College
http://www.anokaramsey.edu/academics/programsofstudy.cfm#degrees

- *Clinical Research Professional Certificate Program for students with a degree in nursing RN (AS, AD, BSN), pharmacology, or biological sciences*

Boston College School of Nursing
http://www.bc.edu/schools/son/ce/clinical_research.html

- *Clinical Research Certificate*

Durham Technical Community College
http://www.durhamtech.edu/distancelearning/degrees.htm

- *Clinical Trials Research Associate (CTRA) and Associate in Applied Science*
- *Data Management Certificate*

Gateway-Maricopa Community College
http://healthcare.maricopa.edu

- *Associate in Applied Science in Clinical Research*
- *Coordinating degree track*
- *Certificate of Completion in Clinical Research*
- *CRA Certificate Program*

Gwinnett Technical College
http://www.gwinnetttech.edu

- *Clinical Research Professional (CRP) Certificate (online)*
- *Certificate in CR (on campus)*
- *AAS in Bioscience Technology*

Johns Hopkins Research Coordinator Training
http://www.ijhn.jhmi.edu

Kansas University School of Nursing
http://www2.kumc.edu/son/academicinformation/clinicalresearchmanagement.html

- *Research clinical trial coordinator*

Louisiana State University School of Nursing
http://nursing.lsuhsc.edu

- *Certificate, Clinical Research Coordinator (in collaboration with Aureus Research Consultants http://www.aureusresearch.com)*

Mercer County Community College
http://www.mccc.edu/programs_noncreditcert_drug.shtml

- *Certificate in Drug Development and Clinical Research*

Mid-State Technical College
http://www.mstc.edu/academics/index.htm

- *Associate in Applied Science (AAS) Degree in Clinical Research Coordinator*

Northwest Vista College
http://www.alamo.edu/nvc/programs/area_jump/program_plans/clinical_research_coord_aas.htm

- *Clinical research coordinator*
- *Associates of Applied Science Degree Program*

Northwestern University (NUCATS)
http://www.nucats.northwestern.edu/education/CRPT/CRC%20Basic%20Live/index.html

- *CRC Basic Training—A Practical Introduction to the Clinical Research Coordinator Role*

Partners Healthcare (Brigham and Women's and Massachusetts General Hospitals)
http://www.partners.org/researchcores/clinical/CCI_education_BWH.html

- *Study Coordinator/Research Nurse Orientation*
- *Introduction to Clinical Research*
- *Statistics Courses*

Pima Community College
http://www.pima.edu/program/clinicaltrial/

- *Clinical research trial coordinator*
- *Certificate or Associate of Applied Science Degree*

Raritan Valley Community College
http://www.raritanval.edu/

- *Clinical Research Associate (CRA)/Clinical Research and Coordinator (CRC) course*

Rochester Community and Technical College/Mayo Clinic
http://www.rctc.edu/catalog/overviews/crsc.html

- *Associate in Applied Science Degree and a diploma option as a clinical research study coordinator*

Rutgers College of Nursing
http://nursing.rutgers.edu/professional_development/Clinical_Research_Certificate_Courses

- *CRA/CRC preparation*

San Francisco State University's College of Extended Learning
http://www.cel.sfsu.edu/clinical-trials/

- *Clinical Trials Design and Management Certificate*

Temple University School of Pharmacy

http://www.temple.edu/pharmacy_qara/pdf/brochure_certificateinclinicaltrialmanagement.pdf

- *Certificate in Clinical Trial Management (CRC/CRA, too)*

University of Alabama
Research Coordinators Building Capacity

http://www.uab.edu/nursing/international-affairs/global-activities/educational-prog/research-coordinators-capacity-bldg

- *Master of Science in Nursing in Clinical Research Management*
- *Noncredit certificate program*

University of California, Irvine

http://unex.uci.edu/certificates/life_sciences/medical_products/

- *Medical Product Development Certificate*

University of California, San Diego

http://extension.ucsd.edu/programs/index.cfm?vAction=certDetail&vCertificateID=25&vStudyAreaID=12

- *Certificate in Clinical Trial and Design Management*

University of Chicago, Graham School of General Studies

https://grahamschool.uchicago.edu/php/clinicaltrialsmanagement/

- *Certificate in Clinical Trials Management and Regulatory Compliance (or nondegree individual courses)*

University of North Carolina Office of Clinical Trials

http://research.unc.edu/oct/training/index.php

- *Nondegree for coordinators and administrators*

University of Pittsburgh

http://www.clinicalresearch.pitt.edu/irs/education/rco.cfm

- *Research Coordinator Orientation course*

University of Rochester

http://www.rochester.edu/ohsp/coordinators/advancedClinicalResearch.html

- *Workshop: "Managing a Clinical Study—Beyond Study Start-Up"*

University of Texas, Houston

http://www.uth.tmc.edu/ctrc/training/clincoord.html

- *Clinical Trials Resource Center*

Vancouver Coastal Health Research Institute
http://www.vchri.ca/s/Workshops.asp

- *Workshops*

Clinical Research or Trial Management

Arizona State University College of Nursing and Health Innovation (online)
http://nursingandhealth.asu.edu/programs/nursing/

- *Master of Science Degree in Clinical Research Management (MSCRM)*
- *Graduate Certificate in Clinical Research Management*

Drexel University
http://www.drexel.com/online-degrees/biomedical-degrees/ms-crom/index.aspx

- *Master of Science in Clinical Research Organization and Management (online)*

Duke University, Graduate School of Nursing
http://nursing.duke.edu

- *Clinical Research Management Specialty*
- *Master of Science in Nursing in Clinical Research Management (CRM)*
- *Nondegree certificate*

Kansas University School of Nursing
http://www2.kumc.edu/son/academicinformation/clinicalresearchmanagement.html

- *MSN clinical research management track*
- *Postmaster's Certificate in Clinical Research Management*

National Council of University Research Administrators (NCURA)
http://www.ncura.edu/content/educational_programs/online/clinical_trials/

- *A Primer on Clinical Trials (online tutorial on clinical trials management)*

NIH Clinical Center Sabbatical in Clinical Research Management
http://www.cc.nih.gov/training/sabbatical/

Northeastern University
http://www.cps.neu.edu/gradcert_clinic/

- *Graduate Certificate in Clinical Trial Design and Project Management*

San Francisco State University
http://www.cel.sfsu.edu/clinical-trials/certificate.cfm

- *Certificate in Clinical Trials Design and Management*

Temple University School of Pharmacy
http://www.temple.edu/pharmacy_qara

- *Clinical Trial Management Certificate and Postmaster's Certificate*
- *Quality Assurance/Regulatory Affairs Graduate Program*

Texas Tech University School of Nursing
http://www.ttuhsc.edu

- *Master or Postmaster in Clinical Practice Management*
- *Nondegree certificate*

Thomas Edison State College
http://www.tesc.edu/2248.php

- *Graduate Certificate in Clinical Trials Management*

University of Alabama at Birmingham (UAB) School of Nursing
http://www.uab.edu/nursing/

- *Certificate in Clinical Research Management*

University of California, Berkeley Extension
http://extension.berkeley.edu/cert/clinical.html

- *Certificate Program in Clinical Research Conduct and Management*

University of California San Diego, Extension
http://extension.ucsd.edu/programs/index.cfm?vAction=certDetail&vCertificateID=25&vStudyAreaID=12

- *Certificate in Clinical Trial and Design Management*

University of California, Santa Cruz, Extension, Silicon Valley (ongoing)
http://www.ucsc-extension.edu

- *Certificate in Clinical Trials Design and Management*

University of Delaware
http://www.pcs.udel.edu/ctm/

- *Clinical Trials Management Certificate*

University of Chicago, Department of Health Studies
http://health.bsd.uchicago.edu/Education/CRTP

- *Clinical Research Training Program (CRTP) (postdoctoral)*

University of Chicago, Graham School of General Studies
https://grahamschool.uchicago.edu/php/clinicaltrialsmanagement/

- *Certificate in Clinical Trials Management and Regulatory Compliance*

University of Delaware
http://www.pcs.udel.edu/ctm/

- *Clinical Trials Management Certificate*

University of Georgia
http://www.rx.uga.edu/main/home/clinicaltrials/index.htm

- *Clinical Trials Design and Regulatory Affairs Certificate*

University of North Texas Health Sciences Center
http://www.hsc.unt.edu/gsbs/clinicalresearch.cfm

- *Clinical research management*

University of Southern California
http://regulatory.usc.edu/

- *Certificate in Clinical Research Design and Management*

University of Western Ontario
http://www.westerncalendar.uwo.ca/2009/pg285.html

- *Certificate in Clinical Trials Management*

Vanderbilt University
http://www.nursing.vanderbilt.edu/msn/crm.html

- *Master of Science in Nursing in Clinical Research Management (distance learning)*

Washington University in St. Louis
http://ucollege.wustl.edu/

- *Certificate in Clinical Research Management*
- *Bachelor of Science in Clinical Research Management*
- *Master of Science in Clinical Research Management*

Dentistry

New York University College of Dentistry
http://www.nyu.edu/dental/advanceded/clinicalresearch/index.html

- *Graduate Program in Clinical Research*
- *Certificate in Clinical Research Program*
- *Master of Science in Clinical Research*

Ohio State University College of Dentistry Clinical Research Curriculum
http://ctoc.osu.edu/k30.php

- *DDS/PhD program*

University of Minnesota
http://www.dentistry.umn.edu/programs_admissions/advanced_programs/home.html

- *Master of Science in Dentistry*

University of Texas Health Science Center at San Antonio
http://dental.uthscsa.edu/research/ResearchGrantOpportunities.pdf

- *Extramural Research Training and Career Development Program*

Virginia Commonwealth University School of Dentistry
http://www.dentistry.vcu.edu/about/research/crcpd.aspx

- *Clinical Research Center for Periodontal Diseases*

Epidemiology

Michigan State University
http://healthteam.msu.edu/medicine/about/about_devopp.htm

- *Certificate in Biostatistics or Clinical Nursing Research*
- *Master's or Certificate in Epidemiology or related field*
- *Training Clinical Researchers in Community Settings (TRECOS)*

Stanford School of Medicine
http://med.stanford.edu/epidemiology/degree.html

- *Master of Science (MS) Degree in Clinical Epidemiology.*

University of Iowa, College of Public Health Summer Institute
http://www.continuetolearn.uiowa.edu/phsi/about.htm

- *Certificate in Emerging Infectious Disease Epidemiology*

University of Pennsylvania Center for Clinical Epidemiology and Biostatistics
http://cceb.med.upenn.edu/main/education/epiGraduate.html

- *Master of Science in Clinical Epidemiology*
- *PhD or MD/PhD*
- *Clinical Research Certificate Program*
- *Master of Science in Translational Research (MTR)*

University of Tennessee
http://www.uthsc.edu/prevmed/pm/msepiprogram.html

- *Master of Science Program in Epidemiology*

Medical Device and Product Development

University of California, Irvine
http://unex.uci.edu/certificates/life_sciences/

- *Medical Product Development Certificate*
- *Clinical Trials, Medical Device and Drug Development Certificate*

University of Southern California
http://regulatory.usc.edu/

- *Certificate in Clinical Research Design and Management*
- *Certificate in Patient and Product Safety*
- *Certificate in Preclinical Drug Development*
- *Certificate in Regulatory and Clinical Affairs*
- *Master of Regulatory Science*
- *Doctor of Regulatory Science (DRSc)*

University of St. Thomas
http://www.stthomas.edu/engineering/graduate/programs/certificates/medical/default.html

- *Certificate in Medical Devices*
- *Certificate in Clinical Studies*

Public Health

Tulane University
http://www.som.tulane.edu/crca/

- *Clinical Research Master of Public Health*
- *Executive Master of Public Health in Clinical Research*

University of Alabama, Birmingham, Center for Clinical and Translational Science (CTSA)
http://www.ccts.uab.edu

- *Certificate and graduate programs*
- *Master of Science in Public Health (MSPH) in Clinical and Translational Science*

University of Kentucky College of Public Health
http://www.mc.uky.edu/publichealth/

- *Career training in therapeutics and translational research*
- *Clinical and experimental therapeutics*
- *Advanced training for doctors of pharmacy (Pharm Ds)*
- *Graduate certificate in Clinical Research Skills*
- *Master's Degree in Public Health*
- *Master of Science in Clinical Research Design*

University of North Carolina
http://www.med.unc.edu/www/education

- *Master of Science in Clinical Research (MSCR)*
- *Master's Public Health Master of Public Health—Health Care and Prevention*

University of Texas Southwestern Medical Center at Dallas
http://www3.utsouthwestern.edu/clinicalresearch/

- *Proficiency certificate in Clinical Investigation (PCCI)*
- *Master of Public Health (MPH)*

University of Washington
http://www.washington.edu/medicine/education/k30/

- *Master's Degree from the School of Public Health and Community Medicine*
- *Nondegree training programs*

University of Wisconsin
http://www.pophealth.wisc.edu/Research

- *Master of Public Health*
- *Master of Science in Population Health*
- *PhD in Population Health*

Regulatory Affairs

Campbell University School of Pharmacy/Research Triangle Park
http://www.campbell.edu/pharmacy/index.html

- *Master's in Clinical Research, course in regulatory affairs*

California State University, East Bay
http://www.ce.csueastbay.edu/certificate/regulatory_affairs/index.shtml

- *Certificate in Regulatory Affairs*

Duke University, Graduate School of Nursing (classroom or online)
http://nursing.duke.edu.

- *Certificate in Clinical Research Regulatory Affairs*

Fairleigh Dickinson University, Silberman College of Business
http://view.fdu.edu/default.aspx?id=108

- *MBA with a track for regulatory affairs*

Hood College
http://www.hood.edu

- *Master's in Biomedical Science*
- *Certificate in Regulatory Compliance*

Johns Hopkins University
http://www.biotechnology.jhu.edu/concentration.html

- *Master of Science Degree in Biotechnology, concentration in Regulatory Affairs*

Kansas University School of Medicine
http://www2.kumc.edu/crcp/

- *Clinical Research Curriculum Program (CRCP)*

http://ph.kumc.edu/mscr.html

- *Preventive medicine and public health*
- *Master of Science in Clinical Research (MS-CR)*

Keck Graduate Institute
http://www.kgi.edu/x1598.xml

- *Master of Bioscience*

Long Island University, Arnold and Marie Schwarz College of Pharmacy
http://www.brooklyn.liu.edu/pharmacy/graduate_programs.htm

- *Master of Science Degree with specialization in drug regulatory affairs*

Massachusetts College of Pharmacy and Health Sciences
http://www.mcphs.edu/academics/programs/pharmaceutical_sciences/regulatory_affairs/

- *Master's in Regulatory Affairs and Health Policy*
- *Graduate Certificate in Regulatory Affairs*
- *Graduate Certificate in Health Policy*

Northeastern University
http://www.cps.neu.edu/programs

- *Graduate Certificate in Biopharmaceutical Domestic Regulatory Affairs*
- *Graduate Certificate in Biopharmaceutical International Regulatory Affairs*
- *Master of Science in Regulatory Affairs for Drugs, Biologics, and Medical Devices*

Northwestern University
http://www.scs.northwestern.edu/grad/crra/professional_graduate.cfm

- *Master of Science in Clinical Research and Regulatory Administration*
- *Graduate Certificate in Clinical Research and Regulatory Administration*
- *Master of Science in Quality Assurance and Regulatory Science*
- *Graduate Certificate in Quality Assurance and Regulatory Science*

Purdue University
http://www.ipph.purdue.edu/graduateprogram/cert-rqc/

- *Certificate in Regulatory Affairs*

San Diego State University Center for Bio/Pharmaceutical and Biodevice Development
http://www.cbbd.sdsu.edu/regaffairs/raprograms.html

- *Master's in Regulatory Affairs*
- *Master's in Biomedical Quality Systems*
- *MBA specialization in biomedical regulatory affairs and management*
- *Postbaccalaureate certificate*

Temple University School of Pharmacy
www.temple.edu/pharmacy/programs/QARA.html

- *Postmaster's Certificate in Quality Assurance/Regulatory Affairs*
- *Master's in Quality Assurance/Regulatory Affairs*

University of California, San Diego, Extension
http://regulatory.usc.edu/

- *Courses and certificates in regulatory affairs*

University of Florida
http://pharmreg.dce.ufl.edu/ethics.html

- *Master of Science in Pharmacy with major in Clinical Research Regulation and Ethics*

University of Georgia College of Pharmacy
http://www.rx.uga.edu/academics.html

- *Regulatory Affairs Graduate Education Program*
- *Regulatory Affairs Certificate*
- *Master of Science in Pharmacy with an emphasis in Regulatory Affairs*

University of Maryland, Baltimore County
http://www.umbc.edu/

- *Graduate Certificate in Biochemical Regulatory Engineering (credit and noncredit options)*

University of Rhode Island Pharmaceutics and Pharmacokinetics Specialty
http://www.uri.edu/pharmacy/programs/graduate/ppk.shtml

- *PhD program in Pharmaceutical Sciences*

University of Southern California
http://regulatory.usc.edu/

- *Master's in Regulatory Science*
- *Certificate in Regulatory and Clinical Affairs*
- *Master of Regulatory Science*
- *Doctor of Regulatory Science (DRSc)*

University of Washington
http://www.outreach.washington.edu/biomedreg/

- *Noncredit Program in Biomedical Regulatory Affairs*
- *Master of Science in Biomedical Regulatory Affairs*

Clinical Research Management—Nursing

Arizona State University College of Nursing and Health Innovation
http://nursingandhealth.asu.edu/programs/nursing/

- *Master of Science Degree in Clinical Research Management (MSCRM)*
- *Graduate Certificate in Clinical Research Management*

Duke University Graduate School of Nursing
http://nursing.duke.edu/modules/son_academic/index.php?id=94

- *Master of Science in Nursing in Clinical Research Management*
- *Nondegree certificate*

Texas Tech University School of Nursing
http://www.ttuhsc.edu/son

- *Master's or Postmaster's in clinical research management*
- *Nondegree certificate*

University of California, Santa Cruz, Extension, Silicon Valley (ongoing)
http://www.ucsc-extension.edu

- *Certificate in Clinical Trials Design and Management*

Vanderbilt University
http://www.nursing.vanderbilt.edu/msn/crm.html

- *Master of Science in Nursing in Clinical Research Management (distance learning)*

International Programs

Europe and the UK

Anglia Ruskin University and the British Association of Research Quality Assurance (BARQA), Cambridge, UK, and other provincial centers.
http://www.anglia.ac.uk/ruskin/en/home.html

- *Master of Science in Quality Management*

Cardiff University Welsh School of Pharmacy (Wales)
http://www.cardiff.ac.uk/phrmy

- *Diploma or Master of Science in Clinical Research*
- *Courses in regulatory affairs*

City University London School of Informatics (UK)
http://www.soi.city/ac.uk

- *Postgraduate Diploma in Pharmaceutical Information Management*
- *Course in regulatory affairs*

Imperial College London (UK)
http://www3.imperial.ac.uk/

- *Clinical Research Design and Management Research Master's (MRes)*

Liverpool John Moores University (UK)
http://www.ljmu.ac.uk/

- *Applied Chemical and Pharmaceutical Sciences Bachelor of Science*
- *Pharmaceutical science and clinical research*

Liverpool School of Tropical Medicine (UK)
http://www.lstmliverpool.ac.uk/groups/clinic_group.htm

- *Master of Philosophy (MPhil)*
- *Doctor in Philosophy (PhD)*

London School of Hygiene and Tropical Medicine (UK)
http://www.lshtm.ac.uk/prospectus/masters/dmsct.html

- *Postgraduate Diploma and Master of Science in Clinical Trials (online)*

The Organization for Professionals in Regulatory Affairs
http://www.cf.ac.uk
http://www.topra.org/postgraduate-qualifications/msc-regulatory-affairs

- *Diploma and Master of Science in Regulatory Affairs in conjunction with the University of Wales*

University of Bonn (Germany)
http://www3.uni-bonn.de/

- *Master of Drug Regulatory Affairs*

University of Glamorgan (UK)
http://www.glam.ac.uk

- *Master of Science Clinical Research*

University of Liverpool (UK)
http://www.liv.ac.uk

- *Master of Science in Clinical Research Administration (MSc)*
- *Master of Science in Clinical Research online*
- *Master of Science in Clinical Research Administration*

University of Southampton (UK)
http://www.southampton.ac.uk/healthsciences/research/awards/mres.html

- *Research Master's Degree in Clinical Research (MRes)*

University of Surrey (UK) Postgraduate Medical School
http://www2.surrey.ac.uk/pgms

- *Master of Science in Pharmaceutical Medicine*

Vienna School of Clinical Research, Medical University of Vienna
http://www.vscr.at/proj_coop/int_up.php

- *Master of Science in Clinical Research*

Australia

Monash University
http://www.monash.us

- *Graduate Certificate in Clinical Research Methods*

University of Canberra
http://www.canberra.edu.au/courses/index.cfm?action=detail&courseid=463AA

- *Graduate Certificate in Clinical Trials Management (online)*

University of Melbourne
http://www.mccp.unimelb.edu.au/courses/award-courses/specialist-certificate/BRM

- *Specialist Certificate in Clinical Research (Clinical Trials Monitoring)*
- *Specialist Certificate in Clinical Research (Clinical Trials Coordination)*

University of New South Wales
http://www.unsw.edu.au/

- *Postgraduate courses in regulatory affairs*

University of Western Australia
http://www.uwa.edu.au/

- *Master of Clinical Research (thesis and coursework)*

Canada

Academy of Applied Pharmaceutical Sciences
http://www.aaps.ca/diplomaprgs.html

- *Pharmaceutical Regulatory Affairs Diploma*
- *Clinical Research Diploma*
- *Pharmaceutical Quality Control Diploma*
- *Pharmaceutical Quality Control and Quality Assurance Diploma*

Humber College
http://www.healthsciences.humber.ca/programs

- *Postgraduate Certificate in Regulatory Affairs*
- *Part-time regulatory affairs program*
- *Postgraduate Certificate in Clinical Research (postbaccalaureate)*

McMaster University
http://fhs.mcmaster.ca/cip

- *Clinician Investigator Program (CIP)*

Michener Institute for Applied Health Sciences
http://www.michener.ca/ce/postdiploma/clinical_research_associate.php

- *Clinical Research Associate Graduate Certificate Program (CRA)*

McGill Department of Medicine, Division of Experimental Medicine
http://www.medicine.mcgill.ca/expmed/default.htm

- *Graduate Diploma in Clinical Research*
- *Master of Science in Experimental Medicine*
- *Master of Science, Bioethics Option*
- *Master of Science, Family Medicine Option*
- *Master of Science, Environment Option*
- *PhD in Experimental Medicine*

Red River College
http://me.rrc.mb.ca/catalogue

Seneca College
http://www.senecac.on.ca/program/index.html

- *Certificate in Pharmaceutical Regulatory Affairs and Quality Operations*
- *Postdiploma program in pharmaceutical RA and quality operations*

University of Montreal, Faculty of Pharmacy
http://www.pharm.umontreal.ca/english/English.html

- *Master of Science and first year program (in French)*

University of Western Ontario
http://www.westerncalendar.uwo.ca/2009/pg285.html

- *Certificate in Clinical Trials Management*

India

Academy for Clinical Excellence, Bombay College of Pharmacy
http://www.aceindia.org

- *Diploma in Clinical Research*
- *Certificate programs (variety for different levels)*
- *Postgraduate Diploma in Pharmaceutical Management under the aegis of APM is available at Bombay College of Pharmacy (two-year full-time program)*

Other International

Universidad de Buenos Aires (Argentina)
http://www.pinclifa.net/index.html

- *Postgrado en Investigación Clínico-Farmacológica*

King Faisal Specialist Hospital and Research Center (Jeddah)
http://www.kfshrcj.org/KFSHRCJ/Research+Center/Research+Departments/

Kriger Research Center (various countries including the United States)
http://www.krigerinternational.com

- *Clinical Research Coordinator Training Program*
- *Clinical Research Associate Program*
- *Data Management Program*
- *Quality Assurance Program*
- *Biopharmaceutical Marketing and Management Program*
- *Clinical Investigator Program*

Notes

Introduction

1. Sumit R. Majumdar et al., "Better Outcomes for Patients Treated at Hospitals That Participate in Clinical Trials," *Archives of Internal Medicine* 168, no. 6 (2008), doi:10.1001/archinternmed.2007.124, http://archinte.ama-assn.org/cgi/content/abstract/168/6/657 (accessed February 9, 2010).

Chapter 1

1. "Maslow's Hierarchy of Needs," http://en.wikipedia.org/wiki/Maslow's_hierarchy_of_needs (accessed November 29, 2005).

2. Association of American Medical Colleges, "Breaking the Scientific Bottleneck: Report of the Graylyn Consensus Development Conference," 1990, http://www.aamc.org/research/calltoaction.htm (accessed January 15, 2006).

3. Alan N. Schechter, "The Crisis in Clinical Research: Endangering the Half-Century National Institutes of Health Consensus," *Journal of the American Medical Association* 280, no. 16 (1998): 1440–42.

4. U.S. Food and Drug Administration (FDA), "Food and Drugs: Investigational New Drug Application," *Code of Federal Regulations*, Title 21, Part 312.60, http://www.gpoaccess.gov/cfr/index.html (accessed November 28, 2005).

5. International Conference on Harmonisation, *E8: Guidance on General Considerations for Clinical Trials*, 1997, http://www.fda.gov/cder/guidance/1857fnl.pdf (accessed February 7, 2004).

6. Bill Mann, "The Life Cycle of a Drug," The Motley Fool, October 25, 1999, http://www.fool.com (accessed January 21, 2002).

7. Cutting Edge Information, *Streamlining Clinical Trials Report*, 2008, 35, http://www.cuttingedgeinfo.com/clinical-trials/?overview.

8. Sarah Robertson, "Clinical Pharmacology 1: Phase 1 Studies and Early Drug Development" (presentation at the FDA Clinical Investigator Course, Silver Spring, MD, November 16, 2009).

9. Cullen T. Vogelson, "Seeking the Perfect Protocol," *Modern Drug Discovery* 4, no. 7 (July 2001): 21–24, http://pubs.acs.org/subscribe/journals/mdd/v04/i07/html/07clinical.html (accessed January 21, 2002).

10. Gardiner Harris, "Where Cancer Progress Is Rare, One Man Says No," *New York Times*, September 16, 2009, sec. Health/Health Care Policy, http://www.nytimes.com/2009/09/16/health/policy/16cancer.html? (accessed February 9, 2010).

11. Melody Petersen, "Madison Avenue Has Growing Role in the Business of Drug Research," *New York Times*, November 22, 2002, A1, also available at http://www.nytimes.com (accessed January 2, 2004); and Melody Petersen, "Documents Show Effort to Promote Unproven Drug," *New York Times*, October 29, 2002, C1, also available at http://www.nytimes.com (accessed January 2, 2004).

12. Donna Young, "FDA's Monitoring of Postmarketing Studies Probed," *American Journal of Health-System Pharmacists' News*, August 15, 2006, http://www.ashp.org/import/News/HealthSystemPharmacyNews/newsarticle.aspx?id=2273 (accessed February 9, 2010).

13. Suzanne Barone, "FDA Amendments Act of 2007 (FDAAA) and Risk Evaluation and Mitigation Strategies (REMS)" (presentation at the Ninth Annual Pharmaceutical Regulatory Congress, October 28, 2008), http://www.ehcca.com/presentations/pharmacongress9/barone_t1_pm.ppt (accessed February 9, 2010).

14. King & Spalding Law Firm, "Postmarketing Studies and Clinical Trials," Client Alert, http://www.kslaw.com/Library/publication/ca081109.pdf (accessed February 9, 2010).

15. Mwango Kashoki, "Drug Safety and Clinical Trials" (presentation at the FDA Clinical Investigator Course, Silver Spring, MD, November 18, 2009).

16. Laurie Tarkan, "FDA Increases Efforts to Avert Drug-Induced Liver Damage," *New York Times*, August 14, 2001, F5, also available at http://www.nytimes.com (accessed February 8, 2003).

17. FDA, Center for Drug Evaluation and Research, *CDER 2002 Report to the Nation: Drug Safety and Quality*, 2002, http://www.fda.gov/cder/reports/rtn/2002/rtn2002-3.HTM#DrugRecallsandWithdrawals (accessed January 16, 2006).

18. FDA, Center for Drug Evaluation and Research, *CDER 2005 Report to the Nation*, 2005, http://www.fda.gov/downloads/AboutFDA/CentersOffices/CDER/WhatWeDo/UCM078935.pdf (accessed February 9, 2010).

19. Tufts Center for the Study of Drug Development, "Drug Safety Withdrawals in the U.S. Not Linked to Speed of FDA Approval," Tufts University, *Impact Report* 7, no. 5 (2005), http://csdd.tufts.edu/InfoServices/ImpactReportPDFs/impactReportSeptemberOctober2005.pdf (accessed September 17, 2009).

20. Institute of Medicine, Committee on the Assessment of the U.S. Drug Safety System, *The Future of Drug Safety*, ed. Alina Baciu, Kathleen Stratton, and Sheila P. Burke (Washington, DC: National Academies Press, 2007), http://www.nap.edu/catalog.php?record_id=11750 (accessed February 9, 2010).

21. Alastair J. J. Wood, "The Safety of New Medicines: The Importance of Asking the Right Questions," *Journal of the American Medical Association* 281, no. 18 (1999), doi:10.1001/jama.281.18.1753, http://jama.ama-assn.org/cgi/content/full/281/18/1753 (accessed February 9, 2010).

22. Daniel B. Klein and Alexander Tabarrok, "Theory, Evidence and Examples of FDA Harm," FDAReview.org, http://www.fdareview.org/harm.shtml (accessed February 9, 2010).

23. National Academies of Science, Office of News and Public Information, "Fixing Drug Safety System Will Require 'New Drug' Symbol on Labels, Major Boost in FDA Staff and Funding, and Increased Public Access to Information," September 22, 2006, http://www8.nationalacademies.org/onpinews/newsitem.aspx?RecordID=11750; and Institute of Medicine, Committee on the Assessment of the U.S. Drug Safety System, *The Future of Drug Safety*, ed. Alina Baciu, Kathleen Stratton, and Sheila P. Burke (Washington, DC: National Academies Press, 2007), http://www.nap.edu/catalog.php?record_id=11750 (accessed February 9, 2010).

24. FDA, *Guidance for Industry: Special Protocol Assessment*, 2002, http://www.fda.gov/cder/guidance/3764fnl.htm (accessed January 23, 2004).

25. Gina Kolata, "Study Is Halted over Rise Seen in Cancer Risk," *New York Times*, July 9, 2002, also available at http://www.nytimes.com (accessed January 2, 2004); and Writing Group for the Women's Health Initiative Investigators, "Risks and Benefits of Estrogen plus Progestin in Healthy Postmenopausal Women: Principal Results from the Women's Health Initiative Randomized Controlled Trial," *Journal of the American Medical Association* 288, no. 3 (2002): 321–33.

26. Jane E. Brody, "Ferreting for Facts in the Realm of Clinical Trials," *New York Times*, October 15, 2002, also available at http://www.nytimes.com (accessed February 8, 2003).

27. Darrell Huff, *How to Lie with Statistics* (New York: W. W. Norton & Company, 1954).

28. James Lind Library, "Documenting the Evolution of Fair Tests," http://www.jameslindlibrary.org/index.html (accessed February 9, 2010).

29. FDA, *Federal Food, Drug, and Cosmetic Act* (FD&C Act), *U.S. Code* 21 (2004), §321, chapter II, "Definitions," http://www.fda.gov/RegulatoryInformation/Legislation/FederalFoodDrugandCosmeticActFDCAct/FDCActChaptersIandIIShortTitleandDefinitions/ucm086297.htm (accessed February 9, 2010).

30. FDA, Center for Devices and Radiological Health, "Learn If a Medical Device Has Been Cleared by FDA for Marketing," April 30, 2009, http://www.fda.gov/MedicalDevices/ResourcesforYou/Consumers/ucm142523.htm (accessed February 9, 2010).

31. FDA, "Investigational Device Exemptions," *Code of Federal Regulations*, Title 21, Part 812, http://www.accessdata.fda.gov/scripts/cdrh/cfdocs/cfcfr/CFRSearch.cfm (accessed February 5, 2010).

32. FDA, Center for Devices and Radiological Health, *Information Sheet Guidance for IRBs, Clinical Investigators, and Sponsors: Significant Risk and Nonsignificant Risk Medical Device Studies*, January 2006, http://www.fda.gov/ScienceResearch/SpecialTopics/RunningClinicalTrials/GuidancesInformationSheetsandNotices/ucm118082.htm (accessed February 9, 2010).

33. Brad Zuckerman, "Medical Device Development and Regulation: An FDA Perspective," Duke Clinical Research Institute, 2007, http://comm.dcri.duke.edu/video/ctn/acc07_zuckerman/ (accessed February 9, 2010).

34. Arundhati Datye and Rachel Holley, "Medical Device Regulation" (presentation at the MAGI Clinical Research Conference–West, San Diego, CA, October 2009).

35. Barry Meier, "Study Finds More Failure of Heart Device," *New York Times*, February 24, 2009, sec. Business, http://www.nytimes com/2009/02/24/business/24device.html (accessed February 9, 2010).

36. Gregory D. Curfman, Stephen Morrissey, and Jeffrey M. Drazen, "The Medical Device Safety Act of 2009," *New England Journal of Medicine* 360, no. 15 (2009), doi:10.1056/NEJMe0902377, http://content.nejm.org/cgi/content/full/360/15/1550 (accessed February 9, 2010).

37. Jules T. Mitchel et al., "The Critical Path Initiative Meets Medical Devices," *Applied Clinical Trials* 16 (2007): 48–55, http://appliedclinicaltrialsonline.findpharma.com/appliedclinicaltrials/article/articleDetail.jsp?id=410607 (accessed February 9, 2010).

38. Paul Below and Barbara Westrum, "Similarities and Differences in Conducting Medical Device and Pharmaceutical Clinical Trials," Minnesota Chapter, Association of Clinical Research Professionals, http://www.mnacrp.org/assets/slides/socra_02-26-03.ppt (accessed February 9, 2009).

39. John Linehan and Jan B. Pietzsch, "Study on Medical Device Development Models," American Institute for Medical and Biological Engineering, http://www.aimbe.org/assets/787_linehanpresentation.pdf (accessed February 9, 2010).

40. Victoria Burt, "A Model for Device Development," *Medical Design*, September 1, 2008, http://medicaldesign.com/mag/model_device_development_0908 (accessed February 9, 2010).

41. Sarah Sorrel, "Medical Device Development: U.S. and E.U. Differences," *Applied Clinical Trials Online*, August 1, 2006, http://appliedclinicaltrialsonline.findpharma.com/appliedclinicaltrials/Regulatory/Medical-Device-Development-US-and-EU-Differences/ArticleStandard/Article/detail/363640 (accessed February 9, 2010).

42. Guy Chamberland, "Developing Drug-Device Combination Products with Unapproved Components," chap. 9 in *Clinical Evaluation of Medical Devices: Principles and Case Studies*, 2nd ed., ed. Karen M. Becker and John J. Whyte (Totowa, NJ: Humana Press, 2006). Chamberland gives an excellent

discussion of the implications of the division assignment (turf) decision and the complexities of combination-device development.

43. U.S. Department of Health and Human Services, Centers for Medicare and Medicaid Services, "Medical Devices," chap. 14 in *Medicare Benefit Policy Manual*, http://www.cms.hhs.gov/manuals/downloads/bp102c14.pdf (accessed February 9, 2010).

44. Barry Meier, "Costs Surge for Medical Devices, but Benefits Are Opaque," *New York Times*, November 5, 2009, sec. Business, http://www.nytimes.com/2009/11/05/business/05device.html (accessed February 9, 2010).

45. Kathleen Kioussopoulos, "Device Clinical Trials: Regulatory Issues and Challenges" (presentation to the Study Coordinator Advisory Committee, March 11, 2006), https://www.ctnbestpractices.org/sites/devicespecific/device/kathy-k-acc-presentation-to-scac-on-devices/view (accessed November 4, 2009).

46. Karen Midthun, "Biologicals: A Vision for the Future of Clinical Investigators in Evaluations of New Biological Products" (presentation at the FDA Clinical Investigator Course, Silver Spring, MD, November 16, 2009).

47. J. R. McGhee and J. Mestecky, "Induction of Secretory Antibodies in Humans Following Ingestion of Streptococcus Mutans," *Advances in Experimental Medicine and Biology* 107 (1977): 177–284.

48. R. H. Waldman et al., "Secretory Antibody Following Oral Influenza Immunization," *American Journal of the Medical Sciences* 292, no. 6 (1986): 367–371.

49. Richard M. Schwartz, "Product Development: Moving from the Bench to the Clinic," http://www.nihtraining.com/cc/ippcr/current/downloads/RSchwartz031609(C).pdf (accessed February 9, 2010).

50. Jon R. Daugherty, "Regulatory Considerations for the Manufacture of Investigational Vaccines for Clinical Trials," October 30, 2007, http://www.fda.gov/downloads/BiologicsBloodVaccines/NewsEvents/WorkshopsMeetingsConferences/UCM106627.pdf (accessed February 10, 2010).

51. Bruce Patsner, "Getting New Influenza Vaccines Developed and Marketed," *Health Law Perspectives*, May 2009, http://www.law.uh.edu/Healthlaw/perspectives/2009/(BP)%20Vaccines.pdf (accessed February 10, 2010).

52. Margaret A. Scuderi, "What Are DNA Vaccines?" May 2003, http://biology.kenyon.edu/slonc/bio38/scuderi/partii.html (accessed February 10, 2010).

53. Institute of Medicine, Board on Population Health and Public Health Practice, *Immunization Safety Review: Vaccines and Autism*, 2004, http://www.iom.edu/Reports/2004/Immunization-Safety-Review-Vaccines-and-Autism.aspx (accessed February 10, 2010).

54. PATH, "Our Work in Vaccine Technologies," PATH.org, http://www.path.org/projects/vaccine-technologies-overview.php (accessed February 10, 2010).

55. FDA, Center for Biologics Evaluation and Research, Division of Vaccines and Related Products Applications, "Regulatory Perspective on Development of Preventive Vaccines for Global Infectious Diseases," by Rosemary Tiernan, October 30, 2007, http://www.fda.gov/downloads/BiologicsBloodVaccines/NewsEvents/WorkshopsMeetingsConferences/UCM106632.pdf (accessed February 10, 2010).

56. Centers for Disease Control, "History of Vaccine Safety," January 15, 2010, http://www.cdc.gov/vaccinesafety/Vaccine_Monitoring/history.html (accessed February 10, 2010).

57. Editorial, "An Influenza Vaccine Debacle," *New York Times*, October 24, 2004, http://www.nytimes.com/2004/10/20/opinion/20wed1.html (accessed February 10, 2010).

58. Mark Senak, "The Swine Flu Vaccine Is Approved—If You Build It Will They Come?" Eye on FDA, September 16, 2009, http://www.eyeonfda.com/eye_on_fda/2009/09/the-swine-flu-vaccine-is-approved-if-you-build-it-will-they-come.html (accessed November 10, 2009).

59. Ketan Desai, "Clinical Trials for Bioterrorism Agents," *Journal of Clinical Research Best Practices* 2, no. 4 (2006), http://firstclinical.com/journal/2006/0604_Bioterrorism.pdf (accessed February 9, 2010).

60. FDA, Center for Biologics Evaluation and Research, Division of Vaccines and Related Products Applications, "Regulatory Perspective on Development of Preventive Vaccines for Global Infectious Diseases," by Rosemary Tiernan, October 30, 2007, http://www.fda.gov/downloads/BiologicsBloodVaccines/NewsEvents/WorkshopsMeetingsConferences/UCM106632.pdf (accessed February 10, 2010).

61. Children's Hospital of Philadelphia, "How Are Vaccines Made?" Chop.edu, http://www.chop.edu/service/vaccine-education-center/vaccine-science/how-are-vaccines-made.html (accessed February 10, 2010).

62. Children's Hospital of Philadelphia, "Vaccine Safety FAQs," Chop.edu, 2008, http://www.chop.edu/service/vaccine-education-center/vaccine-safety/ (accessed February 10, 2010).

63. Robert Chen, "Vaccine (+ Drug) Development Process: A Historical Review of Successes and Failures," 2008, http://www.avac.org/pdf/aidsvax08.pdf (accessed October 20, 2009).

64. Children's Hospital of Philadelphia, "Vaccines Changed Medicine," Chop.edu, 2008, http://www.chop.edu/service/vaccine-education-center/home.html (accessed 11/9/09).

65. Robert Chen, "Vaccine (+ Drug) Development Process: A Historical Review of Successes and Failures," 2008, http://www.avac.org/pdf/aidsvax08.pdf (accessed October 20, 2009).

66. U.S. Department of Health and Human Services, Health Resources and Services Administration, National Vaccine Injury Compensation Program, http://www.hrsa.gov/vaccinecompensation/ (accessed February 10, 2010).

67. Robert Chen, "Vaccine (+ Drug) Development Process: A Historical Review of Successes and Failures," 2008, http://www.avac.org/pdf/aidsvax08.pdf (accessed October 20, 2009).

68. Daniel DeNoon, "Swine Flu Vaccine Timeline: Key Decisions, Key Milestones," WebMD, July 20, 2009, http://www.webmd.com/cold-and-flu/news/20090720/swine-flu-vaccine-when (accessed February 9, 2010).

69. Leonard Horowitz, "Swine Flu Pandemic, 2009, Part II, Baxter Corporation's 'Accident,'" YouTube video, http://www.youtube.com/watch?v=IcVDok5LrAg&NR=1 (accessed February 9, 2010).

70. Dipity, "H1N1 Swine Flu Vaccine Will Be Used for Mass Depopulation—Baxter's Man Made Flu," August 19, 2009, http://www.dipity.com/timeline/H1n1-Vaccine-Safety (accessed February 9, 2010).

71. Zandocomm, "Swine Flu Pandemic, 2009: Anglo-American Genocide Part I and Part II," News Worldwide blog posted June 23, 2009, http://newsworldwide.wordpress.com/2009/06/23/swine-flu-pandemic-2009-anglo-american-genocide-part-i-and-part-ii/ (accessed February 9, 2010).

72. Mark Senak, "The Swine Flu Vaccine Is Approved—If You Build It Will They Come?" Eye on FDA, September 16, 2009, http://www.eyeonfda.com/eye_on_fda/2009/09/the-swine-flu-vaccine-is-approved-if-you-build-it-will-they-come.html (accessed February 9, 2010).

73. Christine Peloquin, "Key Dates in the Development of H1N1 Vaccine," CBC News, November 9, 2009, http://www.cbc.ca/health/story/2009/11/06/f-swine-flu-vaccine-rollout-timeline.html (accessed February 9, 2010).

74. John P. Swann, *History of the FDA* (New York: Oxford University Press, 1998), http://www.fda.gov/oc/history/historyoffda/default.htm (accessed February 9, 2004).

75. Rohit K. Singla, "Missed Opportunities: The Vaccine Act of 1813," Harvard Law School, May 1, 1998, http://leda.law.harvard.edu/leda/data/229/rsingla.pdf (accessed February 12, 2004).

76. FDA, Center for Food Safety and Applied Nutrition, *The Story of the Laws behind the Labels*, June 1981, http://vm.cfsan.fda.gov/~lrd/history1.html#toc (accessed November 28, 2005).

77. FDA, Center for Food Safety and Applied Nutrition, *The Story of the Laws Behind the Labels*; and Thomas Hazlet, "Drug Development and the FDA," 2000, http://depts.washington.edu/pharm543/documents/schedule/3309drugreg.pdf (accessed February 9, 2004).

78. FDA, "The Evolution of U.S. Drug Law," 1988, http://www.fda.gov/fdac/special/newdrug/benlaw.html (accessed February 7, 2004).

79. Thomas Szasz, *Our Right to Drugs* (New York: Praeger Publishers, 1992), http://www.druglibrary.org/schaffer/Library/szasz1.htm (accessed February 8, 2004).

80. FDA, "The Evolution of U.S. Drug Law."

81. National Institutes of Health, Office of Human Subjects Research, "Directives for Human Experimentation: Nuremberg Code," http://www.nihtraining.com/ohsrsite/guidelines/nuremberg.html (accessed June 30, 2006).

82. FDA, "Is the FDA Safe and Effective?" 2001, http://www.fdareview.org/ (accessed February 7, 2004).

83. Rufus King, "Drug Abuse Control, 1965," chap. 26 in *The Drug Hang Up: America's Fifty-Year Folly* (Springfield, IL: Charles C. Thomas, 1972), http://www.druglibrary.net/special/king/dhu/dhu26.htm (accessed September 12, 2005).

84. Tamara Kaplan, "The Tylenol Crisis: How Effective Public Relations Saved Johnson & Johnson," Pennsylvania State University, 1998, http://www.personal.psu.edu/users/w/x/wxk116/tylenol/crisis.html (accessed April 26, 2004).

85. Douglas Throckmorton, "Overview and Introduction to Drug Regulation" (presentation at the FDA Clinical Investigator Course, Silver Spring, MD, November 16, 2009).

86. Joel Sparks, "Timeline of Laws Related to the Protection of Human Subjects," National Institutes of Health, June 2002, http://history.nih.gov/01Docs/historical/2020b.htm (accessed December 5, 2005); and FDA, "The Evolution of U.S. Drug Law."

87. Richard P. Wenzel, "The Antibiotic Pipeline—Challenges, Costs, and Values," *New England Journal of Medicine* 351 (2004): 523–26.

88. Joseph R. Dalovisio, "IDSA Outlines the Problem/Solutions for FDA," Infectious Diseases Society of America, November 10, 2003, http://www.idsociety.org/Template.cfm?Section=News_Releases1&CONTENTID=7444&TEMPLATE=/ContentManagement/ContentDisplay.cfm (accessed November 30, 2003).

89. Infectious Diseases Society of America, "'Bad Bugs, No Drugs': Defining the Antimicrobial Availability Problem," 2003, http://www.idsociety.org (accessed November 15, 2003).

90. Institute of Medicine, "The Research Agenda: Implications for Therapeutic Countermeasures to Biological Threats," in *Biological Threats and Terrorism: Assessing the Science and Response Capabilities: Workshop Summary*, ed. Stacey L. Knobler, Adel A. F. Mahmoud, and Leslie A. Pray (Washington, DC: National Academy Press, 2002), http://www.nap.edu/books/0309082536/html/ (accessed September 14, 2005).

91. Robert Moellering and David Shlaes, "The United States Food and Drug Administration and the End of Antibiotics," *Clinical Infectious Diseases* 34 (2002): 420–22.

92. David N. Gilbert and John E. Edwards, Jr., "Is There Hope for the Prevention of Future Antimicrobial Shortages?" *Clinical Infectious Diseases* 35 (2002): 215–16.

93. Dalovisio, "IDSA Outlines the Problem."

94. Helen W. Boucher et al., "Bad Bugs, No Drugs: No ESKAPE! An Update from the Infectious Diseases Society of America," *Clinical Infectious Diseases* 48, no. 1 (2009), doi:10.1086/595011.

95. Dan Weiner and Mark Hovde, "Critical Mass for Critical Path?" *Pharmaceutical Executive*, May 1, 2007, http://pharmexec.findpharma.com/pharmexec/Regulatory+Articles/Critical-Mass-for-Critical-Path/ArticleStandard/Article/detail/423202 (accessed February 10, 2010).

96. Justin Gillis, "Once-a-Day AIDS Pill Could Be Ready Soon," *Washington Post*, January 19, 2006, A1, http://www.washingtonpost.com/wp-dyn/content/article/2006/01/18/AR2006011802428.html (accessed January 19, 2006).

Chapter 2

1. FDA, "Investigational New Drug Application."

2. Samuel Shem, *The House of God* (Itasca, IL: Putnam Publishing Group, 1984).

3. Joe A. Bollert, "How to Use Study Brokers to Find Sites and Studies" (presentation at the MAGI Clinical Research Conference–West, San Diego, CA, October 2009).

4. Ron Montgomery, site and investigator assessment, personal communication, 2002.

5. Harold Glass, personal communication, February 3, 2003.

6. Trialytics, "About Us," http://trialytics.com/about.aspx (accessed February 11, 2010).

7. Malcolm Bohm, "Applying Healthcare Data to Site Selection and Patient Recruitment" (presentation at the MAGI Clinical Research Conference–West, San Diego, CA, October 2009).

8. Trialytics, "About Us," http://trialytics.com/about.aspx (accessed February 11, 2010).

9. Harold E. Glass, "Investigators in the US: The Quest for Quality," *Scrip Magazine*, March 1, 1997.

10. Kenneth A. Getz, "The Elusive Sponsor-Site Relationship," *Applied Clinical Trials*, February 1, 2009, http://appliedclinicaltrialsonline.findpharma.com/appliedclinicaltrials/Project+Management/The-Elusive-Sponsor-Site-Relationship/ArticleStandard/Article/detail/579328 (accessed February 11, 2010).

11. CenterWatch Industry Reports, "Proportion of New Investigators to New Trials," *CenterWatch Monthly*, October 2007, 13, http://www.vscr.at/news/objects/press/cwm1410_October.pdf (accessed February 11, 2010).

12. Mark Hovde and Robert Seskin, "Selecting U.S. Clinical Investigators," *Applied Clinical Trials* 6 (February 1997): 34–42.

13. Cutting Edge Information, *Streamlining Clinical Trials Report*, 2009, http://www.cuttingedgeinfo.com/clinical-trials/?overview.

14. Carleen Hawn, "The Man Who Sees around Corners," *Forbes Magazine*, January 21, 2002, http://www.forbes.com/forbes/2002/0121/072sidebar_print.html (accessed October 30, 2003).

15. Data Edge, "Compressing Development Times with Better Investigator Selection," Data Edge DataLines, Spring 1996, http://www.fast-track.org (accessed February 4, 2003).

16. Ibid.

17. Linda Meyerson and Tracy Harmon Blumenfeld, "Rethinking the Sponsor-Investigator Relationship," *Pharmaceutical Executive*, January 6, 2009, http://pharmexec.findpharma.com/pharmexec/R&D+Articles/Rethinking-the-Sponsor-Investigator-Relationship/ArticleStandard/Article/detail/574030 (accessed February 11, 2010).

18. Tracy H. Blumenfeld and Darren Zinner, PhD research study at RapidTrials and Harvard Business School, cited in Sarah O'Neil, April Lewis, and Jo Sorgi-Gendreau, "CRAs and Site Performance in the U.S.," *The Monitor*, September 2009, 51, http://www.nxtbook.com/nxtbooks/acrp/monitor_200909/index.php#/51/ (accessed February 12, 2010).

19. Glass, personal communication.

20. Duke Clinical Research Institute, Clinical Trials Networks Best Practices, "Keys to Building a Successful Research Site," https://www.ctnbestpractices.org/edu/keys-to-building-a-successful-research-site (accessed February 11, 2010).

21. Ken Getz, Foreword to *An Industry in Evolution*, Thomson CenterWatch, 2003, http://www.centerwatch.org/bookstore/samples/sample_ind_foreword.html (accessed January 27, 2004); and Dan Vergano, "Drug Trials Vex Medical Ethics: Academic Experts Put Testing by Private Companies under a Microscope," *USA Today*, August 8, 2000.

22. Norman M. Goldfarb, review of *State of the Clinical Trials Industry 2009: A Sourcebook of Charts and Statistics*, CenterWatch, 2009, in *Journal of Clinical Research Best Practices* 5, no. 9 (2009), http://firstclinical.com/journal/2009/0909_Sourcebook_2010.pdf (accessed February 11, 2010).

23. Phyllis Maguire, *Community-Based Trials under Scrutiny*, American College of Physicians, 1999, http://www.acponline.org/journals/news/jul-aug99/cbtrials.htm (accessed Novemer 4 2003).

24. Mark Hovde, "Integrating Protocol Design and Financial Planning," Data Edge DataLines, 2001, http://www.fast-track.org (accessed February 12, 2003).

25. Sean R. Tunis, Daniel B. Stryer, and Carolyn M. Clancy, "Practical Clinical Trials," *Journal of the American Medical Association* 290 (2003): 1624–32.

Chapter 3

1. Laurie Johnson, "Design of Epidemiologic Studies" (presentation at NIH Clinical Center: Introduction to the Principles and Practice of Clinical Research, October 22, 2007), http://www.nihtraining.com/cc/ippcr/current/downloads/Johnson%2010-22-07.pdf, February 11, 2010).

2. Duke Clinical Research Institute, Clinical Trials Networks Best Practices, "Keys to Building a Successful Research Site," https://www.ctnbestpractices.org/edu/keys-to-building-a-successful-research-site (accessed February 11, 2010).

3. FDA, "Investigational New Drug Application," *Code of Federal Regulations*, Title 21, Part 312, https://www.accessdata.fda.gov/scripts/cdrh/cfdocs/cfCFR/CFRSearch.cfm?fr=312.23 (accessed February 11, 2010).

4. Montgomery, site and investigator assessment.

5. Jane Green, "Should We Outsource Our IRB?" *Journal of Clinical Research Best Practices* 4, no. 4 (2008), http://firstclinical.com/journal/2008/0804_Outsource_IRB.pdf (accessed February 11, 2010).

6. Norman M. Goldfarb, "What Am I Missing Here? Thought-Provoking Questions for the Clinical Research Industry," *Journal of Clinical Research Best Practices* 5, no. 8 (2009), http://firstclinical.com/journal/2009/0908_What55.pdf (accessed February 11, 2010).

7. U.S. Department of Health and Human Services, Centers for Medicare and Medicaid Services, "Coverage Determinations," *Medicare National Coverage Determinations Manual*, chapter 1, part 4 (sections 200–310.1), http://www.cms.hhs.gov/manuals/downloads/ncd103c1_part4.pdf (accessed February 11, 2010).

8. James B. Pfadenhauer, "Navigating the Clinical Trial Billing Maze," *Journal of Oncology Practice* 2, no. 6 (2006): 280, http://jop.ascopubs.org/cgi/content/full/2/6/280 (accessed February 11, 2010).

9. Lisa R. Pitler and Philip D. Bonomi, "Developing an Effective and Compliant Plan for Billing Clinical Trials," *Journal of Oncology Practice* 2, no. 6 (2006), doi:10.1200/JOP.2.6.265, http://jop.ascopubs.org/cgi/content/full/2/6/265 (accessed February 11, 2010).

10. Jill Weschler, "Fraud, Abuse, and Consent," *Applied Clinical Trials* 11 (2002): 28, http://appliedclinicaltrialsonline.findpharma.com/appliedclinicaltrials/View+from+Washington/Fraud-Abuse-and-consent/ArticleStandard/Article/detail/87048 (accessed February 11, 2010).

11. Debbie K. McAllister, "Gimme Shelter: Anti-Kickback Safe Harbors and Clinical Trial Agreements," *Journal of Clinical Research Best Practices* 4, no. 5 (2008), http://firstclinical.com/journal/2008/0805_Anti-Kickback.pdf (accessed February 11, 2010).

12. Norman M. Goldfarb and Jill Petro, "Accounting for Study Costs," *Journal of Clinical Research Best Practices* 2, no. 10 (2006), http://firstclinical.com/journal/2006/0610_Accounting.pdf (accessed February 11, 2010).

13. Norman M. Goldfarb, "Clinical Research Terminology Codes: What We Do and How Much It Costs," *Journal of Clinical Research Best Practices* 2, no. 3 (2006), http://firstclinical.com/journal/2006/0603_CRT.pdf (accessed February 11, 2010).

14. Guy P. Johnson, "Part 1: Budget Tool Helps Investigative Sites Calculate the Cost of a Coordinator's Time for a Typical Outpatient Study Visit," Society of Clinical Research Associates, http://www.socra.org/pdf/Investigative_Site_Budget_Tool_by_Guy_Johnson.pdf (accessed February 10, 2010) or https://www.ctnbestpractices.org/sites/budgets-contracts.

15. Guy P. Johnson "Part 2: Budget Tool Helps Investigative Sites Calculate the Cost of a Coordinator's Time for a Typical Outpatient Study Visit," Society of Clinical Research Associates, http://www.socra.org/pdf/Investigative_Site_Budget_Tool_by_Guy_Johnson_Part_2.pdf (accessed February 11, 2010).

16. Duke Clinical Research Institute, Clinical Trials Networks Best Practices, "Budget Template," https://www.ctnbestpractices.org/sites/budgets-contracts/ (accessed February 11, 2010).

17. MAGI, "Budget Template," Magiworld.org, http://www.magiworld.org/documents/FCR_Budget_Template.pdf (accessed February 11, 2010).

18. Medidata Solutions Worldwide, "Best Practice Clinical Trial Pricing Using Benchmark Data," June 23, 2009, http://www.mdsol.com/ (accessed February 11, 2010).

19. K. I. Kaitin, "Number of Active Investigators in FDA-Regulated Clinical Trials Drops," *Tufts CSDD Impact Report* (2005), cited in Kenneth A. Getz et al., "Assessing the Impact of Protocol Design Changes on Clinical Trial Performance," *American Journal of Therapeutics* 15 (2008): 450–457, http://journals.lww.com/americantherapeutics/Abstract/2008/09000/Assessing_the_Impact_of_Protocol_Design_Changes_on.7.aspx (accessed February 10, 2010).

20. Harold E. Glass and Rebecca A. Kane, "Why Investigators Take Part in Clinical Trials," *Applied Clinical Trials* 9 (2000): 46–54.

21. University of Utah Health Sciences Center, "Clinical Trials Management: Budgeting and Project Set-up," 2004, http://uuhsc.utah.edu/clinicalTrials/finanAdmin/index.html#setup (accessed January 28, 2004); University of Washington, "Clinical Trials Administrative Start-up Handbook," 2003, http://www.hscer.washington.edu/clinicaltrialshandbook/ (accessed January 16, 2003); and Research Roundtable, "Budget Corner: Request Separate Payments for End of Study's Clinical Phase and for Completion of CRF's," *Research Roundtable*, December 1999: 1–5, http://www.researchroundtable.com/ (accessed February 7, 2002).

22. Duke Clinical Research Institute, Clinical Trials Networks Best Practices, "Budgets and Contracts," https://www.ctnbestpractices.org/sites/budgets-contracts/ (accessed February 11, 2010).

23. Norman M. Goldfarb, "What Is Killing Off the Investigators? A Clinical Research Mystery," *Journal of Clinical Research Best Practices* 1, no. 7 (2005),

http://firstclinical.com/journal/2005/0507_Mystery.pdf (accessed February 10, 2010).

24. Norman M. Goldfarb, "Clinical Research Terminology Codes: What We Do and How Much It Costs," *Journal of Clinical Research Best Practices* 2, no. 3 (2006), http://firstclinical.com/journal/2006/0603_CRT.pdf (accessed February 10, 2010).

25. U.S. Department of Labor, Occupational Safety and Health Administration, "Bloodborne Pathogens and Needlestick Prevention," http://www.osha.gov/SLTC/bloodbornepathogens/ (accessed January 4, 2006).

26. FDA regulations state that records must be retained for "a period of 2 years following the date a marketing application is approved for the drug for the indication for which it is being investigated; or, if no application is to be filed or if the application is not approved for such indication, until 2 years after the investigation is discontinued and FDA is notified"; FDA, "Investigational New Drug Application," *Code of Federal Regulations*, Title 21, Part 312, https://www.accessdata.fda.gov/scripts/cdrh/cfdocs/cfCFR/CFRSearch.cfm?fr=312.23 (accessed February 11, 2010).

27. Kate Leonard and Shawn Gibbs, "Sensible Payment Terms" (presentation at the MAGI Clinical Research Conferencc–West, San Diego, CA, October 2009).

28. Ibid.

29. Hovde, "Integrating Protocol Design."

30. Ibid.

31. Cullen T. Vogelson, "Happy Trials to You," *Modern Drug Discovery* 4, no. 12 (December 2001): 21–22, 24, http://pubs.acs.org/subscribe/journals/mdd/v04/i12/html/12clinical.html (accessed January 9, 2002).

32. Hovde, "Integrating Protocol Design."

33. Hovde and Seskin, "Selecting U.S. Clinical Investigators."

34. Mark Hovde, "Choosing and Using CROs," *Scrip Magazine*, July/August 1995.

35. Ibid.

36. Research Roundtable, "Budget Corner: Request Separate Payments."

37. University of Washington, "Clinical Trials Administrative Start-up Handbook."

38. Norman M. Goldfarb, "What is Killing Off the Investigators? A Clinical Research Mystery," *Journal of Clinical Research Best Practices* 1, no. 7 (2005), http://firstclinical.com/journal/2005/0507_Mystery.pdf (accessed February 10, 2010).

39. Ibid.

40. Larry Brownstein and Kate Leonard, "Collecting Payments: Financial Viability of Sponsors" (presentation at the MAGI Clinical Research Conference–West, San Diego, CA, October 2009).

41. Michael McCarthy, "Company Sought to Block Paper's Publication," *Lancet* 356 (2000): 1659.

42. University of Iowa, "IRB Forms/Templates," 2001, http://research.uiowa.edu/hso/index.php?get=forms02 (accessed February 23, 2003); and K. A. Schulman et al., "Contract Language for Clinical Research Agreements between Academic Medical Centers and Industry Sponsors," Center for Clinical and Genetic Economics, Duke Clinical Research Institute, 2003, http://www.dcri.duke.edu/ccge/contracts/ (accessed January 14, 2004).

43. Ralph T. King Jr., "Bitter Pill: How a Drug Firm Paid for University Study, Then Undermined Its Research on Thyroid Tablets," *Wall Street Journal*, April 25, 1996, also available at http://www.wsj.com; B. J. Dong et al., "Bioequivalence of Levothyroxine Preparations for Treatment of Hypothyroidism," *Journal of the American Medical Association* 277 (1997): 1199–200; and Drummond Rennie, "Thyroid Storm," *Journal of the American Medical Association* 227, no. 15 (April 16, 1997): 1238–43.

44. *Grant and Kahn v. Pharmacia and Upjohn*, No. 99-N-285 (US Ct. App. Dec. 23, 2002), http://www.kscourts.org/ca10/cases/2002/12/01-1509.htm (accessed January 19, 2004).

45. Norman M. Goldfarb and Aylin Regulski, "18 Subject Injury and Indemnification CTA Loopholes," *Journal of Clinical Research Best Practices* 4, no. 1 (2008), http://firstclinical.com/journal/2008/0801_Loopholes.pdf (accessed February 12, 2010).

46. MAGI, "MAGI Model Clinical Trial Agreement," version 1.26, July 2009, http://www.magiworld.org/documents/ (accessed February 11, 2010).

47. John Ervin, "Opinions: Should Clinical Research Sites Unionize? or We're Mad as #$%& and We're Not Going to Take It Anymore!" *AAPP Rx* 3, no. 2, (2001), 13–14, http://www.aapp.org/pdf/summer2001.pdf (accessed September 14, 2005).

48. John F. Kouten, "A Ten Step Trial Crisis Plan," *Applied Clinical Trials*, July 1, 2009.

49. Joint Commission, *What Did the Doctors Say? Improving Health Literacy to Protect Patient Safety*, 2007, http://www.jointcommission.org/NewsRoom/PressKits/Health_Literacy/ (accessed February 12, 2010).

50. Todd E. Betanzos, "The People vs. Amgen: Study Subjects Sue to Receive Investigational Drugs," *Pharmaceutical Executive*, June 2006, http://www.sdma.com/Publications/detail.aspx?pub=4478 (accessed February 12, 2010).

51. Darwin National Assurance Company, "Clinical Research Liability, 2007," http://www.darwinpro.com/mkt/pdf/med_crli.pdf (accessed February 12, 2010).

52. Norman M. Goldfarb, "Two New Insurance Policies for Clinical Investigators," *Journal of Clinical Research Best Practices* 2, no. 1 (2006), http://firstclinical.com/journal/2006/0601_New_Insurance.pdf (accessed February 12, 2010).

53. Nutter McClennen & Fish, LLP, "Subject Injury Issues in Clinical Research" (presentation to the Massachusetts Biotechnology Council, June 26, 2008), http://www.massbio.org/writable/committees/presentations/june_26_2008_mbc_injury_slides_copy1.ppt (accessed February 12, 2010).

54. Robert Steinbrook, "Compensation for Injured Research Subjects," *New England Journal of Medicine* 354, no. 18 (2006), doi:10.1056/NEJMp068080, http://content.nejm.org/cgi/content/full/354/18/1871 (accessed February 12, 2010).

55. Elisabeth Rosenthal, "Inquiries in Britain Uncover Loopholes in Drug Trials," *New York Times*, August 3, 2006, sec. World, http://www.nytimes.com/2006/08/03/world/europe/03britain.html (accessed February 12, 2010).

56. National Bioethics Advisory Commission, "Summary," *Ethical and Policy Issues in Research Involving Human Participants* (Bethesda, MD: National Bioethics Advisory Commission, August 2001), http://bioethics.georgetown.edu/nbac/human/oversumm.html.

57. Nutter McClennen & Fish, LLP, "Subject Injury Issues in Clinical Research" (presentation to the Massachusetts Biotechnology Council, June 26, 2008), http://www.massbio.org/writable/committees/presentations/june_26_2008_mbc_injury_slides_copy1.ppt (accessed February 12, 2010).

58. Institute of Medicine, Committee on Assessing the System for Protecting Human Research Participants, *Responsible Research: A Systems Approach to Protecting Research Participants*, ed. Daniel D. Federman, Kathi E. Hanna, and Laura Lyman Rodriguez (Washington, DC: National Academies Press, 2002), http://www.nap.edu/booksearch.php?record_id=10508 (accessed February 12, 2010).

59. Robert Steinbrook, "Compensation for Injured Research Subjects," *New England Journal of Medicine* 354, no. 18 (2006), doi:10.1056/NEJMp068080, http://content.nejm.org/cgi/content/full/354/18/1871 (accessed February 12, 2010).

60. Norman M. Goldfarb, "Treatment Reimbursement in Informed Consent Forms and Clinical Trial Agreements," *Journal of Clinical Research Best Practices* 2, no. 5 (2006), http://firstclinical.com/journal/2006/0605_Reimbursement.pdf (accessed February 12, 2010).

61. Norman M. Goldfarb and Aylin Regulski, "18 Subject Injury and Indemnification CTA Loopholes," *Journal of Clinical Research Best Practices* 4, no. 1 (2008), http://firstclinical.com/journal/2008/0801_Loopholes.pdf (accessed February 12, 2010).

62. Nutter McClennen & Fish, LLP, "Subject Injury Issues in Clinical Research" (presentation to the Massachusetts Biotechnology Council, June 26, 2008), http://www.massbio.org/writable/committees/presentations/june_26_2008_mbc_injury_slides_copy1.ppt (accessed February 12, 2010).

63. MAGI, "MAGI Model Clinical Trial Agreement," version 1.26, July 2009, http://www.magiworld.org/documents/ (accessed February 11, 2010).

64. Norman M. Goldfarb, "What Am I Missing Here? Thought-Provoking Questions for the Clinical Research Industry," *Journal of Clinical Research Best Practices* 5, no. 8 (2009), http://www.firstclinical.com/journal/2009/0908_What55.pdf (accessed February 12, 2010).

65. Sheryl Gay Stolberg, "The Biotech Death of Jesse Gelsinger," *New York Times*, November 28, 1999, http://www.nytimes.com/library/magazine/home/19991128mag-stolberg.html (accessed January 15, 2004); Larry Thompson, "Human Gene Therapy—Harsh Lessons, High Hopes," *FDA Consumer*, September–October 2000, http://www.fda.gov/fdac/features/2000/500_gene.html (accessed January 6, 2006); and Dale Keiger and Sue De Pasquale, "Trials and Tribulation," *Johns Hopkins Magazine*, February 1, 2002, also available at http://www.jhu.edu/~jhumag/0202web/trials.html (accessed January 16, 2006).

66. Cutting Edge Information, *Streamlining Clinical Trials Report*, 2009, http://www.cuttingedgeinfo.com/clinical-trials/?overview.

67. Hassan Movahhed, e-mail message to author, October 30, 2003. https://www.accessdata.fda.gov/scripts/cdrh/cfdocs/cfCFR/CFRSearch.cfm?fr=312.23 (accessed February 11, 2010).

68. Bill Jackson and Michael Pfitzmann, "Win-Win Sourcing," *Strategy and Business* 47 (May 29, 2007), http://www.strategy-business.com/article/07207?gko=dblda (accessed February 12, 2010).

69. Tracy H. Blumenfeld and Darren Zinner, PhD research study at RapidTrials and Harvard Business School, cited in Sarah O'Neil, April Lewis, and Jo Sorgi-Gendreau, "CRAs and Site Performance in the U.S.," *The Monitor*, September 2009, 51, http://www.nxtbook.com/nxtbooks/acrp/monitor_200909/index.php#/51/ (accessed February 12, 2010).

70. MAGI, "MAGI Model Clinical Trial Agreement," version 1.26, July 2009, http://www.magiworld.org/documents/ (accessed February 11, 2010).

Chapter 4

1. World Health Organization, "The Impact of Implementation of ICH Guidelines in Non-ICH Countries," 2001, http://www.who.int/medicines/library/qsm/who-edm-qsm-2002-3/who-edm-qsm-2002-3.pdf (accessed July 14, 2005).

2. Paula Waterman, "Institutional Review Boards," IRB Forum 2001, http://www.irbforum.org/documents/documents/FDAvICH56.rtf (accessed July 15, 2005).

3. Kate Maloney, "Good Clinical Practice (GCP) & Clinical Trial Registries," Health Care Conference Administrators, LLC, 2004, http://www.ehcca.com/presentations/pharmacongress5/2_03_2.pdf (accessed July 14, 2005).

4. Kay Dickersin, "Clinical Trials Registration: Overdue yet Elusive," Johns Hopkins Bloomberg School of Public Health, July 7, 2005, http://www

.jhsph.edu/publichealthnews/articles/2005/dickersin.html (accessed July 17, 2005).

5. David Vulcano, "Healthcare Reform: Opportunities and Challenges for the Clinical Research Enterprise" (presentation at the MAGI Clinical Research Conference–West 2009, San Diego, CA, October 2009).

6. National Institutes of Health, Office of Extramural Research, "FAQs—Clinical Trials Registration in ClinicalTrials.gov," Grants Policy, December 17, 2008, http://www.grants.nih.gov/grants/policy/hs/faqs_aps_clinical_trials.htm (accessed February 12, 2010).

7. Ibid.

8. Janet Raloff, "Cancer Data: Burying Bad News," *Science News*, September 24, 2008, http://www.sciencenews.org/view/generic/id/36805/title/Cancer_data_Burying_bad_news (accessed February 12, 2010).

9. U.S. Department of Health and Human Services, Office for Human Research Protections, "Assurances," http://www.hhs.gov/ohrp/assurances/assurances_index.html (accessed February 12, 2010).

10. FDA, "Acceptance of Foreign Clinical Studies—Information Sheet," http://www.fda.gov/RegulatoryInformation/Guidances/ucm126426.htm site updated May 22, 2009, (accessed February 12, 2010).

11. U.S. Department of Health and Human Services, Office of Inspector General, *The Globalization of Clinical Trials: A Growing Challenge in Protecting Human Subjects*, OEI-01-00-00190 (Washington, DC: September 2001), http://www.oig.hhs.gov/oei/reports/oei-01-00-00190.pdf (accessed February 12, 2010).

12. European Medicines Agency, *ICH Topic E5: Ethnic Factors in the Acceptability of Foreign Clinical Data*, 1998, http://www.emea.europa.eu/pdfs/human/ich/028995en.pdf (accessed February 12, 2010).

13. Ibid.

14. W. Thomas Smith, "FDA Requires Foreign Clinical Studies Be in Accordance with Good Clinical Practice to Better Protect Human Subjects," *ABA Health eSource* 5, no. 2 (October 2008), http://www.abanet.org/health/esource/Volume5/02/smith.html#_ftnref19 (accessed February 12, 2010).

15. European Medicines Agency, *Reflection Paper on the Extrapolation of Results from Clinical Studies Conducted Outside Europe to the E.U. Population*, 2009, http://www.emea.europa.eu/pdfs/human/ewp/69270208en.pdf (accessed February 12, 2010).

16. Bruce Binkowitz, "An Overview of Issues Surrounding Multi-Regional Clinical Trials" (presentation at the Harvard Schering-Plough 17th Annual Workshop, Boston, MA, May 28, 2009), http://www.hsph.harvard.edu/schering-plough-workshop/program/index.html (accessed February 12, 2010).

17. FDA, *Guidance for Industry: Collection of Race and Ethnicity Data in Clinical Trials*, September 2005, http://www.fda.gov/downloads/RegulatoryInformation/Guidances/ucm126396.pdf (accessed February 12, 2010).

18. Adriana Petryna, "When Experiments Travel: Clinical Trials and the Global Search for Human Subjects," in *When Experiments Travel: Clinical Trials and the Global Search for Human Subjects* (Princeton University Press, 2009), http://press.princeton.edu/chapters/i8916.html (accessed February 12, 2010).

19. European Medicines Agency, *ICH Topic E5: Ethnic Factors in the Acceptability of Foreign Clinical Data*, 1998, http://www.emea.europa.eu/pdfs/human/ich/028995en.pdf (accessed February 12, 2010).

20. Toshiyoshi Tominaga, "Global Clinical Development—Reducing Japan's Drug Lag," Pharma Focus Asia, 2008, http://www.pharmafocusasia.com/clinical_trials/global_clinical_development_japan_druglag.htm (accessed February 12, 2010).

21. David Vulcano, "Healthcare Reform: Opportunities and Challenges for the Clinical Research Enterprise" (presentation at the MAGI Clinical Research Conference–West 2009, San Diego, CA, October 2009).

22. Centers for Medicare and Medicaid Services and the Joint Commission, "Performance Measurement Initiatives," *Specifications Manual for National Hospital Inpatient Quality Measures*, October 2, 2009, http://www.jointcommission.org/performancemeasurement/performancemeasurement/current+nhqm+manual.htm (accessed February 12, 2010).

23. National Cancer Institute, Clinical Research Information Exchange, "Welcome to the CRIX Web site," http://crix.nci.nih.gov/.

24. David Vulcano, "Healthcare Reform: Opportunities and Challenges for the Clinical Research Enterprise," (presentation at the MAGI Clinical Research Conference–West 2009, San Diego, CA, October 2009).

25. FDA, "Investigational New Drug Application," *Code of Federal Regulations*, Title 21, Part 312, https://www.accessdata.fda.gov/scripts/cdrh/cfdocs/cfCFR/CFRSearch.cfm?fr=312.23 (accessed February 12, 2010).

26. Barnett International, *The Form FDA 1572: A Reference Guide for Clinical Researchers, Sponsors, and Monitors*, 2008, http://www.barnettinternational.com/EducationalServices_Publication.aspx?p=6659 (accessed February 12, 2010).

27. FDA, *Guidance for Institutional Review Boards and Clinical Investigators: 21 CFR Part 50—Protection of Human Subjects*, 1998, http://www.fda.gov/oc/ohrt/irbs/appendixb.html (accessed January 25, 2004).

28. University of Iowa, "Informed Consent and Related Issues," December 31, 2003, http://research.uiowa.edu/hso/index.php?get=inv_guide_toc (accessed January 25, 2004).

29. Keiger and De Pasquale, "Trials and Tribulation"; and R. Weiss, "U.S. Halts Research on Humans at Duke; University Can't Ensure Safety, Probers Find," *Washington Post*, May 12, 1999, http://www.washingtonpost.com (accessed January 7, 2004).

30. Donald F. Phillips, "IRB's Search for Answers and Support during a Time of Institutional Change," *Journal of the American Medical Association* 283,

no. 6 (2000): 729–730, also available at http://jama.ama-assn.org (accessed February 7, 2002).

31. U.S. Department of Health and Human Services, Office for Civil Rights, "HIPPA Medical Privacy—National Standards to Protect the Privacy of Personal Health Information," 2003, http://www.hhs.gov/ocr/hipaa/ (accessed January 25, 2004).

32. See U.S. Department of Health and Human Services, Office for Human Research Protections, "Public Welfare," *Code of Federal Regulations*, Title 45, Part 160—General Administrative Requirements, Part 162—Administrative Requirements, and Part 164—Security and Privacy.

33. Mindy J. Steinberg and Elaine R. Rubin, *The HIPAA Privacy Rule: Lacks Patient Benefit, Impedes Research Growth* (Washington, DC: Association of Academic Health Centers, 2009), http://www.aahcdc.org/policy/reddot/AAHC_HIPAA_Privacy_Rule_Impedes_Research_Growth.pdf (accessed February 12, 2010).

34. Association of Academic Health Centers, "HIPAA Creating Barriers to Research and Discovery," 2008, http://www.aahcdc.org/policy/reddot/AAHC_HIPAA_Creating_Barriers.pdf (accessed February 12, 2010).

35. Ibid.

36. Ibid.

37. Norman M. Goldfarb, "HIPAA Complaints in Clinical Research," *Journal of Clinical Research Best Practices* 4, no. 2 (2008), http://firstclinical.com/journal/2008/0802_complaint.pdf (accessed February 12, 2010).

38. Institute of Medicine, *Beyond the HIPAA Privacy Rule: Enhancing Privacy, Improving Health through Research*, January 27, 2009, http://www.iom.edu/CMS/3740/43729/61796/61836.aspx (accessed February 12, 2010).

39. U.S. Department of Health and Human Services, "Uses and Disclosures to Carry Out Treatment, Payment, or Health Care Operations," *Code of Federal Regulations*, Title 45, Part 164.506.

40. HIPAA Advisory, "Standards for Privacy of Individually Identifiable Health Information," Phoenix Health Systems, 2001, http://www.hipaadvisory.com/regs/finalprivacy/gconsent.htm (accessed January 25, 2004).

41. National Institutes of Health, "HIPPA Privacy Rule—Information for Researchers," January 23, 2004, http://privacyruleandresearch.nih.gov/ (accessed September 15, 2005); University of California, San Francisco, Human Subjects Protection Program, "HIPPA and Human Research, 2003," http://www.research.ucsf.edu/chr/HIPAA/chrHIPAA.asp (accessed January 25, 2004); and University of Iowa, "IRB Forms/Templates."

42. FDA, "Financial Disclosure by Clinical Investigators," *Code of Federal Regulations*, Title 21, Part 54, http://www.accessdata.fda.gov/scripts/cdrh/cfdocs/cfcfr/CFRSearch.cfm?CFRPart=54 (accessed February 12, 2010).

43. FDA, "Financial Interest Form: Certification: Financial Interests and Arrangements of Clinical Investigations," Form FDA 3454, http://www.fda.gov/opacom/morechoices/fdaforms/FDA-3454.pdf (accessed February 12, 2010).

44. FDA, "Financial Interest Form: Disclosure: Financial Interests and Arrangements of Clinical Investigators," Form FDA 3455, http://www.fda.gov/opacom/morechoices/fdaforms/FDA-3455.pdf (accessed February 12, 2010).

45. Norman M. Goldfarb, "Investigator Disclosures of Financial Conflicts" *Journal of Clinical Research Best Practices* 4, no. 10 (2008), http://firstclinical.com/journal/2008/0810_Conflicts.pdf (accessed February 12, 2010).

46. Michael Swit, "FDA Inspections: Handling the Consequences" (presentation at the MAGI Clinical Research Conference–West, San Diego, CA, October 2009).

47. Ali F. Sonel and Kelly Willenberg, "Creating a Strategic Clinical Research Compliance Plan" (presentation at the MAGI Clinical Research Conference–West, San Diego, CA, October 2009).

48. FDA, *Guidance for Industry: Protecting the Rights, Safety, and Welfare of Study Subjects—Supervisory Responsibilities of Investigators*, 2007, http://www.fda.gov/RegulatoryInformation/Guidances/ucm127697.htm (accessed February 12, 2010).

49. Ibid.

50. Michael Swit, "FDA Inspections: Handling the Consequences" (presentation at the MAGI Clinical Research Conference–West, San Diego, CA, October 2009).

51. FDA, Center for Drug Evaluation and Research, *CDER 2001 Report to the Nation: Improving Public Health through Human Drugs*, 2001, http://www.fda.gov/cder/reports/rtn/2001/rtn2001.pdf (accessed January 28, 2004).

52. Michael Swit, "FDA Inspections: Handling the Consequences" (presentation at the MAGI Clinical Research Conference–West, San Diego, CA, October 2009).

53. Joseph P. Salewski, "An FDA Audit: What the Investigator and Sponsor Need to Know," American Society of Gene Therapy, 2001, http://www.asgt.org/recent_course_materials/training_course/salewski.ppt (accessed February 17, 2003).

54. Department of Health and Human Services, Office for Human Research Protections, *Guidance on Reviewing and Reporting Unanticipated Problems Involving Risks to Subjects or Others and Adverse Events*, January 15, 2007, http://www.hhs.gov/ohrp/policy/AdvEvntGuid.htm.

55. FDA, Warning Letter to John M. Kirkwood, MD, September 15, 2009, http://www.fda.gov/ICECI/EnforcementActions/WarningLetters/ucm183577.htm (accessed February 12, 2010).

56. Institute of Medicine, Committee on Assessing the System for Protecting Human Research Participants, *Responsible Research: A Systems Approach to Protecting Research Participants* (Washington, DC: National Academy

Press, 2002), http://www.nap.edu/openbook/0309084881/html/ (accessed February 18, 2004); and FDA, Center for Drug Evaluation and Research, *CDER 2002 Report to the Nation: Drug Safety and Quality.*

57. Cullen T. Vogelson, "Investigators Gone Bad," *Modern Drug Discovery* 4, no. 4 (April 2001): 27–30, http://pubs.acs.org/subscribe/journals/mdd/v04/i04/html/MDD04DeptRules.html (accessed January 31, 2002).

58. Stan W. Woollen, "Misconduct in Research—Innocent Ignorance or Malicious Malfeasance?" FDA, 2003, http://www.fda.gov/oc/gcp/slideshows/2003/gcp2003.ppt, http://www.uvu.edu/irb/documents/gcp2003.ppt (accessed October 17, 2009).

59. U.S. House Committee on Energy and Commerce, Subcommittee on Oversight and Investigations, "Ketek Fact Chronology," U.S. Food and Drug Administration Office of Criminal Investigations Investigative Work Product in Ketek Hearing Exhibit Binder, August 23, 2009, http://archives.energycommerce.house.gov/Investigations/KetekExhibitBinder/12001.pdf (accessed October 17, 2009).

60. Citizens for Responsible Care and Research, "Ketek Clinical Trials and FDA Approval," August 23, 2009, http://www.circare.org/foia5/ketek.htm (accessed February 12, 2010).

61. Ed Silverman, "Clinical-Trial Fraud: The Case of Ketek," Pharmalot, May 29, 2007, http://www.pharmalot.com/2007/05/clinical-trial-fraud-the-case-of-ketek/ (accessed February 12, 2010).

62. U.S. House Committee on Energy and Commerce, Subcommittee on Oversight and Investigations, "Ketek Fact Chronology," U.S. Food and Drug Administration Office of Criminal Investigations Investigative Work Product in Ketek Hearing Exhibit Binder, August 23, 2009, http://archives.energycommerce.house.gov/Investigations/KetekExhibitBinder/12001.pdf (accessed February 12, 2010).

63. Keiger and De Pasquale, "Trials and Tribulation"; Michael D. Lemonick and Andrew Goldstein, "At Your Own Risk," *Time*, April 22, 2002, http://www.time.com/time/health/article/0,8599,230358,00.html (accessed May 2, 2002); and Phillips, "IRB's Search for Answers."

64. Stan W. Woollen and Antoine El Hage, "Scientific Misconduct—the 'F' Word," FDA, October 1, 2001, http://www.fda.gov/oc/gcp/slideshows/misconduct2001/misconduct.html (accessed February 17, 2003); David Lepay, "GCP Compliance: Emerging Issues in Worldwide Clinical Trials," FDA, 1999, http://www.fda.gov/cder/present/dia-699/lepay-dia99/lepay-dia99.PPT (accessed January 27, 2004); and Pyotr G. Platonov and Sergei Varshavsky, "FDA Inspections outside the USA: An Eastern European Perspective," *Applied Clinical Trials* (September 2004), http://www.actmagazine.com/appliedclinicaltrials/article/articleDetail.jsp?id=121811 (accessed July 25, 2005).

65. Marjorie Speers, "AAHRPP Accreditation for Your Human Research Protection Program" (presentation at the MAGI Clinical Research Conference–West, San Diego, CA, October 2009).

66. FDA, Office of Regulatory Affairs, "Disqualified/Restricted/Assurances Lists for Clinical Investigators," November, 21, 2001, http://www.fda.gov/ora/compliance_ref/bimo/dis_res_assur.htm (accessed September 14, 2003).

67. FDA, Warning Letter to Johnson & Johnson Pharmaceutical Research & Development, LLC, August 10, 2009, http://www.fda.gov/ICECI/EnforcementActions/WarningLetters/ucm177398.htm (accessed February 12, 2010).

68. International Conference on Harmonisation, *Guideline for Good Clinical Practice*, ICH E.6, Step 5, Guideline 1.5.96, Section 1.50, http://www.fda.gov/cber/ich/ichguid.htm (accessed January 25, 2004).

69. *Gelsinger v. Trustees of University of Pennsylvania* (Philadelphia County, Ct. Com. Pl., filed September 18, 2000), available at http://www.sskrplaw.com/lawyer-attorney-1475659.html (accessed February 12, 2010).

70. *Grimes v. Kennedy Krieger Institute*, 782 A.2d 807 (Md. 2001), http://biotech.law.lsu.edu/cases/research/grimes_v_KKI.htm (accessed February 12, 2010).

71. Platonov and Varshavsky, "FDA Inspections outside the USA."

72. Michael Swit, "FDA Inspections: Handling the Consequences" (presentation at the MAGI Clinical Research Conference–West, San Diego, CA, October 2009).

73. FDA, *Inspections, Compliance, Enforcement, and Criminal Investigations*, "Bioresearch Monitoring," http://www.fda.gov/ICECI/EnforcementActions/BioresearchMonitoring/default.htm (accessed February 12, 2010).

74. Ibid.

75. FDA, Center for Drug Evaluation and Research, "Dr. Woodcock Provides Highlights of Her Detail: Implementing Quality Systems, Collaboration with NIH Top List," Janet Woodcock, *News along the Pike* 10, no. 1 (2004), http://www.fda.gov/ohrms/dockets/dockets/04p0171/04p-0171-cp00001-04-exhibit-3.pdf (accessed October 18, 2009).

76. Michael Swit, "FDA Inspections: Handling the Consequences" (presentation at the MAGI West Conference, San Diego, CA, October 2009), citing "Compliance and Enforcement" (presentation by David K. Elder, Director, FDA Office of Enforcement, at the Orange County Regulatory Affairs/FDA Joint Educational Conference, June 2005).

Chapter 5

1. Mark Peters, "Thought Identification and Other Potential Future Feelings," Visual Thesaurus: Evasive Maneuvers—Euphemisms Old and New, February 4, 2009, http://www.visualthesaurus.com/cm/evasive/1688/ (accessed February 12, 2010).

2. FDA, *Guidance for Institutional Review Boards: Protection of Human Subjects.*

3. Kathy Schulz, "Phantom of the Oprr," PRIM&R, IRB Follies, http://www.geocities.com/ (site now discontinued).

4. University of Michigan, "Informed Consent," 2003, http://www.med.umich.edu/irbmed/InformationalDocuments/consent/consenttoc.html (accessed February 7, 2003); and University of Southern California, "IRB Forms," 2003, http://ccnt.hsc.usc.edu/irb/docs/instruction.htm (accessed February 7, 2003).

5. University of Michigan, "Tips on Preparing Understandable Informed Consent Documents," 2002, http://www.med.umich.edu/irbmed/InformationalDocuments/consent/investigator.html (accessed February 7, 2003).

6. Claudette Dalton, "Health Literacy Basic Lecture," University of Virginia, 2006, http://www.healthsystem.virginia.edu/internet/som-hlc/Lecture.cfm (accessed November 5, 2009).

7. John Burke, "ICH-GCP and FDA Regulations Differences," April 1, 2009, http://louisville.edu/research/humansubjects/ICH%20GCP%20-%20FDA%20Regulations%20Differences_4-20-09.ppt (accessed February 12, 2010).

8. Institute of Medicine, "Public Confidence and Involvement in Clinical Research," 2001, http://www.iom.edu/report.asp?id=4891 (accessed January 6, 2004).

9. Montgomery, site and investigator assessment.

10. Jacquie Mardell, "Informed Consent/Assent/HIPAA" (presentation at the MAGI Clinical Research Conference–West, San Diego, CA, October 2009); and Linda Rudolph, "Human Subject Protection: Role of the IRB and the Clinical Investigator" (presentation at the MAGI Clinical Research Conference–West, San Diego, CA, October 2009).

11. Jon Hart, "Unapprovable," PRIM&R, IRB Follies, http://www.geocities.com/ (site now discontinued).

12. Limited English Proficiency: A Federal Interagency Website, "Overview of Executive Order 13166," http://www.lep.gov/13166/eo13166.html (accessed February 12, 2010).

13. Institute of Medicine, Committee on Health Literacy, Board on Neuroscience and Behavioral Health, *Health Literacy: A Prescription to End Confusion*, ed. Lynn Nielsen-Bohlman, Allison Panzer, and David A. Kindig (Washington, DC: National Academy Press, 2004), cited in "National Quality Forum, Safe Practices for Better Healthcare 2006," http://www.qualityforum.org/Publications/2007/03/Safe_Practices_for_Better_Healthcare%E2%80%932006_Update.aspx (accessed February 12, 2010).

14. Claudette Dalton, "Health Literacy Basic Lecture," University of Virginia, 2006, http://www.healthsystem.virginia.edu/internet/som-hlc/Lecture.cfm (accessed November 5, 2009).

15. Joint Commission, *What Did the Doctors Say? Improving Health Literacy to Protect Patient Safety*, 2007, http://www.jointcommission.org/NewsRoom/PressKits/Health_Literacy/ (accessed February 12, 2010).

16. Institute of Medicine, Committee on Health Literacy, Board on Neuroscience and Behavioral Health, *Health Literacy: A Prescription to End Confusion*, ed. Lynn Nielsen-Bohlman, Allison Panzer, and David A. Kindig (Washington, DC: National Academy Press, 2004), http://www.qualityforum.org/Publications/2007/03/Safe_Practices_for_Better_Healthcare%E2%80%932006_Update.aspx (accessed February 12, 2010).

17. Dalton, "Health Literacy Basic Lecture," citing Dean Schillinger et al., "Association of Health Literacy with Diabetes Outcomes," *Journal of the American Medical Association* 288 (2002): 475–482, http://jama.ama-assn.org/cgi/content/abstract/288/4/475 (accessed February 12, 2010).

18. U.S. Department of Health and Human Services, Agency for Healthcare Research and Quality, "30 Safe Practices for Better Health Care," fact sheet, http://www.ahrq.gov/qual/30safe.htm (accessed February 12, 2010).

19. Jeffrey Driver, "Informed Consent: It's Not Just a Form, It's a Process," *Health Leaders Media*, June 24, 2008, http://www.healthleadersmedia.com/print/content/213995/topic/WS_HLM2_TEC/Informed-Consent-Its-Not-Just-a-Form-Its-a-Process.html (accessed February 12, 2010).

20. James Henry, Barton Palmer, et al., "Reformed Consent—Adapting to New Media and Research Participant Preferences: Multimedia Consent Aids," Medscape, http://www.medscape.com/viewarticle/704025 (accessed February 12, 2010).

21. Jovianna DiCarlo, "Technology Showcase" (presentation at the MAGI Clinical Research Conference–West, San Diego, CA, October 2009).

22. Dilip v. Jeste et al., "Multimedia Consent for Research in People with Schizophrenia and Normal Subjects: A Randomized Controlled Trial," *Schizophrenia Bulletin* 35, no. 4 (2009), doi:10.1093/schbul/sbm148, http://schizophreniabulletin.oxfordjournals.org/cgi/content/abstract/35/4/719 (accessed February 12, 2010).

23. Vincanne Adams et al., "The Challenge of Cross-Cultural Clinical Trials Research: Case Study from Tibet," *Medical Anthropology Quarterly* 19 (2005): 267–289, http://www.onehearttibet.org/docs/Challenge_of_CrossCultural.pdf (accessed February 12, 2010).

24. Andrew Sporle and Jonathan Koea, "Maori Responsiveness in Health and Medical Research: Key Issues for Researchers (Part 1)," *Journal of the New Zealand Medical Association* 117, no. 1199 (2004): 997, http://www.nzma.org.nz/journal/117-1199/997/ (accessed February 12, 2010).

25. Rawiri Taonui, "Tribal Organisation," in *Te Ara: The Encyclopedia of New Zealand*, 2009, http://www.teara.govt.nz/en/tribal-organisation (accessed February 12, 2010).

26. Jill Wechsler, "Health Information Technology Offers Both Promise and Problems: Biomedical Research Community Finds Privacy Policies Add Cost and

Complexity to Clinical Studies," *Applied Clinical Trials*, April 1, 2009, http://appliedclinicaltrialsonline.findpharma.com/appliedclinicaltrials/US/Health-IT-Offers-Both-Promise-and-Problems/ArticleStandard/Article/detail/591990 (accessed February 12, 2010).

27. Julian Teixeira, "Research Partnership Will Study How Electronic Medical Records Can Address Genetics of Drug Safety," Eurekalert, October 21, 2009, http://www.eurekalert.org/pub_releases/2009-10/zg-rpw102109.php (accessed February 12, 2010).

28. Richard L. Tannen, Mark G. Weiner, and Dawei Xie, "Use of Primary Care Electronic Medical Record Database in Drug Efficacy Research on Cardiovascular Outcomes: Comparison of Database and Randomised Controlled Trial Findings," *British Medical Journal* 338 (2009), doi:10.1136/bmj.b81, http://www.bmj.com/cgi/content/full/338/jan27_1/b81#otherarticles (accessed February 12, 2010).

29. Lawrence B. Afrin et al., "Leveraging of Open EMR Architecture for Clinical Trial Accrual," in *American Medical Informatics Association (AMIA) Annual Symposium Proceedings*, 2003: 16–20, http://www.ncbi.nlm.nih.gov/pmc/articles/PMC1480210/ (accessed February 12, 2010).

30. Peter J. Embi et al., "Development of an Electronic Health Record-Based Clinical Trial Alert System to Enhance Recruitment at the Point of Care," in *American Medical Informatics Association (AMIA) Annual Symposium Proceedings*, 2005: 231–235, http://www.ncbi.nlm.nih.gov/pmc/articles/PMC1560758/ (accessed February 12, 2010).

31. FDA, *Guidance for Industry: Computerized Systems Used in Clinical Investigations*, May 2007, http://www.fda.gov/OHRMS/DOCKETS/98fr/04d-0440-gdl0002.pdf (accessed February 12, 2010).

32. FDA, *Guidance for Industry Part 11, Electronic Records: Electronic Signatures—Scope and Application*, 2003, http://www.fda.gov/downloads/Drugs/GuidanceComplianceRegulatoryInformation/Guidances/UCM072322.pdf (accessed February 12, 2010).

33. Carl Anderson, "The Ins and Outs of Electronic Medical Records," *Applied Clinical Trials*, September 1, 2008, http://appliedclinicaltrialsonline.findpharma.com/appliedclinicaltrials/IT+Articles/The-Ins-and-Outs-of-Electronic-Medical-Records/ArticleStandard/Article/detail/546113 (accessed February 12, 2010).

34. U.S. Department of Health and Human Services, National Institutes of Health, "Health Services Research and the HIPAA Privacy Rule," 2005, http://privacyruleandresearch.nih.gov/healthservicesprivacy.asp (accessed February 12, 2010).

35. Atul Gawande, "A Lifesaving Checklist," *New York Times*, December 30, 2007, sec. Opinion, http://www.nytimes.com/2007/12/30/opinion/30gawande.html (accessed February 12, 2010).

36. Diana Anderson, "Patient Recruitment Strategies," drugdev123.com, January 1, 2002, http://www.drugdev123.com/editorial/PatientRecruitment/87.shtml (accessed November 13, 2002; site now discontinued).

37. Linda Lillington, "Patient Recruitment in Clinical Trials," http://uscnurse.usc.edu/class/461/USClecture701revised.htm (accessed January 19, 2003).

38. Cutting Edge Information, *Streamlining Clinical Trials Report*, 2009, 199, http://www.cuttingedgeinfo.com/clinical-trials/?overview.

39. CenterWatch, "2009 Patient Experience Survey," cited in Veronica Legge, "2009 Subject and Physician Survey Results: Understanding the Relationship to Maximize Study Referrals" (presentation at the MAGI Clinical Research Conference–West, San Diego, CA, October 2009).

40. Ibid.

41. Gardiner Harris, "Student, 19, in Trial of New Antidepressant Commits Suicide," *New York Times*, February 12, 2004, also available at http://www.nytimes.com (accessed September 20, 2004).

42. CenterWatch, "2009 Patient Experience Survey," cited in Veronica Legge, "2009 Subject and Physician Survey Results: Understanding the Relationship to Maximize Study Referrals" (presentation at the MAGI Clinical Research Conference–West, San Diego, CA, October 2009).

43. Institute of Medicine, "Public Confidence and Involvement in Clinical Research."

44. CenterWatch, "2009 Patient Experience Survey," cited in Veronica Legge, "2009 Subject and Physician Survey Results: Understanding the Relationship to Maximize Study Referrals" (presentation at the MAGI Clinical Research Conference–West, San Diego, CA, October 2009).

45. "NCI: Cancer Trial News—Maryland Law Covers Clinical Trials," *Clinical Rounds* 1, no. 1 (2000), http://www.clinicalrounds.com/html/articles/1198-19.htm.

46. Cutting Edge Information, *Streamlining Clinical Trials Report*, 2009, 177, http://www.cuttingedgeinfo.com/clinical-trials/?overview.

47. FDA, *Guidance for Institutional Review Boards and Clinical Investigators: Recruiting Study Subjects*, 1998 update, http://www.fda.gov/oc/ohrt/irbs/toc4.html#recruiting (accessed December 24, 2005).

48. Ibid.

49. Cutting Edge Information, *Streamlining Clinical Trials Report*, 2009, 82, http://www.cuttingedgeinfo.com/clinical-trials/?overview.

50. Jeff Cooper, "Wondercillin Commercial" (presentation at the PRIM&R annual meeting, 1998), http://www.geocities.com/ (accessed January 1, 2006; site now discontinued).

51. Dana-Farber Cancer Institute, "Entering a Clinical Trial: Is It Right for You?" December 17, 2007, http://www.dana-farber.org/res/clinical/trials-info/default.html (accessed February 12, 2010).

52. Center for Information and Study on Research Participation, "Participating in a Clinical Trial," http://www.ciscrp.org/patient/videos.html (accessed February 14, 2010).

53. International Federation of Pharmaceutical Manufacturers and Associations, Clinical Trials Portal, http://clinicaltrials.ifpma.org/en/myportal/index.htm (accessed February 12, 2010).

54. Deborah Borfitz, "Social Networking Sites Have Myriad Trial-Related Uses," eCliniqua, March 2, 2009, http://www.ecliniqua.com/2009/03/02/social-networking-recruitment-sites.html (accessed February 12, 2010).

55. Deb Borfitz and Allison Proffitt, "Social Networking Sites Embrace Clinical Trials," Bio-ITWorld.com, May 19, 2009, http://www.bio-itworld.com/issues/2009/may-jun/social-networking-clinical-trials.html (accessed February 12, 2010).

56. U.S. Department of Health and Human Services, Office of Inspector General, *Clinical Trial Web Sites: A Promising Tool to Foster Informed Consent*, by Janet Rehnquist, OEI-01-97-00198 (Washington, DC: May 2002), http://oig.hhs.gov/oei/reports/oei-01-97-00198.pdf (accessed February 12, 2010).

57. Ibid.

58. Norman M. Goldfarb, "What Is Killing Off the Investigators? A Clinical Research Mystery," *Journal of Clinical Research Best Practices* 1, no. 7 (2005), http://firstclinical.com/journal/2005/0507_Mystery.pdf (accessed February 10, 2010), citing Harris Interactive, "Public Awareness of Clinical Trials Increases: New Survey Suggests Those Conducting Trials Are Doing a Better Job of Informing Potential Participants of Opportunities," http://www.harrisinteractive.com/news/printerfriend/index.asp?NewsID=812.

59. Edward Shin and Jean-Luc Neptune, "Why Should We Participate in Clinical Trials?" mAssKickers, http://www.masskickers.com/main/cancer-info/articles/77-why-should-we-participate-in-clinical-trials, August 12, 2009 (accessed May 2, 2010), citing Harris Interactive, " Misconceptions and Lack of Awareness Greatly Reduce Recruitment for Cancer Clinical Trials," http://www.harrisinteractive.com/news/printerfriend/index.asp?NewsID=222.

Chapter 6

1. Norman M. Goldfarb, "Something for Everyone: Standard Operating Procedure Products for the Investigative Site," *Journal of Clinical Research Best Practices* 1, no. 4 (2005), http://firstclinical.com/journal/2005/0504_SOPReview.pdf.

2. Duke Clinical Research Institute, Clinical Trials Networks Best Practices, "SOP Guidelines for Writers," https://www.ctnbestpractices.org/sites/sops/sop-guidelines-for-writers-word/view (accessed February 13, 2010).

3. Advanced Clinical Software, "Study Manager," 2003, http://www.acs-world.com/ (accessed January 27, 2004).

4. Jack Byrd, Jr., *Operations Research Models for Public Administration* (Lexington, MA: D. C. Heath & Company, 1975); and Martin E. Modell, 1996. "PERT, CPM, and Gantt," in *A Professional's Guide to Systems Analysis*, 2nd ed. (New York: McGraw Hill, 1996), http://studentweb.tulane.edu/~mtruill/dev-pert.html (accessed January 27, 2004).

5. Advanced Clinical Software, "Study Manager."

6. TrialTrac, "Sitetrac," 2004, http://www.trialtrac.com/ (accessed January 29, 2004; now called TrialWorks by ClinPhone, accessed December 26, 2005); and Oracle, "Clinical SiteMinder and TrialMinder Solutions for Clinical Trials Management," 2005, http://www.oracle.com/industries/life_sciences/siteminder_trialminder_data_sheet.pdf (accessed September 15, 2005).

7. U.S. Department of Health and Human Services, Centers for Medicare and Medicaid Services, "Medicare Clinical Trial Policies Overview," http://www.cms.hhs.gov/clinicaltrialpolicies/ (accessed February 13, 2010).

8. Healthcare Billing Compliance Solution, "Regulation and Reimbursement Suite," MediRegs, http://www.mediregs.com/medical-billing-compliance-solution (accessed February 13, 2010).

9. FDA, Center for Drug Evaluation and Research, *CDER 2001 Report to the Nation: Improving Public Health through Human Drugs.*

10. Julie Morganstern, *Organizing from the Inside Out* (New York: Henry Holt and Company, LLC, 1998).

11. Jon Hart, "My Favorite Things," PRIM&R, IRB Follies, http://www.geocities.com (site now discontinued).

12. Cutting Edge Information, *Streamlining Clinical Trials Report*, 2009, 162, http://www.cuttingedgeinfo.com/clinical-trials/?overview.

13. Elizabeth Moench, "The Partially Involved Principal Investigator," *Applied Clinical Trials* 1, no.1 (2002): 30.

14. Cutting Edge Information, *Streamlining Clinical Trials Report*, 2009, 197–202, http://www.cuttingedgeinfo.com/clinical-trials/?overview.

15. Kenneth Getz, *The Gift of Participation: A Guide to Making Informed Decisions about Volunteering for a Clinical Trial* (Bar Harbor, ME: Jerian Publishing, 2007).

16. S. Eric Ceh, "Documenting Concomitant Medications in Clinical Trials," *Journal of Clinical Research Best Practices* 3, no. 7 (2007), http://www.firstclinical.com/journal/2007/0707_Concomitant.pdf (accessed February 13, 2010).

17. E. Maheu et al., "Design and Conduct of Clinical Trials in Patients," *Osteoarthritis Cartilage* 14, no. 4 (2006): 303–22, http://www.ncbi.nlm.nih.gov/pubmed/16697937 (accessed February 13, 2010).

18. Joseph R. Dalovisio, "Hurricane Katrina: Lessons Learned in Disaster Planning for Hospitals, Medical Schools, and Communities," *Current Infectious Disease Reports* 8 (2006): 171–173, http://www.springerlink.com/index/K831155M2437K878.pdf (accessed February 13, 2010).

19. Fran Simon, "Tulane Reaches Out to Clinical Trial Participants," *The New Wave*, November 17, 2005, http://www.tulane.edu/newwave/111705_clinicaltrial.html (accessed February 13, 2010).

20. Joseph R. Dalovisio, "Hurricane Katrina: Lessons Learned in Disaster Planning for Hospitals, Medical Schools, and Communities," *Current Infectious Disease Reports* 8 (2006): 171–173, http://www.springerlink.com/index/K831155M2437K878.pdf (accessed February 13, 2010).

21. Larry H. Hollier, "The Impact of Hurricane Katrina on Louisiana State University Health Sciences Center, New Orleans," Testimony for the United States Senate, htpp://help.senate.gov/Hearings/2006_07_14_b/Hollier.pdf; also available through http://books.google.com (accessed February 13, 2010).

22. Fran Simon, "Tulane Reaches Out to Clinical Trial Participants," *The New Wave*, November 17, 2005, http://www.tulane.edu/newwave/111705_clinicaltrial.html (accessed February 13, 2010).

23. Alicia Pouncey, "Hurricane Katrina: What Have We Learned?" *Applied Clinical Trials*, October 1, 2006, http://appliedclinicaltrialsonline.findpharma.com/appliedclinicaltrials/article/Article/detail/377745 (accessed February 13, 2010).

24. Cullen T. Vogelson, "The Book of Knowledge," *Modern Drug Design* 4, no. 8 (August 2001): 25–26.

25. Katherine L. Monti, "Save Time and Money through Data Management," *Applied Clinical Trials* (October 2001): 54–62.

26. John Clay, cited in Neil McKenna, "Internet-Based Tools to Facilitate Clinical Trials," *Genetic Engineering News* 21, no. 1 (2001): 11.

27. U.S. Department of Health and Human Services, Office for Human Research Protections, "OHRP Policy Guidance," *Guidance on Reviewing and Reporting Unanticipated Problems Involving Risks to Subjects or Others and Adverse Events*, January 15, 2007, http://www.hhs.gov/ohrp/policy/AdvEvntGuid.htm#Q1 (accessed February 3, 2010).

28. International Conference on Harmonisation, *Guideline for Good Clinical Practice*.

29. FDA, "What Is a Serious Adverse Event?" Safety, updated February 9, 2010, http://www.fda.gov/Safety/MedWatch/HowToReport/ucm053087.htm (accessed February 13, 2010).

30. FDA, "New Drug and Biological Drug Products," *Code of Federal Regulations*, Title 21, Parts 312.55(b) and 312.32(c), http://www.gpoaccess.gov/cfr/index.html (accessed September 15, 2005).

31. U.S. Department of Health and Human Services, Office for Human Research Protections, "OHRP Policy Guidance," *Guidance on Reviewing and Reporting Unanticipated Problems Involving Risks to Subjects or Others and Adverse Events*, January 15, 2007, http://www.hhs.gov/ohrp/policy/AdvEvntGuid.htm (accessed February 3, 2010).

32. Anne A. Gershon, IDSA Letter to Dr. Peggy Hamburg Regarding Adverse Event Reporting, September 10, 2009, http://www.idsociety.org/WorkArea/DownloadAsset.aspx?id=15310 (accessed February 13, 2010).

33. U.S. Department of Health and Human Services, Office for Human Research Protections, "OHRP Policy Guidance," *Guidance on Reviewing and Reporting Unanticipated Problems Involving Risks to Subjects or Others and Adverse Events*, January 15, 2007, http://www.hhs.gov/ohrp/policy/AdvEvntGuid.htm (accessed February 3, 2010).

34. FDA, *Guidance for Clinical Investigators, Sponsors, and IRBs: Adverse Event Reporting—Improving Human Subject Protection*, January 2009, http://www.fda.gov/downloads/RegulatoryInformation/Guidances/ucm127346.pdf (accessed February 13, 2010).

35. U.S. Department of Health and Human Services, Office for Human Research Protections, "OHRP Policy Guidance," *Guidance on Reviewing and Reporting Unanticipated Problems Involving Risks to Subjects or Others and Adverse Events*, January 15, 2007, http://www.hhs.gov/ohrp/policy/AdvEvntGuid.htm (accessed February 3, 2010).

36. Ibid.

37. Ibid.

38. Ibid.

39. Ibid.

40. FDA, *Guidance for Clinical Investigators, Sponsors, and IRBs: Adverse Event Reporting—Improving Human Subject Protection*, January 2009, http://www.fda.gov/downloads/RegulatoryInformation/Guidances/ucm127346.pdf (accessed February 13, 2010).

41. U.S. Department of Health and Human Services, Office for Human Research Protections, "OHRP Policy Guidance," *Guidance on Reviewing and Reporting Unanticipated Problems Involving Risks to Subjects or Others and Adverse Events*, January 15, 2007, http://www.hhs.gov/ohrp/policy/AdvEvntGuid.htm (accessed February 3, 2010).

Chapter 7

1. Tufts Center for the Study of Drug Development, "Outlook 2003," Tufts University, 2003, http://csdd.tufts.edu/InfoServices/OutlookReports.asp (accessed September 9, 2003).

2. Tufts Center for the Study of Drug Development, "New Drugs Are Taking Longer to Bring to Market in the U.S," Tufts University, 2005, http://csdd.tufts.edu/NewsEvents/NewsArticle.asp?newsid=58 (accessed January 20, 2005).

3. Tufts Center for the Study of Drug Development, "Backgrounder: How New Drugs Move through the Development and Approval Process," Tufts University, November 2004, http://csdd.tufts.edu/NewsEvents/RecentNews.asp?newsid=4 (accessed September 15, 2003); and Diedtra Henderson, "FDA Rules Aim to Speed Drug Tests and Trim Costs," *Boston Globe*, January 13, 2006, http://www.boston.com/business/healthcare/articles/2006/01/13/fda_rules_aim_to_speed_drug_tests_and_trim_costs/.

4. National Institutes of Health, "NIH Announces New Program to Develop Therapeutics for Rare and Neglected Diseases," NIH News, May 20, 2009, http://www.nih.gov/news/health/may2009/nhgri-20.htm (accessed February 9, 2010).

5. Milton Zall, "The Pricing Puzzle," *Modern Drug Discovery* 4, no. 3 (March 2001): 36–42, http://pubs.acs.org/subscribe/journals/mdd/v04/i03/html/03zall.html (accessed January 31, 2002).

6. Mark Hovde, "Comparing Costs in CRO Contracts," *International Journal of Pharmaceutical Medicine* 11 (1997): 249–53; and Mark Hovde, "Integrating Protocol Design and Financial Planning," Data Edge DataLines, 2001, http://www.fast-track.org (accessed February 12, 2003).

7. Hassan Movahhed, cited in Neil McKenna, "Internet-Based Tools to Facilitate Clinical Trials," *Genetic Engineering News* 21, no. 1 (2001): 10–11.

8. Data from *An Evolution in Industry*, 4th ed. (Boston: Thomson CenterWatch, 2003), cited in Ronald P. Evens, *Drug and Biological Development: From Molecule to Product and Beyond* (New York: Springer, 2007): 15.

9. Frank S. Kilpatrick and Adelle Ricci, "Reducing Clinical Research Time," *Drug & Market Development*, 1999, http://pharmalicensing.com/features/disp/939893414_3805a2a6f2ca2 (accessed January 21, 2002); and Data Edge, "Compressing Development Times with Better Investigator Selection," Data Edge DataLines, Spring 1996, http://www.fast-track.org (accessed February 4, 2003).

10. Zall, "The Pricing Puzzle."

11. Ibid.

12. Harold Glass and Joann Sullivan, "Managing Clinical Grant Costs through the Use of Unaffiliated Investigators," *Drug Information Journal* 29, no. 2 (April–June 1995); and Harold Glass, "Clinical Grant Costs," *Scrip Magazine*, April 1, 1995.

13. Andrew Pollack, "Despite Billions for Discovery, Pipeline of Drugs Is Far from Full," *New York Times*, April 19, 2002, also available at http://www.nytimes.com (accessed February 8, 2003).

14. Tufts Center for the Study of Drug Development, "Backgrounder."

15. Christopher P. Adams and Van V. Brantner, "Estimating the Cost of New Drug Development: Is It Really $802 Million?" *Health Affairs* 25, no. 2 (2006), doi:10.1377/hlthaff.25.2.420, http://content.healthaffairs.org/cgi/reprint/25/2/420 (accessed February 9, 2010).

16. Public Citizen, "Tufts Drug Study Sample Is Skewed; True Figure of R&D Costs Likely Is 75% Lower," December 4, 2001, http://www.citizen.org/pressroom/release.cfm?ID=954 (accessed January 14, 2004).

17. Donald W. Light and Rebecca N. Warburton, "Extraordinary Claims Require Extraordinary Evidence," *Journal of Health Economics* 24, no. 5 (2005), doi:10.1016/j.jhealeco.2005.07.001, http://www.ncbi.nlm.nih.gov/pubmed/16087260 (accessed February 9, 2010).

18. PhRMA, *Pharmaceutical Industry Profile 2009* (Washington, DC: PhRMA, April 2009), http://www.phrma.org/files/attachments/PhRMA%20 2009%20Profile%20FINAL.pdf (accessed October 20, 2009).

19. Tufts Center for the Study of Drug Development, "Outlook 2003."

20. Data from *An Evolution in Industry*, 4th ed. (Boston: Thomson CenterWatch, 2003), cited in Ronald P. Evens, *Drug and Biological Development: From Molecule to Product and Beyond* (New York: Springer, 2007): 15.

21. Christopher P. Adams and Van V. Brantner, "Estimating the Cost of New Drug Development: Is It Really $802 Million?" *Health Affairs* 25, no. 2 (2006), doi:10.1377/hlthaff.25.2.420, http://content.healthaffairs.org/cgi/reprint/25/2/420 (accessed February 9, 2010).

22. Center for Information and Study on Research Participation, "101 Facts about Clinical Research," July 2005, http://www.scribd.com/doc/9768708/101-Facts-About-Clinical-Research (accessed February 10, 2010).

23. J. A. DiMasi, "Measuring Trends in the Development of New Drugs: Time, Costs, Risks and Returns" (presentation to the SLA Pharmaceutical & Health Technology Division Spring Meeting, Boston, MA, 2007); and Tufts Center for the Study of Drug Development, "Growing Protocol Design Complexity Stresses Investigators, Volunteers," *Impact Report* 10, no. 1 (January/February 2008), cited in PhRMA, Pharmaceutical Industry Profile 2009 (Washington, DC: PhRMA, 2009), http://www.phrma.org/files/attachments/PhRMA%202009%20 Profile%20FINAL.pdf (accessed February 9, 2010).

24. Tufts Center for the Study of Drug Development, "Growing Protocol Design Complexity Stresses Investigators, Volunteers," *Impact Report* 10, no. 1 (2008), cited in PhRMA, *Pharmaceutical Industry Profile 2009* (Washington, DC: PhRMA, 2009), http://www.phrma.org/files/attachments/PhRMA%202009%20 Profile%20FINAL.pdf (accessed February 9, 2010).

25. Infectious Diseases Society of America, "'Bad Bugs, No Drugs': Defining the Antimicrobial Availability Problem," 2003, http://www.idsociety.org (accessed November 15, 2003).

26. Scott Hensley, "New Antibiotic Could Boost Besieged Aventis," *Wall Street Journal*, March 4, 2004.

27. Richard P. Wenzel, "The Antibiotic Pipeline—Challenges, Costs, and Values," *New England Journal of Medicine* 351 (2004): 523–26.

28. Sheryl Gay Stolberg and Jeff Gerth, "Drug Makers Design Studies with Eye to Competitive Edge," *New York Times*, December 23, 2000, http://www.nytimes.com (accessed February 8, 2003).

29. Henderson, "FDA Rules Aim to Speed Drug Tests and Trim Costs."

30. FDA, *Guidance for Industry, Investigators, and Reviewers: Exploratory IND Studies*, January 2006, http://www.fda.gov/downloads/Drugs/GuidanceComplianceRegulatoryInformation/Guidances/ucm078933.pdf (accessed February 9, 2010).

31. National Cancer Institute, Division of Cancer Treatment and Diagnosis, "NCI Experimental Therapeutics Program (NExT)," Major Initiatives, February 12, 2009, http://dctd.cancer.gov/MajorInitiatives/02NExT.htm (accessed February 10, 2010).

32. National Cancer Institute, "New Approaches to Cancer Drug Development and Clinical Trials: Questions and Answers," Questions and Answers, June 4, 2007, http://www.cancer.gov/newscenter/pressreleases/PhaseZeroNExTQandA/ (accessed February 10, 2010).

33. National Cancer Institute, "New Study Heralds Shortened Timeline for Anticancer Drug Development," News, June 4, 2007, http://www.cancer.gov/newscenter/pressreleases/PhaseZeroNExT/ (accessed February 10, 2010).

34. FDA, *Guidance for Industry, Investigators, and Reviewers: Exploratory IND Studies*, January 2006, http://www.fda.gov/downloads/Drugs/GuidanceComplianceRegulatoryInformation/Guidances/ucm078933.pdf (accessed February 9, 2010).

35. National Institutes of Health, "NIH Announces New Program to Develop Therapeutics for Rare and Neglected Diseases," NIH News, May 20, 2009, http://www.nih.gov/news/health/may2009/nhgri-20.htm (accessed February 9, 2010).

36. Stephanie Saul and Gardiner Harris, "Diabetes Drug Still Has Heart Risks, Doctors Warn," *New York Times*, June 6, 2007, sec. Health, http://www.nytimes.com/2007/06/06/health/06fda.html (accessed February 9, 2010).

37. Derek Lowe, "Avandia: Trouble or Not?" *In the Pipeline*, May 24, 2007, http://pipeline.corante.com/archives/2007/05/24/avandia_trouble_or_not.php (accessed February 9, 2010).

38. Bruce M. Psaty and Curt D. Furberg, "The Record on Rosiglitazone and the Risk of Myocardial Infarction," *New England Journal of Medicine* 357, no. 1 (2007), doi:10.1056/NEJMe078116, http://content.nejm.org/cgi/content/full/NEJMe078116 (accessed February 10, 2010).

39. Martin Guttierrez, "Recruitment Experience in a Phase 0 Trial of ABT-888, an Inhibitor of Poly (ADP-ribose) Polymerase (PARP), in Patients with Advanced Malignancies" (presentation, National Cancer Institute, Division of Cancer Treatment and Diagnosis), http://dctd.cancer.gov/MajorInitiatives/Sep0507Phase0Workshop/DrGutierrez090507.pps (accessed February 10, 2010).

40. Hermann Mucke, *Microdosing in Translational Medicine: Pros and Cons*, Advances Reports (Cambridge Healthtech Associates, May 2006), http://www.hmpharmacon.com/downloadPharma/CHA%20Microdosing%20Report%20Executive%20Summary%20(May%202006).pdf (accessed February 10, 2010).

41. Derek Lowe, "Adaptive Trials: What You Need to Know about Adaptive Trials," *Pharmaceutical Executive*, July 1, 2006, http://pharmexec.findpharma.com/pharmexec/article/articleDetail.jsp?id=352793 (accessed February 10, 2010).

42. Paul Gallo, Christy Chuang-Stein, et al., "Adaptive Designs in Clinical Drug Development—An Executive Summary of the PhRMA Working Group," *Journal of Biopharmaceutical Statistics* 16, no. 3 (2006): 275–283, http://dx.doi.org/10.1080/10543400600614742 (accessed February 10, 2010).

43. Mark Senak, "FDA's Dr. Janet Woodcock Discusses Adaptive Clinical Trials," Eye on FDA, September 4, 2007, http://www.eyeonfda.com/eye_on_fda/2007/09/fdas-dr-janet-w.html (accessed February 10, 2010).

44. Dan Weiner and Mark Hovde, "Critical Mass for Critical Path?" *Pharmaceutical Executive*, May 1, 2007, http://pharmexec.findpharma.com/pharmexec/Regulatory+Articles/Critical-Mass-for-Critical-Path/ArticleStandard/Article/detail/423202 (accessed February 10, 2010).

45. FDA, Armando Oliva et al., "Bioinformatics Modernization and the Critical Path to Improved Benefit-Risk Assessment of Drugs" (presentation at the 25th annual DIA Clinical Data Management Meeting, Medical Informatics Opportunities to Improve the Benefit-Risk Assessment of Drugs, March 19, 2007), http://www.fda.gov/ScienceResearch/SpecialTopics/CriticalPathInitiative/ArticlesandPresentations/ucm077542.htm (accessed February 10, 2010).

46. FDA, "Critical Path Initiative," http://www.fda.gov/ScienceResearch/SpecialTopics/CriticalPathInitiative/default.htm (accessed February 10, 2010).

47. Lawrence Lesko, "Model-Based Drug Development: A Critical Path Innovation to Integrate Data Analysis," 2005, http://www.fda.gov/ohrms/dockets/ac/05/slides/2005-4194S2_02_Lesko.ppt (accessed February 10, 2010).

48. Institute of Medicine, Committee on Comparative Effectiveness Research Prioritization, *Initial National Priorities for Comparative Effectiveness Research* (Washington, DC: National Academy Press, 2009), http://books.nap.edu/catalog/12648.html (accessed February 10, 2010).

49. Randall S. Stafford, Todd H. Wagner, and Philip W. Lavori, "New, but Not Improved? Incorporating Comparative-Effectiveness Information into FDA Labeling," *New England Journal of Medicine* 361, no. 13 (2009), doi:10.1056/

NEJMp0906490, http://content.nejm.org/cgi/content/full/361/13/1230 (accessed February 10, 2010).

50. Alicia Mundy, "Drug Makers Fight Stimulus Provision," *Wall Street Journal*, February 10, 2009, sec. Politics and Policy, http://online.wsj.com/article/SB123423024203966081.html (accessed February 10, 2010).

51. Barry Meier, "Opponents Line Up Against U.S. Effort to Compare Medical Treatments," *New York Times*, May 7, 2009, sec. Business, http://www.nytimes.com/2009/05/07/business/07compare.html (accessed February 10, 2010).

52. Peter Grier, "Is Comparing Medical Treatments Akin to 'Rationing' Care?" *Christian Science Monitor*, August 28, 2009, http://features.csmonitor.com/politics/2009/08/28/is-comparing-medical-treatments-akin-to-rationing-care/ (accessed February 10, 2010).

53. Randall S. Stafford, Todd H. Wagner, and Philip W. Lavori, "New, but Not Improved? Incorporating Comparative-Effectiveness Information into FDA Labeling," *New England Journal of Medicine* 361, no. 13 (2009), doi:10.1056/NEJMp0906490, http://content.nejm.org/cgi/content/full/361/13/1230 (accessed February 10, 2010).

54. Tracy Staton, "NEJM: Put Comparative Effectiveness on Drug Labels," Fierce Pharma, August 13, 2009, http://www.fiercepharma.com/story/nejm-put-comparative-effectiveness-drug-labels/2009-08-13 (accessed February 10, 2010).

55. Association of American Medical Colleges, "Breaking the Scientific Bottleneck."

56. Ibid.

57. Mark Hovde, "Integrating Protocol Design and Financial Planning," Data Edge DataLines, 2001, http://www.fast-track.org (accessed February 12, 2003).

58. Tufts–New England Medical Center, "The Renewal of Clinical Research," November 20, 2003, http://www.nemc.org/dccr/clinical_research_information.htm (accessed January 16, 2006).

59. Joan F. Bachenheimer, "Good Recruitment Practice: Working to Create the Bond Between Study and Subject," Applied Clinical Trials, April 1, 2004, http://appliedclinicaltrialsonline.findpharma.com/appliedclinicaltrials/article/articleDetail.jsp?id=89626 (accessed October 13, 2009), citing Steve Zisson, "Anticipating a Clinical Investigator Shortfall," CenterWatch 1 (2001): 1.

60. Kenneth A. Getz, "The Elusive Sponsor-Site Relationship," *Applied Clinical Trials*, February 1, 2009, http://appliedclinicaltrialsonline.findpharma.com/appliedclinicaltrials/Project+Management/The-Elusive-Sponsor-Site-Relationship/ArticleStandard/Article/detail/579328 (accessed August 2, 2009).

61. Tufts Center for the Study of Drug Development, "Current Investigator Landscape Poses a Growing Challenge for Sponsors," *Impact Report* 11, no. 1

(January/February 2009), http://csdd.tufts.edu/reports/description/ir_summaries (accessed February 10, 2010).

62. Barnett Educational Services, "2009–2010 Statistical Sourcebook Data Presented at DIA," press release, http://www.barnettinternational.com/EducationalServices_Content.aspx?id=93134 (accessed August 29, 2009).

63. Mary Pat Flaherty, Deborah Nelson, and Joe Stephens, "The Body Hunters, Part 2: Overwhelming the Watchdogs," *Washington Post*, December 18, 2000, A1, http://www.washingtonpost.com (accessed March 4, 2003).

64. Emily Anthes and Scott Allen, "U.S. Scientists Go Abroad to Find Patients for Cancer Studies," *Boston Globe*, December 29, 2007, http://www.boston.com/news/nation/articles/2007/12/29/us_cancer_researchers_go_abroad_for_trials/ (accessed February 10, 2010).

65. Diana Anderson, "Patient Recruitment Strategies," drugdev123.com, January 1, 2002, http://www.drugdev123.com/editorial/PatientRecruitment/87.shtml (accessed November 13, 2002; site now discontinued).

66. "From Bug to Drug," *Washington Post*, August 9, 2003, A14.

67. Association of American Medical College and FDA, *Drug Development Science: Obstacles and Opportunities for Collaboration among Academia, Industry and Government*, Report of an Invitational Conference (Association of American Medical Colleges and FDA, 2005), 5, http://www.aamc.org/drugdevelopmentscience (accessed February 10, 2010).

68. Cutting Edge Information, *Streamlining Clinical Trials Report*, 2009, 169, http://www.cuttingedgeinfo.com/clinical-trials/?overview.

69. Norman M. Goldfarb, "What Is Killing Off the Investigators? A Clinical Research Mystery," *Journal of Clinical Research Best Practices* 1, no. 7 (2005), http://firstclinical.com/journal/2005/0507_Mystery.pdf (accessed February 10, 2010).

70. Ibid.

71. Cutting Edge Information, *Streamlining Clinical Trials Report*, 2009, 176, http://www.cuttingedgeinfo.com/clinical-trials/?overview.

72. Harris Interactive, "Public Awareness of Clinical Trials Increases: New Survey Suggests Those Conducting Trials Are Doing a Better Job of Informing Potential Participants of Opportunities," June 11, 2004, http://www.harrisinteractive.com/news/printerfriend/index.asp?NewsID=812 (accessed February 12, 2010).

73. Harris Interactive, "Nationwide Survey Reveals Public Support of Clinical Research Studies on the Rise," June 27, 2001, http://www.harrisinteractive.com/news/allnewsbydate.asp?NewsID=323 (accessed February 13, 2010).

74. Center for Information and Study on Research Participation, "101 Facts about Clinical Research," July 2005, http://www.scribd.com/doc/9768708/101-Facts-About-Clinical-Research (accessed February 10, 2010).

75. Philippa Smit-Marshall, "Recruitment Strategies in Clinical Trials—A European Perspective," Pharmanet, white paper, http://www.pharmanet.com/pdf/whitepapers/Recruitment.pdf.

76. Kenneth A. Getz, "Protocol Design Trends and Their Effect on Clinical Trial Performance," *Regulatory Affairs Journal Pharma* 19, no. 5 (2008): 315–6, http://csdd.tufts.edu./_documents/www/Doc_233_7875_826.pdf (accessed February 10, 2010).

77. Kenneth A. Getz et al., "Assessing the Impact of Protocol Design Changes on Clinical Trial Performance," *American Journal of Therapeutics* 15, no. 5 (2008), doi:10.1097/MJT.0b013e31816b9027.

78. Kenneth A. Getz, "Protocol Design Trends and Their Effect on Clinical Trial Performance," *Regulatory Affairs Journal Pharma* 19, no. 5 (2008): 315–6, http://csdd.tufts.edu./_documents/www/Doc_233_7875_826.pdf (accessed February 10, 2010).

79. Cutting Edge Information, *Streamlining Clinical Trials Report*, 2009, http://www.cuttingedgeinfo.com/clinical-trials/?overview.

80. National Institutes of Health, Office of Extramural Research, "FAQs—Clinical Trials Registration in ClinicalTrials.gov," Grants Policy, December 17, 2008, http://www.grants.nih.gov/grants/policy/hs/faqs_aps_clinical_trials.htm (accessed February 10, 2010).

81. Jonathan Peachey et al., *The eClinical Equation, Part 1, Electronic Data Capture*, IBM Institute for Business Value, 2005, http://www.mdsol.com/sites/default/files/documents/library/wp/ibm_edc.pdf (accessed February 10, 2010).

82. Arthur A. Stone et al., "Patient Non-Compliance with Paper Diaries," *British Medical Journal* 324 (2002): 1193–4, http://www.bmj.com/cgi/reprint/324/7347/1193 (accessed February 10, 2010).

83. Deborah Borfitz, "Site Gripes and Solutions for EDC," Bio-ITWorld.com, September 15, 2009, http://www.bio-itworld.com/BioIT_Article.aspx?id=94288.

84. Linda Meyerson and Tracy Harmon Blumenfeld, "Rethinking the Sponsor-Investigator Relationship," *Pharmceutical Executive*, January 6, 2009, http://pharmexec.findpharma.com/pharmexec/R&D+Articles/Rethinking-the-Sponsor-Investigator-Relationship/ArticleStandard/Article/detail/574030 (accessed February 10, 2010).

85. Deborah Borfitz, "Site Gripes and Solutions for EDC," Bio-ITWorld.com, September 15, 2009, http://www.bio-itworld.com/BioIT_Article.aspx?id=94288.

86. Norman M. Goldfarb, "eSource: The Future is Here," *Journal of Clinical Research Best Practices* 1, no. 11 (2005), http://firstclinical.com/journal/2005/0511_eSource.pdf (accessed February 10, 2010).

87. Cutting Edge Information, *Streamlining Clinical Trials Report*, 2009, 131, http://www.cuttingedgeinfo.com/clinical-trials/?overview.

88. FDA, Center for Drug Evaluation and Research, "A Tool to Help You Decide: Detect Potentially Serious Liver Injury," Ted Guo, Kate Gelperin,

and John Senior, June 4, 2008, http://www.fda.gov/downloads/Drugs/ScienceResearch/ResearchAreas/ucm076777.pdf (accessed February 10, 2010).

89. National Cancer Institute, Federal Investigator Registry, Federal Investigator Registry of Biomedical Informatics Research Data (FIREBIRD), https://firebird.nci.nih.gov/Firebird/.

90. Dalovisio, "IDSA Outlines the Problem."

91. Ibid.

92. FDA, *Guidance for Industry: Special Protocol Assessment.*

93. Cutting Edge Information, *Streamlining Clinical Trials Report*, 2009, http://www.cuttingedgeinfo.com/clinical-trials/?overview.

94. Andrew Pollack, "Imclone Rejection Focuses Debate on Testing of Cancer Drugs," *New York Times*, February 8, 2002, also available at http://www.nytimes.com (accessed February 8, 2002).

95. Cutting Edge Information, *Streamlining Clinical Trials Report*, 2009, http://www.cuttingedgeinfo.com/clinical-trials/?overview.

96. David M. Dilts and Alan B. Sandler, "Invisible Barriers to Clinical Trials: The Impact of Structural, Infrastructural, and Procedural Barriers to Opening Oncology Clinical Trials," *Journal of Clinical Oncology* 24, no. 28 (2006): 4545-4552, http://www.jcojournal.org/cgi/reprint/24/28/4545 (accessed February 10, 2010).

97. Jennifer Peterson, "Improving the Site Start-up Process" (presentation at the MAGI Clinical Research Conference–West, San Diego, CA, October 2009).

98. Barnett Educational Services, "2009–2010 Statistical Sourcebook Data Presented at DIA," press release, http://www.barnettinternational.com/EducationalServices_Content.aspx?id=93134 (accessed February 10, 2010).

99. Seth Glickman et al., "Ethical and Scientific Implications of the Globalization of Clinical Research," *New England Journal of Medicine* 360, no. 26 (2009): 816–823, http://content.nejm.org/cgi/content/full/360/26/2792 (accessed February 10, 2010).

100. Center for Information and Study on Research Participation, "101 Facts about Clinical Research," July 2005, http://www.scribd.com/doc/9768708/101-Facts-About-Clinical-Research (accessed February 10, 2010).

101. U.S. Department of Health and Human Services, Office of Inspector General, *The Globalization of Clinical Trials: A Growing Challenge in Protecting Human Subjects*, OEI-01-00-00190 (Washington, DC: September 2001), http://www.oig.hhs.gov/oei/reports/oei-01-00-00190.pdf (accessed February 10, 2010).

102. Ted Agres, "Clinical Trials Trickling Away," *Drug Discovery and Development*, July 5, 2005, http://www.dddmag.com/clinical-trials-trickling-away.aspx (accessed February 10, 2010).

103. PhRMA, *Pharmaceutical Industry Profile 2009* (Washington, DC: PhRMA, April 2009), http://www.phrma.org/files/attachments/PhRMA%202009%20Profile%20FINAL.pdf (accessed October 20, 2009).

104. Kenneth A. Getz et al., "Assessing the Impact of Protocol Design Changes on Clinical Trial Performance," *American Journal of Therapeutics* 15, no. 5 (2008), doi:10.1097/MJT.0b013e31816b9027.

105. Kenneth A. Getz, "Tufts Data: Veteran P.I.s Drop Out," ClinPage, July 19, 2007, http://www.clinpage.com/article/tufts_data_veteran_pis_drop_out/ (accessed February 10, 2010).

106. Wynn Bailey, Carol Cruickshank, and Nikhil Sharma, "Make Your Move: Taking Clinical Trials to the Best Location," Pharmafocusasia.com, 2006, http://www.pharmafocusasia.com/knowledge_bank/white_papers/clinicaltrials_bestlocation.htm (accessed February 10, 2010).

107. Emily Anthes and Scott Allen, "U.S. Scientists Go Abroad to Find Patients for Cancer Studies," *Boston Globe*, May 6, 2009, http://www.boston.com/news/nation/articles/2007/12/29/us_cancer_researchers_go_abroad_for_trials/ (accessed February 10, 2010).

108. Wikipedia, "List of Countries by Population," http://en.wikipedia.org/wiki/List_of_countries_by_population (accessed February 17, 2010).

109. Patrick McGee, "Clinical Trials on the Move," *Drug Discovery and Development*, June 12, 2006, http://www.dddmag.com/clinical-trials-on-the-move.aspx (accessed February 10, 2010).

110. Dennis Normile, "The Promise and Pitfalls of Clinical Trials Overseas," *Science* 322, no. 5899 (2008), doi:10.1126/science.322.5899.214, http://www.sciencemag.org/cgi/content/full/322/5899/214?ijkey=UKfYGybirpqQM&keytype=ref&siteid=sci (accessed February 10, 2010).

111. Suz Redfearn, "Trials Thriving in Brazil," ClinPage, December 1, 2008, http://www.clinpage.com/article/trials_thriving_in_brazil/ (accessed February 10, 2010).

112. Toshiyoshi Tominaga, "Global Clinical Development—Reducing Japan's Drug Lag," Pharmafocusasia.com, 2008, http://www.pharmafocusasia.com/clinical_trials/global_clinical_development_japan_druglag.htm (accessed February 10, 2010).

113. David G. Passov, "Optimizing Time and Money in Clinical Trials: Russia and Ukraine" (presentation at the Next Generation Pharmaceutical Summit, Scottsdale, AZ, September 2008), http://www.ngpsummit.com/pdf/Clinstar.pdf (accessed May 6, 2009).

114. Administrator, "Big Pharma Moving More Work Offshore," July 7, 2004, citing Fast Track 2006 data, http://www.amreteckpharma.com/index.php?option=com_content&task=view&id=6&Itemid=40 (accessed October 20, 2009).

115. Samiran Nundy and Chandra Gulhati, "A New Colonialism? Conducting Clinical Trials in India," *New England Journal of Medicine* 352, no. 16 (2005): 1633–6, http://content.nejm.org/cgi/content/short/352/16/1633 (accessed February 10, 2010).

116. U.S. Department of Health and Human Services, Office of Inspector General, *The Globalization of Clinical Trials: A Growing Challenge in Protecting Human Subjects*, OEI-01-00-00190 (Washington, DC: September 2001), http://www.oig.hhs.gov/oei/reports/oei-01-00-00190.pdf (accessed February 10, 2010).

117. Mindy J. Steinberg and Elaine R. Rubin, *The HIPAA Privacy Rule: Lacks Patient Benefit, Impedes Research Growth* (Washington, DC: Association of Academic Health Centers, 2009), http://www.aahcdc.org/policy/reddot/AAHC_HIPAA_Privacy_Rule_Impedes_Research_Growth.pdf (accessed February 10, 2010).

118. Guy P. Johnson, "Part 1: Budget Tool Helps Investigative Sites Calculate the Cost of a Coordinator's Time for a Typical Outpatient Study Visit," Society of Clinical Research Associates, http://www.socra.org/pdf/Investigative_Site_Budget_Tool_by_Guy_Johnson.pdf (accessed February 10, 2010), or https://www.ctnbestpractices.org/sites/budgets-contracts.

119. Lisa R. Pitler and Philip D. Bonomi, "Developing an Effective and Compliant Plan for Billing Clinical Trials," *Journal of Oncology Practice* 2, no. 6 (2006), doi:10.1200/JOP.2.6.265, http://www.jop.ascopubs.org/cgi/content/full/2/6/265 (accessed February 11, 2010).

120. Gardiner Harris, "Drug Making's Move Abroad Stirs Concerns," *New York Times*, January 20, 2009, sec. Health, http://www.nytimes.com/2009/01/20/health/policy/20drug.html (accessed February 11, 2010).

121. Wellcome Trust, *Opinion Formers' Conference on Counterfeit Medicines: Perspectives and Action* (conference report and briefing, Wellcome Trust, 2009), http://www.wellcome.ac.uk/About-us/Policy/Spotlight-issues/Counterfeit-medicines/index.htm (accessed February 11, 2010).

Chapter 8

1. Gina Kolata, "Ethics 101: A Course about the Pitfalls," *New York Times*, October 21, 2003, http://www.nytimes.com/2003/10/21/science/21ETHI.html?ex=1067820478&ei=1&en=3c2e352500777940 (accessed January 2, 2004).

2. National Institutes of Health, "Human Participant Protections Education for Research Teams," 2002, http://cme.cancer.gov/c01/intro_01.htm (accessed January 12, 2004).

3. Jeff Levine, Associated Press, and CNN, "Sour Legacy of Tuskegee Syphilis Study Lingers," 1997, http://www.cnn.com/HEALTH/9705/16/nfm.tuskegee/index.html (accessed February 24, 2004).

4. *Trials of War Criminals before the Nuremberg Military Tribunals under Control Council Law* 10 (Washington, DC: U.S. Government Printing Office, 1949), http://www.nihtraining.com/ohsrsite/guidelines/nuremberg.html (accessed November 28, 2005).

5. Saul Krugman, "The Willowbrook Hepatitis Studies Revisited: Ethical Aspects," *Review of Infectious Disease* 15, no. 1 (January–February 1986): 157–62.

6. World Medical Association, “International Code of Medical Ethics,” 1949, http://history.nih.gov/laws/pdf/ICME.pdf (accessed February 7, 2004).

7. National Commission for the Protection of Human Subjects of Biomedical and Behavioral Research, *The Belmont Report: Ethical Principles and Guidelines for the Protection of Human Subjects of Research*, 1979, http://ohsr.od.nih.gov/guidelines/belmont.html (accessed December 21, 2005).

8. FDA, *Guidance for Industry: E6 Good Clinical Practice, Consolidated Guidance*, 1996, http://www.fda.gov/cder/guidance/959fnl.pdf (accessed July 11, 2005).

9. Stolberg, “The Biotech Death of Jesse Gelsinger”; and Thompson, “Human Gene Therapy.”

10. National Bioethics Advisory Committee, “Ethical and Policy Issues in Research Involving Human Participants,” http://www.georgetown.edu/research/nrcbl/nbac/pubs.html (accessed January 2, 2006).

11. National Commission for the Protection of Human Subjects of Biomedical and Behavioral Research, *The Belmont Report*.

12. Denise Grady, “Liver Donors Face Perils Known and Unknown,” *New York Times*, March 19, 2002, F1, http://www.nytimes.com (accessed October 30, 2003).

13. National Commission for the Protection of Human Subjects of Biomedical and Behavioral Research, *The Belmont Report*.

14. U.S. Senate Committee on Veterans’ Affairs, “Is Military Research Hazardous to Veterans?” 1994, http://www.datafilter.com/mc/militaryHumanExperimentationReport94.html (accessed January 16, 2006).

15. Institute of Medicine, Committee to Survey the Health Effects of Mustard Gas and Lewisite, *Veterans at Risk: The Health Effects of Mustard Gas and Lewisite*, ed. Constance M. Pechura and David P. Rall (Washington, DC: National Academy Press, 1993), http://www.nap.edu/books/030904832X/html/ (accessed January 15, 2006); and U.S. Senate Committee on Veterans’ Affairs, “Is Military Research Hazardous to Veterans?”

16. Advisory Committee on Human Radiation Experiments, “DOE Openness: Human Radiation Experiments,” 1994, http://www.eh.doe.gov/ohre/index.html (accessed September 6, 2005).

17. Federation of American Scientists, “Building Public Trust: Actions to Respond to the Advisory Committee on Human Radiation Experiments,” 1967, http://www.fas.org/sgp/library/humexp/ (accessed July 22, 2005).

18. Advisory Committee on Human Radiation Experiments, *Final Report of the Advisory Committee on Human Radiation Experiments*, 1994, http://www.eh.doe.gov/ohre/roadmap/achre/preface.html (accessed September 6, 2005).

19. Glenn O’Neal, “Behind the Biowarfare ‘Eight Ball,’” *USA Today*, December 19, 2001, http://www.usatoday.com/news/healthscience/health/bioterrorism/2001-12-20-whitecoat-usat.htm (accessed September 14, 2003).

20. FDA, "Pediatric Drug Studies: Protecting Pint-Sized Patients," in *From Test Tube to Patient: Improving Health through Human Drugs* (September 1999), http://www.fda.gov/cder/about/whatwedo/testtube-13.pdf (accessed November 1, 2003).

21. Ibid.

22. U.S. Department of Health and Human Services, Press Office, "Bush Administration Will Seek New Legislation for Mandatory Pediatric Drug Testing," press release, December 16, 2002, http://www.hhs.gov/news/press/2002pres/20021216c.html.

23. U.S. Department of Health and Human Services, National Institutes of Health, "List of Drugs for Which Pediatric Studies Are Needed," *Federal Register* 71, no. 79 (April 25, 2006), http://www.gpo.gov/fdsys/pkg/FR-2006-04-25/html/E6-6122.htm (accessed February 14, 2010).

24. National Center for Biotechnology Innovation Bookshelf, *Addressing the Barriers to Pediatric Drug Development: Workshop Summary,* Institute of Medicine (Washington, DC: National Academy Press, 2008), http://www.ncbi.nlm.nih.gov/bookshelf/br.fcgi?book=nap11911&part=a2001563fddd00018 (accessed February 14, 2010).

25. Government Accountability Office, *Pediatric Drug Research: Studies Conducted under Best Pharmaceuticals for Children Act,* report to Congressional Committees, GAO-07-557 (March 2007), http://www.gao.gov/new.items/d07557.pdf (accessed February 14, 2010).

26. Sandra Kweder, "Considerations for Special Populations" (presentation at the FDA's Clinical Investigator Course, Silver Spring, MD, November 17, 2009).

27. European Medicines Agency, *ICH Topic E11: Clinical Investigation of Medicinal Products in the Pediatric Population,* 2000, http://www.emea.europa.eu/pdfs/human/ich/271199en.pdf (accessed February 14, 2010).

28. FDA, "Pediatric Ethics Working Group Consensus Statement on the Pediatric Advisory Subcommittee's April 24, 2001 Meeting," 2003, http://www.fda.gov/cder/pediatric/ethics-statement-Apr2001.htm (accessed January 4, 2004); American Academy of Pediatrics, "Guidelines for the Ethical Conduct of Studies to Evaluate Drugs in Pediatric Populations," *Pediatrics* 95, no. 2 (1995): 286–94, also available at http://www.aap.org/policy/00655.html; and International Conference on Harmonisation, *E8: Guidance on General Considerations for Clinical Trials.*

29. Mark W. Kline, "Foster Children Were Helped by Medical Trials," *Toledo Blade,* May 21, 2005, http://toledoblade.com/apps/pbcs.dll/article?AID=/20050521/OPINION04/50521038 (accessed July 1, 2005); and Mary Otto, "Drugs Tested on HIV-Positive Foster Children," *Washington Post,* May 19, 2005, http://www.washingtonpost.com/wp-dyn/content/article/2005/05/18/AR2005051802154.html (accessed July 10, 2005).

30. Janny Scott and Leslie Kaufman, "Belated Charge Ignites Furor over AIDS Drug Trial," *New York Times*, July 17, 2005, http://www.nytimes.com/2005/07/17/nyregion/17trials.html (accessed July 17, 2005).

31. Mary C. Ruof, "Vulnerability, Vulnerable Populations, and Policy," Scope Note 44, *Kennedy Institute of Ethics Journal*, December, 2004.

32. Emma Wilkinson, "Teens 'Miss Out' on Cancer Trials," BBC News, Health, November 28, 2008, http://news.bbc.co.uk/2/hi/health/7753283.stm (accessed February 14, 2010).

33. J. M. Birch et al., "Survival from Cancer in Teenagers and Young Adults in England, 1979–2003," *British Journal of Cancer* 99, no. 5 (2008): 830–835, http://www.ncbi.nlm.nih.gov/pmc/articles/PMC2528159/ (accessed February 14, 2010).

34. A. Bleyer, T. Budd, and M. Montello, "Older Adolescents and Young Adults with Cancer and Clinical Trials: Lack of Participation and Progress in North America," chap. 5 in *Cancer in Adolescents and Young Adults* (New York: Springer, 2007), cited in J. M. Birch et al., "Survival from Cancer in Teenagers and Young Adults in England, 1979–2003," *British Journal of Cancer* 99, no. 5 (2008): 830–835.

35. Lilia Talarico, Gang Chen, and Richard Pazdur, "Enrollment of Elderly Patients in Clinical Trials for Cancer Drug Registration: A 7-Year Experience by the U.S. Food and Drug Administration," *Journal of Clinical Oncology* 22, no. 22 (2004), doi:10.1200/JCO.2004.02.175, http://jco.ascopubs.org/cgi/content/abstract/22/22/4626 (accessed February 14, 2010).

36. Matti S. Aapro et al., "Never Too Old? Age Should Not Be a Barrier to Enrollment in Cancer Clinical Trials," *Oncologist* 10, no. 3 (2005), doi:10.1634/theoncologist.10-3-198, http://theoncologist.alphamedpress.org/cgi/content/abstract/10/3/198 (accessed February 14, 2010).

37. European Medicines Agency, *ICH Topic E7: Studies in Support of Special Populations: Geriatrics: Questions & Answers*, 2009, http://www.fda.gov/Drugs/GuidanceComplianceRegulatoryInformation/Guidances/ucm121568.htm (accessed February 14, 2010).

38. Arya M. Sharma, "Obesity: Managing Weighty Issues on Lean Evidence—The Challenges of Bariatric Medicine," *Canadian Medical Association Journal* 172, no. 1 (2005), doi:10.1503/cmaj.1041722., http://www.ncbi.nlm.nih.gov/pmc/articles/PMC543938/ (accessed February 14, 2010).

39. Douglas Brunette, "Hidden Mystery," Agency for Healthcare Research and Quality, Web Morbidity and Mortality Rounds: Case & Commentary, March 2005, http://www.webmm.ahrq.gov/printview.aspx?caseID=88 (accessed February 14, 2010).

40. National Institutes of Health, "Oseltamivir Pharmacokinetics in Morbid Obesity," ClinicalTrials.gov, http://www.clinicaltrials.gov/ct2/show/NCT01002729 (accessed February 14, 2010).

41. Cullen T. Vogelson, "Research Practices and Ethics," *Modern Drug Discovery* 4, no. 4 (April 2001): 23–24, http://pubs.acs.org/subscribe/journals/mdd/v04/i04/html/MDD04DeptClinical.html (accessed January 21, 2002).

42. FDA, *Guidance for Industry: Protecting the Rights, Safety, and Welfare of Study Subjects—Supervisory Responsibilities of Investigators*, 2007, http://www.fda.gov/RegulatoryInformation/Guidances/ucm127697.htm (accessed February 14, 2010).

43. Institute of Medicine, *Conflict of Interest in Medical Research, Education, and Practice* (Washington, DC: National Academy Press, 2009), http://www.iom.edu/CMS/3740/47464/65721.aspx (accessed February 14, 2010).

44. David Willman, "Stealth Merger: Drug Companies and Government Medical Research," *Los Angeles Times*, December 7, 2003, http://www.sunspot.net/business/la-na-nih7dec07,1,7031831.story (accessed September 12, 2004).

45. Robert Steinbrook, "Conflicts of Interest at the NIH—Resolving the Problem," *New England Journal of Medicine* 351, no. 10 (2004): 955–57; and R. Weiss, "NIH Clears Most Researchers in Conflict-of-Interest Probe," *Washington Post*, February 22, 2005, also available at http://www.washingtonpost.com.

46. Evan G. DeRenzo, "Conflict-of-Interest Policy at the National Institutes of Health: The Pendulum Swings Wildly," *Kennedy Institute of Ethics Journal* 15, no. 2 (2005): 199–210, http://muse.jhu.edu/login?uri=/journals/kennedy_institute_of_ethics_journal/v015/15.2derenzo.html (accessed February 14, 2010).

47. Sheila Fleischhaker and Mark Cohen, "The ABCs of Drug Safety: Accountability, Balance, and Citizen Empowerment," Government Accountability Project, April 2009, http://www.whistleblower.org/doc/2008/ABCFinal040709.pdf.

48. Willman, "Stealth Merger."

49. National Institutes of Health, Office of Extramural Research, "Conflict of Interest," Grants Policy, http://grants.nih.gov/grants/policy/coi/ or access at http://grants.nih.gov/grants/policy/coi/tutorial/fcoi.pdf (accessed February 14, 2010).

50. U.S. Department of Health and Human Services, Office of Inspector General, *National Institutes of Health: Conflicts of Interest in Extramural Research*, OEI-03-06-00460 (January 2008), http://oig.hhs.gov/oei/reports/oei-03-06-00460.pdf (accessed February 14, 2010).

51. U.S. Department of Health and Human Services, Office of Inspector General, *How Grantees Manage Financial Conflicts of Interest in Research Funded by the National Institutes of Health*, November 2009, http://oig.hhs.gov/oei/reports/oei-03-07-00700.pdf (accessed February 14, 2010).

52. Weinfurt et al., "Disclosure of Financial Relationships to Participants in Clinical Research," *New England Journal of Medicine* 361, no. 9 (2009): 916–921, http://content.nejm.org/cgi/content/full/361/9/916 (accessed February 14, 2010).

53. Institute of Medicine, *Conflict of Interest in Medical Research, Education, and Practice* (Washington, DC: National Academy Press, 2009), http://www.iom.edu/CMS/3740/47464/65721.aspx (accessed February 14, 2010).

54. Marcia Angell, "Is Academic Medicine for Sale?" *New England Journal of Medicine* 342, no. 20 (2000): 1516–1518.

55. U.S. Department of Health and Human Services, Office of Inspector General, "Recruiting Human Subjects: Pressures in Industry-Sponsored Clinical Research," 2000, http://www.researchroundtable.com/oigreports.htm (accessed January 4, 2004).

56. Temple University Office of Clinical Trials, "Good Clinical Research Practices," 2005, http://www.research.temple.edu/oct/doc/lectures/goodpract.ppt (accessed July 15, 2005).

57. DataEdge, "Patient Treatment Data: The Hidden Key to Faster Studies," Data Edge DataLines, 1998, http://www.fast-track.com (accessed February 17, 2003).

58. Rebecca Skloot, "Taking the Least of You: The Tissue-Industrial Complex," *New York Times*, April 16, 2006, http://www.nytimes.com/2006/04/16/magazine/16tissue.html (accessed February 14, 2010).

59. Ibid.

60. E. Haavi Morreim, "Medical Research Litigation and Malpractice Tort Doctrines: Courts on a Learning Curve," *Houston Journal of Health Law and Policy* 4, no. 1 (2003), http://www.allbusiness.com/legal/3587152-1.html (accessed February 14, 2010).

61. Rebecca Skloot, "Taking the Least of You: Thc Tissue-Industrial Complex," *New York Times*, April 16, 2006, http://www.nytimes.com/2006/04/16/magazine/16tissue.html (accessed February 14, 2010).

62. Ibid.

63. Rebecca Skloot, "Culture Dish: Tissue Ownership Update: *William Catalona v. Washington University*, the Ruling," Culture Dish blog, April 17, 2006, http://rebeccaskloot.blogspot.com/2006/04/tissue-ownership-update-william.html (accessed February 14, 2010).

64. E. Haavi Morreim, "Medical Research Litigation and Malpractice Tort Doctrines: Courts on a Learning Curve," *Houston Journal of Health Law and Policy* 4, no. 1 (2003), http://www.allbusiness.com/legal/3587152-1.html (accessed February 14, 2010).

65. McDermott Will & Emery, "Ownership of Biological Samples and Clinical Data II: U.S. Supreme Court Denies Certiorari in the Catalona Decision," *McDermott Newsletters*, February 21, 2008, http://www.mwe.com/index.cfm/fuseaction/publications.nldetail/object_id/10776f46-f953-4921-9b40-c3dc1fd6ed60.cfm (accessed February 14, 2010).

66. McDermott Will & Emery, "Increasing FDA Oversight Over Clinical Research," *McDermott Newsletters*, November 4, 2004, http://www.mwe.com/

index.cfm/fuseaction/publications.nldetail/object_id/753fb582-f9c7-41fd-aab0-0f18980b10e5.cfm (accessed February 14, 2010).

67. R. Alta Charo, "Body of Research—Ownership and Use of Human Tissue," *New England Journal of Medicine* 355, no. 15 (2006), doi:10.1056/NEJMp068192, http://content.nejm.org/cgi/content/full/355/15/1517 (accessed February 14, 2010).

68. National Cancer Institute, Office of Biorepositories and Biospecimen Research, "Ethical, Legal, and Policy Best Practices," NCI Best Practices for Biospecimen Resources, http://www.biospecimens.cancer.gov/bestpractices/elp/ (accessed February 14, 2010).

69. Prostate SPORE National Biospecimen Network (NBN) Pilot, "NBN Blueprint," http://prostatenbnpilot.nci.nih.gov/blue_app_n.asp (accessed February 14, 2010).

70. Jimmie B. Vaught et al., "Ethical, Legal, and Policy Issues: Dominating the Biospecimen Discussion," *Cancer Epidemiology, Biomarkers & Prevention* 16, no. 12 (2007), http://cebp.aacrjournals.org/content/16/12/2521.full (accessed February 14, 2010).

71. Public Responsibility in Medicine and Research, *Report of the PRIM&R Human Tissue/Specimen Banking Working Group*, white paper, March 2007, http://www.primr.org/uploadedFiles/PRIMR_Site_Home/Public_Policy/Recently_Files_Comments/Tissue%20Banking%20White%20Paper%203-7-07%20final%20combined.pdf (accessed February 14, 2010).

72. Lori Andrews et al., "When Patents Threaten Science," *Science* 314, no. 5804 (2006): 1395, http://www.kentlaw.edu/islat/pdf/WhenPatentsThreatenScience.pdf (accessed February 14, 2010).

73. Julie Burger and Justin Bruner, "A Court's Dilemma: When Patents Conflict with Public Health," *Virginia Journal of Law & Technology* 12, no. 4 (2007): 1–41, http://www.kentlaw.edu/islat/publications.html (accessed February 14, 2010).

74. Ibid.

75. David B. Resnik and Kenneth A. De Ville, "Bioterrorism and Patent Rights: 'Compulsory Licensure' and the Case of Cipro," *American Journal of Bioethics* 2, no. 3 (2002):29–39, http://muse.jhu.edu/login?uri=/journals/american_journal_of_bioethics/v002/2.3resnik.html (accessed February 14, 2010).

76. Edward G. Brightly, "Bird Flu Vaccine Patent," *IPMed*, August 20, 2008, http://ipmed.blogspot.com/2008/08/bird-flu-vaccine-patent.html (accessed February 14, 2010).

77. Martin Ensirink, "The Challenge of Getting Swine Flu Vaccine to Poor Nations," *Science Insider*, November 3, 2009, http://blogs.sciencemag.org/scienceinsider/2009/11/the-challenge-o.html (accessed February 14, 2010).

78. Pauline W. Chen, "Bending the Rules of Clinical Trials," *New York Times*, October 29, 2009, sec. Health, http://www.nytimes.com/2009/10/29/health/29chen.html (accessed February 14, 2010).

79. Charles W. Lidz et al., "Competing Commitments in Clinical Trials," *IRB: Ethics & Human Research* 31, no. 5 (2009): 1–6, http://www.medscape.com/viewarticle/712097 (accessed February 14, 2010).

80. Stephen Straus, "Unanticipated Risk in Clinical Research," chap. 8 in *Principles and Practice of Clinical Research*, ed. John I. Gallin (San Diego: Elsevier, 2002).

81. James Wilson, "Lessons Learned from the Gene Therapy Trial for Ornithine Transcarbamylase Deficiency," *Molecular Genetics and Metabolism* 96, no. 4 (2009), doi:10.1016/j.ymgme.2008.12.016, http://linkinghub.elsevier.com/retrieve/pii/S109671920800499X (accessed February 14, 2010).

82. Ibid.

83. Vogelson, "Research Practices and Ethics."

84. Thompson, "Human Gene Therapy."

85. Molecule of the Day, "Sutent/Sunitinib (Cheer up!)," Science Blogs, March 12, 2009, http://scienceblogs.com/moleculeoftheday/2009/03/sutentsunitinib_cheer_up.php (accessed February 14, 2010).

86. Dennis O. Dixon, "Data and Safety Monitoring," February 2, 2009, http://www.nihtraining.com/cc/ippcr/current/downloads/Dixon020209(C).pdf (accessed February 14, 2010).

87. National Cancer Institute, Executive Committee, "Policy of the NCI for Data and Safety Monitoring of Clinical Trials," June 22, 1999, http://deainfo.nci.nih.gov/grantspolicies/datasafety.htm (accessed February 14, 2010).

88. Holly Presley, "Vioxx and the Merck Team Effort," *Business Ethics* (Kenan Institute for Ethics, 2009), http://www.duke.edu/web/kenanethics/CaseStudies/Vioxx.pdf (accessed February 14, 2010).

89. Snigdha Prakash, "Conflicted Safety Panel Let Vioxx Study Continue," NPR News, Health, June 8, 2006, http://www.npr.org/templates/story/story.php?storyId=5462419 (accessed February 14, 2010).

90. Duff Wilson and Natasha Singer, "Ghostwriting Is Called Rife in Medical Journals," *New York Times*, September 11, 2009, sec. Business, http://www.nytimes.com/2009/09/11/business/11ghost.html (accessed February 14, 2010).

91. International Committee of Medical Journal Editors, "Uniform Requirements for Manuscripts Submitted to Biomedical Journals: Writing and Editing for Biomedical Publication," ICMJE Web site, http://www.icmje.org/urm_main.html (accessed February 14, 2010).

92. Laurence J. Hirsch, "Conflicts of Interest, Authorship, and Disclosures in Industry-Related Scientific Publications: The Tort Bar and Editorial Oversight of Medical Journals," *Mayo Clinic Proceedings* 84, no. 9 (2009), doi:10.4065/

84.9.811, http://www.mayoclinicproceedings.com/content/84/9/811.full (accessed February 14, 2010).

93. Kristin Rising, Peter Bacchetti, and Lisa Bero, "Reporting Bias in Drug Trials Submitted to the Food and Drug Administration: Review of Publication and Presentation," *PLoS Medicine* 5, no. 11 (2008), doi:10.1371/journal.pmed.0050217 (accessed February 14, 2010).

94. An-Wen Chan et al., "Empirical Evidence for Selective Reporting of Outcomes in Randomized Trials: Comparison of Protocols to Published Articles," *Journal of the American Medical Association* 291, no. 20 (2004): 2457–2465, http://jama.ama-assn.org/cgi/content/full/291/20/2457 (accessed February 14, 2010).

95. Anna Wilde Mathews, "Worrisome Ailment in Medicine: Misleading Journal Articles," *Wall Street Journal*, May 10, 2005, sec. A1, http://online.wsj.com/article/SB111567633298328568.html (accessed February 14, 2010).

96. World Health Organization, "International Clinical Trials Registry Platform (ICTRP)," http://www.who.int/ictrp/network/trds/en/index.html (accessed February 14, 2010).

97. CONSORT Group, "The CONSORT (CONsolidated Standards of Reporting Trials) Statement," 2009, http://www.consort-statement.org/consort-statement/ (accessed February 14, 2010).

98. Udo Schuklenk, "JAMA Shenanigans Continue," UdoSchuklenk's Ethx Blog, July 8, 2009, http://ethxblog.blogspot.com/2009/07/jama-shenanigans-continue.html (accessed February 14, 2010).

99. Larry Husten, "Down the Memory Hole: JAMA Editors Rewrite History and Remove Original Editorial," CardioBrief, July 10, 2009, http://cardiobrief.org/2009/07/10/down-the-memory-hole-jama-editors-rewrite-history-and-remove-original-editorial/ (accessed February 14, 2010).

100. R. Taylor and J. Giles, "Cash Interests Taint Drug Advice," *Nature* 437 (2005): 1070–1, cited in editorial, "Clinical Practice Guidelines and Conflict of Interest," *Canadian Medical Association Journal* 173, no. 11 (2005), doi:10.1503/cmaj.051423., http://www.cmaj.ca (accessed February 14, 2010).

101. Institute of Medicine, Board on Health Sciences Policy, *Conflict of Interest in Medical Research, Education, and Practice*, ed. Bernard Lo and Marilyn J. Field, April 21, 2009, http://www.iom.edu/en/Reports/2009/Conflict-of-Interest-in-Medical-Research-Education-and-Practice.aspx (accessed February 14, 2010).

102. Sarah Rubenstein, "Justice Department Beats Chest over Zyprexa Settlement," *Wall Street Journal*, Health Blog, January 15, 2009, http://blogs.wsj.com/health/2009/01/15/justice-department-beats-chest-over-zyprexa-settlement/tab/ (accessed February 14, 2010).

103. David Evans, "Pfizer Broke the Law by Promoting Drugs for Unapproved Uses," Bloomberg.com, November 9, 2009, http://www.bloomberg.com/apps/news?pid=20670001&sid=a4yV1nYxCGoA (accessed February 14, 2010).

104. Ibid.

105. U.S. Department of Justice, "Federal Statutes Imposing Collateral Consequences upon Conviction," November 2000, http://www.justice.gov/pardon/collateral_consequences.pdf (accessed February 14, 2010).

106. John Abramson and Barbara Starfield, "The Effect of Conflict of Interest on Biomedical Research and Clinical Practice Guidelines: Can We Trust the Evidence in Evidence-Based Medicine?" *Journal of the American Board of Family Practice* 18, no. 5 (2005), doi:10.3122/jabfm.18.5.414, http://www.jabfm.org (accessed February 14, 2010); Sarah Rubenstein, "Justice Department Beats Chest over Zyprexa Settlement," Wall Street Journal Health Blog, January 15, 2009, http://blogs.wsj.com/health/2009/01/15/justice-department-beats-chest-over-zyprexa-settlement/tab/ (accessed February 14, 2010); and David Evans, "Pfizer Broke the Law by Promoting Drugs for Unapproved Uses," Bloomberg.com, November 9, 2009, http://www.bloomberg.com/apps/news?pid=20670001&sid=a4yV1nYxCGoA (accessed February 14, 2010).

107. Cullen T. Vogelson, "The Investigational Review Process," *Modern Drug Discovery* 4, no. 5 (May 2001): 27–31, http://pubs.acs.org/subscribe/journals/mdd/v04/i05/html/05clinical.html (accessed January 31, 2002).

108. PRIM&R, "Public Responsibility in Medicine and Research," 2004, http://www.primr.org.

109. Association for the Accreditation of Human Research Protection Programs, Inc., "Pfizer First Pharma Company to Receive Accreditation for Study Subject Protections," April 2, 2009, http://www.aahrpp.org/www.aspx?PageID=287.

110. Alicia Mundy, "Coast IRB, Caught in Sting, to Close," *Wall Street Journal*, April 22, 2009, sec. Business, http://online.wsj.com/article/SB124042341694744375.html (accessed February 14, 2010).

111. BusinessWire, "Congressional 'Sting' Operation Uncovered by Coast IRB," November 3, 2009, http://www.businesswire.com/portal/site/google/?ndmViewId=news_view&newsId=20090311006356&newsLang=en (accessed February 14, 2010).

112. T. Lemmens and B. Freedman, "Ethics Review for Sale? Conflict of Interest and Commercial Review Boards," *Milbank Quarterly* 78, no. 4 (2000), http://www.utoronto.ca/jcb/Research/publications/lemmens_mq00.pdf (accessed September 14, 2003).

113. Ezekiel J. Emanuel, Trudo Lemmens, and Carl Elliot, "Should Society Allow Research Ethics Boards to Be Run as For-Profit Enterprises?" *PLoS Medicine* 3, no. 7 (2006): e309, http://dx.doi.org/10.1371/journal.pmed.0030309 (accessed February 14, 2010).

114. David Evans, Michael Smith, and Liz Willen, "Big Pharma's Shameful Secret," *Bloomberg Markets Special Report*, http://dcscience.net/pharma-bloomberg.pdf (accessed February 14, 2010).

115. Ezekiel J. Emanuel, Trudo Lemmens, and Carl Elliot, "Should Society Allow Research Ethics Boards to Be Run as For-Profit Enterprises?" *PLoS*

Medicine 3, no. 7 (2006): e309, http://dx.doi.org/10.1371/journal.pmed.0030309 (accessed February 14, 2010).

116. U.S. Department of Health and Human Services, Office of Inspector General, "Institutional Review Boards: Time for Reform," 1998, http://oig.hhs.gov/oei/reports/oei-01-97-00193.pdf (accessed September 14, 2003).

117. Robert Steinbrook, "Protecting Research Subjects—The Crisis at Johns Hopkins," *New England Journal of Medicine* 346, no. 9 (2002): 716–720, http://content.nejm.org/cgi/content/full/346/9/716 (accessed February 14, 2010).

118. Michael Goodyear, "Learning from the TGN1412 Trial," *British Medical Journal*, March 2006, doi:10.1136/bmj.38797.635012.47, http://www.bmj.com/cgi/content/full/332/7543/677 (accessed February 17, 2010).

119. Expert Scientific Group on Phase One Clinical Trials, *Final Report*, Chair, Gordon Duff (London: TSO, November 30, 2006), http://www.dh.gov.uk/prod_consum_dh/groups/dh_digitalassets/@dh/@en/documents/digitalasset/dh_073165.pdf (accessed February 17, 2010).

120. Citizens for Responsible Care and Research, *Tegenero Medicines and Healthcare Products Regulatory Agency Clinical Trial Suspension*, interim report, http://www.circare.org/foia5/clinicaltrialsuspension_interimreport.pdf (accessed February 17, 2010).

121. Expert Scientific Group on Phase One Clinical Trials, *Final Report*, Chair, Gordon Duff (London: TSO, November 30, 2006), http://www.dh.gov.uk/prod_consum_dh/groups/dh_digitalassets/@dh/@en/documents/digitalasset/dh_073165.pdf (accessed February 17, 2010).

122. Barbara Rellahan, "The TeGenero Incident March 13, 2006 UK: TGN1412—a Superagonist Anti-CD28 Antibody" (presentation at the FDA Clinical Investigator's Course, Silver Spring, MD, November 17, 2009).

123. Michael Goodyear, "Learning from the TGN1412 Trial," *British Medical Journal,* March 2006, doi:10.1136/bmj.38797.635012.47, http://www.bmj.com/cgi/rapidpdf/bmj.38797.635012.47v1.pdf (accessed February 17, 2010).

124. Norman M. Goldfarb, "Informed Consent in the Tegenero TGN1412 Trial," *Journal of Clinical Research Best Practices* 2, no. 5 (2006), http://www.firstclinical.com/journal/2006/0605_TeGenero.pdf (accessed February 17, 2010).

125. PAREXEL International, "Informed Consent Form" and "Information Sheet," project no. 68419, protocol no. TGN1412-HV, February 9, 2008, http://www.circare.org/foia5/tgn1412_consentform.pdf.

126. Institute of Medicine, Committee to Review the Fialuridine Clinical Trials, *Review of the Fialuridine Clinical Trials*, ed. Frederick Manning and Morton Swartz (Washington, DC: National Academies Press, 1995): 88, http://books.nap.edu/openbook.php?record_id=4887 (accessed February 17, 2010).

127. Ibid.

128. Ibid.

129. Ibid.

130. National Institutes of Health, *Unanticipated Risk*, video of Stephen Straus's presentation for the Introduction to the Principles and Practices of Clinical Research, Unit 8, October 16, 2006–February 26, 2007, http://www.nihtraining.com/cc/ippcr/archive06f/menu.html, slide presentation available at http://www.nihtraining.com/cc/ippcr/current/downloads/Straus111306pdf (accessed February 17, 2010). Straus notes that the gene therapy trial in which Jesse Gelsinger died had been approved by the institution's IRB, the NIH, and the FDA and that the investigator, Dr. James Wilson, who was pilloried, hardly acted on his own.

131. Shem, *The House of God*.

132. National Institutes of Health, Clinical Research Training module, "What Makes Clinical Research Ethical?" http://www.nihtraining.com (accessed November 23, 2009).

Chapter 9

1. Centers for Disease Control, "Condoms and Their Use in Preventing HIV Infection and Other STDS," September 1999, http://www.house.gov/reform/min/pdfs/pdf_inves/pdf_admin_hhs_info_condoms_fact_sheet_orig.pdf; Centers for Disease Control, "Male Latex Condoms and Sexually Transmitted Diseases," fact sheet, October 2003, http://www.cdc.gov/condomeffectiveness/latex.htm (accessed February 15, 2010) and Centers for Disease Control, "Programs That Work," http://www.cdc.gov/nccdphp/dash/rtc/, archived version available at http://web.archive.org/web/20010606142729/www.cdc.gov/nccdphp/dash/rtc/index.htm) (accessed February 17, 2010).

2. Heather Boonstra, "Health Advocates Say Campaign to Disparage Condoms Threatens STD Prevention Efforts," *The Guttmacher Report on Public Policy* 6, no. 1 (2003), http://www.guttmacher.org/pubs/tgr/06/1/gr/060101.html (accessed February 15, 2010).

3. David Wahlberg, "Public Health Tailored to Bush Line, Critics Charge," *Atlanta Journal and Constitution*, August 3, 2003, http://www.allbusiness/government/government-bodies-offices/10369712-1.html (accessed February 15, 2010).

4. Union of Concerned Scientists, *An Investigation into the Bush Administration's Misuse of Science* (Cambridge, MA: Union of Concerned Scientists, 2004), http://stephenschneider.stanford.edu/Publications/PDF_Papers/RSI_final_fullreport.pdf (accessed February 15, 2010).

5. HIV Medicine Association, Infectious Diseases Society of America, "Preventing HIV and Other Sexually Transmitted Infections: A Call for Science-Based Government Policies," HIVMA, 2005, http://www.hivma.org/Content.aspx?id2784 (accessed February 15, 2010).

6. Committee on HIV Prevention Strategies in the United States, *No Time to Lose: Getting More from HIV Prevention* (Washington, DC: National Academy Press, 2001).

7. Erica Goode, "Certain Words Can Trip Up AIDS Grants, Scientists Say," *New York Times*, April 18, 2003, http://www.nytimes.com/2003/04/18/national/18GRAN.html?pagewanted=1 (accessed February 15, 2010).

8. Paul A. Volberding and Joseph R. Dalovisio, "The Impact of Ideology on NIH Research," letter to Tommy G. Thompson, Secretary of Health and Human Services, U.S. Department of Health and Human Services from the Infectious Diseases Society of America, 2003, http://www.idsociety.org/Content.aspx?id=4474 (accessed February 17, 2010).

9. HIV Medicine Association, Infectious Diseases Society of America, "Preventing HIV and other Sexually Transmitted Infections: A Call for Science-Based Government Policies," HIVMA, 2005, http://www.hivma.org/Content.aspx?id=2784 (accessed February 15, 2010).

10. Elizabeth Blackburn, "Bioethics and the Political Distortion of Biomedical Science," *New England Journal of Medicine* 350, no. 14 (2004): 1379, http://www.nejm.org/cgi/content/short/350/14/1379 (accessed February 15, 2010).

11. Alex Gordon, "The Delicate Dance of Immersion and Insulation: The Politicization of the FDA Commissioner," April 29, 2003, http://leda.law.harvard.edu/leda/data/536/Gordon.pdf (accessed February 17, 2010).

12. Ibid.

13. Karen Tumulty, "Jesus and the FDA," *Time*, October 5, 2002, http://www.time.com/time/nation/article/0,8599,361521,00.html (accessed February 15, 2010).

14. Marc Kaufman, "Abortion Foe to Be Reappointed to FDA Panel," *Washington Post*, June 28, 2004, sec. A, 6, http://www.washingtonpost.com/ac2/wp-dyn/A13192-2004Jun28 (accessed December 1, 2009).

15. Gardiner Harris, "Ex-Head of FDA Faces Criminal Inquiry," *New York Times*, April 29, 2006, sec. Washington, http://www.nytimes.com/2006/04/29/washington/29fda.html (accessed February 15, 2010).

16. Marc Kaufman, "FDA Official Quits Over Delay on Plan B," *Washington Post*, September 1, 2005, sec. Health, http://www.washingtonpost.com/wp-dyn/content/article/2005/08/31/AR2005083101271_pf.html (accessed February 15, 2010); Center for Constitutional Rights, "Tummino, et al. v. von Eschenbach," March 2009, http://ccrjustice.org/ourcases/current-cases/tummino,-et-al.-v.-von-eschenbach (accessed February 17, 2010); and U.S. District Court, Eastern District of New York, *Tummino, et al. v. Torti*, 427 F. Supp. 2d 212, 231–34 (E.D.N.Y. 2006); Oct. 11, 2006 Hr'g Tr. 20; July 26, 2006 Hr'g Tr. 9:1, http://www.nyed.uscourts.gov/pub/rulings/cv/2005/05cv366mofinal.pdf (accessed February 15, 2010).

17. Center for Constitutional Rights, "Tummino, et al. v. von Eschenbach," March 2009, http://ccrjustice.org/ourcases/current-cases/tummino,-et-al.-v.-von-eschenbach (accessed February 17, 2010).

18. Center for Reproductive Law and Policy, "Citizen's Petition," submitted to the FDA on February 14, 2001, http://www.crlp.org/pdf/EC_petition.pdf (accessed February 15, 2010).

19. Union of Concerned Scientists, *Voices of Scientists at the FDA: Protecting Public Health Depends on Independent Science*, 2006, http://www.ucsusa.org/scientific_integrity/abuses_of_science/summary-of-the-fda-scientist.html (accessed February 17, 2010).

20. U.S. Senate Committee on Finance, Memorandum from Senator Chuck Grassley regarding the Union of Concerned Scientists Survey of FDA Scientists, July 20, 2006, http://www.ucsusa.org/assets/documents/scientific_integrity/FDA-7-20-06-Grassley-press-statement.pdf (accessed February 17, 2010).

21. Gardiner Harris, "Antidepressant Study Seen to Back Expert," *New York Times*, August 20, 2004, http://www.nytimes.com/2004/08/20/us/antidepressant-study-seen-to-back-expert.html (accessed February 17, 2010).

22. David J. Graham, testimony before the United States Senate, November 18, 2004, http://finance.senate.gov/hearings/testimony/2004test/111804dgtest.pdf (accessed February 17, 2010).

23. Sean Hennessy and Brian L. Strom, "PDUFA Reauthorization—Drug Safety's Golden Moment of Opportunity?" *New England Journal of Medicine* 356, no. 17 (April 26, 2007), doi:10.1056/NEJMp078048, http://content.nejm.org/cgi/content/full/NEJMp078048 (accessed February 17, 2010).

24. Christopher Moraff, "Safety First," *American Prospect*, April 3, 2007, http://www.prospect.org/cs/articles?articleId=12616 (accessed February 17, 2010).

25. John Dingell, Chairman of U.S. House of Representatives Committee on Energy and Commerce, letter to Michael Leavitt, Secretary, U.S. Department of Health and Social Security, March 28, 2007, http://archives.energycommerce.house.gov/.../DrugSafety.032807.HHS.ltr.pdf (accessed February 17, 2010).

26. Kaiser Health News Daily Report, "Bush Administration Fails to Comply with Subpoena for Documents on Testimony about FDA Approval of Ketek," Kaiser Health News, February 13, 2008, http://www.kaiserhealthnews.org/Daily-Reports/2008/February/13/dr00050393.aspx (accessed February 17, 2010).

27. Gardiner Harris and David M. Halbfinger, "F.D.A. Reveals It Fell to a Push by Lawmakers," *New York Times*, September 25, 2009, sec. Health/Health Care Policy, http://www.nytimes.com/2009/09/25/health/policy/25knee.html (accessed February 17, 2010).

28. John Schwartz, "And Then the Patients Suddenly Started Dying: How NIH Missed Warning Signs in Drug Test," *Washington Post*, September 7, 1993, sec. A, http://pqasb.pqarchiver.com/washingtonpost/access/72184201 (accessed February 17, 2010).

29. Philip Hilts, "U.S. Doctor Drops Patient for Criticizing Drug Trial," *New York Times*, October 23, 1993, sec. 1, http://www.nytimes.com/1993/10/23/us/

us-doctor-drops-patient-for-criticizing-drug-trial.html (accessed February 17, 2010).

30. Stephen Straus, "Unanticipated Risk in Clinical Research" chap. 8 in *Principles and Practice of Clinical Research*, ed. John I. Gallin (San Diego: Elsevier, 2002).

31. Ibid.

32. Institute of Medicine, Committee to Review the Fialuridine Clinical Trials, *Review of the Fialuridine Clinical Trials*, ed. Frederick Manning and Morton Swartz (Washington, DC: National Academies Press, 1995), 152, http://books.nap.edu/openbook.php?record_id=4887 (accessed February 17, 2010).

33. Ibid.

34. Tracy Johnson and Elizabeth Fee, "Women's Participation in Clinical Research: From Protectionism to Access," in *Women and Health Research: Ethical and Legal Issues of Including Women in Clinical Studies*, ed. Anna C Mastroianni, Ruth Faden, and Daniel Federman, Institute of Medicine (Washington, DC: National Academy Press, 1994), http://books.nap.edu/books/0309050405/html/ (accessed January 16, 2006); and Beryl Lieff Benderly, "Research on Women, Women in Research," in *In Her Own Right: The Institute of Medicine's Guide to Women's Health Issues* (Washington, DC: National Academy Press, 1997), also available at http://books.nap.edu/books/0309053277/html (accessed September 14, 2003).

35. FDA, "Women's Health Initiatives," 2003, http://www.fda.gov/cder/audiences/women/default.htm (accessed February 27, 2003).

36. Johnson and Fee, "Women's Participation in Clinical Research."

37. Benderly, "Research on Women," 182.

38. Carol S. Weisman and Sandra D. Cassard, "Health Consequences of Exclusion or Underrepresentation of Women in Clinical Studies, in *Women and Health Research: Ethical and Legal Issues of Including Women in Clinical Studies*, vol. 2, 35–36, ed. Anna C Mastroianni, Ruth Faden, and Daniel Federman, Institute of Medicine (Washington, DC: National Academy Press, 1994), http://books.nap.edu/books/0309050405/html/ (accessed January 16, 2006).

39. Benderly, "Research on Women," 195.

40. B. Evelyn et al., "Participation of Racial/Ethnic Groups in Clinical Trials and Race-Related Labeling: A Review of New Molecular Entities Approved 1995–1999," *Journal of the National Medicine Association*, Supplement (December 2001), http://www.fda.gov/cder/reports/race_ethnicity/race_ethnicity_report.htm (accessed September 14, 2003).

41. Weisman and Cassard, "Health Consequences of Exclusion," 37.

42. Reproductive Health Technologies Project, *The Quinacrine Debate and Beyond*, 2001, also available at http://www.rhtp.org/news/publications/default.asp (accessed January 16, 2006).

43. Susan Sherwin, "Women in Clinical Studies: A Feminist View," in *Women and Health Research: Ethical and Legal Issues of Including Women*

in Clinical Studies, vol. 2, ed. Anna C Mastroianni, Ruth Faden, and Daniel Federman, Institute of Medicine (Washington DC: National Academy Press, 1994), http://books.nap.edu/catalog/2343.html (accessed January 16, 2006).

44. Florence P. Haseltine and Beverly Greenberg Jacobson, *Women's Health Research: A Medical and Policy Primer* (Washington, DC: American Psychiatric Press, 1997), cited in Lori Mosca et al., "Setting a Local Research Agenda for Women's Health: The National Centers of Excellence in Women's Health," *Journal of Women's Health and Gender-Based Medicine* 10, no. 10 (2001): 927–35, http://www.4woman.gov/COE/journals/local.pdf (accessed September 15, 2005).

45. National Institutes of Health, "Human Participant Protections Education for Research Teams," 22.

46. Benderly, "Research on Women."

47. *Trials of War Criminals before the Nuremberg Military Tribunals.*

48. National Institutes of Health, "Human Participant Protections Education for Research Teams," 22.

49. Johnson and Fee, "Women's Participation in Clinical Research."

50. Board on Health Sciences Policy, Committee on Understanding the Biology of Sex and Gender Differences, *Exploring the Biological Contributions to Human Health: Does Sex Matter?* ed. Theresa Wizemann and Mary-Lou Pardue (Washington, DC: National Academy Press, 2001), 25, http://www.nap.edu/books/0309072816/html/ (accessed January 24, 2004).

51. Benderly, "Research on Women."

52. Board on Health Sciences Policy, Committee on Understanding the Biology of Sex and Gender Differences, *Exploring the Biological Contributions to Human Health.*

53. FDA, Press Office, "FDA Proposes Rule on Women in Clinical Trials," FDA Talk Paper, September 23, 1997, http://www.fda.gov/bbs/topics/ANSWERS/ANS00822.html (accessed May 3, 2004).

54. Evelyn et al., "Racial/Ethnic Groups in Clinical Trials."

55. Society for Women's Health Research, "Understanding Research—Milestones in the Inclusion of Women in Clinical Research," 2003, http://www.womenshealthresearch.org (accessed February 12, 2003); and U.S. General Accounting Office, *Report to Congressional Requesters: Women's Health—Women Sufficiently Represented in New Drug Testing, but FDA Oversight Needs Improvement* (Washington, DC: U.S. General Accounting Office, 2001), GAO-01-754, also available at: http://www.gao.gov/new.items/d01754.pdf.

56. Robert Pear, "Sex Differences Called Key in Medical Studies," *New York Times*, April 25, 2001, also available at http://www.nytimes.com (accessed February 8, 2003).

57. Diane B. Stoy, "Recruitment and Retention of Women in Clinical Studies: Theoretical Perspectives and Methodological Considerations," in *Women and Health Research: Ethical and Legal Issues of Including Women in Clinical Studies*, vol. 2, 45–64, ed. Anna C. Mastroianni, Ruth Faden, and

Daniel Federman, Institute of Medicine (Washington, DC: National Academy Press, 1994), http://www.nap.edu/books/0309050405/html/45.html (accessed September 14, 2003).

58. Johnson and Fee, "Women's Participation in Clinical Research."

59. Society for Women's Health Research, "Funding Research," 2002, http://www.womens-health.org (accessed January 26, 2004).

60. Cynthia M. Farquhar, "Extracts from "Clinical Evidence: Endometriosis," *British Medical Journal* 320, no. 7247 (2000), doi:10.1136/bmj.320.7247.1449, http://www.bmj.com/cgi/content/abstract/320/7247/1449 (accessed February 17, 2010).

61. Tamar Lewin, "Court Says Health Coverage May Bar Birth-Control Pills," *New York Times*, March 17, 2007, sec. Health, http://www.nytimes.com/2007/03/17/health/17pill.html (accessed February 17, 2010).

62. Carolyn Y. Johnson, "Scientist Takes Aim at Her Longtime Silent Scourge," *Boston Globe*, December 4, 2009, http://www.boston.com/news/local/massachusetts/articles/2009/12/04/scientist_takes_aim_at_her_longtime_silent_scourge/ (accessed December 4, 2009).

63. Ibid.

64. Lois Uttley and Ronnie Pawelko, "No Strings Attached: Public Funding of Religiously Sponsored Hospitals in the U.S.," MergerWatch Project of Family Planning Advocates of N.Y.S., 2001, also available at http://www.mergerwatch.org/briefing_papers.html.

65. The Catholic Health Association of the U.S., "Catholic Healthcare in the United States," January 2009, http://www.chausa.org/NR/rdonlyres/68B7C0E5-F9AA-4106-B182-7DF0FC30A1CA/0/FACTSHEET.pdf (accessed February 17, 2010).

66. Catholics for a Free Choice, "Caution: Catholic Health Restrictions May Be Hazardous to Your Health," 1999, also available at http://www.cath4choice.org/healthmergers.htm.

67. Lisa Ikemoto, "Doctrine at the Gate: Religious Restrictions in Health Care," *Journal of Gender-Specific Medicine* 4, no. 4 (April 2001): 8–12, http://www.mmhc.com/jgsm/articles/JGSM0104/law.html (accessed September 14, 2003); and Jane Lampman, "Different Faiths, Different Views on Stem Cells," *Christian Science Monitor*, July 23, 2001, http://search.csmonitor.com/durable/2001/07/23/p1s2.htm (accessed January 5, 2004).

68. Ikemoto, "Doctrine at the Gate."

69. National Conference of Catholic Bishops/U.S. Conference of Catholic Bishops, *Ethical and Religious Directives for Catholic Health Care Services*, 4th ed., 2003, http://www.nccbuscc.org/bishops/directives.htm (accessed September 17, 2004).

70. Maureen Dobie, "Clinical Drug Tests: Women Need Not Apply," *Indianapolis Business Journal*, January 22, 1996, cited in Lisa Ikemoto, "When a Hospital Becomes Catholic," *Mercer Law Review* 47, no. 4 (April 1996):

1087–1134, http://review.law.mercer.edu/old/fr47308.htm (accessed January 16, 2006); and Lisa Ikemoto, "When a Hospital Becomes Catholic," *Mercer Law Review* 47, no. 4 (April 1996): 1087–1134, http://review.law.mercer.edu/old/fr47308.htm (accessed January 15, 2006).

71. Amy Argetsinger and Avram Goldstein. "GU to Continue Controversial Research," *Washington Post*, January 30, 2004, http://www.washingtonpost.com/ (accessed February 1, 2004).

72. Edward J. Furton, "Vaccines Originating in Abortion," *Ethics & Medics* 24, no. 3 (1999), http://www.immunize.org/concerns/furton.pdf (accessed April 5, 2004).

73. Nancy Frazier O'Brien, "Bishops Approve Revised Directives on Withdrawal of Food, Water," *Catholic News Service*, November 19, 2009, http://www.catholicnews.com/data/stories/cns/0905131.htm (accessed February 17, 2010).

74. Evelyn et al., "Racial/Ethnic Groups in Clinical Trials."

75. U.S. Food and Drug Administration et al., "Deadly Diseases and People of Color: Are Clinical Trials an Option?" 1996, http://www.fda.gov/oashi/patrep/howard.html (accessed January 25, 2004).

76. Evelyn et al., "Racial/Ethnic Groups in Clinical Trials."

77. Ibid.

78. G. Corbie-Smith, S. Thomas, and D. St. George, "Distrust, Race, and Research," *Archives of Internal Medicine* 162 (2002): 2458–63.

79. Scott and Kaufman, "Belated Charge Ignites Furor over AIDS Drug Trial."

80. Chidi Chike Achebe, "The Polio Epidemic in Nigeria: A Public Health Emergency," The Nigerian Village Square, July 14, 2004, http://www.nigeriavillagesquare1.com/Articles/CCAchebe4.htm (accessed July 18, 2005).

81. National Institutes of Health, Office of AIDS Research, *HIV/AIDS Research at NIH: Racial and Ethnic Minorities*, 2001, http://www.nih.gov/od/oar/about/research/racial/oarrace.htm (accessed January 16, 2006).

82. Ibid.

83. Janet L. Mitchell, "Recruitment and Retention of Women of Color in Clinical Studies," in *Women and Health Research: Ethical and Legal Issues of Including Women in Clinical Studies*, ed. Anna C Mastroianni, Ruth Faden, and Daniel Federman, Institute of Medicine (Washington, DC: National Academy Press, 1994), http://www.nap.edu/books/030904992X/html/R1.html (accessed January 16, 2006).

84. Institute of Medicine, Committee on Understanding and Eliminating Racial and Ethnic Disparities in Health Care, *Unequal Treatment: Confronting Racial and Ethnic Disparities in Health Care*, ed. Brian D. Smedley, Adrienne Y. Stith, and Alan R. Nelson (Washington, DC: National Academy Press, 2003), http://www.nap.edu/books/030908265X/html/ (accessed January 16, 2006).

85. Reproductive Health Technologies Project, "Quinacrine Debate."

86. B. Hartmann, *Reproductive Rights and Wrongs: The Global Politics of Population Control* (Boston: South End Press, 1995), cited in Reproductive Health Technologies Project, "Quinacrine Debate."

87. Reproductive Health Technologies Project, "Quinacrine Debate."

88. Ibid.

89. Hartmann, *Reproductive Rights and Wrongs*; and Laura Marks, *Sexual Chemistry: A History of the Contraceptive Pill* (New Haven, CT: Yale University Press, 2001), cited in Reproductive Health Technologies Project, "Quinacrine Debate."

90. Mary Jo Lamberti, "Going Global," *Applied Clinical Trials* (June 2004).

91. Nisha Das, "On the Clinical Trial Trail," Domain-b.com, March 11, 2005, http://www.domain-b.com/industry/pharma/2005/20050311_clinical.html (accessed July 14, 2005).

92. South African Department of Health, "Ethical Considerations for HIV/AIDS Clinical and Epidemiological Research," in *Guidelines for Good Clinical Practice in the Conduct of Trials in Human Participants in South Africa* (2000), chap. 9, http://www.doh.gov.za/docs/policy/trials/trials_09.html (accessed March 4, 2003).

93. John Pomfret and Deborah Nelson, "The Body Hunters, Part 4: In Rural China, a Genetic Mother Lode," *Washington Post*, December 20, 2000, also available at http://www.washingtonpost.com (accessed March 3, 2003).

94. FDA, *Guidance for Industry: Acceptance of Foreign Clinical Studies*, 2001, http://www.fda.gov/cder/guidance/fstud.htm (accessed March 3, 2003).

95. PATH (Program for Appropriate Technology in Health), "Background Information on the Meningitis Vaccine Project," 2004, http://www.path.org/resources/meningitis-background.htm (accessed March 3, 2003).

96. World Health Organization, "Epidemic Meningitis in Africa," 1997, http://www.who.int/archives/inf-pr-1997/en/pr97-11.html (accessed March 3, 2003).

97. Joe Stephens, "The Body Hunters, Part 1: As Drug Testing Spreads, Profits and Lives Hang in Balance," *Washington Post*, December 17, 2000, http://www.washingtonpost.com (accessed September 13, 2003).

98. Xavier Saez-Llorens et al., "Quinolone Treatment for Pediatric Bacterial Meningitis: A Comparative Study of Trovafloxacin and Ceftriaxone with or without Vancomycin," *Pediatric Infectious Disease Journal* 21, no. 1 (2002): 14–22.

99. Pfizer, "Trovan Fact Sheet-Final," http://media.pfizer.com/files/news/trovan_fact_sheet_final.pdf (accessed February 17, 2010).

100. Ed Silverman, "Supreme Court Seeks Pfizer Trovan Comment," Pharmalot, http://www.pharmalot.com/2009/11/supreme-court-seeks-comment-on-pfizer-trovan-case/ (accessed February 17, 2010).

101. Joe Stephens, "Pfizer to Pay $75 Million to Settle Nigerian Trovan Drug-Testing Suit," *Washington Post*, July 31, 2009, http://www.washingtonpost.com/wp-dyn/content/article/2009/07/30/AR2009073001847.html (accessed February 17, 2010).

102. Association for the Accreditation of Human Research Protection Programs, Inc., "Pfizer First Pharma Company to Receive Accreditation for Study Subject Protections," April 2, 2009, http://www.aahrpp.org/www.aspx?PageID=287 (accessed November 9, 2009).

103. Gambia Government/Medical Research Council Joint Ethical Committee, "Ethical Issues Facing Medical Research in Developing Countries," *Lancet*, no. 351 (1998): 286–87.

104. S. Woolhandler, T. Campbell, and D.U. Himmelstein, "Costs of Health Care Administration in the United States and Canada," *New England Journal of Medicine* 349, no. 8 (2003): 768–75.

105. Gambia Government/Medical Research Council Joint Ethical Committee, "Ethical Issues in Developing Countries."

106. Harold Varmus and David Satcher, "Ethical Complexities of Conducting Research in Developing Countries," *New England Journal of Medicine* 337, no. 14 (1997): 1003–5.

107. R. K. Lie et al., "The Standard of Care Debate: The Declaration of Helsinki versus the International Consensus Opinion," *Journal of Medical Ethics* 30 (2004): 190–93, also available at http://www.bioethics.nih.gov/international/readings/intresearch/helsinki.pdf (accessed July 11, 2005).

108. Ruth Macklin, "The Declaration of Helsinki: Another Revision," *Indian Journal of Medical Ethics* 6, no. 1 (March 2009), http://www.ijme.in/171ed2 (accessed February 17, 2010).

109. Michael Goodyear, "Fresh Thinking about the Declaration of Helsinki," *British Medical Journal* 337 (October 17, 2008): a2128, http://www.bmj.com/cgi/content/extract/337/oct17_2/a2128 (accessed February 17, 2010).

110. John R. Williams, "Helsinki Declaration 2008" (presentation at Witwatersrand Medical University, March 19, 2009), http://web.wits.ac.za/NR/rdonlyres/9A4CDFCC-9E5A-4DB9-ADC4-0CD165D1DEE5/0/Helsinkideclaration2008.pdf (accessed February 17, 2010).

111. International Conference on Harmonisation, *Guideline for Good Clinical Practice*, ICH E.6, step 5, guideline 1.5.96, section 1.50, 1996, http://www.ich.org/LOB/media/MEDIA482.pdf.

112. Michael Goodyear, "Fresh Thinking about the Declaration of Helsinki," *British Medical Journal* 337 (October 17, 2008): a2128, http://www.bmj.com/cgi/content/extract/337/oct17_2/a2128 (accessed February 17, 2010).

113. W. Thomas Smith, "FDA Requires Foreign Clinical Studies Be in Accordance with Good Clinical Practice to Better Protect Human Subjects," *ABA Health eSource* 5, no. 2 (October 2008), http://www.abanet.org/health/esource/Volume5/02/smith.html#_ftnref19 (accessed February 17, 2010).

114. Ibid.

115. Sandhya Srinivasan, *Ethical Concerns in Clinical Trials in India: An Investigation* (Mumbai, India: Centre for Studies in Ethics and Rights, February 2009), http://www.fairdrugs.org/uploads/files/Ethical_concerns_in_clinical_trials_in_India_An_investigation.pdf (accessed February 8, 2010).

116. Ibid.

117. Arijit Chadraborty, "Are Phase I Clinical Trials of Foreign Drugs Permitted in India?" Legal Service India (cached September 4, 2009), http://www.legalserviceindia.com/medicolegal/clinicaltrial.htm (accessed February 17, 2010).

118. Samiran Nundy and Chandra Gulhati, "A New Colonialism? Conducting Clinical Trials in India," *New England Journal of Medicine* 352, no. 16 (April 21, 2005): 1633–6, http://content.nejm.org/cgi/content/short/352/16/1633 (accessed February 17, 2010).

119. Sandhya Srinivasan, "Bodies for Hire: The Outsourcing of Clinical Trials," *Himal Southasian*, August 2009, http://www.himalmag.com/Bodies-for-hire;-The-outsourcing-of-clinical-trials_nw3213.html (accessed November 7, 2009); Sandhya Srinivasan, "Trial by Fire," Infochange, September 2009, http://infochangeindia.org/index2.php?option=com_content&task=view&id=7947&pop=1&page=0&Itemid=44 (accessed February 17, 2010).

120. United Nations, "HIV/AIDS in Africa," 2003, http://www.unaids.org/en/media/fact+sheets.asp (accessed May 18, 2003).

121. Sharon LaFraniere, Mary Pat Flaherty, and Joe Stephens, "The Body Hunters, Part 3: The Dilemma: Submit or Suffer," *Washington Post*, December 19, 2000, also available at http://www.washingtonpost.com (accessed March 4, 2003).

122. Hovde, "Integrating Protocol Design."

123. U.S. Department of Health and Human Services, Office of Inspector General, "The Globalization of Clinical Trials: A Growing Challenge in Protecting Human Subjects," 2001, http://oig.hhs.gov/oei/reports/oei-01-00-00190.pdf.

124. LaFraniere, Flaherty, and Stephens, "The Body Hunters, Part 3."

125. Marcia Angell, "Investigators' Responsibilities for Human Subjects in Developing Countries," *New England Journal of Medicine* 342, no. 13 (2000): 967–68; and Mary Pat Flaherty and Joe Stephens, "PA Firm Asks FDA to Back Experiment Forbidden in U.S.," *Washington Post*, February 23, 2001, also available at http://www.washingtonpost.com (accessed March 4, 2003).

126. Public Agenda, "Medical Research: Discussion Guides—The Perspectives in Brief," 2002, http://www.publicagenda.org/issues/debate.cfm?issue_type=medical_research (accessed 2003).

127. John Santa, "The Real Cost of Free Antibiotics," Consumer Reports Health, January 9, 2009, http://blogs.consumerreports.org/health/2009/01/free-antibiotic.html (accessed February 17, 2010).

128. Editorial, "Viagra for Seniors," *Washington Post*, February 4, 2005, sec. A, http://www.washingtonpost.com/ac2/wp-dyn/A62098-2005Feb3? (accessed February 17, 2010).

129. Janet Maslin, "The Truth about the Drug Companies: Indicting the Drug Industry's Practices," *New York Times*, September 6, 2004, sec. Books, http://www.nytimcs.com/2004/09/06/books/06masl.html (accessed February 17, 2010).

130. Ed Silverman, "Come Again? A Spray for Premature Ejaculation," Pharmalot, November 23, 2009, http://www.pharmalot.com/2009/11/come-again-a-spray-for-premature-ejaculation/ (accessed February 17, 2010).

131. TheFreeDictionary.com, s.v. "lifestyle drug," http://medical-dictionary.thefreedictionary.com/lifestyle+drug.

132. Diana Zuckerman, "There's No Such Thing as Free Viagra," National Research Center for Women and Families, January 2006, http://www.center4research.org/news/viagra.html (accessed February 17, 2010).

133. Allergan, "Allergan Announces U.S. Food and Drug Administration Approval of LATISSE—First and Only Treatment Approved by the FDA for Hypotrichosis of Eyelashes," December 26, 2008, http://agn.client.shareholder.com/releasedetail.cfm?ReleaseID=356159 (accessed February 17, 2010).

134. Stephen Heuser, "One Girl's Hope, a Nation's Dilemma," *Boston Globe*, June 14, 2009, http://www.boston.com/news/world/latinamerica/articles/2009/06/14/one_girls_hope_a_nations_dilemma/ (accessed February 17, 2010).

135. Global Network for Neglected Tropical Disease Control, "NTDs and Poverty," GNNTDC, January 6, 2007, http://web.archive.org/web/20070106123443re_/www.gnntdc.org/what/poverty.html (accessed February 17, 2010).

136. World Bank, "Poverty—Overview," PovertyNet, 2009, http://go.worldbank.org/RQBDCTUXW0 (accessed February 17, 2010).

137. "Rapid Impact: Integrating the Neglected Tropical Diseases with Malaria and HIV/AIDS Control," Conference, George Washington University, Washington, DC, October 26–27, 2006.

138. Global Network for Neglected Tropical Disease Control, "NTDs and Poverty," GNNTDC, January 6, 2007, http://web.archive.org/web/20070106123443re_/www.gnntdc.org/what/poverty.html (accessed February 17, 2010).

139. David H. Molyneux, Peter J. Hotez, and Alan Fenwick, "'Rapid-Impact Interventions': How a Policy of Integrated Control for Africa's Neglected Tropical Diseases Could Benefit the Poor," *PLoS Medicine* 2, no. 11 (2005), doi:10.1371/journal.pmed.0020336, http://dx.doi.org/10.1371/journal.pmed.0020336 (accessed February 17, 2010).

140. Ibid.

141. Peter J. Hotez et al., "Incorporating a Rapid-Impact Package for Neglected Tropical Diseases with Programs for HIV/AIDS, Tuberculosis, and Malaria," *PLoS Medicine* 3, no. 5 (2006), doi:10.1371/journal.pmed.0030102, http://dx.doi.org/10.1371/journal.pmed.0030102 (accessed December 5, 2009).

142. Global Network for Neglected Tropical Disease Control, "NTDs and Poverty," GNNTDC, January 6, 2007, http://web.archive.org/web/20070106123443re_/www.gnntdc.org/what/poverty.html (accessed February 17, 2010).

143. Bill and Melinda Gates Foundation, "Disability-Adjusted-Life-Years Lost for Other Health Conditions Addressed by the Foundation (2002 Estimates)," http://web.archive.org/web/20071019181718/www.gatesfoundation.org/NR/rdonlyres/92577317-E8F9-443D-99B2-DD421E76D043/0/DALYS_lowfruit.gif (accessed December 5, 2009); Global Network, "The Impact of NTDS," http://globalnetwork.org/about-ntds/impact-ntds (accessed March 2, 2010); Peter Hotez et al., "Rescuing the Bottom Billion through Control of Neglected Tropical Diseases," *Lancet* 373 (2009): 1570–75 (accessed March 2, 2010).

144. Ibid.

145. Ibid.

146. Ibid.

147. Sheila Davey, ed., *The 10/90 Report on Health Research 2001–2002* (Geneva: Global Forum for Health Research, 2002), http://www.globalforumhealth.org/Media-Publications/Publications/10-90-Report-on-Health-Research-2001-2002 (accessed February 17, 2010).

148. Carlos M. Morel, "Neglected Diseases: Under-funded Research and Inadequate Health Interventions: Can We Change This Reality?" *EMBO Reports* 4, Supplement (June 2003), doi:10.1038/sj.embor.embor851, http://www.ncbi.nlm.nih.gov/pubmed/12789404 (accessed February 17, 2010).

149. Anup Shah, "World Military Spending," *Global Issues*, citing Center for Arms Control and Non-Proliferation, "U.S. Military Spending vs. the World," February 6, 2006, http://www.globalissues.org/Geopolitics/ArmsTrade/Spending.asp (accessed February 17, 2010).

150. Richard L. Guerrant, "Why America Must Care about Tropical Medicine: Threats to Global Health and Security from Tropical Infectious Diseases," *American Journal of Tropical Medicine and Hygiene* 59 no. 1 (1998): 3–16. Also available at http://www.ajtmh.org/cgi/reprint/59/1/3 (accessed July 14, 2005).

151. Peter J. Hotez, "Gandhi's Hookworms," *Foreign Policy*, January 21, 2010, http://www.foreignpolicy.com/articles/2010/01/21/gandhis_hookworms?page=0,0.

152. David H. Molyneux, Peter J. Hotez, and Alan Fenwick, "'Rapid-Impact Interventions': How a Policy of Integrated Control for Africa's Neglected Tropical Diseases Could Benefit the Poor," *PLoS Medicine* 2, no. 11 (2005), doi:10.1371/journal.pmed.0020336, http://dx.doi.org/10.1371/journal.pmed.0020336 (accessed February 17, 2010).

153. Vaniqa Web site, November 9, 2004, http://www.vaniqa.com (accessed with Wayback Machine, web.archive.org, February 21, 2007).

154. Jim Edwards, "Price of Viagra Has Risen 108% Since Launch: 100 Pills Now Cost $1,400," BNET Pharma blog, September 10, 2009, http://industry.bnet.com/pharma/10004198/price-of-viagra-has-risen-98-since-launch-100-pills-now-cost-1400/ (accessed February 17, 2010).

155. FDA, Colors and Cosmetics Technology, *Compliance Program Guidance Manual*, http://www.fda.gov/downloads/Cosmetics/GuidanceComplianceRegulatoryInformation/ComplianceEnforcement/UCM073356.pdf (accessed February 17, 2010).

156. Peter Singer and Solomon R. Benatar, "Beyond Helsinki: A Vision for Global Health Ethics," *British Medical Journal* 322, no. 3 (2001): 747–48, http://www.bmj.org/cgi/content/full/322/7289/747 (accessed July 14, 2005).

157. PhRMA, "Pharmaceutical Companies Lead the Way in Corporate Philanthropy," 2003, http://www.phrma.org/publications/policy_papers/pharmaceutical_companies_lead_the_way_in_corporate_philanthropy/ (accessed February 17, 2010).

158. Medecins Sans Frontieres, "Take the Patent Pool Plunge!" Access and Patents, Campaign for Access to Essential Medicines, http://www.msfaccess.org/main/access-patents/take-the-patent-pool-plunge/ (accessed February 2, 2010); and Medecins Sans Frontieres, "Over 300,000 Messages of Support Help Realise Creation of UNITAID's Patent Pool," Access and Patents, Make It Happen Campaign, http://www.msfaccess.org/main/access-patents/make-it-happen-campaign/campaign-updates/december-16-2009/.

159. Julie George, "Concerns Regarding the UNITAID Patent Pool Implementation Plan," letter to UNITAID Chair Philippe Douste-Blazy, WorldCareCouncil.org, December 10, 2009, http://www.worldcarecouncil.org/content/unitaid-chair-douste-blazy-patent-pool-scope (accessed February 4, 2010).

160. Andrew Witty, "Open Labs, Open Minds: Breaking Down Barriers to Innovation and Access to Medicines and Vaccines in the Developing World" (speech, Council on Foreign Relations, New York, January 20, 2010), http://www.gsk.com/media/Open-innovation-strategy-transcript-English-20jan2010.pdf.

161. Mary Moran et al., "Neglected Disease Research and Development: How Much Are We Really Spending?" *PLoS Medicine* 6, no. 2 (2009), doi:10.1371/journal.pmed.1000030, http://dx.doi.org/10.1371/journal.pmed.1000030 (accessed February 17, 2010).

162. Mary Moran, *The New Landscape of Neglected Disease Drug Development* (London: Wellcome Trust, 2005), http://www.wellcome.ac.uk/News/2007/Features/WTX037099.htm (accessed February 17, 2010).

163. Sherwin, "Women in Clinical Studies."

164. National Institute of Allergy and Infectious Diseases, "Strategic Plan 2000," Emerging Infectious Diseases and Global Health, http://www3.niaid

.nih.gov/about/overview/planningpriorities/strategicplan/emerge.htm (accessed February 17, 2010).

165. International Federation of Pharmaceutical Manufacturers and Associations, "Nifurtimox-Eflornithine for Sleeping Sickness with Training in Tropical Diseases," Health Partnerships: Developing World—2009, http://www.ifpma.org/index.php?id=2223 (accessed April 6, 2010).

166. Donald G. McNeil, Jr., "Low-Cost Antimalarial Pill Available," *New York Times*, March 1, 2007, http://www.nytimes.com/2007/03/01/health/01malaria.html?scp=2&sq=Donald+G.+McNeil+malaria&st=nyt (accessed February 17, 2010).

167. United Nations, "Secretary-General Calls for Concerted Action in Message Marking International Day for Eradication of Poverty," press release issued by U.N. Secretary-General Kofi Annan, November 10, 2002, http://www.un.org/News/Press/docs/2002/sgsm8431.doc.htm (accessed February 17, 2010).

Chapter 10

1. U.S. Department of Labor, Bureau of Labor Statistics, *Career Guide to Industries, 2010–11 Edition*, Pharmaceutical and Medicine Manufacturing, http://www.bls.gov/oco/cg/cgs009.htm; Medical Scientists, http://www.bls.gov/oco/ocos309.htm; Scientific Research and Development Services, http://www.bls.gov/oco/cg/cgs053.htm (accessed February 27, 2010).

2. Carol G. Duane, et al., "Study Coordinators' Perceptions of Their Work Experiences," *The Monitor*, September 2008, 39–42.

3. CenterWatch, "Distribution of Investigative Site Operating Income" in *An Industry in Evolution*, 2002, http://www.centerwatch.com/bookstore/samples/sample_ind_is.html (accessed January 16, 2006).

4. Cullen T. Vogelson, "Participating in Clinical Research," *Modern Drug Discovery* 4 no. 1 (January 2001): 15–16, http://pubs.acs.org/subscribe/journals/mdd/v04/i01/html/clinical.html (accessed January 21, 2002).

5. Ibid.

6. National Institutes of Health, "Human Participant Protections Education for Research Teams."

7. National Institutes of Health, "Introduction to the Principles and Practice of Clinical Research," video, http://www.nihtraining.com/cc/ippcr/archive03s/menu.html.

8. Tufts–New England Medical Center, "The Renewal of Clinical Research."

9. Thomas R. Cech et al., "The Biomedical Research Bottleneck." *Science* 293 (2001): 573.

10. David G. Kaufman, "Testimony before the Subcommittee on Labor, Health and Human Services, Education and Related Agencies," 2000, http://www.faseb.org/opa/govttest/2000test.html (accessed January 16, 2006).

11. Tufts–New England Medical Center, "The Renewal of Clinical Research"; and N. S. Sung et al., "Central Challenges Facing the National Clinical Research Enterprise," *Journal of the American Medical Association* 289 (2003): 1278–87.

12. NIH Common Fund, "Re-engineering the Clinical Research Enterprise," http://nihroadmap.nih.gov/clinicalresearch/ (accessed February 27, 2010).

13. National Institutes of Health, "The NIH Almanac: National Center for Research Resources," http://www.nih.gov/about/almanac/organization/NCRR.htm (accessed February 27, 2010).

14. National Institutes of Health, National Institute of Biomedical Imaging and Bioengineering, "Clinical Research Training Opportunities & Resources," http://www.nibibl.nih.gov/Training/Clinical (accessed February 27, 2010).

Epilogue

1. Julia Bess Frank, "Laments of a Clinical Clerk," *New England Journal of Medicine* 298, no. 18 (1978): 1009.

Appendix A

1. Sparks, "Timeline of Laws"; and FDA, "The Evolution of U.S. Drug Law.

2. Ibid.

3. FDA, *From Test Tube to Patient: Improving Health through Human Drugs*, 1999, http://www.fda.gov/cder/about/whatwedo/testtube.pdf (accessed November 1, 2003).

4. *Trials of War Criminals before the Nuremberg Military Tribunals.*

5. World Medical Association, "International Code of Medical Ethics."

6. FDA, "The Evolution of U.S. Drug Law."

7. Ibid.

8. W. G. McBride, "Thalidomide and Congenital Anomalies," *Lancet*, no. 2 (1961): 1358, http://www.mindfully.org/Health/Thalidomide-Back.htm (accessed February 7, 2004).

9. King, "Drug Abuse Control 1965."

10. McBride, "Thalidomide and Congenital Anomalies."

11. U.S. Department of Health and Human Services, Office for Human Research Protections, "Protection of Human Subjects," *Code of Federal Regulations*, Title 45, Part 46, 2005, http://www.hhs.gov/ohrp/humansubjects/guidance/45cfr46.htm (accessed January 2, 2006).

12. National Commission for the Protection of Human Subjects of Biomedical and Behavioral Research, *The Belmont Report.*

13. FDA, "Expanded Access and Expedited Approval of New Therapies Related to HIV/AIDS," http://www.fda.gov/oashi/aids/expanded.html (accessed January 2, 2006).

14. Advisory Committee on Human Radiation Experiments, *Final Report of the Advisory Committee on Human Radiation Experiments.*

15. President's Council on Bioethics, "Council Publications," http://www.bioethics.gov/reports/ (accessed January 2, 2006).

16. World Health Organization, *Operational Guidelines for Ethics Committees That Review Biomedical Research*, 2000, http://www.who.int/tdr/publications/publications/ethics.htm (accessed February 7, 2004).

17. FDA, *Best Pharmaceuticals for Children Act*, 2001, http://www.fda.gov/opacom/laws/pharmkids/contents.html (accessed February 7, 2004).

18. Ceci Connolly, "U.S. Food and Drug Administration to Suspend a Rule on Child Drug Testing," *Washington Post*, March 19, 2002, http://www.washingtonpost.com/ac2/wp-dyn/A47229-2002Mar18 (accessed February 7, 2004).

19. FDA, "Significant Dates in U.S. Drug Law History," updated April 2009, http://www.fda.gov/AboutFDA/WhatWeDo/History/Milestones/ucm128305.htm (accessed March 25, 2010).

20. FDA, "Critical Path 2010 Update," updated March 2010, http://www.fda.gov/ScienceResearch/SpecialTopics/CriticalPathInitiative/ucm204289.htm (accessed March 25, 2010)

21. Cornell University Law School, "Riegel v. Medtronic, Inc. (No. 06-179) 451 F. 3d 104, Affirmed," http://www.law.cornell.edu/supct/html/06-179.ZS.html.

22. Mark Senak, "The Supremes and the Pre-emption Thing," Eye on FDA, March 5, 2009, http://www.eyeonfda.com/eye_on_fda/2009/03/the-supremes-and-the-preemption-thing.html (accessed April 13, 2009).

23. Norman M. Goldfarb, "Informed Consent in the Tegenero TGN1412 Trial," *Journal of Clinical Research Best Practices* 2, no. 5 (2006), http://www.firstclinical.com/journal/2006/0605_TeGenero.pdf (accessed February 17, 2010).

24. PAREXEL International, "Informed Consent Form" and "Information Sheet," project no. 68419, protocol no. TGN1412-HV, February 9, 2008, http://www.circare.org/foia5/tgn1412_consentform.pdf.

25. Expert Scientific Group on Phase One Clinical Trials, *Final Report*, Chair, Gordon Duff (London: TSO, November 30, 2006), http://www.dh.gov.uk/prod_consum_dh/groups/dh_digitalassets/@dh/@en/documents/digitalasset/dh_073165.pdf (accessed February 17, 2010).

26. Ibid.

27. Barbara Rellahan, "The TeGenero Incident March 13, 2006 UK: TGN1412—a Superagonist Anti-CD28 Antibody" (presentation at the FDA Clinical Investigator's Course, Silver Spring, MD, November 17, 2009).

28. Ibid.

29. Expert Scientific Group on Phase One Clinical Trials, *Final Report*, Chair, Gordon Duff (London: TSO, November 30, 2006), http://www.dh.gov.uk/prod_consum_dh/groups/dh_digitalassets/@dh/@en/documents/digitalasset/dh_073165.pdf (accessed February 17, 2010).

30. Ibid.

31. Ibid.

32. Norman M. Goldfarb, "Informed Consent in the Tegenero TGN1412 Trial," *Journal of Clinical Research Best Practices* 2, no. 5 (2006), http://www.firstclinical.com/journal/2006/0605_TeGenero.pdf (accessed February 17, 2010).

33. Ibid.

34. PAREXEL International, "Informed Consent Form" and "Information Sheet," project no. 68419, protocol no. TGN1412-HV, February 9, 2008, http://www.circare.org/foia5/tgn1412_consentform.pdf.

35. Norman M. Goldfarb, "Informed Consent in the Tegenero TGN1412 Trial," *Journal of Clinical Research Best Practices* 2, no. 5 (2006), http://www.firstclinical.com/journal/2006/0605_TeGenero.pdf (accessed February 17, 2010).

36. PAREXEL International, "Informed Consent Form" and "Information Sheet," project no. 68419, protocol no. TGN1412-HV, February 9, 2008, http://www.circare.org/foia5/tgn1412_consentform.pdf.

37. Norman M. Goldfarb, "Informed Consent in the Tegenero TGN1412 Trial," *Journal of Clinical Research Best Practices* 2, no. 5 (2006), http://www.firstclinical.com/journal/2006/0605_TeGenero.pdf (accessed February 17, 2010).

38. Ibid.

39. Ibid.

40. Ibid.

41. Ibid.

42. PAREXEL International, "Informed Consent Form" and "Information Sheet," project no. 68419, protocol no. TGN1412-HV, February 9, 2008, http://www.circare.org/foia5/tgn1412_consentform.pdf.

43. Norman M. Goldfarb, "Informed Consent in the Tegenero TGN1412 Trial," *Journal of Clinical Research Best Practices* 2, no. 5 (2006), http://www.firstclinical.com/journal/2006/0605_TeGenero.pdf (accessed February 17, 2010).

44. Ibid.

45. Ibid.

46. Ibid.

47. National Commission for the Protection of Human Subjects of Biomedical and Behavioral Research, *The Belmont Report.*

48. *Trials of War Criminals before the Nuremberg Military Tribunals.*

Glossary

1. Association of American Medical Colleges, "Breaking the Scientific Bottleneck."

2. Tufts–New England Medical Center, "The Renewal of Clinical Research."

3. Schechter, "The Crisis in Clinical Research."

4. FDA, "Investigational New Drug Application."

5. FDA, Establishment of Prescription Drug User Fee Rates for Fiscal Year 2010," August 3, 2009, http://www.fda.gov/forindustry/userfees/prescriptiondruguserfee/default.htm (accessed April 3, 2010).

6. International Conference on Harmonisation, *Guideline for Good Clinical Practice.*

7. Ibid.

Glossary and Acronym Guide

adverse event (AE). Any potential side effect—any new, untoward sign or symptom or lab test abnormality that develops while a subject is on a study, whether or not you believe it is related to the investigational medication.

AE. *See* adverse event.

Apache. A scoring system commonly used to assess a patient's severity of illness in an attempt to standardize data for study.

approval (by an institutional review board). The decision of the IRB, after review, that the clinical trial protocol may be conducted at the site under consideration, if it is done in accordance with good clinical practice, institutional, and regulatory requirements.

arm. One of the different treatment groups being compared on a study.

audit. A review by the sponsor or FDA to examine a site's conduct of trial-related activities and its documents. This review is to determine whether the study activities were conducted properly and if the data were obtained accurately, assessed, and reported according to the protocol, the sponsor's standard operating procedures, good clinical practice, and other regulatory requirements.

baseline evaluation. The assessment of subjects at study entry, before they receive any treatment.

Belmont Report. *Ethical Principles and Guidelines for the Protection of Human Subjects of Research.* This report concerns the conduct of research with human subjects. It is known as the "Belmont Report" because it came out of a series of discussions originally held in 1976 at the Smithsonian Institution's Belmont Conference Center.

biological agents. Materials originating from living organisms that can cause disease, including bacteria, viruses, and toxins.

biologics. Compounds derived from living sources (animals or microorganisms) and manufactured into drugs or therapies.

biopharmaceuticals. Drugs produced from biotechnology and living sources. These include human insulin, drugs made from recombinant (genetically engineered) proteins, recombinant vaccines, and monoclonal antibodies.

blinded study. A study structured so that one or more parties to a trial are kept unaware of the treatment assignments. Single-blinding usually refers to the subjects being unaware, and double-blinding usually refers to the subjects, investigators, monitor, and, in some cases, data analysts being unaware of the treatment assignments.

blinded study medications. Different (or active and inactive) drugs that are made to appear identical in size, shape, color, and flavor. Medications are blinded to make it very hard for subjects or investigators to determine which medication is being administered, to avoid introducing bias into a study.

budget. An itemized account of the estimated time and expense required to complete a project. An investigator's best guess of the cost of conducting a study versus the amount allowed per subject by the drug company (the grant).

case report form (CRF). The biography, or life history, of a volunteer's participation on a trial in an encodable format. The data-capture form designed to record all of the protocol-required information from the source documents or raw data for submission to a sponsor in the sponsor's preferred format.

cbc. *See* complete blood count.

CBER. *See* Center for Biologics Evaluation and Research.

CDER. *See* Center for Drug Evaluation and Research.

CDRH. *See* Center for Devices and Radiological Health.

Center for Biologics Evaluation and Research (CBER). The division of the FDA responsible for vaccines, blood and tissue products, and cellular or gene therapies.

Center for Devices and Radiological Health (CDRH). The division of the FDA that oversees products such as intravenous catheters, pacemakers, implantable pumps for insulin or other medications, synthetic grafts, and breast implants.

Center for Drug Evaluation and Research (CDER). The division of the FDA responsible for the safety of chemically synthesized drugs.

central lab. A specific laboratory selected by a trial sponsor to do the testing for all of the sites conducting the trial protocol. This eliminates any variations in test results that might occur between different laboratories. Special, sophisticated lab tests that are not routinely available at local laboratories can also be sent to such a reference lab.

clinical hold. An order issued by the FDA to a trial sponsor to delay or suspend the clinical investigation.

clinical research. "A component of medical and health research intended to produce knowledge valuable for understanding human disease, preventing and treating illness, and promoting health."[1]

Or the NIH definition: "Patient-oriented clinical research conducted with human subjects, or research on the causes and consequences of disease in human populations involving material of human origin (such as tissue specimens and cognitive phenomena) for which an investigator or colleague directly interacts with human subjects in an outpatient or inpatient setting to clarify a problem in human physiology, pathophysiology or disease, or epidemiologic or behavioral studies, outcomes research or health services research, or developing new technologies, therapeutic interventions, or clinical trials."[2]

My favorite definition is that of the NIH's Dr. Alan N. Schechter: "research performed by a scientist and a human subject working together, both being warm and alive."[3]

clinical research associate (CRA). This person works as an agent of the drug company sponsoring a clinical trial and manages the details of the trial at the study sites for the sponsor, along with the MRA. The CRA also monitors the data from the study sites for accuracy and veracity. CRAs are often referred to as "monitors"; they visit the study sites to make sure that everything is being done by the books—the protocol, federal regulations, and good clinical practice guidelines.

clinical research coordinator (CRC). aka **study coordinator.** The person in charge of "keeping it together," managing a clinical study on a day-to-day basis at the study site.

clinical study. *See* clinical trial.

clinical trial or **clinical study.** A planned, systematic investigation (as opposed to after the fact discovery by trial and error) of the effects of a drug, treatment, or device on a group of volunteers.

clinical trial agreement (CTA). A contract between an investigator and/or institution and the sponsor of a clinical trial defining the terms and conditions associated with the conduct of the clinical trial.

closeout visit. The final visit the CRA makes to a site to finalize paperwork, review outstanding queries, reconcile drug shipments, and return necessary supplies to the sponsor.

coinvestigator. Subinvestigator.

comparator. The product used as a reference or standard in a clinical study.

compassionate use. An experimental drug or treatment made available outside of a trial protocol to a (usually dying) patient for whom no alternative therapies exist.

complete blood count (cbc). Routine hematology lab tests, including red blood cell count, white blood cell count, and platelets.

contract research organization (CRO). A company hired by a trial sponsor to conduct some of the sponsor's duties. CROs act as middlemen or subcontractors on the trial, carrying out specific tasks such as finding appropriate sites and administrating the study for the sponsor. One CRO works for many different drug companies.

control. A point of reference. For example, a volunteer may serve as his or her own control in a study so that any changes seen in a given volunteer can be attributed to the study intervention, rather than person-to-person variability.

CPM. *See* Critical Path Method.

CRA. *See* clinical research associate.

CRC. *See* clinical research coordinator.

CRF. *See* case report form.

critical path method (CPM). A project management technique that allows you to identify constraints in a sequence of events.

CRO. *See* contract research organization.

CRO Capability Assessment Service (CROCAS). A commercial, proprietary database available to sponsors to provide them with information about the experience of specific CROs with different types of trials.

CROCAS. *See* CRO Capability Assessment Service.

crossover study. An investigation in which each subject receives both treatments being compared, during different time periods.

CTA. *See* clinical trial agreement.

Data Safety Monitoring Board (DSMB). An independent board of experts in the field, statisticians, and other specialists (e.g., ethicists) who may help evaluate a clinical trial. The DSMB evaluates a trial at periodic intervals, assessing both safety and outcomes. It can end the trial at any time, either because of safety concerns or because the DSMB's analysis of outcomes shows that one treatment group is faring significantly better than the other and therefore it would be unethical to continue the trial.

Dear Doctor Letter. A letter from a drug manufacturer or others addressed to doctors and other health professionals regarding new product issues, such as new warnings, safety information, or changes to prescribing information.

Declaration of Helsinki. A code of ethics developed by the World Medical Association in 1964 and widely adopted by medical associations in various countries. It was revised in 1975, 1989, and 2000, most recently requiring a worldwide standard of care that many feel is not attainable in developing countries.

Department of Health, Education, and Welfare (DHEW). A cabinet-level department of the U.S. government from 1953 to 1979, when it was restructured.

DHEW. *See* Department of Health, Education, and Welfare.

documentation. All records, in any form, that describe or record the methods, conduct, and/or results of a trial.

double-blinded study. A study in which neither the volunteer nor the study personnel making the assessments are aware of the treatment group to which the volunteer has been assigned. The pharmacist generally knows which medicine is which. No matter who is blinded to the study, an emergency code is always available explaining which treatment a particular subject has received.

double-dummy. A type of procedure used to compare two medications in such a way as to eliminate bias. A fake (placebo) study medication is made to appear identical to one of the active medications being studied. Some patients receive Study Drug A, with active medication, and also a look-alike placebo (fake) Drug B. Others receive a placebo for Drug A and active medication for Drug B. In each case, the volunteers receive an active drug—they just can't tell which one by the appearance.

DSMB. *See* Data Safety Monitoring Board.

early escape. The provision allowing for a volunteer's early withdrawal from participation in a trial.

efficacy. Whether and how well a drug or device works for its intended purpose.

electronic health record. *See* electronic medical record.

electronic medical record (EMR), aka electronic health record. A computerized collection of a patient's medical information, previously known as a patient's "chart."

EMR. *See* electronic medical record.

end of therapy (EOT) visit. Study visit performed just as a study subject is completing the course of investigational medicine.

end point. Outcome or criteria for ending the study.

enrollment. The commitment of a patient to a study; "signing on the dotted line."

EOT. *See* end of therapy.

evaluable patient. A patient who meets the inclusion and exclusion enrollment criteria for a study and who completes all the requirements of the protocol successfully.

exclusion criteria. Those characteristics (age, sex, lab test results, underlying disease, etc.) that exclude a potential subject from a study.

facilities letter. A letter of understanding between a study site and sponsor acknowledging that the site (e.g., a hospital) has given permission to the investigators to conduct the trial and outlining the responsibilities of the site and investigators.

FDA. *See* Food and Drug Administration.

FDAMA. *See* FDA Modernization Act.

FDA Modernization Act (FDAMA). A 1997 law that gave huge incentives to pharmaceutical manufacturers to extend studies to include children, among other changes.

finder's fees. A reward or bonus for identifying and referring a patient to a study.

Food and Drug Administration (FDA). The U.S. government agency that is responsible for the conduct of clinical trials involving the manufacture, testing, and use of drugs and medical devices.

formulary. The list of drugs a hospital or insurance company allows to be used by their participants. Often, only one drug in a group, or class, of drugs is allowed; e.g., one statin type of medicine for elevated cholesterol or one proton pump inhibitor for ulcer therapy. Among similar agents, which drug is allowed is generally decided by cost.

f/u. Follow-up.

Gantt chart. A planning tool that can be used to illustrate the timing of tasks needed to complete a specific project and to identify potential bottlenecks. This chart graphically displays tasks versus time and shows the progress of a project. This type of chart is named for Henry Laurence Gantt, an early twentieth century mechanical engineer and management consultant.

GCP. *See* good clinical practice.

good clinical practice (GCP). Guidelines, or the Golden Rule, bureaucratized. A standard for designing and conducting a clinical trial, which provides assurances regarding the accuracy of the data and reported results and, most importantly, that the rights of the volunteer subjects are protected.

Health Insurance Portability and Accountability Act, 42 USC § 201 (HIPAA). Very restrictive privacy regulations enacted in 1996; see "HIPAA Highlights for Researchers" in appendix C.

HIPAA. *See* Health Insurance Portability and Accountability Act.

ICH. *See* International Conference on Harmonisation.

IDE. *See* Investigational Device Exemption.

inclusion criteria. Those characteristics that potential subjects *must* meet to be eligible for a study (depending on the study and how bad enrollment is, the medical monitor may be able to make exceptions).

IND. *See* investigational new drug.

indemnification. The act of insuring, or holding harmless. A letter or agreement assuring that a trial sponsor will provide legal and financial coverage for adverse events resulting from a volunteer's participation on the sponsor's trial. Increasingly, sponsors want the study sites to indemnify them!

indication. The illness being treated or targeted.

IND safety report. *See* Investigational New Drug safety report.

informed consent. An agreement between an investigator and a subject, which outlines the purpose of a clinical trial and all of the procedures, benefits, risks, and alternatives to participation. The subject must review and sign this agreement before any study procedures are performed, indicating his or her voluntary agreement to participate.

initiation (meeting). The meeting of the monitor (CRA), investigator, and site personnel, after all the regulatory documents for a study are approved. The protocol and procedures are reviewed, and then enrollment can begin.

inpt. Inpatient.

inservice. A training session at the site, targeting a particular audience. This session may occur for a specific nursing unit, for example, to teach about a new medicine or procedure. It is a brief, on-the-job, training experience.

Institute of Medicine (IOM). A division of the National Academy of Sciences whose purpose is to provide unbiased, authoritative guidance regarding health issues. The IOM is an independent, nongovernmental group.

Institutional Review Board (IRB). An independent committee, usually composed of members from an investigator's institution as well as from the local community. This board must scrutinize all clinical trials performed at the institution, provide oversight, and issue approvals or requests for actions. It is the IRB's task to make sure that a study is following all FDA regulations. The IRB grants or denies approval for a proposed research study and for the methods and materials used in obtaining and documenting informed consent.

intent to treat analysis. A examination of data from all patients in the groups they were randomized to, whether or not they actually received treatment.

interactive voice response system (IVRS). A centralized call (dial-in) system that provides treatment randomization. Study site personnel enter information about a subject (demographics, etc.) over a phone via touch tones or voice. The centralized computer then randomizes the volunteer to a treatment group and provides coded information back to the site. The system can also be used to reorder supplies.

intercurrent illness. An illness that occurs coincidentally and simultaneously to the condition being studied.

International Conference on Harmonisation (ICH). International Conference on Harmonisation of the Technical Requirements for Registration of Pharmaceuticals for Human Use, which established good clinical practice guidance. Note that the FDA, HHS (Health and Human Services), and ICH have somewhat different definitions of "good clinical practice."

Investigational Device Exemption (IDE). An application and authorization from the FDA allowing a sponsor to use an unapproved medical device for investigational purposes. This is the device equivalent of an IND application.

investigational new drug (IND). A new drug or biological agent that is used in a clinical investigation and not yet approved by the FDA. An IND approval allows an experimental drug to be tested for safety and efficacy.

Investigational New Drug (IND) application. The application from a trial sponsor to the FDA requesting permission from the FDA to begin human testing in the United States and allowing the experimental drug to be shipped legally across state lines.

Investigational New Drug safety report. A report reflecting new adverse events with a study drug. These reports are sent to all investigators and study sites involved with that drug.

investigational product. An active ingredient being tested or a placebo being used as a reference in a clinical trial. An investigational product may also include a product that is already approved and marketed for other indications.

investigator. The person who "is responsible for ensuring that an investigation is conducted according to the signed investigator statement (Form FDA 1570), the investigational plan (protocol), and applicable regulations; for protecting the rights, safety, and welfare of subjects under the investigator's care; and for the control of drugs under investigation."[4]

investigator-initiated study. A clinical trial designed and proposed by an investigator rather than a sponsor drug company. This type of study is generally quite small and conducted at one or two sites.

Investigator's Brochure. A document that provides a study investigator with the relevant preclinical and clinical data about the study drug or device that are known to date.

investigator's meeting. A meeting between the sponsor and study investigators (and coordinators) prior to beginning a trial. The protocol is reviewed and the sponsor attempts to answer any questions or concerns.

IOM. *See* Institute of Medicine.

IRB. *See* Institutional Review Board.

IVRS. *See* interactive voice response system.

K30 awards. NIH grants to universities to develop or improve training programs in clinical research and to promote career development of clinical investigators.

long-term follow-up (LTFU). A follow-up visit often occurring 30–60 days after the subject completes taking the investigational medicine, to see if there have been any delayed reactions that might pose safety concerns, and to confirm the continued efficacy of the therapy.

LTFU. *See* long-term follow-up.

manual of operations (MOO). Standard operating procedures, or SOPs.

manual of procedures (MOP). Standard operating procedures, or SOPs.

MAR. *See* medicine administration record.

medical monitor. The MD on call for protocol questions or safety issues. The medical monitor should know something about the area of investigation. If not experienced, a good medical monitor will be willing to learn on the job.

medical research associate (MRA). Like a CRA, only "in-house" at the sponsor company. The MRA helps manage the details of the trial at the study sites but works at the sponsor company.

medicine administration record (MAR). A record of all medications a patient receives, including the name, dose, route, and time of administration. For some medications, the MAR also includes the duration of individual infusions of medications.

monitor. Generally refers to the CRA.

monitoring. Overseeing the progress of a clinical trial and ensuring that it is conducted, recorded, and reported in accordance with the protocol, standard operating procedures, GCP, and other regulatory requirements.

MOO. *See* manual of operations.

MOP. *See* manual of procedures

MRA. *See* medical research associate.

multicenter trial. A clinical trial that is conducted at multiple sites, usually covering a wide geographic area. A different investigator works at each site, but all investigators follow one uniform protocol.

multivariate analysis. A statistical technique intended to evaluate the relative contribution that multiple variables make to an end result.

National Academies. The umbrella oversight organization for the National Academy of Sciences, the National Academy of Engineering, the Institute of Medicine (IOM), and the National Research Council.

National Academy of Sciences. A private society of well-respected academic scientists. It was granted a charter by Congress in 1863, requiring it to advise the federal government on scientific and technical matters.

National Commission for the Protection of Human Subjects of Biomedical and Behavioral Research. The commission, formed by Congress, that issued the

Belmont Report recommendations (*see* Belmont Report) in 1979, outlining basic ethical principles to guide research.

National Institutes of Health (NIH). The primary biomedical research agency of the federal government; the NIH is officially part of the Department of Health and Human Services. It has an extensive campus in Bethesda, Maryland.

National Research Act. A law passed by Congress in 1974 requiring IRBs to review all DHEW-funded research. This act also authorized the creation of the National Commission for the Protection of Human Subjects of Biomedical and Behavioral Research.

NDA. *See* New Drug Application.

New Drug Application (NDA). The application to the FDA by a trial sponsor for a license to market a new drug. An approved NDA allows the drug to be sold in the United States.

NIH. *See* National Institutes of Health.

NOAEL. *See* no observable adverse effect level.

no observable adverse effect level (NOAEL). The maximal concentration of a drug at which no increased harmful effects are seen compared to an unexposed control.

Occupational Safety and Health Administration (OSHA). The part of the U.S. government's Department of Labor responsible for overseeing the safety and health of workers in most U.S. businesses and industries.

on-treatment. The period during which a volunteer is actually taking an investigational medicine.

open label study. A study in which both the subject and the investigator know which drug or device the subject is receiving.

orphan drug. A drug targeted to rare illnesses affecting fewer than 200,000 people.

OSHA. *See* Occupational Safety and Health Administration.

over-the-counter drug. A drug that is available for purchase without a prescription.

parallel study. A study in which each participant is assigned to a specific treatment arm but all study activities are the same for all participants.

pathophysiology. The study of how physiologic functions (of animals or people) change due to illness or injury.

PD. *See* pharmacodynamics.

PDUFA. *See* Prescription Drug User Fee Act.

Pediatric Studies Rule. A 1998 regulation requiring specific pediatric labeling information for some drugs.

PERT. *See* Program Evaluation and Review Technique.

Pharmaceutical Information Cost Assessment Service (PICAS). A commercial database available to trial sponsors that provides extensive cost-related data and can be used to develop trial budgets.

pharmacist. A person trained to prepare and dispense medicines.

pharmacodynamics (PD). The study of reactions between drugs and living beings, including the physiology of responses to drugs or other therapeutic interventions.

pharmacoeconomics. The study of the cost benefit or cost effectiveness in comparing drug therapies or other treatments.

pharmacokinetics (PK). The study of the absorption, distribution, metabolism, and excretion of drugs.

phases. The development cycle of a drug; stages of testing that each drug goes through before becoming eligible for FDA approval.

PHI. *See* protected health information.

phlebotomist. The lab worker trained to draw blood from patients.

PI. *See* Principal Investigator.

PICAS. *See* Pharmaceutical Information Cost Assessment Service.

PK. *See* pharmacokinetics.

placebo. An inactive substance used in studies to help determine the effectiveness of the (investigational) medicine. Comparisons are made between the responses to the active and inactive drugs.

PO. *Per os*, or "by mouth."

postmarketing study. A clinical study conducted after a drug has received FDA approval and is on the market or available by prescription.

Prescription Drug User Fee Act (PDUFA). A law that imposes fees on drug, biologic, or device sponsors. This is used to help fund the FDA and expedite product reviews. Fee rates for FY 2010 include those "for application fees for an application requiring clinical data ($1,405,500), for an application not requiring clinical data or a supplement requiring clinical data ($702,750), for establishment fees ($457,200), and for product fees ($77,720)."[5]

pretreatment. The period of study activities performed before a volunteer receives the investigational product.

primary efficacy studies. Trials that are pivotal in demonstrating a drug's efficacy.

Principal Investigator (PI). Top dog, or "the buck stops here." Usually, but not always, a physician; the lead person responsible for the conduct of a clinical trial at a study site. *See* investigator.

prn. On an "as needed" basis. Usually refers to administration of medications or treatments.

Program Evaluation and Review Technique (PERT). A list of tasks with length and prerequisites (previous tasks on which a task is dependent).

protected health information (PHI). According to privacy rules under HIPAA, information that allows someone to be individually identified, including name, social security number, and address.

protocol. The plan for a clinical study, with rationale, background information, and objectives. The protocol also includes inclusion and exclusion criteria, laboratory requirements, a schedule of activities for each subject visit, drug administration information, and planned study analysis methods.

pts. Patients.

QOL. *See* quality of life.

quality of life (QOL). A person's social and psychological well-being. QOL is evaluated by surveys that try to assess whether a subject can be more active, can manage "activities of daily living" better, or generally feels better after treatment. Often used as an important marketing tool.

query. A request for clarification regarding data entry. It may relate to an obviously implausible figure being entered in a data field on a case report form or to inconsistencies between data submitted in different sections of the report.

randomization. The assignment of patients to treatment groups without bias (like rolling dice).

recruitment. The process used to identify and enroll volunteers on a clinical trial.

Rx. Treatment or therapy.

SAE. *See* serious adverse event.

screening. Identifying patients who may be eligible to enter a study and then sorting through enrollment criteria to see if there are obvious contraindications.

screening fee. Reimbursement to a site for going through the application of inclusion and exclusion criteria to evaluate a potential study volunteer to assess if that person is eligible for a trial.

serious adverse event (SAE). An adverse event defined as death, a life-threatening event, or an event leading to or prolonging hospitalization, resulting in persistent or significant disability or incapacity, or resulting in a congenital anomaly or birth defect. Cancer and overdose were previously required in SAE reports, too, and may still be required by a trial sponsor; the ICH worldwide standards do not include them.[6]

short-term follow-up (STFU). A study visit often occurring 2–7 days after the subject completes an investigational treatment. This visit assesses the short-term efficacy and safety of the treatment.

single-blinded study. A study design in which the volunteers do not know which treatment they are receiving, but the investigator and sponsor do.

site management organization (SMO). Similar to, though less common than, a CRO, an SMO often provides a study site with the staff to conduct a trial protocol. SMOs often try to manage a group or network of sites and market to drug companies for trials.

SMO. *See* site management organization.

SOP. *See* standard operating procedure.

source document. All of the *original* data collected from each study subject at a study site. Source documents may include worksheets, the medical chart, x-rays, laboratory reports, and EKGs. They are used to verify all data submitted to the sponsor and the FDA.

sponsor. A pharmaceutical company or device manufacturer whose product is being investigated by a clinical trial; the overall developer of the drug.

standard operating procedure (SOP). A too-formal term for a checklist. Procedures that should be followed routinely.

standard treatment. The FDA-approved treatment for a particular disease that is currently in use or is the standard of care. For trials of novel treatments, no standard treatment may be available as a comparator, and a placebo might be used.

STFU. *See* short-term follow-up.

study coordinator. *See* clinical research coordinator.

study site. A place at which a clinical trial is conducted.

subinvestigator. Second billing. Someone designated and supervised by the Principal Investigator at a study site to perform critical trial-related procedures and/or to make important trial-related decisions.

subject. A participant who volunteers to receive treatment in a clinical trial. Many people prefer the more respectful terms *patient* or *volunteer* to the clinical term *subject*. Occasionally referred to as a "guinea pig" by the press or the public.

subject identification code. A unique identifier assigned by the investigator to each trial subject to protect the subject's identity. The subject identification code is used in lieu of the subject's name when the investigator reports adverse events and other trial-related data.

superbugs. Bacteria that are resistant to most, if not all, antibiotics. Superbugs are increasingly difficult to treat.

symptomatic treatment. A therapy intended to help someone feel better but that may not benefit their underlying disease.

teratogenic. Causing developmental abnormalities in fetuses.

treatment IND. An FDA approval that enables a pharmaceutical company to provide investigational drugs to patients with serious or immediately life-threatening diseases for which no comparable or satisfactory alternate therapy exists (and who do not qualify for clinical trial participation). These drugs are given as "compassionate use." Regulations were enacted by the FDA in 1987.

Tuskegee experiment. A study of men (mostly African American) with syphilis. These men were followed between 1932 and 1972, without medical intervention, to study the natural history of the disease, even after good treatments became available for their disease.

UADE. *See* unanticipated adverse device effect.

unanticipated adverse device effect (UADE). Device equivalent of an AE; any serious adverse effect on health or safety or any life-threatening problem or death caused by or associated with a device.

unexpected adverse drug reaction (or event). An adverse reaction to a product when that reaction has not been previously described or when the severity of the reaction is not consistent with the currently available product information (i.e., the Investigator's Brochure for an unapproved investigational product or package insert or summary of product characteristics for an approved product).

vulnerable subjects. Potential clinical trial subjects whose willingness to participate may be less voluntary than the norm, either because of an expectation of great benefit or because of a fear of retaliation for refusal. "Examples are members of a group with a hierarchical structure, such as medical, pharmacy, dental and nursing students, subordinate hospital and laboratory personnel, employees of the pharmaceutical industry, members of the armed forces, and persons kept in detention. Other vulnerable subjects include patients with incurable diseases, persons in nursing homes, unemployed or impoverished persons, patients in emergency situations, ethnic minority groups, homeless persons, nomads, refugees, minors, and those incapable of giving consent."[7]

washout period. The period in which a trial volunteer receives no treatment for the indication being studied in order to eliminate the effects of previous treatment before beginning the experimental phase. This period reduces the chance of a previous drug treatment interfering with the assessment of the response to the drug being studied.

Bibliography

Aapro, Matti S., Claus-Henning Köhne, Harvey Jay Cohen, and Martine Extermann. et al. "Never Too Old? Age Should Not Be a Barrier to Enrollment in Cancer Clinical Trials." *Oncologist* 10, no. 3 (2005), doi:10.1634/theoncologist.10-3-198. http://theoncologist.alphamedpress .org/cgi/content/abstract/10/3/198 (accessed November 9, 2009).

Abramson, John, and Barbara Starfield. "The Effect of Conflict of Interest on Biomedical Research and Clinical Practice Guidelines: Can We Trust the Evidence in Evidence-Based Medicine?" *Journal of the American Board of Family Practice* 18, no. 5 (2005), doi:10.3122/jabfm.18.5.414. http://www .jabfm.org (accessed December 3, 2009).

Achebe, Chidi Chike. "The Polio Epidemic in Nigeria: A Public Health Emergency." The Nigerian Village Square, July 14, 2004. http://www .nigeriavillagesquare1.com/Articles/CCAchebe4.htm (accessed July 18, 2005).

Adams, Christopher P., and Van V. Brantner. "Estimating the Cost of New Drug Development: Is It Really $802 Million?" *Health Affairs* 25, no. 2 (2006), doi:10.1377/hlthaff.25.2.420. http://content.healthaffairs.org/cgi/ reprint/25/2/420 (accessed February 9, 2010).

Adams, Vincanne, Suellen Miller, Sienna Craig, et al. "The Challenge of Cross-Cultural Clinical Trials Research: Case Study from Tibet." *Medical Anthropology Quarterly* 19 (2005): 267–289. http://www.oneheartibet.org/ docs/Challenge_of_CrossCultural.pdf (accessed October 21, 2009).

Administrator. "Big Pharma Moving More Work Offshore." July 7, 2004. Citing Fast Track 2006 data. http://www.amreteckpharma.com/index .php?option=com_content&task=view&id=6&Itemid=40 (accessed October 20, 2009).

Advanced Clinical Software. "Study Manager." 2003. http://www.acs-world.com (accessed January 27, 2004).

Advisory Committee on Human Radiation Experiments. "DOE Openness: Human Radiation Experiments." 1994. http://www.eh.doe.gov/ohre/index .html (accessed September 6, 2005).

Advisory Committee on Human Radiation Experiments. *Final Report of the Advisory Committee on Human Radiation Experiments.* 1994. http://www .eh.doe.gov/ohre/roadmap/achre/preface.html (accessed September 6, 2005).

Afrin, Lawrence B., James C. Oates, Caroline K. Boyd, and Mark S. Daniels. "Leveraging of Open EMR Architecture for Clinical Trial Accrual." *American Medical Informatics Association (AMIA) Annual Symposium Proceedings.* (2003): 16–20. http://www.ncbi.nlm.nih.gov/pmc/articles/PMC1480210/ (accessed November 5, 2009).

Agres, Ted. "Clinical Trials Trickling Away." *Drug Discovery and Development,* July 5, 2005. http://www.dddmag.com/clinical-trials-trickling-away.aspx (accessed October 20, 2009).

AIDS Treatment Activists Coalition (including the National Minority AIDS Council) Letter to President Bush. July 31, 2003. http://www.hivma.org/Content.aspx?id=3776 (accessed February 15, 2010).

Allergan. "Allergan Announces U.S. Food and Drug Administration Approval of LATISSE—First and Only Treatment Approved by the FDA for Hypotrichosis of Eyelashes." December 26, 2008. http://agn.client.shareholder.com/releasedetail.cfm?ReleaseID=356159.

American Academy of Pediatrics. "Guidelines for the Ethical Conduct of Studies to Evaluate Drugs in Pediatric Populations." *Pediatrics* 95, no. 2 (1995): 286–94. Also available at http://www.aap.org/policy/00655.html (accessed January 4, 2004).

Anderson, Carl. "The Ins and Outs of Electronic Medical Records." *Applied Clinical Trials,* September 1, 2008. http://appliedclinicaltrialsonline.findpharma.com/appliedclinicaltrials/IT+Articles/The-Ins-and-Outs-of-Electronic-Medical-Records/ArticleStandard/Article/detail/546113 (accessed November 4, 2009).

Anderson, Dianna. "Budgeting for International Subject Recruiting." Presentation at the MAGI Clinical Research Conference–West, San Diego, CA, October 2009.

Andrews, Lori, Jordan Paradise, Timothy Holbrook, and Danielle Bochneak. "When Patents Threaten Science." *Science* 314, no. 5804 (2006): 1395. http://www.kentlaw.edu/islat/pdf/WhenPatentsThreatenScience.pdf (accessed November 27, 2009).

Angell, Marcia. "Investigators' Responsibilities for Human Subjects in Developing Countries." *New England Journal of Medicine* 342, no. 13 (2000): 967–68.

Angell, Marcia. "Is Academic Medicine for Sale?" *New England Journal of Medicine* 342, no. 20 (2000): 1516–18.

Anthes, Emily, and Scott Allen. "U.S. Scientists Go Abroad to Find Patients for Cancer Studies." *Boston Globe,* December 29, 2007. http://www.boston.com/news/nation/articles/2007/12/29/us_cancer_researchers_go_abroad_for_trials/ (accessed May 6 2009).

Argetsinger, Amy, and Avram Goldstein. "GU to Continue Controversial Research." *Washington Post,* January 30, 2004. http://www.washingtonpost.com/ (accessed February 1, 2004).

Ascension Health. "Healthcare Ethics." http://www.ascensionhealth.org.

Asherman, Ira G. "Language, Culture, and the Drug Development Process." *Drug Information Association Today*. 2005. http://www.asherman.com/downloads/asherman_1.04.06.pdf (accessed October 22, 2009).

Asherman, Ira G. "The Regulatory Affairs Manager: Management Training for the Multicultural Workforce." *Regulatory Affairs Focus* 9 (2004): 39–41. http://www.asherman.com/images1/RAManager.pdf (accessed October 22, 2009).

Association for the Accreditation of Human Research Protection Programs, Inc. "Pfizer First Pharma Company to Receive Accreditation for Study Subject Protections." *Medical Research Law & Policy Report*, 8 MRLR 276, April 15, 2009. http://www.aahrpp.org/www.aspx?PageID=287 (accessed November 9, 2009).

Association of Academic Health Centers. "HIPAA Creating Barriers to Research and Discovery." 2008. http://www.aahcdc.org/policy/reddot/AAHC_HIPAA_Creating_Barriers.pdf (accessed October 14, 2009).

Association of American Medical Colleges. "Breaking the Scientific Bottleneck: Report of the Graylyn Consensus Development Conference." 1990. http://www.aamc.org/research/calltoaction.htm (accessed January 16, 2006).

Association of American Medical College and FDA. *Drug Development Science: Obstacles and Opportunities for Collaboration among Academia, Industry and Government*. Report of an Invitational Conference, Association of American Medical Colleges and FDA, 2005, http://www.aamc.org/drugdevelopmentscience (accessed October 13, 2009).

Bachenheimer, Joan F. "Good Recruitment Practice: Working to Create the Bond Between Study and Subject." *Applied Clinical Trials*, April 1, 2004. http://appliedclinicaltrialsonline.findpharma.com/appliedclinicaltrials/article/articleDetail.jsp?id=89626 (accessed October 13, 2009).

Bailey, Wynn, Carol Cruickshank, and Nikhil Sharma. "Make Your Move: Taking Clinical Trials to the Best Location." 2006. http://www.pharmafocusasia.com/knowledge_bank/white_papers/clinicaltrials_bestlocation.htm (accessed May 5, 2009).

Barnett Educational Services. "2009–2010 Statistical Sourcebook Data Presented at DIA." Press release. http://www.barnettinternational.com/EducationalServices_Content.aspx?id=93134 (accessed August 29, 2009).

Barnett International. *The Form FDA 1572: A Reference Guide for Clinical Researchers, Sponsors, and Monitors*. 2008. http://www.barnettinternational.com/EducationalServices_Publication.aspx?p=6659 (accessed November 12, 2009).

Barone, Suzanne. "FDA Amendments Act of 2007 (FDAAA) and Risk Evaluation and Mitigation Strategies (REMS)." Presentation at the Ninth Annual Pharmaceutical Regulatory Congress, October 28, 2008. http://www.ehcca.com/presentations/pharmacongress9/barone_t1_pm.ppt (accessed February 9, 2010).

Below, Paul, and Barbara Westrum. "Similarities and Differences in Conducting Medical Device and Pharmaceutical Clinical Trials." Minnesota Chapter,

Association of Clinical Research Professionals, http://www.mnacrp.org/assets/slides/socra_02-26-03.ppt (accessed February 9, 2009).

Benderly, Beryl Lieff. "Research on Women, Women in Research." In *In Her Own Right: The Institute of Medicine's Guide to Women's Health Issues.* Washington, DC: National Academy Press, 1997. Also available at http://books.nap.edu/books/0309053277/html (accessed September 14, 2003).

Berenson, Alex. "Drugs in '05: Much Promise, Little Payoff." *New York Times*, January 11, 2006. http://www.nytimes.com/2006/01/11/business/11drug.html (accessed January 30, 2006).

Betanzos, Todd E. "The People vs. Amgen: Study Subjects Sue to Receive Investigational Drugs." *Pharmaceutical Executive*, June 2006. http://www.sdma.com/Publications/detail.aspx?pub=4478 (accessed September 20, 2009).

Bill and Melinda Gates Foundation. "Disability-Adjusted-Life-Years Lost for Other Health Conditions Addressed by the Foundation (2002 Estimates)." http://web.archive.org/web/20071019181718/www.gatesfoundation.org/NR/rdonlyres/92577317-E8F9-443D-99B2-DD421E76D043/0/DALYS_lowfruit.gif (accessed December 5, 2009).

Binkowitz, Bruce. "An Overview of Issues Surrounding Multi-Regional Clinical Trials." Presentation at the Harvard Schering-Plough 17th Annual Workshop, Boston, May 28, 2009. http://www.hsph.harvard.edu/schering-plough-workshop/program/index.html (accessed November 8, 2009).

Birch, J. M., D. Pang, R. D. Alston, et al. "Survival from Cancer in Teenagers and Young Adults in England, 1979–2003." *British Journal of Cancer* 99, no. 5 (2008): 830–835. http://www.ncbi.nlm.nih.gov/pmc/articles/PMC2528159/ (accessed November 9, 2009).

Blackburn, Elizabeth. "Bioethics and the Political Distortion of Biomedical Science." *New England Journal of Medicine* 350 (2004): 1379. http://www.nejm.org/cgi/content/short/350/14/1379 (accessed February 15, 2010).

Bleyer, A., T. Budd, and M. Montello. "Older Adolescents and Young Adults with Cancer and Clinical Trials: Lack of Participation and Progress in North America." Chapter 5 in *Cancer in Adolescents and Young Adults.* New York: Springer, 2007, 71–81. Cited in Birch, J. M., D. Pang, R. D. Alston, et al. "Survival from Cancer in Teenagers and Young Adults in England, 1979–2003." *British Journal of Cancer* 99, no. 5 (2008): 830–835. http://www.ncbi.nlm.nih.gov/pmc/articles/PMC2528159/ (accessed November 9, 2009).

Blumenfeld, T. H., and D. Zinner. PhD research study at RapidTrials and Harvard Business School. Cited in Sarah O'Neil, April Lewis, and Jo Sorgi-Gendreau. "CRAs and Site Performance in the U.S." *The Monitor*, September 2009, p. 51.

Bohm, Malcolm. "Applying Healthcare Data to Site Selection and Patient Recruitment." Presentation at the MAGI Clinical Research Conference–West, San Diego, CA, October 2009.

Bollert, Joe A. "How to Use Study Brokers to Find Sites and Studies." Presentation at the MAGI Clinical Research Conference–West, San Diego, CA, October 2009.

Boonstra, Heather. "Health Advocates Say Campaign to Disparage Condoms Threatens STD Prevention Efforts." *The Guttmacher Report on Public Policy* 6, no. 1 (2003). http://www.guttmacher.org/pubs/tgr/06/1/gr060101.html (accessed February 15, 2010).

Borfitz, Deborah. "Site Gripes and Solutions for EDC." Bio-IT World.com, September 15, 2009. http://www.bio-itworld.com/BioIT_Article.aspx?id=94288 (accessed September 15, 2009).

Borfitz, Deborah. "Social Networking Sites Have Myriad Trial-Related Uses." eCliniqua, March 2, 2009. http://www.ecliniqua.com/2009/03/02/social-networking-recruitment-sites.html (accessed September 27, 2009).

Borfitz, Deborah, and Allison Proffitt. "Social Networking Sites Embrace Clinical Trials." Bio-ITWorld.com, May 19, 2009. http://www.bio-itworld.com/issues/2009/may-jun/social-networking-clinical-trials.html (accessed September 27, 2009).

Boucher, Helen W., George H. Talbot, John S. Bradley, et al. "Bad Bugs, No Drugs: No ESKAPE! An Update from the Infectious Diseases Society of America." *Clinical Infectious Diseases* 48, no. 1 (2009), doi:10.1086/595011.

Brightly, Edward G. "Bird Flu Vaccine Patent." IPMed, August 20, 2008. http://www.ipmed.blogspot.com/2008/08/bird-flu-vaccine-patent.html (accessed November 28, 2009).

Brody, Jane E. "Ferreting for Facts in the Realm of Clinical Trials." *New York Times*, October 15, 2002. Also available at http://www.nytimes.com (accessed February 8, 2003).

Brownstein, Larry, and Kate Leonard. "Collecting Payments: Financial Viability of Sponsors." Presentation at the MAGI Clinical Research Conference–West, San Diego, CA, October 2009.

Brunette, Douglas. "Hidden Mystery." Agency for Healthcare Research and Quality. Web Morbidity and Mortality Rounds: Case & Commentary, March 2005. http://www.webmm.ahrq.gov/printview.aspx?caseID=88 (accessed November 9, 2009).

Bureau of National Affairs. "Pfizer First Pharma Company to Receive Accreditation for Study Subject Protections." *Medical Research Law & Policy Report*, April 15, 2009. http://www.aahrpp.org/www.aspx?PageID=242 (accessed October 14, 2009).

Burger, Julie, and Justin Bruner. "A Court's Dilemma: When Patents Conflict with Public Health." *Virginia Journal of Law & Technology* 12, no. 4 (2007): 1–41. http://www.kentlaw.edu/islat/publications.html (accessed November 28, 2009).

Burke, John. "ICH-GCP & FDA Regulations Differences." April 1, 2009. http://louisville.edu/research/humansubjects/ICH%20GCP%20-%20FDA%20Regulations%20Differences_4-20-09.ppt (accessed October 18, 2009).

Burt, Victoria. "A Model for Device Development." *Medical Design*, September 1, 2008. http://www.medicaldesign.com/mag/model_device_development_0908 (accessed February 9, 2010).

BusinessWire. "Congressional 'Sting' Operation Uncovered by Coast IRB." November 3, 2009. http://www.businesswire.com/portal/site/google/?ndmViewId=news_view&newsId=20090311006356&newsLang=en (accessed October 14, 2009).

Byrd, Jack, Jr. *Operations Research Models for Public Administration*. Lexington, MA: D. C. Heath & Company, 1975.

Catholic Health Association of the U.S. "Catholic Healthcare in the United States." January 2009. http://www.chausa.org/NR/rdonlyres/68B7C0E5-F9AA-4106-B182-7DF0FC30A1CA/0/FACTSHEET.pdf (accessed November 30, 2009).

Catholics for a Free Choice. "Caution: Catholic Health Restrictions May Be Hazardous to Your Health." 1999. Also available at http://www.cath4choice.org/healthmergers.htm.

Cech, Thomas R., Lorraine W. Egan, Carolyn Doyle, et al. "The Biomedical Research Bottleneck." *Science* 293 (2001): 573.

Ceh, S. Eric. "Documenting Concomitant Medications in Clinical Trials." *Journal of Clinical Research Best Practices* 3, no. 7 (2007). http://www.firstclinical.com/journal/2007/0707_Concomitant.pdf (accessed February 13, 2010).

Center for Constitutional Rights. "Tummino, et al. v. von Eschenbach." March 23, 2009. http://ccrjustice.org/ourcases/current-cases/tummino,-et-al.-v.-von-eschenbach (accessed February 15, 2010).

Center for Information and Study on Research Participation. "101 Facts about Clinical Research." July 2005. http://www.scribd.com/doc/9768708/101-Facts-About-Clinical-Research (accessed February 10, 2010).

Center for Information and Study on Research Participation. "Participating in a Clinical Trial." http://www.ciscrp.org/patient/videos.html (accessed February 14, 2010).

Center for Reproductive Law and Policy. "Citizen's Petition." Submitted to the Food and Drug Administration on February 14, 2001.

Centers for Disease Control. "Condoms and Their Use in Preventing HIV Infection and Other STIS." September 1999. http://house.gov/reform/min/pdfs/pdf_inves/pdf_admin_hhs_info_condoms_fact_sheet_orig.pdf.

Centers for Disease Control. "History of Vaccine Safety." January 15, 2010. http://www.cdc.gov/vaccinesafety/Vaccine_Monitoring/history.html (accessed February 10, 2010).

Centers for Disease Control. "Male Latex Condoms and Sexually Transmitted Diseases." Fact sheet. October 2003. http://www.cdc.gov/nchstp/od/latex.htm.

Centers for Disease Control. "Programs That Work." http://www.cdc.gov/nccdphp/dash/rtc. Original, data-based, archived version online at http://

web.archive.org/web/20010606142729/www.cdc.gov/nccdphp/dash/rtc/index.htm.

Centers for Medicare and Medicaid Services and the Joint Commission. *Specifications Manual for National Hospital Inpatient Quality Measures.* Performance Measurement Initiatives, October 2, 2009. http://www.jointcommission.org/performancemeasurement/performancemeasurement/current+nhqm+manual.htm (accessed October 15, 2009).

CenterWatch. Cited in Ronald P. Evens. *Drug and Biological Development: From Molecule to Product and Beyond.* New York: Springer, 2007, 15. http://www.books.google.com/books?id=aSB4xfVyTSEC (accessed February 9, 2010).

CenterWatch. "Distribution of Investigative Site Operating Income." In *An Industry in Evolution.* 2002. http://www.centerwatch.com/bookstore/samples/sample_ind_is.html (accessed January 16, 2006).

CenterWatch. "Proportion of New Investigators to New Trials." *CenterWatch Monthly*, October 2007, p. 13. http://www.vscr.at/news/objects/press/cwm1410_October.pdf (accessed October 13, 2009).

CenterWatch. "2009 Patient Experience Survey." Cited in Veronica Legge. "2009 Subject and Physician Survey Results: Understanding the Relationship to Maximize Study Referrals." Presentation at the MAGI Clinical Research Conference–West, San Diego, CA, October 2009.

Chadraborty, Arijit. "Are Phase I Clinical Trials of Foreign Drugs Permitted in India?" Legal Service India (cached September 4, 2009). http://www.legalserviceindia.com/medicolegal/clinicaltrial.htm (accessed November 8, 2009).

Chamberland, Guy. "Developing Drug-Device Combination Products with Unapproved Components." Chap. 9 in *Clinical Evaluation of Medical Devices: Principles and Case Studies.* 2nd ed. Edited by Karen M. Becker and John J. Whyte. Totowa, NJ: Humana Press, 2005. http://www.books.google.com/books?id=V9BLgoOv5T4C (accessed February 9, 2010).

Chan, An-Wen, Asbjørn Hróbjartsson, Mette T. Haahr, Peter C. Gøtzsche, and Douglas G. Altman. "Empirical Evidence for Selective Reporting of Outcomes in Randomized Trials: Comparison of Protocols to Published Articles." *Journal of the American Medical Association* 291, no. 20 (2004): 2457–2465. http://www.jama.ama-assn.org/cgi/content/full/291/20/2457 (accessed November 10, 2009).

Charo, R. Alta. "Body of Research—Ownership and Use of Human Tissue." *New England Journal of Medicine* 355, no. 15 (2006), doi:10.1056/NEJMp068192. http://content.nejm.org/cgi/content/full/355/15/1517 (accessed November 27, 2009).

Chen, Pauline W. "Bending the Rules of Clinical Trials." *New York Times*, October 29, 2009, sec. Health. http://www.nytimes.com/2009/10/29/health/29chen.html (accessed November 22, 2009).

Chen, Robert. "Vaccine (+ Drug) Development Process: A Historical Review of Successes and Failures." 2008. http://www.avac.org/pdf/aidsvax08.pdf (accessed October 20, 2009).

Children's Hospital of Philadelphia. "How are Vaccines Made?" http://www.chop.edu/service/vaccine-education-center/vaccine-science/how-are-vaccines-made.html (accessed February 10, 2010).

Children's Hospital of Philadelphia. "Vaccine Safety FAQs." 2008. http://www.chop.edu/service/vaccine-education-center/vaccine-safety/#Was_the_rotavirus (accessed February 10, 2010).

Citizens for Responsible Care and Research. "Ketek Clinical Trials and FDA Approval." August 23, 2009. http://www.circare.org/foia5/ketek.htm (accessed October 17, 2009).

Citizens for Responsible Care and Research. *Tegenero Medicines and Healthcare Products Regulatory Agency Clinical Trial Suspension.* Interim report. http://www.circare.org/foia5/clinicaltrialsuspension_interimreport.pdf (accessed November 29, 2009).

Clay, John. Cited in *Genetic Engineering News* 21, no. 1 (2001): 11.

Collier, Roger. "Drug Development Cost Estimates Hard to Swallow." *Canadian Medical Association Journal* 180, no. 3 (2009), doi:10.1503/cmaj.082040. http://www.pubmedcentral.nih.gov/articlerender.fcgi?artid=2630351 (accessed February 9, 2010).

Committee on HIV Prevention Strategies in the United States. *No Time to Lose: Getting More from HIV Prevention.* Washington, DC: National Academy Press, 2001.

Connolly, Ceci. "U.S. Food and Drug Administration to Suspend a Rule on Child Drug Testing." *Washington Post,* March 19, 2002. http://www.washingtonpost.com/ac2/wp-dyn/A47229-2002Mar18 (accessed February 7, 2004).

CONSORT Group. "The CONSORT (CONsolidated Standards of Reporting Trials) Statement." 2009. http://www.consort-statement.org/consort-statement/ (accessed November 10, 2009).

Corbie-Smith, G., S. Thomas, and D. St. George. "Distrust, Race, and Research." *Archives of Internal Medicine* 162 (2002): 2458–63.

Curfman, Gregory D., Stephen Morrissey, and Jeffrey M. Drazen. "The Medical Device Safety Act of 2009." *New England Journal of Medicine* 360, no. 15 (2009), doi:10.1056/NEJMe0902377. http://content.nejm.org/cgi/content/full/360/15/1550 (accessed February 9, 2010).

Cutting Edge Information. *Streamlining Clinical Trials Report.* 2009. http://www.cuttingedgeinfo.com/clinical-trials/?overview.

Dalovisio, Joseph R. "Hurricane Katrina: Lessons Learned in Disaster Planning for Hospitals, Medical Schools, and Communities." *Current Infectious Disease Reports* 8, no. 3 (2006): 171–173. http://www.springerlink.com/index/K831155M2437K878.pdf (accessed February 13, 2010).

Dalovisio, Joseph. "IDSA Outlines the Problem/Solutions for FDA." Infectious Diseases Society of America, November 10, 2003. http://www.idsociety.org/Template.cfm?Section =News_Releases1&CONTENTID=7444&TEMPLATE=/ContentManagement/ContentDisplay.cfm (accessed November 30, 2003).

Dalton, Claudette. "Health Literacy Basic Lecture." University of Virginia, 2006. http://www.healthsystem.virginia.edu/internet/som-hlc/Lecture.cfm (accessed November 5, 2009).

Dalton, Claudette. "Health Literacy Basic Lecture." University of Virginia, 2006. http://www.healthsystem.virginia.edu/internet/som-hlc/Lecture.cfm. Citing Dean Schillinger, et al. "Association of Health Literacy with Diabetes Outcomes." *Journal of the American Medical Association* 288 (2002): 475–482. http://www.jama.ama-assn.org/cgi/content/abstract/288/4/475 (accessed November 5, 2009).

Dana-Farber Cancer Institute. "Entering a Clinical Trial: Is It Right for You?" December 17, 2007. http://www.dana-farber.org/res/clinical/trials-info/default.html (accessed September 27, 2009).

Darwin National Assurance Company. "Clinical Research Liability. 2007." http://www.darwinpro.com/mkt/pdf/med_crli.pdf (accessed September 20, 2009).

Das, Nisha. "On the Clinical Trial Trail." Domain-b.com, March 11, 2005, http://www.domain-b.com/industry/pharma/2005/20050311_clinical.html (accessed July 14, 2005).

Data Edge. "Compressing Development Times with Better Investigator Selection." Data Edge DataLines, Spring 1996. http://www.fast-track.org (accessed February 4, 2003).

Data Edge. "Patient Treatment Data: The Hidden Key to Faster Studies." Data Edge DataLines, 1998. http://www.fast-track.com (accessed February 17, 2003).

Datye, Arundhati, and Rachel Holley. "Medical Device Regulation." Presentation at the MAGI Clinical Research Conference–West, San Diego, CA, October 2009.

Daugherty, Jon R. "Regulatory Considerations for the Manufacture of Investigational Vaccines for Clinical Trials." October 30, 2007. http://www.fda.gov/downloads/BiologicsBloodVaccines/NewsEvents/WorkshopsMeetingsConferences/UCM106627.pdf (accessed February 10, 2010).

Davey, Sheila, ed. *The 10/90 Report on Health Research 2001–2002*. Geneva: Global Forum for Health Research, 2002. http://www.globalforumhealth.org/Media-Publications/Publications/10-90-Report-on-Health-Research-2001-2002.

David J. Graham. "Testimony before the United States Senate." November 18, 2004. http://finance.senate.gov/hearings/testimony/2004test/111804dgtest.pdf (accessed December 1, 2009).

DeNoon, Daniel. "Swine Flu Vaccine Timeline: Key Decisions, Key Milestones." WebMD, July 20, 2009. http://www.webmd.com/cold-and-flu/news/20090720/swine-flu-vaccine-when (accessed February 9, 2010).

DeRenzo, Evan G. "Conflict-of-Interest Policy at the National Institutes of Health: The Pendulum Swings Wildly." *Kennedy Institute of Ethics Journal* 15, no. 2 (2005): 199–210. http://muse.jhu.edu/login?uri=/journals/kennedy

_institute_of_ethics_journal/v015/15.2derenzo.html (accessed November 24, 2009).

Desai, Ketan. "Clinical Trials for Bioterrorism Agents." *Journal of Clinical Research Best Practices* 2, no. 4 (2006). http://firstclinical.com/journal/2006/0604_Bioterrorism.pdf (accessed October 20, 2009).

DiCarlo, Jovianna. "Planning & Executing Global Trials." Presentation at the MAGI Clinical Research Conference–West, San Diego, CA, October 2009.

DiCarlo, Jovianna. "Technology Showcase." Presentation at the MAGI Clinical Research Conference–West, San Diego, CA, October 2009.

Dickersin, Kay. "Clinical Trials Registration: Overdue yet Elusive." Johns Hopkins Bloomberg School of Public Health, July 7, 2005. http://www.jhsph.edu/publichealthnews/articles/2005/dickersin.html (accessed July 17, 2005).

Dilts, David M., and Alan B. Sandler. "Invisible Barriers to Clinical Trials: The Impact of Structural, Infrastructural, and Procedural Barriers to Opening Oncology Clinical Trials." *Journal of Clinical Oncology* 24, no. 28 (2006): 4545–4552. http://www.jcojournal.org/cgi/reprint/24/28/4545 (accessed October 16, 2009).

DiMasi, J. A. (Tufts Center for the Study of Drug Development) "Measuring Trends in the Development of New Drugs: Time, Costs, Risks and Returns." Presentation to the SLA Pharmaceutical & Health Technology Division Spring Meeting, Boston, MA, 2007. Cited in PhRMA. *Pharmaceutical Industry Profile 2009.* Washington, DC: PhRMA, April 2009. http://www.phrma.org/files/attachments/PhRMA%202009%20Profile%20FINAL.pdf (accessed October 20, 2009).

Dingell, John, Chairman of U.S. House of Representatives Committee on Energy and Commerce. Letter to Michael Leavitt, Secretary, U.S. Department of Health and Social Security, March 28, 2007. http://archives.energycommerce.house.gov/Investigations/DrugSafety.032807.HHS.ltr (accessed December 1, 2009).

Dipity. "H1N1 Swine Flu Vaccine Will Be Used for Mass Depopulation—Baxters Man Made Flu." August 19, 2009. http://www.dipity.com/timeline/H1n1-Vaccine-Safety (accessed November 10, 2009).

Dixon, Dennis O. "Data and Safety Monitoring." February 2, 2009. http://www.nihtraining.com/cc/ippcr/current/downloads/Dixon020209(C).pdf (accessed November 10, 2009).

Dobie, Maureen. "Clinical Drug Tests: Women Need Not Apply." *Indianapolis Business Journal*, January 22, 1996. Cited in Lisa Ikemoto. "When a Hospital Becomes Catholic." *Mercer Law Review* 47, no. 4 (1996): 1087–134. http://review.law.mercer.edu/old/fr47308.htm (accessed January 16, 2006).

Dong, B. J., W. W. Hauk, J. G. Gambertoglio, et al. "Bioequivalence of Levothyroxine Preparations for Treatment of Hypothyroidism." *Journal of the American Medical Association* 277 (1997):1199–200.

Driver, Jeffrey. "Informed Consent: It's Not Just a Form, It's a Process." Health Leaders Media, June 24, 2008. http://www.healthleadersmedia.com/print/

content/213995/topic/WS_HLM2_TEC/Informed-Consent-Its-Not-Just-a-Form-Its-a-Process.html (accessed November 7, 2009).

Duane, Carol G., Stephanie E. Granda, David C. Munz, and Joan C. Cannon. "Study Coordinators' Perceptions of Their Work Experiences." *The Monitor*, September 2008, 39–42.

Duke Clinical Research Institute. Clinical Trials Networks Best Practices. "Budget Template." https://www.ctnbestpractices.org/sites/budgets-contracts/budgettemplate/view.

Duke Clinical Research Institute. Clinical Trials Networks Best Practices. "Budgets and Contracts." https://www.ctnbestpractices.org/sites/budgets-contracts/ (accessed February 11, 2010).

Duke Clinical Research Institute. Clinical Trials Networks Best Practices. "Keys to Building a Successful Research Site." http://www.ctnbestpractices.org/edu/keys-to-building-a-successful-research-site (accessed September 18, 2009).

Duke Clinical Research Institute. Clinical Trials Networks Best Practices. "SOP Guidelines for Writers." https://www.ctnbestpractices.org/sites/sops/sop-guidelines-for-writers-word/view (accessed February 13, 2010).

Duke Clinical Research Institute. "Keys to Building a Successful Research Site." http://www.dcri.duke.edu/investigator/quickref.pdf (accessed September 30, 2009).

Editorial. "An Influenza Vaccine Debacle." *New York Times*, October 20, 2004. http://www.nytimes.com/2004/10/20/opinion/20wed1.html (accessed February 10, 2010).

Editorial. "Viagra for Seniors." *Washington Post*, February 4, 2005, sec. A. http://www.washingtonpost.com/ac2/wp-dyn/A62098-2005Feb3.

Edwards, Jim. "Price of Viagra Has Risen 108% Since Launch: 100 Pills Now Cost $1,400." BNET Pharma blog, September 10, 2009. http://industry.bnet.com/pharma/10004198/price-of-viagra-has-risen-98-since-launch-100-pills-now-cost-1400/.

Emanuel, Ezekiel J., Trudo Lemmens, and Carl Elliot. "Should Society Allow Research Ethics Boards to Be Run as For-Profit Enterprises?" PLoS Medicine 3, no. 7 (2006): e309. http://www.dx.doi.org/10.1371/journal.pmed.0030309.

Embi, Peter J., Anil Jain, Jeffrey Clark, and C. Martin Harris. "Development of an Electronic Health Record-Based Clinical Trial Alert System to Enhance Recruitment at the Point of Care." In *American Medical Informatics Association Annual Symposium Proceedings*, 2005: 231–235. http://www.ncbi.nlm.nih.gov/pmc/articles/PMC1560758/ (accessed November 5, 2009).

Ensirink, Martin. "The Challenge of Getting Swine Flu Vaccine to Poor Nations." *Science Insider*, November 3, 2009. http://blogs.sciencemag.org/scienceinsider/2009/11/the-challenge-o.html (accessed November 28, 2009).

Ervin, John. "Opinions: Should Clinical Research Sites Unionize? or We're Mad as #$%& and We're Not Going to Take It Anymore!" *AAPP Rx* 3, no. 2 (2001): 13–14. http://www.aapp.org/pdf/summer2001.pdf (accessed September 14, 2005).

European Medicines Agency. *ICH Topic E5: Ethnic Factors in the Acceptability of Foreign Clinical Data.* 1998. http://www.emea.europa.eu/pdfs/human/ich/028995en.pdf (accessed November 8, 2009).

European Medicines Agency. *ICH Topic E7: Studies in Support of Special Populations: Geriatrics—Questions & Answers.* 2009. http://www.ema.europa.eu/pdfs/human/ich/60466109en.pdf.

European Medicines Agency. *ICH Topic E11: Clinical Investigation of Medicinal Products in the Pediatric Population.* 2000. http://www.emea.europa.eu/pdfs/human/ich/271199en.pdf (accessed February 14, 2010).

European Medicines Agency. *Reflection Paper on the Extrapolation of Results from Clinical Studies Conducted Outside Europe to the EU Population.* 2009. http://www.emea.europa.eu/pdfs/human/ewp/69270208en.pdf (accessed November 8, 2009).

Evans, David. "Pfizer Broke the Law by Promoting Drugs for Unapproved Uses." Bloomberg.com, November 9, 2009. http://www.bloomberg.com/apps/news?pid=20670001&sid=a4yV1nYxCGoA (accessed December 3, 2009).

Evans, David, Michael Smith, and Liz Willen. "Big Pharma's Shameful Secret." *Bloomberg Markets Special Report*, December 2005. http://dcscience.net/pharma-bloomberg.pdf.

Evelyn, B., T. Toigo, D. Banks, et al. "Participation of Racial/Ethnic Groups in Clinical Trials and Race-Related Labeling: A Review of New Molecular Entities Approved 1995–1999." *Journal of the National Medicine Association*, Supplement (December 2001). http://www.fda.gov/cder/reports/race_ethnicity/race_ethnicity_report.htm (accessed September 14, 2003).

Expert Scientific Group on Phase One Clinical Trials. Gordon Duff, Chair. *Final Report*. London: TSO, November 30, 2006. www.dh.gov.uk/prod_consum_dh/groups/dh_digitalassets/@dh/@en/documents/digitalasset/dh_073165.pdf.

Farquhar, Cynthia M. "Clinical Evidence: Endometriosis." *British Medical Journal* 320, no. 7247 (2000): 1449–1452. http://clinicalevidence.bmj.com/ceweb/conditions/woh/0802/0802_background.jsp#REF3.

Farquhar, Cynthia M. Extracts from "Clinical Evidence: Endometriosis." *British Medical Journal* 320, no. 7247 (2000), doi:10.1136/bmj.320.7247.1449. http://www.bmj.com/cgi/content/abstract/320/7247/1449.

Federation of American Scientists. "Building Public Trust: Actions to Respond to the Advisory Committee on Human Radiation Experiments." 1967. http://www.fas.org/sgp.library/humexp/ (accessed July 22, 2005).

Flaherty, Mary Pat, Deborah Nelson, and Joe Stephens. "The Body Hunters, Part 2: Overwhelming the Watchdogs." *Washington Post*, December 18, 2000, A1. http://www.washingtonpost.com (accessed March 4, 2003).

Flaherty, Mary Pat, and Joe Stephens. “PA Firm Asks FDA to Back Experiment Forbidden in U.S.” *Washington Post*, February 3, 2001, A3. http://www.washingtonpost.com (accessed March 4, 2003).

Fleischhaker, Sheila, and Mark Cohen. “The ABCs of Drug Safety: Accountability, Balance, and Citizen Empowerment.” Government Accountability Project (GAP), April 2009. http://www.whistleblower.org/storage/documents/ABCFinal.pdf.

Frank, Julia Bess. “Laments of a Clinical Clerk.” *New England Journal of Medicine* 298, no. 18 (1978): 1009.

“From Bug to Drug.” *Washington Post*, August 9, 2003, A14.

Furton, Edward J. “Vaccines Originating in Abortion.” *Ethics & Medics* 24, no. 3 (1999). http://www.immunize.org/concerns/furton.pdf (accessed April 5, 2004).

Gallo, Paul, Christy Chuang-Stein, et al. “Adaptive Designs in Clinical Drug Development—An Executive Summary of the PhRMA Working Group.” *Journal of Biopharmaceutical Statistics* 16, no. 3 (2006): 275–283. dx.doi.org/10.1080/10543400600614742 (accessed February 10, 2010).

Gambia Government/Medical Research Council Joint Ethical Committee. “Ethical Issues Facing Medical Research in Developing Countries,” *Lancet*, no. 351 (1998): 286–87.

Gates, Cynthia. “Adverse Events vs. Unanticipated Problems.” Presentation at the MAGI Clinical Research Conference–West, San Diego, CA, October 2009.

Gawande, Atul. “A Lifesaving Checklist.” *New York Times*, December 30, 2007, sec. Opinion. http://www.nytimes.com/2007/12/30/opinion/30gawande.html (accessed November 4, 2009).

Gelsinger v. University of Pennsylvania. Philadelphia County, Ct. Com. Pl., filed September 18, 2000. http://www.sskrplaw.com/lawyer-attorney-1475659.html (accessed October 19, 2009).

George, Julie. “Concerns Regarding the UNITAID Patent Pool Implementation Plan.” Letter to UNITAID Chair Philippe Douste-Blazy, WorldCareCouncil.org, December 10, 2009. http://www.worldcarecouncil.org/content/unitaid-chair-douste-blazy-patent-pool-scope (accessed February 4, 2010).

Gershon, Anne A. IDSA Letter to Dr. Peggy Hamburg Regarding Adverse Event Reporting. September 10, 2009. http://www.idsociety.org/WorkArea/DownloadAsset.aspx?id=15310 (accessed February 13, 2010).

Getz, Kenneth A. Foreword to *An Industry in Evolution*. 4th ed. Boston: Thomson CenterWatch, 2003. http://www.centerwatch.org/bookstore/samples/sample_ind_foreword.html (accessed January 27, 2004).

Getz, Kenneth A. “The Elusive Sponsor-Site Relationship.” *Applied Clinical Trials Online*, February 1, 2009. http://appliedclinicaltrialsonline.findpharma.com/appliedclinicaltrials/Project+Management/The-Elusive-Sponsor-Site-Relationship/ArticleStandard/Article/detail/579328 (accessed August 2, 2009).

Getz, Kenneth A. *The Gift of Participation: A Guide to Making Informed Decisions about Volunteering for a Clinical Trial.* Bar Harbor, ME: Jerian Publishing, 2007.

Getz, Kenneth A. "Protocol Design Trends and Their Effect on Clinical Trial Performance." *Regulatory Affairs Journal Pharma* 19 (2008): 315–6. http://www.csdd.tufts.edu/files/uploads/centerbib_w_links_110509.pdf (accessed September 15, 2009).

Getz, Kenneth A. "Tufts Data: Veteran P.I.s Drop Out." ClinPage, July 19, 2007. http://www.clinpage.com/article/tufts_data_veteran_pis_drop_out/ (accessed April 26, 2009).

Getz, Kenneth A., Julia Wenger, Rafael A. Campo, Edward S. Seguine, and Kenneth I. Kaitin. "Assessing the Impact of Protocol Design Changes on Clinical Trial Performance." *American Journal of Therapeutics* 15, no. 5(2008), doi:10.1097/MJT.0b013e31816b9027.

Gilbert, David N., and John E. Edwards, Jr. "Is There Hope for the Prevention of Future Antimicrobial Shortages?" *Clinical Infectious Diseases* 35 (2002): 215–16.

Gillis, Justin. "Once-a-Day AIDS Pill Could Be Ready Soon." *Washington Post,* January 19, 2006, A1. http://www.washingtonpost.com/wp-dyn/content/article/2006/01/18/AR2006011802428.html (accessed January 19, 2006).

Glass, Harold. "Clinical Grant Costs." *Scrip Magazine,* April 1, 1995.

Glass, Harold. "Investigators in the US: The Quest for Quality." *Scrip Magazine,* March 1, 1997.

Glass, Harold, and Rebecca A. Kane. "Why Investigators Take Part in Clinical Trials." *Applied Clinical Trials* 9, no. 6 (2000): 46–54.

Glass, Harold, and Joann Sullivan. "Managing Clinical Grant Costs through the Use of Unaffiliated Investors." *Drug Information Journal* 29, no. 2 (April–June 1995).

Glickman, Seth, J. G. McHutchison, E. D. Peterson, et al. "Ethical and Scientific Implications of the Globalization of Clinical Research." *New England Journal of Medicine* 360, no. 26 (2009): 816–823. http://www.content.nejm.org/cgi/content/full/360/26/2792 (accessed February 19, 2009).

Global Network, "The Impact of NTDS." http://globalnetwork.org/about-ntds/impact-ntds (accessed March 2, 2010).

Global Network for Neglected Tropical Disease Control. "NTDs and Poverty." GNNTDC, January 6, 2007. http://www.web.archive.org/web/20070106123443re_/www.gnntdc.org/what/poverty.html.

Goldfarb, Norman M. "Clinical Research Terminology Codes: What We Do and How Much It Costs." *Journal of Clinical Research Best Practices* 2, no. 3 (2006). http://www.firstclinical.com/journal/2006/0603_CRT.pdf.

Goldfarb, Norman M. "eSource: The Future Is Here." *Journal of Clinical Research Best Practices* 1, no. 11 (2005). http://firstclinical.com/journal/2005/0511_eSource.pdf (accessed September 17, 2009).

Goldfarb, Norman M. "HIPAA Complaints in Clinical Research." *Journal of Clinical Research Best Practices* 4, no. 2 (2008). http://firstclinical.com/journal/2008/0802_Complaints.pdf (accessed October 14, 2009).

Goldfarb, Norman M. "Informed Consent in the Tegenero TGN1412 Trial." *Journal of Clinical Research Best Practices* 2, no. 5 (2006). http://www.firstclinical.com/journal/2006/0605_TeGenero.pdf.

Goldfarb, Norman M. "Investigator Disclosures of Financial Conflicts." *Journal of Clinical Research Best Practices* 4, no. 10 (2008). http://firstclinical.com/journal/2008/0810_Conflicts.pdf (accessed October 19, 2009).

Goldfarb, Norman M. "Protocol Evaluation Questions." *Journal of Clinical Research Best Practices* 5, no. 4 (2009). http://firstclinical.com/journal/2009/0904_Evaluation.pdf (accessed September 21, 2009).

Goldfarb, Norman M. Review of "State of the Clinical Trials Industry 2009: A Sourcebook of Charts and Statistics." CenterWatch, 2009. *Journal of Clinical Research Best Practices* 5, no. 9 (2009). http://firstclinical.com/journal/2009/0909_Sourcebook_2010.pdf.

Goldfarb, Norman M. "Something for Everyone: Standard Operating Procedure Products for the Investigative Site." *Journal of Clinical Research Best Practices* 1, no. 4 (2005). http://firstclinical.com/journal/2005/0504_SOPReview.pdf.

Goldfarb, Norman M. "Treatment Reimbursement in Informed Consent Forms and Clinical Trial Agreements." *Journal of Clinical Research Best Practices* 2, no. 5 (2006). http://firstclinical.com/journal/2006/0605_Reimbursement.pdf (accessed September 19, 2009).

Goldfarb, Norman M. "Two New Insurance Policies for Clinical Investigators." *Journal of Clinical Research Best Practices* 2, no. 1 (2006). http://firstclinical.com/journal/2006/0601_New_Insurance.pdf.

Goldfarb, Norman M. "What Am I Missing Here? Thought-Provoking Questions for the Clinical Research Industry," *Journal of Clinical Research Best Practices* 5, no. 8 (2009). http://www.firstclinical.com/journal/2009/0908_What55.pdf (accessed February 11, 2010).

Goldfarb, Norman M. "What Is Killing Off the Investigators? A Clinical Research Mystery." *Journal of Clinical Research Best Practices* 1, no. 7 (2005). http://www.firstclinical.com/journal/2005/0507_Mystery.pdf (accessed February 10, 2010).

Goldfarb, Norman M., and Jill Petro. "Accounting for Study Costs." *Journal of Clinical Research Best Practices* 2, no. 10 (2006). http://firstclinical.com/journal/2006/0610_Accounting.pdf.

Goldfarb, Norman M., and Aylin Regulski. "18 Subject Injury and Indemnification CTA Loopholes." *Journal of Clinical Research Best Practices* 4, no. 1 (2008). http://firstclinical.com/journal/2008/0801_Loopholes.pdf (accessed February 12, 2010).

Goode, Erica. "Certain Words Can Trip Up AIDS Grants, Scientists Say." *New York Times*, April 18, 2003. http://www.nytimes.com/2003/04/18/national/18GRAN.html?pagewanted=1 (accessed February 15, 2010).

Goodyear, Michael. "Learning from the TGN1412 Trial." *British Medical Journal*, March 2006, doi:10.1136/bmj.38797.635012.47. http://www.bmj.com/cgi/rapidpdf/bmj.38797.635012.47v1.pdf.

Goodyear, Michael, Lisa A. Eckenwiler, and Carolyn Ells. "Fresh Thinking about the Declaration of Helsinki." *British Medical Journal* 337 (October 17, 2008): a2128. http://www.bmj.com/cgi/content/extract/337/oct17_2/a2128 (accessed November 7, 2009).

Goodyear, Michael, Trudo Lemmens, Dominique Sprumont, and Godfrey Tangwa. "Does the FDA Have the Authority to Trump the Declaration of Helsinki?" *British Medical Journal* 338 (April 21, 2009): b1559. http://www.bmj.com/cgi/content/full/338/apr21_1/b1559?ijkey=NiOv6nqknE9xVPB&keytype=ref (accessed November 7, 2009).

Gordon, Alex. "The Delicate Dance of Immersion and Insulation: The Politicization of the FDA Commissioner." April 29, 2003. http://leda.law.harvard.edu/leda/data/536/Gordon.pdf (accessed February 15, 2010).

Government Accountability Office. *Pediatric Drug Research: Studies Conducted under Best Pharmaceuticals for Children Act.* Report to Congressional Committees. GAO-07-557, March 2007. http://www.gao.gov/new.items/d07557.pdf (accessed February 14, 2010).

Grady, Denise. "Liver Donors Face Perils Known and Unknown." *New York Times*, March 19, 2002, F1. http://www.nytimes.com (accessed October 30, 2003).

Grant and Kahn v. Pharmacia and Upjohn. No. 99-N-285 (US Ct. App. Dec. 23, 2002). http://www.kscourts.org/ca10/cases/2002/12/01-1509.htm (accessed January 19, 2004).

Green, Jane. "Should We Outsource Our IRB?" *Journal of Clinical Research Best Practices* 4, no. 4 (2008). http://firstclinical.com/journal/2008/0804_Outsource_IRB.pdf (accessed November 12, 2009).

Greenberger, Phyllis. "Political Action Based on Science." *XX vs. XY* 1 (2003): 52–56. http://xxvsxy.syr.edu (accessed July 24, 2005).

Grier, Peter. "Is Comparing Medical Treatments Akin to 'Rationing' Care?" *Christian Science Monitor*, August 28, 2009. http://features.csmonitor.com/politics/2009/08/28/is-comparing-medical-treatments-akin-to-rationing-care/ (accessed February 10, 2010).

Grimes v. Kennedy Krieger Institute. 782 A.2d 807 (Md. 2001). http://biotech.law.lsu.edu/cases/research/grimes_v_KKI.htm (accessed October 19, 2009).

Guerrant, Richard L. "Why America Must Care about Tropical Medicine: Threats to Global Health and Security from Tropical Infectious Diseases." *American Journal of Tropical Medicine and Hygiene* 59, no. 1 (1998): 3–16. Also available at http://www.ajtmh.org/cgi/reprint/59/1/3 (accessed July 14, 2005).

Guttierrez, Martin. "Recruitment Experience in a Phase 0 Trial of ABT-888, an Inhibitor of Poly (ADP-ribose) Polymerase (PARP), in Patients with Advanced Malignancies." Presentation, National Cancer Institute, Division of Cancer Treatment and Diagnosis. http://dctd.cancer.gov/MajorInitiatives/

Sep0507Phase0Workshop/DrGutierrez090507.pps (accessed February 10, 2010).

Harris, Gardiner. "Antidepressant Study Seen to Back Expert." *New York Times*, August 20, 2004. http://www.nytimes.com/2004/08/20/us/antidepressant-study-seen-to-back-expert.html.

Harris, Gardiner. "Drug Making's Move Abroad Stirs Concerns." *New York Times*, January 20, 2009, sec. Health. http://www.nytimes.com/2009/01/20/health/policy/20drug.html (accessed January 22, 2009).

Harris, Gardiner. "Ex-Head of FDA Faces Criminal Inquiry." *New York Times*, April 29, 2006, Washington section. http://www.nytimes.com/2006/04/29/washington/29fda.html (accessed February 15, 2010).

Harris, Gardiner. "Student, 19, in Trial of New Antidepressant Commits Suicide." *New York Times*, February 12, 2004, sec. 1. Also available at http://www.nytimes.com/2004/02/12/health/12SUIC.html (accessed September 20, 2004).

Harris, Gardiner. "Where Cancer Progress Is Rare, One Man Says No." *New York Times*, September 16, 2009, sec. Health/Health Care Policy. http://www.nytimes.com/2009/09/16/health/policy/16cancer.html? (accessed February 9, 2010).

Harris, Gardiner and David M. Halbfinger. "FDA Reveals It Fell to a Push by Lawmakers." *New York Times*, September 25, 2009, sec. Health/Health Care Policy. http://www.nytimes.com/2009/09/25/health/policy/25knee.html (accessed December 1, 2009).

Harris Interactive. "Misconceptions and Lack of Awareness Greatly Reduce Recruitment for Cancer Clinical Trials." January 22, 2001. http://www.harrisinteractive.com/news/printerfriend/index.asp?NewsID=222 (accessed September 27, 2009).

Harris Interactive. "Nationwide Survey Reveals Public Support of Clinical Research Studies on the Rise." June 27, 2001. http://www.harrisinteractive.com/news/allnewsbydate.asp?NewsID=323 (accessed February 13, 2010).

Harris Interactive. "Public Awareness of Clinical Trials Increases: New Survey Suggests Those Conducting Trials Are Doing a Better Job of Informing Potential Participants of Opportunities." June 11, 2004. http://www.harrisinteractive.com/news/printerfriend/index.asp?NewsID=812 (accessed October 19, 2009).

Hartmann, B. *Reproductive Rights and Wrongs: The Global Politics of Population Control.* Boston: South End Press, 1995. Cited in Reproductive Health Technologies Project. *The Quinacrine Debate and Beyond.* 2001. Also available at http://www.rhtp.org/news/publications/default.asp (accessed January 16, 2006).

Haseltine, Florence P., and Beverly Greenberg Jacobson. *Women's Health Research: A Medical and Policy Primer.* Washington, DC: American Psychiatric Press, 1997. Cited in Lori Mosca, Catherine Allen, Emma Fernandez-Repollet, et al. "Setting a Local Research Agenda for Women's Health: The National Centers of Excellence in Women's Health." *Journal of Women's Health and Gender-Based Medicine* 10, no. 10 (2001): 927–35. http://www.4woman.gov/COE/journals/local.pdf (accessed September 15, 2005).

Hawn, Carleen. "The Man Who Sees around Corners." *Forbes Magazine*, January 21, 2002. http://www.forbes.com/forbes/2002/0121/072sidebar_print.html (accessed October 30, 2003).

Hazlet, Thomas. "Drug Development and the FDA." 2000. http://depts.washington.edu/pharm543/documents/schedule/3309drugreg.pdf (accessed February 9, 2004).

Helmer-Smith, Christine. "Letter to Novartis Pharmaceuticals: NDA# 21-200." U.S. Food and Drug Administration (FDA). http://www.fda.gov/cder/warn/2003/11577.pdf (accessed January 25, 2004).

Henderson, Diedtra. "FDA Rules Aim to Speed Drug Tests and Trim Costs." *Boston Globe*, January 13, 2006. http://www.boston.com/business/healthcare/articles/2006/01/13/fda_rules_aim_to_speed_drug_tests_and_trim_costs/.

Hennessy, Sean, and Brian L Strom. "PDUFA Reauthorization—Drug Safety's Golden Moment of Opportunity?" *New England Journal of Medicine* 356, no. 17 (April 2007), doi:10.1056/NEJMp078048. http://content.nejm.org (accessed December 1, 2009).

Henry, James, Barton Palmer, et al. "Reformed Consent-Adapting to New Media and Research Participant Preferences: Multimedia Consent Aids." Medscape. http://www.medscape.com/viewarticle/704025 (accessed November 6, 2009).

Hensley, Scott. "New Antibiotic Could Boost Besieged Aventis." *Wall Street Journal*, March 4, 2004.

Heuser, Stephen. "One Girl's Hope, a Nation's Dilemma." *Boston Globe*, June 14, 2009. http://www.boston.com/news/world/latinamerica/articles/2009/06/14/one_girls_hope_a_nations_dilemma/.

Hilts, Philip. "U.S. Doctor Drops Patient for Criticizing Drug Trial." *New York Times*, October 23, 1993, sec. 1. http://www.nytimes.com/1993/10/23/us/us-doctor-drops-patient-for-criticizing-drug-trial.html (accessed December 2, 2009).

HIPAA Advisory. "Standards for Privacy of Individually Identifiable Health Information." Phoenix Health Systems, 2001. http://www.hipaadvisory.com/regs/finalprivacy/gconsent.htm (accessed January 25, 2004).

Hirsch, Laurence J. "Conflicts of Interest, Authorship, and Disclosures in Industry-Related Scientific Publications: The Tort Bar and Editorial Oversight of Medical Journals." *Mayo Clinic Proceedings* 84, no. 9 (2009), doi:10.4065/84.9.811. http://www.mayoclinicproceedings.com/content/84/9/811.full (accessed November 2009).

HIV Medicine Association. Infectious Diseases Society of America. "Preventing HIV and Other Sexually Transmitted Infections: A Call for Science-Based Government Policies." HIVMA, 2005. http://www.hivma.org/Content.aspx?id=2784 (accessed February 15, 2010).

Hollier, Larry H. "The Impact of Hurricane Katrina on Louisiana State University Health Sciences Center, New Orleans." Testimony before the United States Senate. http://help.senate.gov/Hearings/2006_07_14_b/Hollier.pdf (accessed February 13, 2010).

Horowitz, Leonard. "Swine Flu Pandemic, 2009, Part II, Baxter Corporation's 'Accident.'" YouTube video. http://www.youtube.com/watch?v=IcVDok5LrAg&NR=1 (accessed February 9, 2010).

Hotez, Peter J. "Gandhi's Hookworms." *Foreign Policy*, January 21, 2010. http://www.foreignpolicy.com/articles/2010/01/21/gandhis_hookworms?page=0,0.

Hotez, Peter, Alan Fenwick, Lorenzo Savioli, and David H Molyneux. "Rescuing the Bottom Billion through Control of Neglected Tropical Diseases." *Lancet* 373 (2009): 1570–75. (accessed March 2, 2010).

Hotez, Peter J., David H. Molyneux, Alan Fenwick, Eric Ottesen, Sonia Ehrlich Sachs, and Jeffrey D. Sachs. "Incorporating a Rapid-Impact Package for Neglected Tropical Diseases with Programs for HIV/AIDS, Tuberculosis, and Malaria." *PLoS Medicine* 3, no. 5 (2006), doi:10.1371/journal.pmed.0030102. dx.doi.org/10.1371/journal.pmed.0030102 (accessed December 5, 2009).

Hovde, Mark. "Choosing and Using CROs." *Scrip Magazine*, July/August 1995.

Hovde, Mark. "Comparing Costs in CRO Contracts." *International Journal of Pharmaceutical Medicine* 11 (1997): 249–53.

Hovde, Mark. "Integrating Protocol Design and Financial Planning." Data Edge DataLines, 2001. http://www.fast-track.org (accessed February 12, 2003).

Hovde, Mark, and Robert Seskin. "Selecting U.S. Clinical Investigators." *Applied Clinical Trials* 6 (February 1997): 34–42.

Huff, Darrell. *How to Lie with Statistics*. New York: W. W. Norton & Company, 1954.

Husten, Larry. "Down the Memory Hole: *JAMA* Editors Rewrite History and Remove Original Editorial." CardioBrief, July 10, 2009. http://www.cardiobrief.org/2009/07/10/down-the-memory-hole-jama-editors-rewrite-history-and-remove-original-editorial/ (accessed November 10, 2009).

Ikemoto, Lisa C. "Doctrine at the Gate: Religious Restrictions in Health Care." *Journal of Gender-Specific Medicine* 4, no. 4 (April 2001): 8–12. http://www.mmhc.com/jgsm/articles/JGSM0104/law.html (accessed September 14, 2003).

Ikemoto, Lisa C. "When a Hospital Becomes Catholic." *Mercer Law Review* 47, no. 4 (April 1996): 1087–134. http://review.law.mercer.edu/old/fr47308.htm (accessed January 15, 2006).

Infectious Diseases Society of America. "'Bad Bugs, No Drugs': Defining the Antimicrobial Availability Problem." 2003. http://www.idsociety.org (accessed November 15, 2003).

Institute of Medicine. *Beyond the HIPAA Privacy Rule: Enhancing Privacy, Improving Health through Research*, January 27, 2009. http://www.iom.edu/Reports/2009/Beyond-the-HIPAA-Privacy-Rule-Enhancing-Privacy-Improving-Health-Through-Research.aspx (accessed March 15, 2009).

Institute of Medicine. "Public Confidence and Involvement in Clinical Research." 2001. http://www.iom.edu/report.asp?id=4891 (accessed January 6, 2004).

Institute of Medicine. "The Research Agenda: Implications for Therapeutic Countermeasures to Biological Threats." In *Biological Threats and Terrorism: Assessing the Science and Response Capabilities: Workshop Summary*, edited by Stacey L. Knobler, Adel A. F. Mahmoud, and Leslie A. Pray. Washington, DC: National Academy Press, 2002. http://www.nap.edu/books/0309082536/html/ (accessed September 14, 2005).

Institute of Medicine. Board on Health Sciences Policy. *Conflict of Interest in Medical Research, Education, and Practice.* Edited by Bernard Lo and Marilyn J. Field. Washington, DC: National Academy Press, 2009. http://www.iom.edu/en/Reports/2009/Conflict-of-Interest-in-Medical-Research-Education-and-Practice.aspx.

Institute of Medicine. Board on Population Health and Public Health Practice. *Immunization Safety Review: Vaccines and Autism*, 2004. http://www.iom.edu/Reports/2004/Immunization-Safety-Review-Vaccines-and-Autism.aspx (accessed February 10, 2010).

Institute of Medicine. Committee on Assessing the System for Protecting Human Research Participants. *Responsible Research: A Systems Approach to Protecting Research Participants.* Edited by Daniel D. Federman, Kathi E. Hanna, and Laura Lyman Rodriguez. Washington, DC: National Academy Press, 2002. http://www.nap.edu/booksearch.php?record_id=10508 (accessed October 15, 2009).

Institute of Medicine. Committee on the Assessment of the U.S. Drug Safety System. *Future of Drug Safety.* Edited by Alina Baciu, Kathleen Stratton, and Sheila P. Burke. Washington, DC: National Academy Press, 2007. http://www.nap.edu/catalog.php?record_id=11750 (accessed February 9, 2010).

Institute of Medicine. Committee on Comparative Effectiveness Research Prioritization. *Initial National Priorities for Comparative Effectiveness Research.* Washington, DC: National Academy Press, 2009. http://www.books.nap.edu/catalog/12648.html (accessed August 29, 2009).

Institute of Medicine. Committee on Health Literacy. Board on Neuroscience and Behavioral Health. *Health Literacy: A Prescription to End Confusion.* Edited by Lynn Nielsen-Bohlman, Allison Panzer, and David A. Kindig. Washington, DC: National Academy Press, 2004. Cited in "National Quality Forum, Safe Practices for Better Healthcare 2006." http://www.qualityforum.org/Publications/2007/03/Safe_Practices_for_Better_Healthcare%E2%80%932006_Update.aspx (accessed November 5, 2009).

Institute of Medicine. Committee to Review the Fialuridine Clinical Trials. *Review of the Fialuridine Clinical Trials.* Edited by Frederick Manning and Morton Swartz. Washington, DC: National Academy Press, 1995. http://books.nap.edu/openbook.php?record_id=4887 (accessed December 2, 2009).

Institute of Medicine. Committee on Understanding and Eliminating Racial and Ethnic Disparities in Health Care. *Unequal Treatment: Confronting Racial and Ethnic Disparities in Health Care.* Edited by Brian D. Smedley, Adrienne Y. Stith, and Alan R. Nelson. Washington, DC: National Academy Press, 2003. http://www.nap.edu/books/030908265X/html/ (accessed January 16, 2006).

Institute of Medicine. Committee on Understanding the Biology of Sex and Gender Differences. *Exploring the Biological Contributions to Human Health: Does Sex Matter?* Edited by Theresa Wizemann and Mary-Lou Pardue. Washington, DC: National Academy Press, 2001. http://www.nap.edu/books/0309072816/html/ (accessed January 24, 2004).

Institute of Medicine. Committee to Survey the Health Effects of Mustard Gas and Lewisite. *Veterans at Risk: The Health Effects of Mustard Gas and Lewisite.* Edited by Constance M. Pechura and David P. Rall. Washington, DC: National Academy Press, 1993. http://www.nap.edu/books/030904832X/html (accessed January 15, 2006).

International Committee of Medical Journal Editors. "Uniform Requirements for Manuscripts Submitted to Biomedical Journals: Writing and Editing for Biomedical Publication." ICMJE. http://www.icmje.org/urm_main.html (accessed November 2009).

International Conference on Harmonisation. *E6: Good Clinical Practice.* 1996. http://www.ich.org/cache/compo/276-254-1.html (accessed November 7, 2009).

International Conference on Harmonisation. *E8: Guidance on General Considerations for Clinical Trials.* 1997. http://www.fda.gov/cder/guidance/1857fnl.pdf (accessed February 7, 2004).

International Conference on Harmonisation. *Guideline for Good Clinical Practice,* ICH E.6, Step 5, Guideline 1.5.96, Section 1.50. http://www.fda.gov/cber/ich/ichguid.htm (accessed January 25, 2004).

International Federation of Pharmaceutical Manufacturers and Associations. Clinical Trials Portal. http://clinicaltrials.ifpma.org/en/myportal/index.htm.

International Federation of Pharmaceutical Manufacturers and Associations. "Nifurtimox-Eflornithine for Sleeping Sickness with Training in Tropical Diseases." Health Partnerships: Developing World—2009. http://www.ifpma.org/index.php?id=2223 (accessed April 6, 2010).

Jackson, Bill and Michael Pfitzmann. "Win-Win Sourcing." *Strategy and Business* 47, May 29, 2007. http://www.strategy-business.com/article/07207?gko=db1da (accessed September 18, 2009).

James Lind Library. "Documenting the Evolution of Fair Tests." http://www.jameslindlibrary.org/index.html (accessed February 9, 2010).

Jeste, Dilip V., Barton W. Palmer, Shahrokh Golshan. "Multimedia Consent for Research in People with Schizophrenia and Normal Subjects: A Randomized Controlled Trial." *Schizophrenia Bulletin* 35, no. 4 (2009), doi:10.1093/

schbul/sbm148. http://www.schizophreniabulletin.oxfordjournals.org/cgi/content/abstract/35/4/719 (accessed October 22, 2009).

Johnson, Carolyn Y. "Scientist Takes Aim at Her Longtime Silent Scourge." *Boston Globe*, December 4, 2009. http://www.boston.com/news/local/massachusetts/articles/2009/12/04/scientist_takes_aim_at_her_longtime_silent_scourge/ (accessed December 4, 2009).

Johnson, Guy P. "Part 1: Budget Tool Helps Investigative Sites Calculate the Cost of a Coordinator's Time for a Typical Outpatient Study Visit." Society of Clinical Research Associates. http://www.socra.org/pdf/Investigative_Site_Budget_Tool_by_Guy_Johnson.pdf (accessed March 15, 2009).

Johnson, Guy P. "Part 2: Budget Tool Helps Investigative Sites Calculate the Cost of a Coordinator's Time for a Typical Outpatient Study Visit." Society of Clinical Research Associates. http://www.socra.org/pdf/Investigative_Site_Budget_Tool_by_Guy_Johnson_Part_2.pdf (accessed November 12, 2009).

Johnson, Laurie. "Design of Epidemiologic Studies." Presentation at NIH Clinical Center: The Introduction to the Principles and Practice of Clinical Research (IPPCR), October 22, 2007. http://www.nihtraining.com/cc/ippcr/current/downloads/Johnson%2010-22-07.pdf, http://www.nihtraining.com/cc/ippcr/ (accessed August 13, 2009).

Johnson, Tracy, and Elizabeth Fee. "Women's Participation in Clinical Research: From Protectionism to Access." In *Women and Health Research: Ethical and Legal Issues of Including Women in Clinical Studies*, edited by Anna C. Mastroianni, Ruth Faden, and Daniel Federman. Institute of Medicine. Washington, DC: National Academy Press, 1994. http://books.nap.edu/books/0309050405/html/ (accessed January 15, 2006).

Joint Commission. *What Did the Doctors Say? Improving Health Literacy to Protect Patient Safety.* February 2007. http://www.jointcommission.org/NewsRoom/PressKits/Health_Literacy/ (accessed September 20, 2009).

Kaiser Health News Daily Report. "Bush Administration Fails to Comply with Subpoena for Documents on Testimony about FDA Approval of Ketek." Kaiser Health News, February 13, 2008. http://www.kaiserhealthnews.org/Daily-Reports/2008/February/13/dr00050393.aspx (accessed December 1, 2009).

Kaitin, K. I. "Number of Active Investigators in FDA-Regulated Clinical Trials Drops." *Tufts CSDD Impact Report,* (2005). Cited in Kenneth A. Getz, Julia Wenger, Rafael A. Campo, Edward S. Seguine, and Kenneth I Kaitin. "Assessing the Impact of Protocol Design Changes on Clinical Trial Performance." *American Journal of Therapeutics* 15 (2008): 450–457. http://journals.lww.com/americantherapeutics/Abstract/2008/09000/Assessing_the_Impact_of_Protocol_Design_Changes_on.7.aspx (accessed February 10, 2010).

Kaplan, Tamara. "The Tylenol Crisis: How Effective Public Relations Saved Johnson & Johnson." Pennsylvania State University, 1998. http://www.personal.psu.edu/users/w/x/wxk116/tylenol/crisis.html (accessed April 26, 2004).

Kashoki, Mwango. "Drug Safety and Clinical Trials." Presentation at the FDA Clinical Investigator Course, Silver Spring, MD, November 18, 2009.

Kaufman, David G. "Testimony before the Subcommittee on Labor, Health and Human Services, Education and Related Agencies." 2000. http://www.faseb.org/opa/govttest/2000test.html (accessed January 16, 2006).

Kaufman, Marc. "Abortion Foe to Be Reappointed to FDA Panel." *Washington Post*, June 28, 2004, p. A06. http://www.washingtonpost.com/wp-dyn/A13192-2004Jun28.html (accessed February 15, 2010).

Kaufman, Marc. "FDA Official Quits over Delay on Plan B." *Washington Post*, September 1, 2005, sec. Health. http://www.washingtonpost.com/wp-dyn/content/article/2005/08/31/AR2005083101271_pf.html (accessed February 15, 2010).

Keiger, Dale, and Sue De Pasquale. "Trials and Tribulation." *Johns Hopkins Magazine*, February 1, 2002. Also available at http://www.jhu.edu/~jhumag/0202web/trials.html (accessed January 16, 2006).

Kilpatrick, Frank S., and Adelle Ricci. "Reducing Clinical Research Time." *Drug & Market Development*, 1999. http://pharmalicensing.com/features/disp/939893414_3805a2a6f2ca2 (accessed January 21, 2002).

King, Ralph T., Jr. "Bitter Pill: How a Drug Firm Paid for University Study, Then Undermined Its Research on Thyroid Tablets." *Wall Street Journal*, April 25, 1996. Also available at http://www.wsj.com.

King, Rufus. "Drug Abuse Control, 1965." Chap. 26 in *The Drug Hang Up: America's Fifty-Year Folly*. Springfield, IL: Charles C. Thomas, 1972. http://www.druglibrary.org/special/king/dhu/dhu26.htm (accessed September 12, 2005).

King & Spalding Law Firm. "Client Alert: Postmarketing Studies and Clinical Trials." Client Alert, King and Spalding Law Firm, July 31, 2009. http://www.kslaw.com/Library/publication/ca081109.pdf (accessed February 9, 2010).

Kioussopoulos, Kathleen. "Device Clinical Trials: Regulatory Issues and Challenges." Presentation to the Study Coordinator Advisory Committee, March 11, 2006, Clinical Trials Best Practices. www.ctnbestpractices.org/sites/devicespecific/device/kathy-k-acc-presentation-to-scac-on-devices/view (accessed November 4, 2009).

Klein, Daniel B., and Alexander Tabarrok. "Theory, Evidence and Examples of FDA Harm." FDAReview.org. http://www.fdareview.org/harm.shtml (accessed February 9, 2010).

Kline, Mark W. "Foster Children Were Helped by Medical Trials." *Toledo Blade*, May 21, 2005. http://toledoblade.com/apps/pbcs.dll/article?AID=/20050521/OPINION04/50521038 (accessed July 1, 2005).

Kolata, Gina. "Ethics 101: A Course about the Pitfalls." *New York Times*, October 21, 2003, F1. http://www.nytimes.com/2003/10/21/science/21ETHI.html?ex=1067820478&ei=1&en=3c2e352500777940 (accessed January 2, 2004).

Kolata, Gina. "Study Is Halted over Rise Seen in Cancer Risk." *New York Times*, July 9, 2002, A1. Also available at http://www.nytimes.com (accessed January 2, 2004).

Kouten, John F. "A Ten Step Trial Crisis Plan." *Applied Clinical Trials*, July 1, 2009.

Krugman, Saul. "The Willowbrook Hepatitis Studies Revisited: Ethical Aspects." *Review of Infectious Disease* 15, no. 1 (January–February 1986): 157–62.

Kweder, Sandra. "Considerations for Special Populations." Presentation at the FDA Clinical Investigator Course, Silver Spring, MD, November 17, 2009.

LaFraniere, Sharon, Mary Pat Flaherty, and Joe Stephens. "The Body Hunters, Part 3: The Dilemma: Submit or Suffer." *Washington Post*, December 19, 2000, A1. Also available at http://www.washingtonpost.com (accessed March 4, 2003).

Lamberti, Mary Jo. "Going Global." *Applied Clinical Trials* (June 2004).

Lampman, Jane. "Different Faiths, Different Views on Stem Cells." *Christian Science Monitor*, July 23, 2001. http://search.csmonitor.com/durable/2001/07/23/p1s2.htm (accessed January 5, 2004).

Lemmens, T., and B. Freedman. "Ethics Review for Sale? Conflict of Interest and Commercial Review Boards." *Milbank Quarterly* 78, no. 4 (2000). http://www.utoronto.ca/jcb/Research/publications/lemmens_mq00.pdf (accessed September 14, 2003).

Lemonick, Michael D., and Andrew Goldstein. "At Your Own Risk." *Time*, April 22, 2002. http://www.time.com/time/health/article/0,8599,230358,00.html (accessed May 2, 2002).

Leonard, Kate, and Shawn Gibbs. "Sensible Payment Terms." Presentation at the MAGI Clinical Research Conference–West, San Diego, CA, October 2009.

Lepay, David. "GCP Compliance: Emerging Issues in Worldwide Clinical Trials." FDA. 1999. http://www.fda.gov/cder/present/dia-99/lepay-dia99/lepay-dia99.PPT (accessed January 27, 2004).

Lesko, Lawrence. "Model-Based Drug Development: A Critical Path Innovation to Integrate Data Analysis." 2005. http://www.fda.gov/ohrms/dockets/ac/05/slides/2005-4194S2_02_Lesko.ppt (accessed September 16, 2009).

Levine, Jeff, Associated Press, and CNN. "Sour Legacy of Tuskegee Syphilis Study Lingers." 1997. http://www.cnn.com/HEALTH/9705/16/nfm.tuskegee/index.html (accessed February 24, 2004).

Lewin, Tamar. "Court Says Health Coverage May Bar Birth-Control Pills." *New York Times*, March 17, 2007, sec. Health. http://www.nytimes.com/2007/03/17/health/17pill.html (accessed December 4, 2009).

Lidz, Charles W., Paul S. Appelbaum, Steven Joffe, Karen Albert, Jill Rosenbaum, and Lorna Simon. "Competing Commitments in Clinical Trials." *IRB: Ethics & Human Research* 31, no. 5 (2009): 1–6. www.medscape.com/viewarticle/712097 (accessed November 22, 2009).

Lie, R. K., E. Emanuel, C. Grady, and D. Wendler. "The Standard of Care Debate: The Declaration of Helsinki versus the International Consensus Opinion."

Journal of Medical Ethics 30 (2004): 190–93. Also available at http://www.bioethics.nih.gov/international/readings/intresearch/helsinki.pdf (accessed July 11, 2005).

Light, Donald W., and Rebecca N. Warburton. "Extraordinary Claims Require Extraordinary Evidence." *Journal of Health Economics* 24, no. 5 (2005), doi:10.1016/j.jhcalcco.2005.07.001. http://www.ncbi.nlm.nih.gov/pubmed/16087260 (accessed February 9, 2010).

Lillington, Linda. "Patient Recruitment in Clinical Trials." http://uscnurse.usc.edu/class/461/USClecture701revised.htm (accessed January 19, 2003).

Limited English Proficiency: A Federal Interagency. "Overview of Executive Order 13166." http://www.lep.gov/13166/eo13166.html (accessed November 5, 2009).

Linehan, John, and Jan B. Pietzsch. "Study on Medical Device Development Models." American Institute for Medical and Biological Engineering. http://www.aimbe.org/assets/787_linehanpresentation.pdf (accessed February 9, 2010).

Lowe, Derek. "Adaptive Trials: What You Need to Know About Adaptive Trials." *Pharmaceutical Executive*, July 1, 2006. http://pharmexec.findpharma.com/pharmexec/article/articleDetail.jsp?id=352793 (accessed February 10, 2010).

Lowe, Derek. "Avandia: Trouble or Not?" *In the Pipeline*, May 24, 2007. http://www.pipeline.corante.com/archives/2007/05/24/avandia_trouble_or_not.php (accessed February 9, 2010).

Macklin, Ruth. "The Declaration of Helsinki: Another Revision." *Indian Journal of Medical Ethics* 6, no. 1 (March 2009). http://www.ijme.in/171ed2 (accessed November 8, 2009).

MAGI. "Budget Template." Magiworld.org. http://www.magiworld.org/documents/FCR_Budget_Template.pdf.

MAGI. "Model Clinical Trial Agreement." Version 1.26, July 2009. http://www.magiworld.org/documents/ (accessed October 13, 2009).

Maguire, Phyllis. "Community-Based Trials under Scrutiny." American College of Physicians, 1999. http://www.acpon-line.org/journals/news/jul-aug99/cbtrials.htm (accessed November 4, 2003).

Maheu, E., R. D. Altman, D. A. Bloch, et al. "Design and Conduct of Clinical Trials in Patients with Osteoarthritis of the Hand." *Osteoarthritis Cartilage* 14, no. 4 (2006): 303–22. http://www.ncbi.nlm.nih.gov/pubmed/16697937 (accessed February 13, 2010).

Majumdar, Sumit R., Matthew T. Roe, Eric D. Peterson, Anita Y. Chen, Brian Gibler, and Paul W. Armstrong. "Better Outcomes for Patients Treated at Hospitals That Participate in Clinical Trials." *Archives of Internal Medicine* 168, no. 6 (2008), doi:10.1001/archinternmed.2007.124. http://archinte.ama-assn.org/cgi/content/abstract/168/6/657 (accessed February 9, 2010).

Maloney, Kate. "Good Clinical Practice (GCP) & Clinical Trial Registries." Health Care Conference Administrators, LLC, 2004. http://www.ehcca.com/presentations/pharmacongress5/2_03_2.pdf (accessed July 14, 2005).

Mann, Bill. "The Life Cycle of a Drug." The Motley Fool, October 25, 1999. http://www.fool.com (accessed January 21, 2002).

Mardell, Jacquie. "Informed Consent/Assent/HIPAA." Presentation at the MAGI Clinical Research Conference–West, San Diego, CA, October 2009.

Marks, Laura. *Sexual Chemistry: A History of the Contraceptive Pill.* New Haven, CT: Yale University Press, 2001. Cited in Reproductive Health Technologies Project. *The Quinacrine Debate and Beyond.* 2001. Also available at http://www.rhtp.org/news/publications/default.asp (accessed December 26, 2003).

Maslin, Janet. "The Truth about the Drug Companies: Indicting the Drug Industry's Practices." *New York Times*, September 6, 2004, sec. Books. http://www.nytimes.com/2004/09/06/books/06masl.html.

Mathews, Anna Wilde. "Worrisome Ailment in Medicine: Misleading Journal Articles." *Wall Street Journal*, May 10, 2005, sec. A1. http://online.wsj.com/article/SB111567633298328568.html (accessed November 10, 2009).

McAllister, Debbie K. "Gimme Shelter: Anti-Kickback Safe Harbors and Clinical Trial Agreements." *Journal of Clinical Research Best Practices* 4, no. 5 (2008). http://www.firstclinical.com/journal/2008/0805_Anti-Kickback.pdf (accessed October 13, 2009).

McBride, W. G. "Thalidomide and Congenital Anomalies." *Lancet*, no. 2 (1961): 1358. http://www.mindfully.org/Health/Thalidomide-Back.htm (accessed February 7, 2004).

McCarthy, Michael. "Company Sought to Block Paper's Publication." *Lancet* 356 (2000): 1659.

McDermott Will & Emery. "Increasing FDA Oversight Over Clinical Research." *McDermott Newsletters*, November 4, 2004. http://www.mwe.com/index.cfm/fuseaction/publications.nldetail/object_id/753fb582-f9c7-41fd-aab0-0f18980b10e5.cfm (accessed November 8, 2009).

McDermott Will & Emery. "Ownership of Biological Samples and Clinical Data II: U.S. Supreme Court Denies Certiorari in the Catalona Decision." *McDermott Newsletters*, February 21, 2008. http://www.mwe.com/index.cfm/fuseaction/publications.nldetail/object_id/10776f46-f953-4921-9b40-c3dc1fd6ed60.cfm (accessed November 27, 2009).

McGee, Patrick. "Clinical Trials on the Move." *Drug Discovery and Development*, June 12, 2006. http://www.dddmag.com/clinical-trials-on-the-move.aspx (accessed October 19, 2009).

McGhee, J., and J. Mestechy. "Induction of Secretory Antibodies in Humans Following Ingestion of Streptococcus Mutans." *Advances in Experimental Medicine and Biology* 107 (1977): 177–284.

McInnes, John S., and Grant P. Bagley. "Legal Implications of Clinical Trial Sponsor Financial Support for Subject Healthcare Costs in Clinical Trials." *Journal of Clinical Research Best Practices* 3, no. 4 (2007). http://firstclinical

.com/journal/2007/0704_Financial_Support.pdf (accessed February 10, 2010).

McNeil, Donald G, Jr. "Low-Cost Antimalarial Pill Available." *New York Times*, March 1, 2007.

Medecins Sans Frontieres, "Over 300,000 Messages of Support Help Realise Creation of UNITAID's Patent Pool." Access and Patents, Make It Happen Campaign. http://www.msfaccess.org/main/access-patents/make-it-happen-campaign/campaign-updates/december-16-2009/ (accessed February 2, 2010).

Medecins Sans Frontieres. "Take the Patent Pool Plunge!" Access and Patents, Campaign for Access to Essential Medicines. http://www.msfaccess.org/main/access-patents/take-the-patent-pool-plunge/ (accessed February 2, 2010).

Medidata Solutions Worldwide. "Best Practice Clinical Trial Pricing Using Benchmark Data." June 23, 2009. http://www.mdsol.com/ (accessed September 21, 2009).

MediRegs Regulation and Reimbursement Solutions. "Regulation & Reimbursement Suite." MediRegs. http://www.mediregs.com/medical-billing-compliance-solution (accessed February 13, 2010).

Meier, Barry. "Costs Surge for Medical Devices, but Benefits Are Opaque." *New York Times*, November 5, 2009, sec. Business. http://www.nytimes.com/2009/11/05/business/05device.html (accessed February 9, 2010).

Meier, Barry. "Opponents Line Up Against U.S. Effort to Compare Medical Treatments." *New York Times*, May 7, 2009, sec. Business. http://www.nytimes.com/2009/05/07/business/07compare.html (accessed February 10, 2010).

Meier, Barry. "Study Finds More Failure of Heart Device." *New York Times*, February 24, 2009, sec. Business. http://www.nytimes.com/2009/02/24/business/24device.html (accessed February 9, 2010).

Meyerson, Linda, and Tracy Harmon Blumenfeld. "Rethinking the Sponsor-Investigator Relationship." *Pharmaceutical Executive*, January 6, 2009. http://pharmexec.findpharma.com/pharmexec/R&D+Articles/Rethinking-the-Sponsor-Investigator-Relationship/ArticleStandard/Article/detail/574030 (accessed September 18, 2009).

Midthun, Karen. "Biologicals: A Vision for the Future of Clinical Investigators in Evaluations of New Biological Products." Presentation at the FDA Clinical Investigator Course, Silver Spring, MD, November 16, 2009.

Mitchel, Jules T., Vanessa Hays, Mary Shatzoff, and Glen Park. "The Critical Path Initiative Meets Medical Devices." *Applied Clinical Trials* 16 (2007): 48–55. http://appliedclinicaltrialsonline.findpharma.com/appliedclinicaltrials/article/articleDetail.jsp?id=410607 (accessed February 9, 2010).

Mitchell, Janet L. "Recruitment and Retention of Women of Color in Clinical Studies." In *Women and Health Research: Ethical and Legal Issues of Including Women in Clinical Studies*, edited by Anna C. Mastroianni, Ruth Faden, and Daniel Federman. Institute of Medicine. Washington, DC:

National Academy Press, 1994. http://www.nap.edu/books/030904992X/html/R1.html (accessed January 16, 2006).

Modell, Martin E. "PERT, CPM, and Gantt." In *A Professional's Guide to Systems Analysis*, 2nd ed. New York: McGraw Hill, 1996. http://studentweb.tulane.edu/~mtruill/dev-pert.html (accessed January 27, 2004).

Moellering, Robert, and David Shlaes. "The United States Food and Drug Administration and the End of Antibiotics." *Clinical Infectious Diseases* 34 (2002): 420–22.

Moench, Elizabeth. "The Partially Involved Principal Investigator." *Applied Clinical Trials* 1, no. 1 (2002): 30.

Molecule of the Day. "Sutent/Sunitinib (Cheer up!)." Science Blogs, March 12, 2009. http://www.scienceblogs.com/moleculeoftheday/2009/03/sutentsunitinib_cheer_up.php (accessed November 10, 2009).

Molyneux, David H., Peter J. Hotez, and Alan Fenwick. "'Rapid-Impact Interventions': How a Policy of Integrated Control for Africa's Neglected Tropical Diseases Could Benefit the Poor." *PLoS Medicine* 2, no. 11 (2005): e336. doi:10.1371/journal.pmed.0020336. dx.doi.org/10.1371/journal.pmed.0020336.

Monti, Katherine L. "Save Time and Money through Data Management." *Applied Clinical Trials* (October 2001): 54–62.

Moraff, Christopher. "Safety First." *American Prospect*, April 3, 2007. http://www.prospect.org/cs/articles?articleId=12616 (accessed December 1, 2009).

Moran, Mary, Javier Guzman, Anne-Laure Ropars, et al. "Neglected Disease Research and Development: How Much Are We Really Spending?" *PLoS Medicine* 6, no. 2 (2009): e1000030. doi:10.1371/journal.pmed.1000030. dx.doi.org/10.1371/journal.pmed.1000030.

Moran, Mary, Anne-Laure Ropars, Javier Guzman, Jose Diaz, and Christopher Garrison. *The New Landscape of Neglected Disease Drug Development*. London: The Wellcome Trust, 2005. http://www.wellcome.ac.uk/stellent/groups/corporatesite/@msh_publishing_group/documents/web_document/wtx026592.pdf.

Morel, Carlos M. "Neglected Diseases: Under-funded Research and Inadequate Health Interventions: Can We Change This Reality?" *EMBO Reports* 4 Supplement, June 2003, doi:10.1038/sj.embor.embor851. http://www.ncbi.nlm.nih.gov/pubmed/12789404.

Morganstern, Julie. *Organizing from the Inside Out*. New York: Henry Holt and Company, LLC, 1998.

Morreim, E. Haavi. "Medical Research Litigation and Malpractice Tort Doctrines: Courts on a Learning Curve." *Houston Journal of Health Law and Policy* 4, no. 1 (2003). http://www.allbusiness.com/legal/3587152-1.html (accessed November 27, 2009).

Mosca, Lori, Catherine Allen, Emma Fernandez-Repollet, et al. "Setting a Local Research Agenda for Women's Health: The National Centers of Excellence in Women's Health." *Journal of Women's Health and Gender-Based Medicine*

10, no. 10 (2001): 927–35. http://www.4woman.gov/COE/journals/local.pdf (accessed September 15, 2005).

Movahhed, Hassan. Cited in McKenna, Neil. "Internet-Based Tools to Facilitate Clinical Trials." *Genetic Engineering News* 21, no. 1 (2001): 10–11.

Mucke, Hermann. *Microdosing in Translational Medicine: Pros and Cons.* Advances Reports, Cambridge Healthtech Associates, May 2006. http://www.hmpharmacon.com/downloadPharma/CHA%20Microdosing%20Report%20Executive%20Summary%20(May%202006).pdf (accessed February 10, 2010).

Mundy, Alicia. "Coast IRB, Caught in Sting, to Close." *Wall Street Journal*, April 22, 2009, sec. Business. http://online.wsj.com/article/SB124042341694744375.html (accessed October 14, 2009).

Mundy, Alicia. "Drug Makers Fight Stimulus Provision." *Wall Street Journal*, February 10, 2009, sec. Politics and Policy. http://online.wsj.com/article/SB123423024203966081.html (accessed August 29, 2009).

National Academies of Science. Office of News and Public Information. "Fixing Drug Safety System Will Require 'New Drug' Symbol on Labels, Major Boost in FDA Staff and Funding, and Increased Public Access to Information." September 22, 2006. http://www8.nationalacademies.org/onpinews/newsitem.aspx?RecordID=11750.

National Bioethics Advisory Committee. "Summary." *Ethical and Policy Issues in Research Involving Human Participants*, Bethesda, MD: National Bioethics Advisory Commission, August 2001. http://www.georgetown.edu/research/nrcbl/nbac/pubs.html (accessed January 2, 2006).

National Cancer Institute. "New Approaches to Cancer Drug Development and Clinical Trials: Questions and Answers." Questions and Answers, June 4, 2007. http://www.cancer.gov/newscenter/pressreleases/PhaseZeroNExTQandA/ (accessed February 10, 2010).

National Cancer Institute. "New Study Heralds Shortened Timeline for Anticancer Drug Development." News, June 4, 2007. www.cancer.gov/newscenter/pressreleases/PhaseZeroNExT/ (accessed February 10, 2010).

National Cancer Institute. "Simian Virus 40 and Human Cancer." Fact sheet, April 3, 2003. http://www.cancer.gov/cancertopics/factsheet/risk/sv40#r1 (accessed February 9, 2010).

National Cancer Institute. Division of Cancer Treatment and Diagnosis. "NCI Experimental Therapeutics Program (NExT)." Major Initiatives, February 12, 2009. http://dctd.cancer.gov/MajorInitiatives/02NExT.htm (accessed February 10, 2010).

National Cancer Institute. Executive Committee. "Policy of the NCI for Data and Safety Monitoring of Clinical Trials." June 22, 1999. http://deainfo.nci.nih.gov/grantspolicies/datasafety.htm (accessed November 10, 2009).

National Cancer Institute. Office of Biorepositories and Biospecimen Research. "Ethical, Legal, and Policy Best Practices." NCI Best Practices for Biospecimen Resources. http://www.biospecimens.cancer.gov/bestpractices/elp/ (accessed November 28, 2009).

National Center for Biotechnology Innovation Bookshelf. *Addressing the Barriers to Pediatric Drug Development: Workshop Summary.* Institute of Medicine, Washington, DC: National Academy Press, 2008. http://www.ncbi.nlm.nih.gov/bookshelf/br.fcgi?book=nap11911&part=a2001563fddd00018 (accessed February 14, 2010).

National Commission for the Protection of Human Subjects of Biomedical and Behavioral Research. *The Belmont Report: Ethical Principles and Guidelines for the Protection of Human Subjects of Research.* 1979. http://ohsr.od.nih.gov/guidelines/belmont.html (accessed December 21, 2005).

National Conference of Catholic Bishops/U.S. Conference of Catholic Bishops. *Ethical and Religious Directives for Catholic Healthcare Services.* 4th ed. 2003. http://www.nccbuscc.org/bishops/directives.htm (accessed September 17, 2004).

National Institute of Allergy and Infectious Diseases. "Strategic Plan 2000." http://www3.niaid.nih.gov/about/overview/planningpriorities/strategicplan/emerge.htm.

National Institutes of Health. "Health Services Research and the HIPAA Privacy Rule." 2005. http://privacyruleandresearch.nih.gov/healthservicesprivacy.asp (accessed November 4, 2009).

National Institutes of Health. "HIPAA Privacy Rule—Information for Researchers." January 23, 2004. http://privacyruleandresearch.nih.gov/ (accessed September 15, 2005).

National Institutes of Health. "Human Participant Protections Education for Research Teams." 2002. http://ohsr.od.nih.gov/cbt/nonNIHpeople.html (accessed January 12, 2004).

National Institutes of Health. "Insurance Coverage: Maryland." National Cancer Institute, December 19, 2002. http://www.cancer.gov/clinicaltrials/developments/laws-about-clinical-trial-costs-maryland (accessed January 19, 2004).

National Institutes of Health. "Introduction to the Principles and Practice of Clinical Research." Video. http://www.nihtraining.com/cc/ippcr/archive03s/menu.html.

National Institutes of Health. "List of Drugs for Which Pediatric Studies Are Needed." *Federal Register,* 71 no. 79, April 25, 2006. http://www.gpo.gov/fdsys/pkg/FR-2006-04-25/html/E6-6122.htm (accessed February 14, 2010).

National Institutes of Health. "Loan Repayment Programs." 2009. http://www.lrp.nih.gov/about/index.htm.

National Institutes of Health. "National Center for Research Resources: Mission." NIH Almanac. http://www.nih.gov/about/almanac/organization/NCRR.htm (accessed February 27, 2010).

National Institutes of Health. "NIH Announces New Program to Develop Therapeutics for Rare and Neglected Diseases." NIH News, May 20, 2009. http://www.nih.gov/news/health/may2009/nhgri-20.htm (accessed February 9, 2010).

National Institutes of Health. "NIH Research Opportunities: K30 Clinical Research Curriculum Award." 2003. http://grants2.nih.gov/training/k30 .htm (accessed December 31, 2005).

National Institutes of Health. "Oseltamivir Pharmacokinetics in Morbid Obesity (OPTIMO)." ClinicalTrials.gov. http://www.clinicaltrials.gov/ct2/show/ NCT01002729 (accessed November 9, 2009).

National Institutes of Health. *Unanticipated Risk.* Video of Stephen Straus's presentation for the Introduction to the Principles and Practices of Clinical Research, Unit 8, October 16, 2006–February 26, 2007. http://www .nihtraining.com/cc/ippcr/archive06f/menu.html http://www.nihtraining .com/cc/ippcr/current/downloads/Straus111306pdf.

National Institutes of Health. Clinical Research Training module. "What Makes Clinical Research Ethical?" http://www.nihtraining.com (accessed November 23, 2009).

National Institutes of Health. Division of Program Coordination, Planning, and Strategic, Initiatives. "Re-engineering the Clinical Research Enterprise." NIH Common Fund. http://nihroadmap.nih.gov/clinicalresearch/ (accessed February 27, 2010).

National Institutes of Health. National Institute of Biomedical Imaging and Bioengineering. "Clinical Research Training Opportunities and Resources." http://www.nibib1.nih.gov/Training/Clinical (accessed February 27, 2010).

National Institutes of Health. Office of AIDS Research. *HIV/AIDS Research at NIH: Racial and Ethnic Minorities.* 2001. http://www.nih.gov/od/oar/about/ research/racial/oarrace.htm (accessed January 16, 2006).

National Institutes of Health. Office of Extramural Research. "Conflict of Interest." Grants Policy. http://www.grants.nih.gov/grants/policy/coi/, http://www.grants.nih.gov/grants/policy/coi/tutorial/fcoi.pdf (accessed November 23, 2009).

National Institutes of Health. Office of Extramural Research. "FAQs—Clinical Trials Registration in ClinicalTrials.gov." Grants Policy, December 17, 2008. http://www.grants.nih.gov/grants/policy/hs/faqs_aps_clinical_trials.htm (accessed September 16, 2009).

National Institutes of Health. Office of Human Subjects Research. "Directives for Human Experimentation: Nuremberg Code." http://www.nihtraining.com/ ohsrsite/guidelines/nuremberg.html (accessed June 30, 2006).

"NCI: Cancer Trials News—Maryland Law Covers Clinical Trials." *Clinical Rounds* 1, no. 1 (2000). http://www.clinicalrounds.com/html/ articles/1198-19.htm.

Normile, Dennis. "The Promise and Pitfalls of Clinical Trials Overseas." *Science* 322, no. 5899 (2008), doi:10.1126/science.322.5899.214. http://www .sciencemag.org/cgi/content/full/322/5899/214?ijkey=UKfYGybirpqQM& keytype=ref&siteid=sci (accessed October 19, 2009).

Nundy, Samiran and Chandra Gulhati. "A New Colonialism? Conducting Clinical Trials in India." *New England Journal of Medicine* 352, no. 16

(2005): 1633–6. http://content.nejm.org/cgi/content/short/352/16/1633 (accessed October 20, 2009).

Nutter McClennen & Fish, LLP. "Subject Injury Issues in Clinical Research." Presentation to the Massachusetts Biotechnology Council, June 26, 2008. http://www.massbio.org/writable/committees/presentations/june_26_2008_mbc_injury_slides_copy1.ppt (accessed September 19, 2009).

O'Brien, Nancy Frazier. "Bishops Approve Revised Directives on Withdrawal of Food, Water." *Catholic News Service*, November 19, 2009. http://www.catholicnews.com/data/stories/cns/0905131.htm (accessed November 30, 2009).

O'Neal, Glenn. "Behind the Biowarfare 'Eight Ball.'" *USA Today*, December 19, 2001. http://www.usatoday.com/news/healthscience/health/bioterrorism/2001-12-20-whitecoat-usat.htm (accessed September 14, 2003).

Oracle. "Clinical SiteMinder and TrialMinder Solutions for Clinical Trials Management." 2005. http://www.oracle.com/industries/life_sciences/siteminder_trialminder_data_sheet.pdf (accessed September 15, 2005).

Otto, Mary. "Drugs Tested on HIV-Positive Foster Children." *Washington Post*, May 19, 2005, B1. http://www.washingtonpost.com/wp-dyn/content/article/2005/05/18/AR2005051802154.html (accessed July 10, 2005).

PAREXEL International. "Informed Consent Form" and "Information Sheet." Project no. 68419, protocol no. TGN1412-HV, February 9, 2008. http://www.circare.org/foia5/tgn1412_consentform.pdf.

Passov, David G. "Optimizing Time and Money in Clinical Trials: Russia and Ukraine." Presentation at the Next Generation Pharmaceutical Summit, Scottsdale, AZ, September 2008. http://www.ngpsummit.com/pdf/Clinstar.pdf (accessed May 6, 2009).

PATH. "Background Information on the Meningitis Vaccine Project." 2004. http://www.path.org/resources/meningitis-background.htm (accessed March 3, 2003).

PATH. "Our Work in Vaccine Technologies." http://www.path.org/projects/vaccine-technologies-overview.php (accessed February 10, 2010).

Patsner, Bruce. "Getting New Influenza Vaccines Developed and Marketed." *Health Law Perspectives*, May 2009. http://www.law.uh.edu/Healthlaw/perspectives/2009/(BP)%20Vaccines.pdf (accessed February 10, 2010).

Peachey, Jonathan,Colin Spink, Heather E. Fraser, and Stuart Henderson. *The eClinical Equation, Part 1, Electronic Data Capture*. IBM Institute for Business Value, 2005. http://www.mdsol.com/sites/default/files/documents/library/wp/ibm_edc.pdf (accessed September 17, 2009).

Pear, Robert. "Sex Differences Called Key in Medical Studies." *New York Times*, April 25, 2001, A14. Also available at http://www.nytimes.com (accessed February 8, 2003).

Peloquin, Christine. "Key Dates in the Development of H1N1 Vaccine." CBC News, November 9, 2009. http://www.cbc.ca/health/story/2009/11/06/f-swine-flu-vaccine-rollout-timeline.html (accessed February 9, 2010).

Peters, Mark. "Thought Identification and Other Potential Future Feelings." Visual Thesaurus: Evasive Maneuvers—Euphemisms Old and New, February 4, 2009. http://www.visualthesaurus.com/cm/evasive/1688/ (accessed February 12, 2010).

Petersen, Melody. "Documents Show Effort to Promote Unproven Drug." *New York Times*, October 29, 2002, C1. Also available at http://www.nytimes.com (accessed January 2, 2004).

Petersen, Melody. "Madison Avenue Has Growing Role in the Business of Drug Research." *New York Times*, November 22, 2002, A1. Also available at http://www.nytimes.com (accessed January 2, 2004).

Peterson, Jennifer. "Improving the Site Start-up Process." Presentation at the MAGI Clinical Research Conference–West, San Diego, CA, October 2009.

Petryna, Adriana. *When Experiments Travel: Clinical Trials and the Global Search for Human Subjects.* Princeton University Press, 2009. http://www.press.princeton.edu/chapters/i8916.html (accessed February 7, 2010).

Pfadenhauer, James B. "Navigating the Clinical Trial Billing Maze." *Journal of Oncology Practice* 2, no. 6 (2006): 280. http://jop.ascopubs.org/cgi/content/full/2/6/280 (accessed September 20, 2009).

Pfizer. "Trovan Fact Sheet—Final." http://media.pfizer.com/files/news/trovan_fact_sheet_final.pdf (accessed November 9, 2009).

Pharmagossip. "Slumdog Clinical Trials: Big Pharma in India." Blog posted March 12, 2009. http://www.pharmagossip.blogspot.com/2009/03/slumdog-clinical-trials-contd.html (accessed February 8, 2010).

Phillips, Donald F. "IRB's Search for Answers and Support during a Time of Institutional Change." *Journal of the American Medical Association* 283 no. 6 (2000): 729–730. Also available at http://jama.ama-assn.org (accessed February 7, 2002).

PhRMA. "Pharmaceutical Companies Lead the Way in Corporate Philanthropy." 2003. http://www.phrma.org/publications/policy_papers/pharmaceutical_companies_lead_the_way_in_corporate_philanthropy/ (accessed December 5, 2009).

PhRMA. *Pharmaceutical Industry Profile 2009.* Washington, DC: PhRMA, April 2009. http://www.phrma.org/files/attachments/PhRMA%202009%20Profile%20FINAL.pdf (accessed October 20, 2009).

Pitler, Lisa R., and Philip D. Bonomi. "Developing an Effective and Compliant Plan for Billing Clinical Trials." *Journal of Oncology Practice* 2, no. 6 (2006), doi:10.1200/JOP.2.6.265. http://www.jop.ascopubs.org/cgi/content/full/2/6/265 (accessed February 11, 2010).

Platonov, Pyotr G., and Sergei Varshavsky. "FDA Inspections outside the USA: An Eastern European Perspective." *Applied Clinical Trials* (September 2004).

http://www.actmagazine.com/appliedclinicaltrials/article/articleDetail.jsp?id=121811 (accessed July 25, 2005).

Pollack, Andrew. "Despite Billions for Discovery, Pipeline of Drugs Is Far from Full." *New York Times*, April 19, 2002. Also available at http://www.nytimes.com (accessed February 8, 2003).

Pollack, Andrew. "Imclone Rejection Focuses Debate on Testing of Cancer Drugs." *New York Times*, February 8, 2002. Also available at http://www.nytimes.com (accessed February 8, 2002).

Pomfret, John, and Deborah Nelson. "The Body Hunters, Part 4: In Rural China, a Genetic Mother Lode." *Washington Post*, December 20, 2000. Also available at http://www.washingtonpost.com (accessed March 3, 2003).

Pouncey, Alicia. "Hurricane Katrina: What Have We Learned?" *Applied Clinical Trials*, October 1, 2006. http://appliedclinicaltrialsonline.findpharma.com/appliedclinicaltrials/article/Article/detail/377745 (accessed February 13, 2010).

Prakash, Snigdha. "Conflicted Safety Panel Let Vioxx Study Continue." NPR News, Health, June 8, 2006. http://www.npr.org/templates/story/story.php?storyId=5462419 (accessed November 10, 2009).

President's Council on Bioethics. "Council Publications." http://www.bioethics.gov/reports/ (accessed January 2, 2006).

Presley, Holly. "Vioxx and the Merck Team Effort." *Business Ethics*. The Kenan Institute for Ethics, 2009. http://www.duke.edu/web/kenanethics/CaseStudies/Vioxx.pdf (accessed November 10, 2009).

PRIM&R. "Public Responsibility in Medicine and Research." 2004. http://www.primr.org.

Prostate SPORE National Biospecimen Network (NBN) Pilot. "NBN Blueprint." http://www.prostatenbnpilot.nci.nih.gov/blue_app_n.asp (accessed November 28, 2009).

Psaty, Bruce M., and Curt D. Furberg. "The Record on Rosiglitazone and the Risk of Myocardial Infarction." *New England Journal of Medicine* 357, no. 1 (2007), doi:10.1056/NEJMe078116. http://www.content.nejm.org/cgi/content/full/NEJMe078116 (accessed February 10, 2010).

Public Agenda. "Medical Research: Discussion Guides—The Perspectives in Brief." 2002. http://www.publicagenda.org/issues/debate.cfm?issue_type=medical_research (accessed 2003).

Public Citizen, "Tufts Drug Study Sample Is Skewed; True Figure of R&D Costs Likely Is 75% Lower." December 2004. http://www.citizen.org/publications/release.cfm?ID=7065 (accessed January 14, 2004).

Public Responsibility in Medicine and Research. *Report of the PRIM&R Human Tissue/Specimen Banking Working Group*. white paper, March 2007. http://www.primr.org/uploadedFiles/PRIMR_Site_Home/Public_Policy/Recently_Files_Comments/Tissue%20Banking%20White%20Paper%203-7-07%20final%20combined.pdf (accessed November 28, 2009).

Raloff, Janet. "Cancer Data: Burying Bad News." *Science News*, September 24, 2008. http://www.sciencenews.org/view/generic/id/36805/title/Cancer_data_Burying_bad_news (accessed November 8, 2009).

Rapid Impact: Integrating the Neglected Tropical Diseases with Malaria and HIV/AIDS Control. Conference, George Washington University, Washington DC, October 26–27, 2006.

Redfearn, Suz. "Trials Thriving in Brazil." ClinPage, December 1, 2008. http://www.clinpage.com/article/trials_thriving_in_brazil/ (accessed April 25, 2009).

Rellahan, Barbara. "The TeGenero Incident March 13, 2006 UK: TGN1412—a Superagonist anti-CD28 Antibody." Presentation at the FDA Clinical Investigator Course, Silver Spring, MD, November 17, 2009.

Rennie, Drummond. "Thyroid Storm." *Journal of the American Medical Association* 227, no. 15 (April 16, 1997): 1238–43.

Reproductive Health Technologies Project. *The Quinacrine Debate and Beyond*. 2001. Also available at http://www.rhtp.org/news/publications/default.asp (accessed January 16, 2006).

Research Roundtable. "Budget Corner: Request Separate Payments for End of Study's Clinical Phase and for Completion of CRF's." *Research Roundtable*, December 1999, 1–5. http://www.researchroundtable.com/ (accessed February 7, 2002).

Resnik, David B., and Kenneth A. De Ville. "Bioterrorism and Patent Rights: 'Compulsory Licensure' and the Case of Cipro." *American Journal of Bioethics* 2, no. 3 (2002): 29–39. http://muse.jhu.edu/login?uri=/journals/american_journal_of_bioethics/v002/2.3resnik.html (accessed November 28, 2009).

Rising, Kristin, Peter Bacchetti, and Lisa Bero. "Reporting Bias in Drug Trials Submitted to the Food and Drug Administration: Review of Publication and Presentation." *PLoS Medicine* 5, no. 11 (2008), doi:10.1371/journal.pmed.0050217 (accessed November 10, 2009).

Robertson, Sarah. "Clinical Pharmacology 1: Phase 1 Studies and Early Drug Development." Presentation at the FDA Clinical Investigator Course, Silver Spring, MD, November 16, 2009.

Rosenthal, Elisabeth. "Inquiries in Britain Uncover Loopholes in Drug Trials." *New York Times*, August 3, 2006, sec. World. http://www.nytimes.com/2006/08/03/world/europe/03britain.html (accessed August 3, 2006).

Rubenstein, Sarah. "Justice Department Beats Chest over Zyprexa Settlement." Wall Street Journal Health Blog, January 15, 2009. http://www.blogs.wsj.com/health/2009/01/15/justice-department-beats-chest-over-zyprexa-settlement/tab/ (accessed December 3, 2009).

Rubenstein, Sarah. "When Drug Trials Go Wrong, Patients Have Little Recourse." *Wall Street Journal*, January 31, 2008, sec. A. http://online.wsj.com/article/SB120173515260330205.html (accessed September 19, 2009).

Rudolph, Linda. "Human Subject Protection: Role of the IRB and the Clinical Investigator." Presentation at the MAGI Clinical Research Conference–West, San Diego, CA, October 2009.

Ruof, Mary C. "Vulnerability, Vulnerable Populations, and Policy." Scope Note 44, *Kennedy Institute of Ethics Journal*, December 2004.

Saez-Llorens, Xavier, Cynthia McCoig, Jesus M. Feris, et al. "Quinolone Treatment for Pediatric Bacterial Meningitis: A Comparative Study of Trovafloxacin and Ceftriaxone with or without Vancomycin." *Pediatric Infectious Disease Journal* 21, no. 1 (2002): 14–22.

Salewski, Joseph P. "An FDA Audit: What the Investigator and Sponsor Need to Know." American Society of Gene Therapy, 2001. http://www.asgt.org/recent_course_materials/training_course/salewski.ppt (accessed February 17, 2003).

Santa, John. "The Real Cost of Free Antibiotics." Consumer Reports Health, January 9, 2009. http://blogs.consumerreports.org/health/2009/01/free-antibiotic.html (accessed December 6, 2009).

Saul, Stephanie, and Gardiner Harris. "Diabetes Drug Still Has Heart Risks, Doctors Warn." *New York Times*, June 6, 2007, sec. Health. http://www.nytimes.com/2007/06/06/health/06fda.html (accessed February 9, 2010).

Schechter, Alan N. "The Crisis in Clinical Research: Endangering the Half-Century National Institutes of Health Consensus." *Journal of the American Medical Association* 280, no. 16 (1998): 1440–42.

Schuklenk, Udo. "JAMA Shenanigans Continue." UdoSchuklenk's Ethx Blog, July 8, 2009. http://www.ethxblog.blogspot.com/2009/07/jama-shenanigans-continue.html (accessed November 10, 2009).

Schulman, K. A., et al. "Contract Language for Clinical Research Agreements between Academic Medical Centers and Industry Sponsors." Center for Clinical and Genetic Economics. Duke Clinical Research Institute. 2003. http://www.dcri.duke.edu/ccge/contracts/ (accessed January 14, 2004).

Schwartz, John. "And Then the Patients Suddenly Started Dying: How NIH Missed Warning Signs in Drug Test." *Washington Post*, September 7, 1993, sec. A.

Schwartz, Richard M. "Product Development: Moving from the Bench to the Clinic." http://www.nihtraining.com/cc/ippcr/current/downloads/RSchwartz031609(C).pdf (accessed November 11, 2009).

Scott, Janny, and Leslie Kaufman. "Belated Charge Ignites Furor over AIDS Drug Trial." *New York Times*, July 17, 2005. http://www.nytimes.com/2005/07/17/nyregion/17trials.html (accessed July 17, 2005).

Scuderi, Margaret A. "What Are DNA Vaccines?" May 2003. http://biology.kenyon.edu/slonc/bio38/scuderi/partii.html (accessed February 10, 2010).

Senak, Mark. "FDA's Dr. Janet Woodcock Discusses Adaptive Clinical Trials." Eye on FDA, September 4, 2007. http://www.eyeonfda.com/eye_on_FDA/2007/09/FDAs-dr-janet-w.html (accessed February 10, 2010).

Senak, Mark. "The Swine Flu Vaccine Is Approved—If You Build It Will They Come?" Eye on FDA, September 16, 2009. http://www.eyeonfda.com/eye_on_FDA/2009/09/the-swine-flu-vaccine-is-approved-if-you-build-it-will-they-come.html (accessed February 9, 2010).

Shah, Anup. "World Military Spending." *Global Issues*. Citing Center for Arms Control and Non-Proliferation. "U.S. Military Spending vs. the World." February 6, 2006. http://globalissues.org/Geopolitics/ArmsTrade/Spending.asp.

Sharma, Arya M. "Obesity: Managing Weighty Issues on Lean Evidence—The Challenges of Bariatric Medicine." *Canadian Medical Association Journal* 172, no. 1 (2005), doi:10.1503/cmaj.1041722. http://www.ncbi.nlm.nih.gov/pmc/articles/PMC543938/ (accessed November 9, 2009).

Shem, Samuel. *The House of God*. (Itasca, IL: Putnam Publishing Group, 1984).

Sherwin, Susan. "Women in Clinical Studies: A Feminist View." In *Women and Health Research: Ethical and Legal Issues of Including Women in Clinical Studies*, vol. 2, edited by Anna C. Mastroianni, Ruth Faden, and Daniel Federman. Institute of Medicine. Washington, DC: National Academy Press, 1994. http://books.nap.edu/catalog/2343.html (accessed January 16, 2006).

Silverman, Ed. "Clinical-Trial Fraud: The Case of Ketek." Pharmalot, May 29, 2007. http://www.pharmalot.com/2007/05/clinical-trial-fraud-the-case-of-ketek/ (accessed November 2009).

Silverman, Ed. "Come Again? A Spray for Premature Ejaculation." Pharmalot, November 23, 2009. http://www.pharmalot.com/2009/11/come-again-a-spray-for-premature-ejaculation/.

Silverman, Ed. "Supreme Court Seeks Pfizer Trovan Comment." Pharmalot, November 5, 2009. http://www.pharmalot.com/2009/11/supreme-court-seeks-comment-on-pfizer-trovan-case/.

Simon, Fran. "Tulane Reaches Out to Clinical Trial Participants." *The New Wave*, November 17, 2005. http://www.tulane.edu/newwave/111705_clinicaltrial.html (accessed February 13, 2010).

Singer, Peter, and Solomon R. Benatar. 2001. "Beyond Helsinki: A Vision for Global Health Ethics." *British Medical Journal* 322, no. 3 (2001): 747–48. http://www.bmj.org/cgi/content/full/322/7289/747 (accessed July 14, 2005).

Singla, Rohit K. "Missed Opportunities: The Vaccine Act of 1813." Harvard Law School, May 1, 1998. http://leda.law.harvard.edu/leda/data/229/rsingla.pdf (accessed February 12, 2004).

Skloot, Rebecca. "Taking the Least of You: The Tissue-Industrial Complex." *New York Times*, April 16, 2006. http://www.nytimes.com/2006/04/16/magazine/16tissue.html (accessed November 27, 2009).

Skloot, Rebecca. "Tissue Ownership Update: *William Catalona v. Washington University*, the Ruling." Culture Dish blog, April 17, 2006. http://www.rebeccaskloot.blogspot.com/2006/04/tissue-ownership-update-william.html (accessed February 14, 2010).

Smith, W. Thomas. "FDA Requires Foreign Clinical Studies Be in Accordance with Good Clinical Practice to Better Protect Human Subjects." *ABA Health eSource* 5, no. 2 (2008). http://www.abanet.org/health/esource/Volume5/02/smith.html#_ftnref19 (accessed November 8, 2009).

Smit-Marshall, Philippa. "Recruitment Strategies in Clinical Trials—A European Perspective." Pharmanet, white paper. http://www.pharmanet.com/pdf/whitepapers/Recruitment.pdf.

Society for Women's Health Research. "Funding Research." 2002. http://www.womens-health.org (accessed January 26, 2004).

Society for Women's Health Research. "Understanding Research—Milestones in the Inclusion of Women in Clinical Research." 2003. http://www.womens-health.org (accessed February 12, 2003).

Sonel, Ali F., and Kelly Willenberg. "Creating a Strategic Clinical Research Compliance Plan." Presentation at the MAGI Clinical Research Conference–West, San Diego, CA, October 2009.

Sorrel, Sarah. "Medical Device Development: U.S. and E.U. Differences." *Applied Clinical Trials Online*, August 1, 2006. http://appliedclinicaltrialsonline.findpharma.com/appliedclinicaltrials/Regulatory/Medical-Device-Development-US-and-EU-Differences/ArticleStandard/Article/detail/363640 (accessed February 9, 2010).

South African Department of Health. "Ethical Considerations for HIV/AIDS Clinical and Epidemiological Research." Chap. 9 in *Guidelines for Good Clinical Practice in the Conduct of Trials in Human Participants in South Africa*. 2000. http://www.doh.gov.za/docs/policy/trials/trials_09.html (accessed March 4, 2003).

Sparks, Joel. "Timeline of Laws Related to the Protection of Human Subjects." National Institutes of Health, June 2002. http://history.nih.gov/01Docs/historical/2020b.htm (accessed December 5, 2005).

Speers, Marjorie. "AAHRPP Accreditation for your Human Research Protection Program." Presentation at the MAGI Clinical Research Conference–West, San Diego, CA, October 2009.

Sporle, Andrew, and Jonathan Koea. "Maori Responsiveness in Health and Medical Research: Key Issues for Researchers (Part 1)." *Journal of the New Zealand Medical Association* 117, no. 1199 (2004): 997. http://www.nzma.org.nz/journal/117-1199/997/ (accessed October 22, 2009).

Srinivasan, Sandhya. "Bodies for Hire: The Outsourcing of Clinical Trials." *Himal Southasian*, August 2009. http://www.himalmag.com/Bodies-for-hire;-The-outsourcing-of-clinical-trials_nw3213.html (accessed November 7, 2009).

Srinivasan, Sandhya. *Ethical Concerns in Clinical Trials in India: An Investigation*. Mumbai, India: Centre for Studies in Ethics and Rights, February 2009. http://www.fairdrugs.org/uploads/files/Ethical_concerns_in_clinical_trials_in_India_An_investigation.pdf (accessed February 8, 2010).

Srinivasan, Sandhya. "Trial by Fire." *Economic and Political Weekly*, August 29–September 4, 2009, pgs. 29–33. http://infochangeindia.org/200909177947/Health/Analysis/Trial-by-fire.html (accessed February 8, 2010).

Stafford, Randall S., Todd H. Wagner, and Philip W. Lavori. "New, but Not Improved? Incorporating Comparative-Effectiveness Information into FDA Labeling." *New England Journal of Medicine* 361, no. 13 (2009), doi:10.1056/NEJMp0906490. http://content.nejm.org/cgi/content/full/361/13/1230 (accessed August 29, 2009).

Staton, Tracy. "NEJM: Put Comparative Effectiveness on Drug Labels." Fierce Pharma, August 13, 2009. http://www.fiercepharma.com/story/nejm-put-comparative-effectiveness-drug-labels/2009-08-13 (accessed February 10, 2010).

Steinberg, Mindy J., and Elaine R. Rubin. *The HIPAA Privacy Rule: Lacks Patient Benefit, Impedes Research Growth.* Washington, DC: Association of Academic Health Centers, 2009. http://www.aahcdc.org/policy/reddot/AAHC_HIPAA_Privacy_Rule_Impedes_Research_Growth.pdf (accessed March 15, 2009).

Steinbrook, Robert. "Compensation for Injured Research Subjects." *New England Journal of Medicine* 354, no. 18 (2006), doi:10.1056/NEJMp068080. http://content.nejm.org/cgi/content/full/354/18/1871 (accessed September 19, 2009).

Steinbrook, Robert. "Conflicts of Interest at the NIH—Resolving the Problem." *New England Journal of Medicine* 351, no. 10 (2004): 955–57.

Steinbrook, Robert. "Protecting Research Subjects—The Crisis at Johns Hopkins." *New England Journal of Medicine* 346, no. 9 (2002): 716–720. http://content.nejm.org/cgi/content/full/346/9/716 (accessed February 14, 2010).

Stephens, Joe. "The Body Hunters, Part 1: As Drug Testing Spreads, Profits and Lives Hang in Balance." *Washington Post*, December 17, 2000. http://www.washingtonpost.com (accessed September 13, 2003).

Stephens, Joe. "Pfizer Faces Criminal Charges in Nigeria." *Washington Post*, May 29, 2007. http://www.washingtonpost.com/wp-dyn/content/article/2007/05/29/AR2007052902107.html.

Stephens, Joe. "Pfizer to Pay $75 Million to Settle Nigerian Trovan Drug-Testing Suit." *Washington Post*, July 31, 2009. http://www.washingtonpost.com/wp-dyn/content/article/2009/07/30/AR2009073001847.html (accessed November 9, 2009).

Stolberg, Sheryl Gay. "The Biotech Death of Jesse Gelsinger." *New York Times*, November 28, 1999. http://www.nytimes.com/library/magazine/home/19991128mag-stolberg.html (accessed January 15, 2004).

Stolberg, Sheryl Gay, and Jeff Gerth. "Drug Makers Design Studies with Eye to Competitive Edge." *New York Times*, December 23, 2000. http://www.nytimes.com (accessed February 8, 2003).

Stone, Arthur A., Saul Shiffman, Joseph E. Schwartz, Joan E. Broderick, and Michael R. Hufford. "Patient Non-Compliance with Paper Diaries." *British Medical Journal* 324 (2002): 1193–4. http://www.bmj.com/cgi/reprint/324/7347/1193 (accessed September 17, 2009).

Stone, Heather. "Genzyme Puts the Squeeze on Developing Countries." *Boston Globe*, June 21, 2009. http://www.boston.com/bostonglobe/editorial_opinion/letters/articles/2009/06/21/genzyme_puts_the_squeeze_on_developing_countries.

Stoy, Diane B. "Recruitment and Retention of Women in Clinical Studies: Theoretical Perspectives and Methodological Considerations." In *Women and Health Research: Ethical and Legal Issues of Including Women in Clinical Studies*, vol. 2, 45–64, edited by Anna C. Mastroianni, Ruth Faden, and Daniel Federman. Institute of Medicine. Washington, DC: National Academy Press, 1994. http://www.nap.edu/books/0309050405/html/45.html (accessed September 14, 2003).

Straus, Stephen. "Unanticipated Risk in Clinical Research." Chap. 8 in *Principles and Practice of Clinical Research*, edited by John I. Gallin. San Diego: Elsevier, 2002.

St. Vincent's Health. "Participant Information and Guidelines for Research at St. Vincent's Health." 2005. http://www.svhm.org.au/Department_Index/RnG/documents%5CHREC%5CPICF%20Guidelines.pdf (accessed September 6, 2005).

Sung, N. S., W. F. Crowley, M. Genel, et al. "Central Challenges Facing the National Clinical Research Enterprise." *Journal of the American Medical Association* 289 (2003): 1278–87.

Swann, John P. *History of the FDA*. New York: Oxford University Press, 1998. http://www.fda.gov/oc/history/historyoffda/default.htm (accessed February 9, 2004).

Swit, Michael. "FDA Inspections: Handling the Consequences." Presentation at the MAGI Clinical Research Conference–West, San Diego, CA, October 2009.

Swit, Michael. "FDA Inspections: Handling the Consequences." Presentation at the MAGI Clinical Research Conference–West, San Diego, CA, October 2009, citing "Compliance and Enforcement." Presentation by David K. Elder, Director, FDA Office of Enforcement, at the Orange County Regulatory Affairs/FDA Joint Educational Conference, June 2005.

Szasz, Thomas. *Our Right to Drugs*. New York: Praeger Publishers, 1992. http://www.druglibrary.org/schaffer/Library/szasz1.htm (accessed February 8, 2004).

Talarico, Lilia, Gang Chen, and Richard Pazdur. "Enrollment of Elderly Patients in Clinical Trials for Cancer Drug Registration: A 7-Year Experience by the U.S. Food and Drug Administration." *Journal of Clinical Oncology* 22, no. 22 (2004), doi:10.1200/JCO.2004.02.175. http://www.jco.ascopubs.org/cgi/content/abstract/22/22/4626 (accessed November 9, 2009).

Tannen, Richard L., Mark G. Weiner, and Dawei Xie. "Use of Primary Care Electronic Medical Record Database in Drug Efficacy Research on

Cardiovascular Outcomes: Comparison of Database and Randomised Controlled Trial Findings." *British Medical Journal* 338 (2009), doi:10.1136/bmj.b81. http://www.bmj.com/cgi/content/full/338/jan27_1/b81#otherarticles (accessed November 5, 2009).

Taonui, Rawiri. "Tribal Organisation." In *Te Ara: The Encyclopedia of New Zealand*, 2009. http://www.teara.govt.nz/en/tribal-organisation (accessed October 22, 2009).

Tarkan, Laurie. "FDA Increases Efforts to Avert Drug-Induced Liver Damage." *New York Times*, August 13, 2001. Also available at http://www.nytimes.com (accessed February 8, 2003).

Taylor, R., and J. Giles. "Cash Interests Taint Drug Advice." *Nature* 437 (2005): 1070–1. Cited in editorial, "Clinical Practice Guidelines and Conflict of Interest." *Canadian Medical Association Journal* 173, no. 11 (2005), doi:10.1503/cmaj.051423. http://www.cmaj.ca (accessed December 3, 2009).

Teixeira, Julian. "Research Partnership Will Study How Electronic Medical Records Can Address Genetics of Drug Safety." Eurekalert, October 21, 2009. http://www.eurekalert.org/pub_releases/2009-10/zg-rpw102109.php (accessed November 4, 2009).

Temple University Office of Clinical Trials. "Good Clinical Research Practices." 2005. http://www.research.temple.edu/oct/doc/lectures/goodpract.ppt (accessed July 15, 2005).

TheFreeDictionary.com., s.v. "lifestyle drug." http://medical-dictionary.thefreedictionary.com/lifestyle+drug.

Thompson, Larry. "Human Gene Therapy—Harsh Lessons, High Hopes," *FDA Consumer*, September–October 2000. http://www.fda.gov/fdac/features/2000/500_gene.html (accessed January 6, 2006).

Throckmorton, Douglas. "Overview and Introduction to Drug Regulation." Presentation at the FDA Clinical Investigator Course, Silver Spring, MD, November 16, 2009.

Tominaga, Toshiyoshi. "Global Clinical Development—Reducing Japan's Drug Lag." Pharmafocusasia.com, 2008. http://www.pharmafocusasia.com/clinical_trials/global_clinical_development_japan_druglag.htm (accessed March 18, 2009).

Trials of War Criminals before the Nuremberg Military Tribunals under Control Council Law No. 10. 2 vols. Washington, DC: U.S. Government Printing Office, 1949. http://www.nihtraining.com/ohsrsite/guidelines/nuremberg.html (accessed November 28, 2005).

TrialTrac. "Sitetrac." 2004. http://www.trialtrac.com/ (accessed January 29, 2004; now called TrialWorks by ClinPhone, accessed December 26, 2005).

Trialytics. "About Us." http://www.trialytics.com/about.aspx (accessed September 27, 2009).

Tufts Center for the Study of Drug Development. "Backgrounder: How New Drugs Move through the Development and Approval Process." Tufts

University, November 2004. http://csdd.tufts.edu/NewsEvents/RecentNews.asp?newsid=4 (accessed September 15, 2003).

Tufts Center for the Study of Drug Development. "Current Investigator Landscape Poses a Growing Challenge for Sponsors." Tufts University. *Impact Report* 11, no. 1 (2009). http://csdd.tufts.edu/reports/description/ir_summaries (accessed August 23, 2009).

Tufts Center for the Study of Drug Development. "Drug Safety Withdrawals in the U.S. Not Linked to Speed of FDA Approval." Tufts University. *Impact Report* 7, no. 5 (2005). http://csdd.tufts.edu/InfoServices/ImpactReportPDFs/impactReportSeptemberOctober2005.pdf (accessed September 17, 2009).

Tufts Center for the Study of Drug Development. "Growing Protocol Design Complexity Stresses Investigators, Volunteers." Tufts University. *Impact Report* 10, no. 1 (2008). Cited in PhRMA. "Pharmaceutical Industry Profile 2009." http://www.phrma.org/files/PhRMA%202009%20Profile%20FINAL.pdf (accessed August 23, 2009).

Tufts Center for the Study of Drug Development. "New Drugs Are Taking Longer to Bring to Market in the U.S." Tufts University, 2005. http://csdd.tufts.edu/NewsEvents/NewsArticle.asp?newsid=58 (accessed January 20, 2005).

Tufts Center for the Study of Drug Development. "Outlook 2003." Tufts University, 2003. http://csdd.tufts.edu/InfoServices/OutlookReports.asp (accessed September 9, 2003).

Tufts Center for the Study of Drug Development. "Outlook 2009." Tufts University, 2009. http://www.csdd.tufts.edu/InfoServices/OutlookPDFs/Outlook2009.pdf (accessed August 23, 2009).

Tufts–New England Medical Center. "The Renewal of Clinical Research." November 20, 2003, http://www.nemc.org/dccr/clinical_research_information.htm (accessed January 15, 2006).

Tumulty, Karen. "Jesus and the FDA." *Time*, October 5, 2002. http://www.time.com/time/nation/article/0,8599,361521,00.html (accessed February 15, 2010).

Tunis, Sean R., Daniel B. Stryer, and Carolyn M. Clancy, "Practical Clinical Trials." *Journal of the American Medical Association* 290 (2003): 1624–32.

Union of Concerned Scientists. *An Investigation into the Bush Administration's Misuse of Science.* Cambridge, MA: Union of Concerned Scientists, 2004. http://stephenschneider.stanford.edu/Publications/PDF_Papers/RSI_final_fullreport.pdf (accessed February 15, 2010).

Union of Concerned Scientists. *Voices of Scientists at the FDA: Protecting Public Health Depends on Independent Science.* 2006. http://www.ucsusa.org/scientific_integrity/abuses_of_science/summary-of-the-FDA-scientist.html (accessed December 1, 2009).

United Nations. "HIV/AIDS in Africa." 2003. http://www.unaids.org/en/media/fact+sheets.asp (accessed May 18, 2003).

United Nations. "Secretary-General Calls for Concerted Action in Message Marking International Day for Eradication of Poverty." Press release issued by U.N. Secretary-General Kofi Annan, November 10, 2002. http://www.un.org/News/Press/docs/2002/sgsm8431.doc.htm.

University of California, San Francisco. Human Subjects Protection Program. "HIPAA and Human Research, 2003." http://www.research.ucsf.edu/chr/HIPAA/chrHIPAA.asp (accessed January 25, 2004).

University of Iowa. "Informed Consent and Related Issues." December 31, 2003. http://research.uiowa.edu/hso/indes.php?Get=forms02 (accessed January 25, 2004).

University of Iowa. "IRB Forms/Templates." 2001. http://research.uiowa.edu/hso/index.php?get=forms02 (accessed February 23, 2003).

University of Michigan. "Informed Consent." 2003. http://www.med.umich.edu/irbmed/InformationalDocuments/consent/consenttoc.html (accessed February 7, 2003).

University of Michigan. "Tips on Preparing Understandable Informed Consent Documents." 2002. http://www.med.umich.edu/irbmed/InformationalDocuments/consent/investigator.html (accessed February 7, 2003).

University of Southern California "IRB Forms." 2003. http://ccnt.hsc.usc.edu/irb/docs/instruction.htm (accessed February 7, 2003).

University of Utah Health Sciences Center. "Clinical Trials Management:Budgeting and Project Set-up." 2004. http://uuhsc.utah.edu/clinicalTrials/finanAdmin/index.html#setup (accessed January 28, 2004).

University of Washington "Clinical Trials Administrative Start-up Handbook." 2003. http://www.hscer.washington.edu/clinicaltrialshandbook/ (accessed January 16, 2003).

U.S. Department of Health and Human Services. "Uses and Disclosures to Carry Out Treatment, Payment, or Health Care Operations." *Code of Federal Regulations*, Title 45, Part 164.506.

U.S. Department of Health and Human Services. Agency for Healthcare Research and Quality. "30 Safe Practices for Better Health Care." Fact sheet. http://www.ahrq.gov/qual/30safe.htm (accessed November 6, 2009).

U.S. Department of Health and Human Services. Centers for Medicare and Medicaid Services. *Medicare Benefit Policy Manual*. Chapter 14 in publication number 100–02. http://www.cms.hhs.gov/manuals/downloads/bp102c14.pdf (accessed November 3, 2009).

U.S. Department of Health and Human Services. Centers for Medicare and Medicaid Services. "Medicare Clinical Trial Policies Overview." http://www.cms.hhs.gov/clinicaltrialpolicies/ (accessed February 13, 2010).

U.S. Department of Health and Human Services. Centers for Medicare and Medicaid Services. *Medicare National Coverage Determinations Manual*. Chapter 1, part 4 (Sections 200–310.1), Coverage Determinations. http://

www.cms.hhs.gov/manuals/downloads/ncd103c1_part4.pdf (accessed September 20, 2009).

U.S. Department of Health and Human Services. Health Resources and Services Administration. "National Vaccine Injury Compensation Program." http://www.hrsa.gov/vaccinecompensation/ (accessed February 10, 2010).

U.S. Department of Health and Human Services. Office for Civil Rights. "HIPAA Medical Privacy—National Standards to Protect the Privacy of Personal Health Information." 2003. http://www.hhs.gov/ocr/hipaa/ (accessed January 25, 2004).

U.S. Department of Health and Human Services. Office for Human Research Protections. "Assurances." http://www.hhs.gov/ohrp/assurances/assurances_index.html (accessed October 1, 2009).

U.S. Department of Health and Human Services. Office for Human Research Protections. *Guidance on Reviewing and Reporting Unanticipated Problems Involving Risks to Subjects or Others and Adverse Events.* OHRP Policy Guidance, January 15, 2007. http://www.hhs.gov/ohrp/policy/AdvEvntGuid.htm (accessed February 3, 2010).

U.S. Department of Health and Human Services. Office for Human Research Protections. "Protection of Human Subjects." *Code of Federal Regulations,* Title 45, Part 46. 2005. http://www.hhs.gov/ohrp/humansubjects/guidance/45cfr46.htm (accessed January 2, 2006).

U.S. Department of Health and Human Services. Office for Human Research Protections. "Public Welfare." *Code of Federal Regulations,* Title 45. 2001. http://www.hhs.gov/ohrp/humansubjects/guidance/45cfr46.htm (accessed January 25, 2004).

U.S. Department of Health and Human Services. Office of Inspector General. *Clinical Trial Web Sites: A Promising Tool to Foster Informed Consent.* OEI-01-97-00198, Washington DC, May 2002. http://oig.hhs.gov/oei/reports/oei-01-97-00198.pdf (accessed September 27, 2009).

U.S. Department of Health and Human Services. Office of Inspector General. *The Globalization of Clinical Trials: A Growing Challenge in Protecting Human Subjects.* OEI-01-00-00190. Washington, DC, September 2001. http://www.oig.hhs.gov/oei/reports/oei-01-00-00190.pdf (accessed March 18, 2009).

U.S. Department of Health and Human Services. Office of Inspector General. *How Grantees Manage Financial Conflicts of Interest in Research Funded by the National Institutes of Health.* November 2009. http://oig.hhs.gov/oei/reports/oei-03-07-00700.pdf (accessed November 23, 2009).

U.S. Department of Health and Human Services. Office of Inspector General. "Institutional Review Boards: Time for Reform." 1998. http://oig.hhs.gov/oei/reports/oei-01-97-00193.pdf (accessed September 14, 2003).

U.S. Department of Health and Human Services. Office of Inspector General. *National Institutes of Health: Conflicts of Interest in Extramural Research.* OEI-03-06-00460, January 2008. http://oig.hhs.gov/oei/reports/oei-03-06-00460.pdf (accessed November 23, 2009).

U.S. Department of Health and Human Services. Office of Inspector General. "Recruiting Human Subjects: Pressures in Industry-Sponsored Clinical Research." 2000. http://www.researchroundtable.com/oigreports.htm (accessed January 4, 2004).

U.S. Department of Health and Human Services. Press Office. "Bush Administration Will Seek New Legislation for Mandatory Pediatric Drug Testing." Press release, December 16, 2002. http://www.hhs.gov/news/press/2002pres/20021216c.html.

U.S. Department of Justice. "Federal Statutes Imposing Collateral Consequences upon Conviction." November 2000. http://www.justice.gov/pardon/collateral_consequences.pdf (accessed December 4, 2009).

U.S. Department of Labor, Bureau of Labor Statistics. *Career Guide to Industries, 2010–11 Edition.* Pharmaceutical and Medicine Manufacturing, http://www.bls.gov/oco/cg/cgs009.htm; Medical Scientists, http://www.bls.gov/oco/ocos309.htm; Scientific Research and Development Services, http://www.bls.gov/oco/cg/cgs053.htm (accessed February 27, 2010).

U.S. Department of Labor. Occupational Safety and Health Administration. "Bloodborne Pathogens and Needlestick Prevention." http://www.osha.gov/SLTC/bloodbornepathogens/ (accessed January 4, 2006).

U.S. District Court, Eastern District of New York, *Tummino, et al. v. Torti. Tummino v. von Eschenbach*, 427 F. Supp. 2d 212, 231–34 (E.D.N.Y. 2006); Oct. 11, 2006 Hr'g Tr. 20; July 26, 2006 Hr'g Tr. 9:1, http://www.nyed.uscourts.gov/pub/rulings/cv/2005/05cv366mofinal.pdf (accessed February 15, 2010).

U.S. Food and Drug Administration. "Acceptance of Foreign Clinical Studies—Information Sheet." http://www.fda.gov/RegulatoryInformation/Guidances/ucm126426.htm (site update May 22, 2009) (accessed November 8, 2009).

U.S. Food and Drug Administration. *Best Pharmaceuticals for Children Act.* 2001. http://www.fda.gov/opacom/laws/pharmkids/contents.html (accessed February 7, 2004).

U.S. Food and Drug Administration. *Code of Federal Regulations*, Title 21. http://www.accessdata.fda.gov/scripts/cdrh/cfdocs/cfCFR/CFRSearch.cfm?fr=312.62 (accessed September 26, 2009).

U.S. Food and Drug Administration. "Colors and Cosmetics Technology." *Compliance Program Guidance Manual.* http://www.fda.gov/downloads/Cosmetics/GuidanceComplianceRegulatoryInformation/ComplianceEnforcement/UCM073356.pdf (accessed December 5, 2009).

U.S. Food and Drug Administration. "Critical Path Initiative." http://www.fda.gov/ScienceResearch/SpecialTopics/CriticalPathInitiative/default.htm (accessed September 16, 2009).

U.S. Food and Drug Administration. "Draft Warning Letter." 2003. http://www.fda.gov/cder/warn/2003/11577.pdf (accessed January 25, 2004).

U.S. Food and Drug Administration. "Drug Application Forms and Electronic Submissions: FDA 1572 Statement of Investigator." http://www.fda.gov/cder/regulatory/applications/Forms.htm (accessed January 25, 2004).

U.S. Food and Drug Administration. "The Evolution of U.S. Drug Law." http://www.fda.gov/fdac/special/newdrug/benlaw.html (accessed on February 7, 2004).

U.S. Food and Drug Administration. "Expanded Access and Expedited Approval of New Therapies Related to HIV/AIDS." http://www.fda.gov/oashi/aids/expanded.html (accessed January 2, 2006).

U.S. Food and Drug Administration. FDA Warning Letter to John M. Kirkwood, MD. http://www.fda.gov/ICECI/EnforcementActions/WarningLetters/ucm183577.htm (accessed October 19, 2009).

U.S. Food and Drug Administration. *Federal Food, Drug, and Cosmetic Act* (FD&C Act), *U.S. Code* 21 (2004), §321, chapter II, "Definitions." http://www.fda.gov/RegulatoryInformation/LegislationFederalFoodDrugandCosmeticActFDCAct/FDCActChaptersIandIIShortTitleandDefinitions/ucm086297.htm (accessed February 9, 2010).

U.S. Food and Drug Administration. "Financial Disclosure by Clinical Investigators." *Code of Federal Regulations*, Title 21, Part 54. http://www.accessdata.fda.gov/scripts/cdrh/cfdocs/cfcfr/CFRSearch.cfm?CFRPart=54.

U.S. Food and Drug Administration. "Financial Interest Form: Certification: Financial Interests and Arrangements of Clinical Investigations." FDA Form 3454. http://www.fda.gov/opacom/morechoices/FDAforms/FDA-3454.pdf.

U.S. Food and Drug Administration. "Financial Interest Form: Disclosure: Financial Interests and Arrangements of Clinical Investigators." FDA Form 3455. http://www.fda.gov/opacom/morechoices/FDAforms/FDA-3455.pdf.

U.S. Food and Drug Administration. "Food and Drugs: Investigational New Drug Application." *Code of Federal Regulations*, Title 21, Part 312.60. http://www.gpoaccess.gov/cfr/index.html (accessed November 28, 2005).

U.S. Food and Drug Administration. *From Test Tube to Patient: Improving Health through Human Drugs.* 1999. http://www.fda.gov/cder/about/whatwedo/testtube.pdf (accessed November 1, 2003).

U.S. Food and Drug Administration. *Guidance for Clinical Investigators, Sponsors, and IRBs: Adverse Event Reporting—Improving Human Subject Protection.* January 2009. http://www.fda.gov/downloads/RegulatoryInformation/Guidances/ucm127346.pdf (accessed February 13, 2010).

U.S. Food and Drug Administration. *Guidance for Industry: Acceptance of Foreign Clinical Studies.* 2001. http://www.fda.gov/cder/guidance/fstud.htm (accessed March 3, 2003).

U.S. Food and Drug Administration. *Guidance for Industry: Collection of Race and Ethnicity Data in Clinical Trials.* September 2005. http://www.fda.gov/downloads/RegulatoryInformation/Guidances/ucm126396.pdf.

U.S. Food and Drug Administration. *Guidance for Industry: Computerized Systems Used in Clinical Investigations.* May 2007. http://www.fda.gov/OHRMS/DOCKETS/98fr/04d-0440-gdl0002.pdf (accessed November 4, 2009).

U.S. Food and Drug Administration. *Guidance for Industry: E6 Good Clinical Practice, Consolidated Guidance.* 1996. http://www.fda.gov/cder/guidance/959fnl.pdf (accessed July 11, 2005).

U.S. Food and Drug Administration. *Guidance for Industry, Investigators and Reviewers: Exploratory IND Studies.* January 2006. http://www.fda.gov/downloads/Drugs/GuidanceComplianceRegulatoryInformation/Guidances/ucm078933.pdf.

U.S. Food and Drug Administration. *Guidance for Industry Part 11, Electronic Records: Electronic Signatures—Scope and Application.* 2003. http://www.fda.gov/downloads/Drugs/GuidanceComplianceRegulatoryInformation/Guidances/UCM072322.pdf (accessed November 4, 2009).

U.S. Food and Drug Administration. *Guidance for Industry: Protecting the Rights, Safety, and Welfare of Study Subjects—Supervisory Responsibilities of Investigators.* 2007. http://www.fda.gov/downloads/RegulatoryInformation/Guidances/ucm127740.pdf (accessed November 7, 2009).

U.S. Food and Drug Administration. *Guidance for Industry: Special Protocol Assessment.* 2002. http://www.fda.gov/cder/guidance/3764fnl.htm (accessed January 23, 2004).

U.S. Food and Drug Administration. *Guidance for Institutional Review Boards and Clinical Investigators: Recruiting Study Subjects.* 1998 update. http://www.fda.gov/oc/ohrt/irbs/toc4.html#recruiting (accessed December 24, 2005).

U.S. Food and Drug Administration. *Guidance for Institutional Review Boards and Clinical Investigators: 21 CFR Part 50—Protection of Human Subjects.* 1998. http://www.fda.gov/oc/ohrt/irbs/appendixb.html (accessed January 25, 2004).

U.S. Food and Drug Administration. *Inspections, Compliance, Enforcement, and Criminal Investigations—Bioresearch Monitoring.* http://www.fda.gov/ICECI/EnforcementActions/BioresearchMonitoring/default.htm (accessed October 18, 2009).

U.S. Food and Drug Administration. "Investigational Device Exemptions." *Code of Federal Regulations*, Title 21, Part 812. http://www.accessdata.fda.gov/scripts/cdrh/cfdocs/cfcfr/CFRSearch.cfm?CFRPart=812&showFR=1 (accessed February 5, 2010).

U.S. Food and Drug Administration. "Investigational New Drug Application." *Code of Federal Regulations*, Title 21, Part 312. http://www.accessdata.fda.gov/scripts/cdrh/cfdocs/cfCFR/CFRSearch.cfm?CFRPart=312 (accessed November 12, 2009).

U.S. Food and Drug Administration. "Is the FDA Safe and Effective?" 2001. http://www.fdareview.org/ (accessed February 7, 2004).

U.S. Food and Drug Administration. "New Drug and Biological Drug Products." *Code of Federal Regulations*, Title 21, Parts 312.55(b) and 312.32(c). http://www.gpoaccess.gov/cfr/index.html (accessed September 15, 2005).

U.S. Food and Drug Administration. "New Drug and Biological Drug Products; Evidence Needed to Demonstrate Effectiveness of New Drugs When Human

Efficacy Studies Are Not Ethical or Feasible." *Code of Federal Regulations*, Title 21, Parts 314 and 601. 2002. http://www.fda.gov/OHRMS/DOCKETS/98fr/98n-0237-nfr0001-vol1.pdf (accessed February 7, 2004).

U.S. Food and Drug Administration. "Newly Added Guidance Documents." http://www.fda.gov/Drugs/GuidanceComplianceRegulatoryInformation/Guidances/ucm121568.htm (accessed November 10, 2009).

U.S. Food and Drug Administration. "Pediatric Drug Studies: Protecting Pint-Sized Patients." In *From Test Tube to Patient: Improving Health through Human Drugs*. September 1999. http://www.fda.gov/cder/about/whatwedo/testtube-13.pdf (accessed November 1, 2003).

U.S. Food and Drug Administration. "Pediatric Ethics Working Group Consensus Statement on the Pediatric Advisory Subcommittee's April 24, 2001 Meeting." 2003. http://www.fda.gov/cder/pediatric/ethics-statement-Apr2001.htm (accessed January 4, 2004).

U.S. Food and Drug Administration. "Warning Letter to Johnson & Johnson Pharmaceutical Research & Development, LLC." August 10, 2009. http://www.fda.gov/ICECI/EnforcementActions/WarningLetters/ucm177398.htm (accessed October 19, 2009).

U.S. Food and Drug Administration. "What Is a Serious Adverse Event?" Safety, updated February 9, 2010. http://www.fda.gov/Safety/MedWatch/HowToReport/ucm053087.htm (accessed February 13, 2010).

U.S. Food and Drug Administration. "Women's Health Initiatives." 2003. http://www.fda.gov/cder/audiences/women/default.htm (accessed February 27, 2003).

U.S. Food and Drug Administration. Center for Biologics Evaluation and Research. Division of Vaccines and Related Products Applications. "Regulatory Perspective on Development of Preventive Vaccines for Global Infectious Diseases." By Rosemary Tiernan, October 30, 2007. http://www.fda.gov/downloads/BiologicsBloodVaccines/NewsEvents/WorkshopsMeetingsConferences/UCM106632.pdf (accessed February 10, 2010).

U.S. Food and Drug Administration. Center for Devices and Radiological Health. *Information Sheet Guidance for IRBs, Clinical Investigators, and Sponsors: Significant Risk and Nonsignificant Risk Medical Device Studies*. January 2006. http://www.fda.gov/ScienceResearch/SpecialTopics/RunningClinicalTrials/GuidancesInformationSheetsandNotices/ucm118082.htm (accessed February 9, 2010).

U.S. Food and Drug Administration. Center for Devices and Radiological Health. "Learn If a Medical Device Has Been Cleared by FDA for Marketing." April 30, 2009. http://www.fda.gov/MedicalDevices/ResourcesforYou/Consumers/ucm142523.htm (accessed February 9, 2010).

U.S. Food and Drug Administration. Center for Drug Evaluation and Research. *CDER 2001 Report to the Nation: Improving Public Health through Human Drugs*. 2001. http://www.fda.gov/cder/reports/rtn/2001/rtn2001.pdf (accessed January 28, 2004).

U.S. Food and Drug Administration. Center for Drug Evaluation and Research. *CDER 2002 Report to the Nation: Drug Safety and Quality*. 2002. http://www.fda.gov/cder/reports/rtn/2002/rtn2002-3.HTM#DrugRecallsandWithdrawals (accessed January 16, 2006).

U.S. Food and Drug Administration. Center for Drug Evaluation and Research. *CDER 2005 Report to the Nation*. 2005. http://www.fda.gov/downloads/AboutFDA/CentersOffices/CDER/WhatWeDo/UCM078935.pdf (accessed September 17, 2009).

U.S. Food and Drug Administration. Center for Drug Evaluation and Research. "Dr. Woodcock Provides Highlights of Her Detail: Implementing Quality Systems, Collaboration with NIH Top List." By Janet Woodcock, *News along the Pike* 10, no. 1 (2004). http://www.fda.gov/ohrms/dockets/dockets/04p0171/04p-0171-cp00001-04-exhibit-3.pdf (accessed October 18, 2009).

U.S. Food and Drug Administration. Center for Drug Evaluation and Research. "A Tool to Help You Decide: Detect Potentially Serious Liver Injury." By Ted Guo, Kate Gelperin, and John Senior, June 4, 2008. http://www.fda.gov/downloads/Drugs/ScienceResearch/ResearchAreas/ucm076777.pdf (accessed November 19, 2009).

U.S. Food and Drug Administration. Center for Food Safety and Applied Nutrition. *The Story of the Laws behind the Labels*. June 1981. http://vm.cfsan.fda.gov/~lrd/history1.html#toc (accessed November 28, 2005).

U.S. Food and Drug Administration, Howard University, et al. "Deadly Diseases and People of Color: Are Clinical Trials an Option?" 1996. http://www.fda.gov/oashi/patrip/howard.html (accessed January 25, 2004).

U.S. Food and Drug Administration. Office of Regulatory Affairs. "Disqualified/Restricted/Assurances Lists for Clinical Investigators." November 21, 2001. http://www.fda.gov/ora/compliance_ref/bimo/dis_res_assur.htm (accessed September 14, 2003).

U.S. Food and Drug Administration. Oliva, Armando, Randy Levin, Rachel Behrman, and Janet Woodcock. "Bioinformatics Modernization and the Critical Path to Improved Benefit-Risk Assessment of Drugs." Presentation at the 25th Annual DIA Clinical Data Management Meeting, Medical Informatics Opportunities to Improve the Benefit-Risk Assessment of Drugs, March 19, 2007. http://www.fda.gov/ScienceResearch/SpecialTopics/CriticalPathInitiative/ArticlesandPresentations/ucm077542.htm (accessed September 16, 2009).

U.S. Food and Drug Administration. Press Office. "FDA Proposes Rule on Women in Clinical Trials." FDA Talk Paper, September 23, 1997. http://www.fda.gov/bbs/topics/ANSWERS/ANS00822.html (accessed May 3, 2004).

U.S. General Accounting Office. *Report to Congressional Requesters: Women's Health—Women Sufficiently Represented in New Drug Testing, but FDA Oversight Needs Improvement*. Washington, DC: U.S. General Accounting Office, 2001. GAO-01-754. Also available at: http://www.gao.gov/new.items/d01754.pdf.

U.S. House Committee on Energy and Commerce. Subcommittee on Oversight and Investigations. "Ketek Fact Chronology." U.S. Food and Drug Administration Office of Criminal Investigations Investigative Work Product in Ketek Hearing Exhibit Binder, August 23, 2009. http://archives.energycommerce.house.gov/Investigations/KetekExhibitBinder/12001.pdf (accessed October 17, 2009).

U.S. Senate Committee on Finance. Memorandum from Senator Chuck Grassley regarding the Union of Concerned Scientists Survey of FDA Scientists. July 20, 2006. http://www.ucsusa.org/assets/documents/scientific_integrity/FDA-7-20-06-Grassley-press-statement.pdf http://www.ucsusa.org/scientific_integrity/abuses_of_science/summary-of-the-FDA-scientist.html (accessed December 1, 2009).

U.S. Senate Committee on Veterans' Affairs. "Is Military Research Hazardous to Veterans?" 1994. ttp://www.datafilter.com/mc/militaryHumanExperimentationReport94.html (accessed January 16, 2006.)

Uttley, Lois, and Ronnie Pawelko. "No Strings Attached: Public Funding of Religiously Sponsored Hospitals in the U.S." MergerWatch Project of Family Planning Advocates of N.Y.S., 2001. Also available at http://www.edfundfpa.org/publications/briefing_papers.html.

Vaniqa Web site, November 9, 2004. http://www.vaniqa.com (accessed with Wayback Machine, web.archive.org, February 21, 2007).

Varmus, Harold, and David Satcher. "Ethical Complexities of Conducting Research in Developing Countries." *New England Journal of Medicine* 337, no. 14 (1997): 1003–5.

Vaught, Jimmie V., Nicole Lockhart, Karen S. Thiel, and Julie A. Schneider. "Ethical, Legal, and Policy Issues: Dominating the Biospecimen Discussion." *Cancer Epidemiology, Biomarkers & Prevention* 16, no. 12 (2007). http://cebp.aacrjournals.org/content/16/12/2521.full (accessed November 28, 2009).

Vergano, Dan. "Drug Trials Vex Medical Ethics—Academic Experts Put Testing by Private Companies under a Microscope." *USA Today*, August 8, 2000.

Viagra Web site. http://www.viagra.com.

Vogelson, Cullen T. "The Book of Knowledge." *Modern Drug Design* 4, no. 8 (August 2001): 25–26.

Vogelson, Cullen T. "Happy Trials to You." *Modern Drug Discovery* 4, no. 12 (December 2001): 21–22, 24. http://pubs.acs.org/subscribe/journals/mdd/v04/i12/html/12clinical.html (accessed January 9, 2002).

Vogelson, Cullen T. "The Investigational Review Process." *Modern Drug Discovery* 4, no. 5 (May 2001): 27–31. http://pubs.acs.org/subscribe/journals/mdd/v04/i05/html/05clinical.html (accessed January 31, 2002).

Vogelson, Cullen T. "Investigators Gone Bad." *Modern Drug Discovery* 4, no. 4 (April 2001): 27–30. http://pubs.acs.org/subscribe/journals/mdd/v04/i04/html/MDD04DeptRules.html (accessed January 31, 2002).

Vogelson, Cullen T. "Participating in Clinical Research." *Modern Drug Discovery* 4, no. 1 (January 2001): 15–16. http://pubs.acs.org/subscribe/journals/mdd/v04/i01/html/clinical.html (accessed January 21, 2002).

Vogelson, Cullen T. "Research Practices and Ethics." *Modern Drug Discovery* 4, no. 4 (April 2001): 23–24. http://pubs.acs.org/subscribe/journals/mdd/v04/i04/html/MDD04DeptClinical.html (accessed January 21, 2002).

Vogelson, Cullen T. "Seeking the Perfect Protocol." *Modern Drug Discovery* 4, no. 7 (July 2001): 21–24. http://pubs.acs.org/subscribe/journals/mdd/v04/i07/html/07clinical.html (accessed January 21, 2002).

Volberding, Paul A., and Joseph R. Dalovisio. "The Impact of Ideology on NIH Research." Letter to Tommy G. Thompson, Secretary of Health and Human Services, U.S. Department of Health and Human Services from the Infectious Diseases Society of America, 2003. http://www.idsociety.org/Content.aspx?id=4474 (accessed February 17, 2010).

Vulcano, David. "Healthcare Reform: Opportunities and Challenges for the Clinical Research Enterprise." Presentation at the MAGI Clinical Research Conference–West 2009, San Diego, CA, October 2009.

Wahlberg, David. "Public Health Tailored to Bush Line, Critics Charge." *Atlanta Journal and Constitution* (GA), August 3, 2003. http://www.allbusiness/government/government-bodies-offices/10369712-1.html (accessed February 15, 2010).

Waldman, R. H., et al. "Secretory Antibody Following Oral Influenza Immunization." *American Journal of the Medical Sciences* 292, no. 6 (1986): 367–371.

Waterman, Paula. "Institutional Review Boards." IRB Forum 2001. http://www.irbforum.org/documents/documents/FDAvICH56.rtf (accessed July 15, 2005).

Weiner, Dan, and Mark Hovde. "Critical Mass for Critical Path?" *Pharmaceutical Executive*, May 1, 2007. http://pharmexec.findpharma.com/pharmexec/Regulatory+Articles/Critical-Mass-for-Critical-Path/ArticleStandard/Article/detail/423202 (August 22, 2009).

Weisman, Carol, and Sandra D. Cassard. "Health Consequences of Exclusion or Underrepresentation of Women in Clinical Studies." In *Women and Health Research: Ethical and Legal Issues of Including Women in Clinical Studies*, vol. 2, edited by Anna C. Mastroianni, Ruth Faden, and Daniel Federman. Institute of Medicine. Washington, DC: National Academy Press, 1994. http://books.nap.edu/catalog/2343.html (accessed January 16, 2006).

Weiss, R. "NIH Clears Most Researchers in Conflict-of-Interest Probe." *Washington Post*, February 22, 2005, national edition, sec. 1. Also available at http://www.washingtonpost.com.

Weiss, R. "U.S. Halts Research on Humans at Duke; University Can't Ensure Safety, Probers Find." *Washington Post*, May 12, 1999. http://www.washingtonpost.com (accessed January 7, 2004).

Wellcome Trust. *Opinion Formers' Conference on Counterfeit Medicines: Perspectives and Action*. Conference report and briefing, Wellcome Trust,

2009. http://www.wellcome.ac.uk/About-us/Policy/Spotlight-issues/Counterfeit-medicines/index.htm (accessed November 22, 2009).

Wenzel, Richard P. "The Antibiotic Pipeline—Challenges, Costs, and Values." *New England Journal of Medicine* 351 (2004): 523–26.

Wechsler, Jill. "Fraud, Abuse, and Consent." *Applied Clinical Trials* 11 (2002): 28. http://appliedclinicaltrialsonline.findpharma.com/appliedclinicaltrials/View+from+Washington/Fraud-Abuse-and-consent/ArticleStandard/Article/detail/87048 (accessed September 20, 2009).

Wechsler, Jill. "Health Information Technology Offers Both Promise and Problems: Biomedical Research Community Finds Privacy Policies Add Cost and Complexity to Clinical Studies." *Applied Clinical Trials*, April 1, 2009. http://appliedclinicaltrialsonline.findpharma.com/appliedclinicaltrials/US/Health-IT-Offers-Both-Promise-and-Problems/ArticleStandard/Article/detail/591990 (accessed November 4, 2009).

Weinfurt, Mark A. Hall, Nancy M.P. King, Joëlle Y. Friedman, Kevin A. Schulman, and Jeremy Sugarman. "Disclosure of Financial Relationships to Participants in Clinical Research." *New England Journal of Medicine* 361, no. 9 (2009): 916–921. http://content.nejm.org/cgi/content/full/361/9/916 (accessed November 23, 2009).

Wilkinson, Emma. "Teens 'Miss Out' on Cancer Trials." BBC News, Health, November 28, 2008. http://news.bbc.co.uk/2/hi/health/7753283.stm (accessed November 9, 2009).

Williams, John R. "The 2008 Declaration of Helsinki." Presentation at Witwatersrand Medical University, March 19, 2009. http://web.wits.ac.za/NR/rdonlyres/9A4CDFCC-9E5A-4DB9-ADC4-0CD165D1DEE5/0/Helsinkideclaration2008.pdf (accessed November 7, 2009).

Willman, David. "Stealth Merger: Drug Companies and Government Medical Research." *Los Angeles Times*, December 7, 2003. http://www.sunspot.net/business/la-na-nih7dec07,1,7031831.story (accessed September 12, 2004).

Wilson, Duff, and Natasha Singer. "Ghostwriting Is Called Rife in Medical Journals." *New York Times*, September 11, 2009, sec. Business. http://www.nytimes.com/2009/09/11/business/11ghost.html (accessed November 2009).

Wilson, James. "Lessons Learned from the Gene Therapy Trial for Ornithine Transcarbamylase Deficiency." *Molecular Genetics and Metabolism* 96, no. 4 (2009), doi:10.1016/j.ymgme.2008.12.016. http://linkinghub.elsevier.com/retrieve/pii/S109671920800499X (accessed December 3, 2009).

Witty, Andrew. "Open Labs, Open Minds: Breaking Down Barriers to Innovation and Access to Medicines and Vaccines in the Developing World." Speech, Council on Foreign Relations, New York, January 20, 2010. http://www.gsk.com/media/Open-innovation-strategy-transcript-English-20jan2010.pdf.

Wood, Alastair J. J. "The Safety of New Medicines: The Importance of Asking the Right Questions." *Journal of the American Medical Association* 281, no. 18 (1999), doi:10.1001/jama.281.18.1753. http://jama.ama-assn.org/cgi/content/full/281/18/1753 (accessed February 9, 2010).

Woolhandler, S., T. Campbell, and D. U. Himmelstein. "Costs of Health Care Administration in the United States and Canada." *New England Journal of Medicine* 349, no. 8 (2003): 768–75.

Woollen, Stan W. "Misconduct in Research—Innocent Ignorance or Malicious Malfeasance?" FDA, 2003. http://www.fda.gov/oc/gcp/slideshows/2003/gcp2003.ppt (accessed October 17, 2009).

Woollen, Stan W., and Antoine El Hage. "Scientific Misconduct—the 'F' Word." FDA, October 1, 2001. http://www.fda.gov/oc/gcp/slideshows/misconduct2001/misconduct.html (accessed February 17, 2003).

World Bank. "Poverty—Overview." PovertyNet, 2009. http://go.worldbank.org/RQBDCTUXW0.

World Health Organization. "Epidemic Meningitis in Africa." 1997. http://www.who.int/archives/inf-pr-1997/en/pr97-11.html (accessed March 3, 2003).

World Health Organization. "The Impact of Implementation of ICH Guidelines in Non-ICH Countries." 2001. http://www.who.int/medicines/library/qsm/who-edm-qsm-2002-3/who-edm-qsm-2002-3.pdf (accessed July 14, 2005).

World Health Organization. "International Clinical Trials Registry Platform (ICTRP)." http://www.who.int/ictrp/network/trds/en/index.html (accessed November 10, 2009).

World Health Organization. *Operational Guidelines for Ethics Committees That Review Biomedical Research.* 2000. http://www.who.int/tdr/publications/publications/ethics.htm (accessed February 7, 2004).

World Medical Association. "International Code of Medical Ethics." 1949. http://history.nih.gov/history/laws/ICME.html (accessed February 7, 2004).

World Medical Association. *World Medical Association Declaration of Helsinki: Ethical Principles for Medical Research Involving Human Subjects.* 2004 (1964). http://www.wma.net/e/policy/b3.htm (accessed January 2, 2006).

Writing Group for the Women's Health Initiative Investigators. "Risks and Benefits of Estrogen plus Progestin in Healthy Postmenopausal Women: Principal Results from the Women's Health Initiative Randomized Controlled Trial." *Journal of the American Medical Association* 288, no. 3 (2002): 321–33.

Young, Donna. "FDA's Monitoring of Postmarketing Studies Probed." *American Journal of Health-System Pharmacists' News*, August 15, 2006. http://www.ashp.org/import/News/HealthSystemPharmacyNews/newsarticle.aspx?id=2273 (accessed February 9, 2010).

Zall, Milton. "The Pricing Puzzle." *Modern Drug Discovery* 4, no. 3 (March 2001): 36–42. http://pubs.acs.org/subscribe/journals/mdd/v04/i03html/03zall.html (accessed January 31, 2002).

Zandocomm. "Swine Flu Pandemic, 2009: Anglo-American Genocide Part I and Part II." News Worldwide blog posted June 23, 2009. http://newsworldwide.wordpress.com/2009/06/23/swine-flu-pandemic-2009-anglo-american-genocide-part-i-and-part-ii/ (accessed February 9, 2010).

Zisson, Steve. "Anticipating a Clinical Investigator Shortfall." *CenterWatch* 1 (2001): 1.

Zuckerman, Brad. "Medical Device Development and Regulation: An FDA Perspective." Duke Clinical Research Institute, 2007. http://comm.dcri.duke.edu/video/ctn/acc07_zuckerman/ (accessed February 9, 2010).

Zuckerman, Diana. "There's No Such Thing as Free Viagra." National Research Center for Women and Families, January 2006. http://www.center4research.org/news/viagra.html.

Index

A

Abbott, 222
abuse
  allegations of, 104, 118, 248, 312, 375
  by Department of Defense, 251
  of information, 164
access denial, 106
accountability. *See* drug accountability; Health Insurance Portability and Accountability Act (HIPAA)
accreditation systems, 133, 279–280, 319
Achebe, Chidi Chike, 312
ACHRE Report, 252
ACIP (Advisory Committee on Immunization Practices), 32
acquiring your first study
  approaches to, 48–49
  difficulties of, 53–55
  new methods for, 49–51
  requirements for, 45–47
activities. *See* study activities
acts, legislative. *See* legislation
Adams, Vincanne, 157
adaptive clinical trials, 223
adjuvent drugs, 30, 36
administering/dispensing drugs, 70, 129, 130, 183, 202, 213
administrative issues
  costs, 93, 240–241
  IRB fees, 78, 88–89
  starting the study, 236
administrative support, 69
adminstering/dispensing drugs, 70, 129, 130, 183, 202, 213
adverse audits, 141
adverse drug reactions (ADRs)
  in children, 254
  failure to report, 142
  frequency, 239
adverse effects algorithm, 210
adverse events (AEs). *See also* serious adverse events (SAEs)
  adverse experience or effect versus, 207
  attributing causality, 272
  classifying, 258, 261
  disincentives for reporting, 209
  documentation of, 206–211
  ethical issues, 271–274
  International Serious Adverse Events Consortium (SAEC), 161
  missing, 272
  no observable adverse effect level (NOAEL), 12
  reporting, 136, 137, 206–211
  time and budgeting required for, 89–90
  Vaccine Adverse Events Reporting Systems (VAERS), 32–33
advertising. *See also* recruiting participants
  approach to, 177–178
  approval of materials, 78, 170–171
  centralized venues, 172–173
  costs, 92
  deceptive, 278
  direct-to-consumer, 326
  example ads, 172, 173, 283, 284
  FDA warning letters, 173
  online, 175–176
  requirements and regulations, 171–172
Advisory Committee on Human Radiation Experiments, 353
Advisory Committee on Immunization Practices (ACIP), 32
AEs. *See* adverse events (AEs)
Africa, 157, 312, 319
African Americans, 176, 311
AIDS. *See also* HIV
  denial of treatment options with, 302

AIDS (*continued*)
development of treatments, 42
lag in research on, 325
President's Emergency Plan for AIDS Relief (PEPFAR), 331
racial perceptions and, 312
trial participation in South Africa, 323
vaccine research, 29
ALCOA elements, 163, 231
Allergan, 327
allocation of resources, 324–325, 338–339
Altman, Douglas, 276
American Academy of Pediatrics, 254
American Academy of Pharmaceutical Physicians, 341
Amgen, 106
Anan, Kofi, 335
Andrews, Lori, 266
Angell, Marcia, 326
animal testing, 220
announcing your study, 172
antibiotics
appropriate use of, 234
classes of, 41
free programs, 326
generic, 269
indiscriminate prescribing of, 120
overseas trials, 317–318
problems with development of, 41–43, 233–234
resistance to, 179, 326
for resistant organisms, 42, 318
return on investment in researching, 221
safety of approved, 287
side effects of, 259, 287
unnecessary, 210, 288
antidiscrimination laws, 154
antikickback statutes, 82
applications
Biologics License Applications (BLA), 225–227
Investigational Device Exemption (IDE), 24
Investigational New Drug (IND), 11, 24
New Drug Applications (NDAs), 13, 52, 131, 218, 317
submission deadlines, 78
Applied Research Ethics National Association (ARENA), 124–125
apprenticeships, 48, 342
approaching patients, 178–179
approvals
antibiotics approval, 41
approval packages from IRBs, 79
approval process concerns, 16
compassionate use approvals, 22
fast-tracking, 217
H1N1 flu vaccine approval, 36–37
IRB submission packets, 78
approvals (*continued*)
seals of approval, 19–20
TeGenero trial, 360
archiving procedures, 182
ARENA (Applied Research Ethics National Association), 124–125
Asia, 142
assent
ability to give, 370
by children, 254
definition, 246
documentation of, 150
assessing literacy, 155–156
Association for the Accreditation of Human Research Protection Programs (AAHRP), 133, 279–280, 319
Association of Academic Health Centers(AAHC), 126
Association of American Medical Colleges, 225–227, 342
Astra Zeneca, 322
audits
consequences of adverse, 141
FDA, 132–135
for-cause, 140–141
informed consent focus, 135, 137–138
by institutional review boards (IRBs), 142
international, 142
mock compliance, 192
preparing for, 143–145
responding to, 134
sponsor, 141
time required for, 91
triggers for, 56
types of, 132–142
authorization waivers, 125, 126, 128, 129, 151
autonomy, 315
AZT trials, 321–322

B

back-loading costs, 93
bacterial infections, 42, 179, 318, 326. *See also* antibiotics; neglected tropical diseases (NTDs)
bait-and-switch clauses, 95
"balance on hand" logs, 130
bankruptcies, 102
baseline examination findings, 208
Bayer Corporation, 269
Belmont Report *(Ethical Principles and Guidelines for the Protection of Human Subjects of Research)*, 246, 247, 248–257, 251, 301, 373–374, 375–384

beneficence principle, 249–250, 377–378, 382–383
benefit/risk dilemma, 16, 34, 39, 110, 134, 151, 178–180
benefits
as coercion, 167
to community, 340
describing, 176
expectation of, 115, 124, 149
HIPAA rules on, 129
to patients, 18, 123
to sponsors, 100, 104, 131
best practices
best current tests and therapies, 320
Clinical Trials Networks (CTN) Best Practices, 86, 182, 187
NCI Best Practices for Biospecimen Resources, 267–268
Betty Dong affair, 104, 114, 276
biased language, 361
bias in publishing results, 276–277, 301
billing for clinical trials, 80–82, 183, 191–192
binders, study, 159–160
biohazardous materials, shipping, 191
biologics, 10, 28–37, 251
Biologics License Applications (BLA), 225–227
Biomarker Initiative, 224
bioterrorism agents, development of drugs for, 32
BIO Ventures for Global Health, 332
bird flu, 269–270
birth defects, 304
BLA (Biologics License Applications), 225–227
blacklists, 141
blinded studies, 21, 22, 25, 130, 187
Bloomberg Markets, 281
Blumenfeld, Tracy, 111, 231–232
Boots Pharmaceutical, 104
Boston Women's Health Collective, 300
bottlenecks, breaking, 225–228
Brazil, 239
Bristol-Myers Squibb, 42
British cancer trials, 256
British health authorities, 297
British Medical Journal, 277
brokerage fees, 97
brokers, on-line, 49, 51–52
Brownstein, Larry, 102
budget feasibility/costs
by activity, 92–94
advertising, 92
brokerage fees, 97
cost anticipation, 84
data collection, 205
delays in approvals, 218
budget feasibility/costs (*continued*)
equipment/supplies, 88
by evaluability, 94–96
hidden costs, 83
income allocation, 338–339
IRB preparation time, 88–89
laboratory costs, 87, 191
of large trials, 235
Medicare coverage for routine, 80–81
miscellaneous costs, 91–92
overhead costs, 93
overseas trials, 240–241
overview of issues, 83–84
paperwork, 90
paradigm shifts affecting, 109–110
payment schedules, 100–101, 112, 262
per-patient costs, 219
Pharmaceutical Information Cost Assessment Service (PICAS), 84–85
pharmacy costs, 87–88
questions to ask, 70
radiology and special studies costs, 89
reduction of, 229
research and development, 220
site-sponsor meetings, 90–91
staff costs, 96–97
start-up costs, 91, 93–94
worksheets, 96
Bureau of Labor Statistics, 337
Bush, George H. W., 295
Bush, George W., 295
Byrd, Jack, 189

C

Career Guide to Industries, 337
case report forms (CRFs), 90, 135, 142, 143, 187, 203–205, 215, 232
cash flow problems, 101
Castro, Fidel, 39–40
Catalona, William, 266–267
catastrophic outcomes, 106–107
Catholic healthcare institutions, 307–310
Ceh, Eric, 200
Center for Biologics Evaluation and Research (CBER), 28
Center for Cancer Research NCI Experimental Therapeutics (NExT) program, 222
Center for Devices and Radiological Health (CDRH), 10, 25
Center for Drug Evaluation and Research (CDER), 10, 25, 297–298
Center for Gynepathology Research, 307
Center for Information and Study on Clinical Research Participation (CISCRP), 175, 197

Centers for Disease Control (CDC), 32
CenterWatch, 220, 338–339
CER (comparative effective research), 224–225
Certified Physician Investigator examination, 341
checklists
  feasibility, 69
  Informed Consent Form Requirements, 148
  IRB communications, 212
  IRB submission checklist, 77, 78
  Regulatory Binder Contents, 159
  Study Closeout Checklist, 213
chemical agent testing, 251
chemistry and manufacturing controls (CMC), 31
chemotherapy case study, 286–287
"Chicken Man," 212
children as subjects, 245–246, 252–255, 317, 354
Children without Worms program, 335
China, 316, 317
CIOMS (Council of the International Organizations of Medical Sciences), 247
CISCRP (Center for Information and Study on Clinical Research Participation), 175, 197
clauses. *See also* contracts
  bait-and-switch, 95
  confidentiality, 67, 103, 108
  incentives for discoveries, 112
  indemnification, 105–107, 108–109
  inventions, 104
  meaningful use, 119
  no-fault compensation, 108
  patents and inventions, 110
  pay for performance, 119–120
  payment, 101
  publication of studies, 103–105
  rights of ownership, 103–104, 269
  to watch out for, 100
Clay, John, 205
clinical practice
  enhancement of, 338–339
  good clinical practices (GCPs), 59, 113
  individual research practice, 258
  practice guidelines, 277–278
  practice/research boundaries, 375–376
  transferring research findings to, 29
clinical research
  articles explaining, 339
  benefits to community, 340
  definition of, 5
  NIAID-sponsored, 29
  reasons for conducting, 3–4, 338
  requirements for, 26
clinical research associates (CRAs)
  career outlook, 337
  courting, 60
  documentation of visits, 202
  information required by, 61–62
  loss of clout of, 48–49
  meeting with, 57, 340
  roles of, 7
  training for, 99
clinical research (or study) coordinators (CRCs), 6, 45–46, 74–75, 337
Clinical Research Information Exchange (CRIX), 120
Clinical Research Summit report, 225–227
Clinical Research Terminology (CRT), 83
clinical trial agreements (CTAs), 105
clinical trials industry, 236–237, 237–241, 238, 241
Clinical Trials Networks Best Practices (CTNBP), 86, 182, 187
Clinical Trials Registry, 116–117, 355
Clinical Trials Transformation Initiative (CTTI), 116, 117
Clinton, Bill, 153, 252, 295
closing the study, 212–215
clothing, appropriate, 174–175
CMC (chemistry and manufacturing controls), 31
coauthoring a study, 52
Code of Federal Regulations, 5–7, 45, 123–124, 125
coercion, 106, 167, 245–246, 251, 316
collaboration
  among hospitals, 175
  among pharmaceuticals companies, 42–43, 224
  among research programs, 222
  benefits of, 43
  development of, 269, 291
  disincentives for, 266
  funding for, 227
  public/private, 259–260
  reasons for, 111
  research and development (R&D), 332, 333
commercial institutional review boards (IRBs), 76, 123, 124, 280–281
Common Rule (Federal Policy for the Protection of Human Subjects), 248
community clinicians, 63
community versus university sites, 64–65
comparative effective research (CER), 224–225
compassionate use trials, 21–22, 285–286
compensation arrangements with sponsors, 130–131
competing studies, 60, 61, 158
complaint databases, MAUDE, 26

compliance (patient), 43, 69–70, 143, 183, 198, 381
compliance (study)
  audit, 192
  billing, 191
  coding, 191
  Compliance Program Guidance Manual (FDA), 143
  with Declaration of Helsinki, 117, 321
  documentation, 82
  FDA Compliance, Enforcement, and Criminal Investigations, 143
  GCP, 54
  with HIPAA, 54
  ICH, 117, 151
  IRB, 162
  noncompliant data, 118
  penalties and obligations, 81
  plans, 133–134
  SOP, 184
Compliance Program Guidance Manual (FDA), 143
concomitant (con) medications, 199–200
confidentiality, 67, 103, 108
Confidentiality Letter or Nondisclosure Agreement, 67
conflicts of interest (COIs), 131, 258–262, 274–275, 281
consent. *See* informed consent
consistency, 64
Consolidated Standards of Reporting Trials (CONSORT), 276–277
consulting fees, 260
contamination of vaccines, 28, 31, 33, 38, 350
continuation of treatment, 310
contraception/contraceptives, 295, 296, 302, 306, 308–309, 313–315
contract research organizations (CROs), 7, 49, 94, 97–100
contracts. *See also* clauses
  equitable, 111
  facilities letters, 108–109
  fair terms, 112
  grant payment schedules, 100–102
  language, 110
  negotiations, 100, 110
  problems with, 109–110
  subject injuries, 107–108
  terms for start-ups, 102–103
  win-win, 110–111
controversies, mandatory vaccinations, 34, 37
costs. *See also* budget feasibility/costs
  of clinical trials, 217–221
  of delays in development, 56
  of nonproductive sites, 56
Council for Certification of IRB Professionals, 279
Council of the International Organizations of Medical Sciences (CIOMS), 247
Council on Foreign Relations, 332
counterfeit drugs, 38, 241, 350
country attractiveness index, 238
covered entities, 128
cowpox vaccine, 33
CPI (Critical Path Initiative), 25, 221, 354
CPM (Critical Path Method), 189
CPT (Current Procedural Terminology) codes, 83
CRAs. *See* clinical research associates (CRAs)
Crawford, Lester, 295
CRCs (clinical research coordinators), 6
CRFs. *See* case report forms (CRFs)
criteria, 73, 161–162, 239, 264
Critical Path Initiative (CPI), 25, 221, 354
Critical Path Method (CPM), 189
CRIX (Clinical Research Information Exchange), 120
CRO Capability Assessment Service (CROCAS), 85
CROs. *See* contract research organizations (CROs)
cross-cultural issues, 156–157
cross-indemnification, 105
crossover study designs, 20, 21
CTAs (clinical trial agreements), 105
CTTI (Clinical Trials Transformation Initiative), 116, 117
Cuba, 39–40
cued literacy, 155
cultural competency, 312–313
  cultural issues/beliefs
  African cultures, 157
  cross-cultural issues, 156–157
  cultural competency, 312–313
  recruitment and, 240
  staff training in, 313
Current Procedural Terminology (CPT) codes, 83
Cutting Edge, 228, 229
CYPHER Sirolimus-Eluting Coronary Stent, 26

D

Dalton, Claudette, 154
DALY (disability-adjusted life year) metric, 328, 329, 332–333
Data Clarification or Query form, 204
data/databases
  acceptance of foreign, 117–119
  collection procedures, 182
  data mining, 53–55

Data Safety Monitoring Boards (DSMBs), 7, 14, 17, 274–275, 279
electronic data capture (EDC), 230–232
errors of, 232
noncompliant, 118
Pharmaceutical Information Cost Assessment Service (PICAS), 84–85
posting summary results, 275
sharing of, 224
trial registry in public, 320
Davenport, Suzanne, 106, 358
DCTD (Division of Cancer Treatment and Diagnosis), 222
DeAngelis, Catherine, 276, 277
death of patients, 271, 284, 285–290, 299
decision points, 236
Declaration of Helsinki, 108, 238, 246, 247, 317, 320, 321, 322, 351, 362–363, 367–372
delays, 218, 236
delegation of tasks, 110, 121, 133–134, 137, 151, 245, 258
DeRenzo, Evan, 259
designer drugs, 325
developing countries, 113–114, 315–324
development of vaccines, 28–37
devices, 22–24, 25
device (medical) trials, 22–28
Dickersin, Kay, 114
diethylstilbestrol (DES), 304
dilemmas, ethical, 287–290
Dingell, John D., 298
direct-to-consumer (DTC) advertising, 326
disability-adjusted life year (DALY) metric, 328, 329, 332–333
disaster planning, 200–202
disclosures, 130–132, 260–261, 380–381
disease creation, 327
disincentives, 209, 263, 272
dispensing drugs, 70, 129, 130, 183, 202, 213
disposal of drugs/records, 136, 183, 215
distributive justice principle, 250, 253, 302, 315
Division of Cancer Treatment and Diagnosis (DCTD), 222
DNA sequencing study, 316
DNA vaccines, 30
DNDi (Drugs for Neglected Diseases Initiative), 334, 335
Doctors Without Borders, 331, 332, 335
documentation
adverse events, 206–211
of assent, 150
audits of, 136
case report forms (CRFs), 90, 135, 142, 143, 187, 203–205, 215
documentation (*continued*)
collection of forms from patients, 203–204
of consent, 157
CRA visits, 202
dispensing drugs, 213
for drug accountability, 128
Drug Accountability or Dispensing Log, 130
electronic medical records (EMRs), 161–164
exceptions to protocols to, 185–186
falsification of, 139
Form FDA 483, 140
obtaining informed consent, 151–152
other medications taken, 199
outcome logs, 186
paperwork management, 186–188
of patient symptoms, 208
poor, 141
procedures for, 183
regulatory (study) binders, 159–160
retaining study records, 214
safety reports, 212–213
site-sponsor, 184
source documents, 202–203
Specimen Shipping Log, 190
of sponsor-site communications, 213
storage of, 215
worksheets/forms/folders, 186–189
of your experience, 58–59, 60
donations (funds/supplies), 39, 268, 269, 270, 329
donations, tissue, 249, 267, 376
Dong, Betty, 104, 114, 276
dose-finding phase of study, 12–13
double-blind studies, 21, 22
double dipping, 82
double-dummy studies, 20–21
dropping patients from trials, 220, 285
Drug Abuse Control Amendments, 40
drug accountability
auditing of records, 135
in blinded studies, 130
documentation, 128
drug storage, 192–193
recordkeeping, 129
supply inventories, 193–194
verification of shipping, 129
drug development (in general)
compared to device development, 25
historical timeline of, 350–355
phase 0 trials, 222, 223
phase 1 trials, 11–12, 283, 320, 338–339
phase 2 trials, 12–13
phase 3 trials, 13–14
phase 4 trials, 14–16

drug development (in general) (*continued*)
priority drugs, 253
process for, 26
social justice issues of, 325–329
success rates, 218
drug development trial phases
early development, 11
initiation phase, 159
preclinical, 12
summary of, 10, 12
time line of, 11
drug interactions, 199
drugs
access to, 325
dispensing, 70, 129, 130, 183, 202, 213
off-label use, 278–279
patented versus generic, 278
permission to give to humans, 11
side effects, 212
storage of, 192–193
symptom-modifying, 200
tracking difficulties, 130
withdrawn, 15
Drugs and Cosmetics Rules (India), 322
Drugs for Neglected Diseases Initiative (DNDi), 334, 335
Drug Study Announcement Memo, 172
DSMBs (Data Safety Monitoring Boards), 7, 14, 17, 274–275, 279
DTC (direct-to-consumer) advertising, 326
Duff commission, 282–283
Duke University, 238
Durham-Humphrey amendment, 351

E

EDC (electronic data capture), 230–232
eDISH (electronic tool for drug-induced serious hepatotoxicity), 233
efficacy trials, 26, 31
elderly patients, 256–257
electronic data capture (EDC), 230–232
electronic medical records (EMRs), 116, 119, 161–164
electronic tool for drug-induced serious hepatotoxicity (eDISH), 233
Eli Lilly and Company, 316
Emanuel, Ezekiel J., 281
emergency codes, for blinded studies, 21
emergency preparedness, 200–202, 354
emerging infections, 334
employees. *See* staff/team members
end of therapy (EOT) phase of study, 10
enrollment phase of study, 10
enrollment procedures, 183
EOT (end of therapy) phase of study, 10
equipment/supplies, 46, 88, 182, 193–194
equitable contracts, 111
ERDs (Ethical and Religious Directives), 310
errors
billing, 81–82
contracting for too many patients, 73
data, 232
FDA audit findings, 136
fraud versus, 138–139
judgment, 284
liability for, 105–107
signature, 138
e-source documents, 230–231
Ethical and Religious Directives (ERDs), 310
ethical issues
absolute versus situational ethics, 324
access to care/new therapies, 319
adverse events, 271–274
business versus patients, 267–268
challenging/exposing volunteers to infectious agents, 32
chemotherapy case study, 286–287
coercion, 106, 245–246, 251, 316
conflicts/dilemmas, 280, 287–290
conflicts of interest, 258–262
cross-cultural issues, 157
Data Safety Monitoring Boards (DSMBs), 274–275
developing countries, 240, 241, 247, 268, 269, 313, 314, 315–324
ethical development milestones, 247–248
Ethical Principles and Guidelines for the Protection of Human Subjects of Research (Belmont Report), 246, 247, 248–257, 301, 373–374, 375–384
financial incentives, 323
future considerations, 336
historical context, 241–247, 351
individual research practice, 258
IRB-related, 279–281
lack of safeguards, 318
mindfulness of, 68
misconduct and fraud, 182
Mrs. G case study, 285–290
NIH Office of Human Subjects, 243
nonfinancial ethic conflicts, 280
Nuremberg Code (*See* Nuremberg Code of Ethics)
off-label use, 278–279
patents versus public health, 268–270
patient-prompted, 270–271
practice guidelines, 277–278
pressure to cut corners, 263–264
publication-related, 275–277
reproductive technology as political tool, 315

ethical issues (*continued*)
  shifting studies to developing countries, 315–316
  special populations, 255–257
  tissue ownership, 265–267
  unanticipated risks, 281–285
  vulnerable populations, 250–255
Ethnic Factors in the Acceptability of Foreign Clinical Data, 118–119, 239
ethnic groups, 239
European Union, 13, 85, 239
evaluability, 94–96, 102
EVEREST II trial, 28
exceptions to protocols, 185–186
exclusion criteria, 161–162, 239
Executive Order 13505, 120–121
expenses. *See* budget feasibility/costs
experience, documenting your, 58–59, 60
exploratory IND studies, 221
Exploring the Biological Contributions to Human Health (IOM), 305

F

facilities letters, 108–109
failure to warn, 24
false claims, 82, 122
falsification of documents, 139
fast-tracking approvals, 217
fatalities, patient, 271, 284, 285–290, 299
FDA
  acceptance of foreign clinical trial data by, 117–119, 355
  Amendments Act, 14, 40, 230
  antibiotics approval, 41
  approval process concerns, 16
  audits by, 56, 118, 132–135
  Bioresearch Monitoring Program, 141
  BLA examination, 32
  Clinical Trials Registry, 116–117
  Clinical Trials Transformation Initiative (CTTI), 117, 355
  Code of Federal Regulations, 123–124
  compassionate use approvals, 22
  Compliance Program Guidance Manual, 143
  Critical Path Initiative (CPI), 354
  criticism of, 223
  design plan requirements, 26
  electronic medical records regulations, 163
  focus of, 40
  follow-up and enforcement by, 14
  Food and Drug Administration Act, 294
  Food and Drug Administration Amendments Act (FDAAA), 115, 116–117, 354
FDA (*continued*)
  Food and Drug Administration Modernization Act (FDAMA), 248, 253
  Food and Drugs Act, 38
  Form FDA 483, 140
  Form FDA 1572 (Statement of Investigator), 54, 78, 121–122, 130, 136, 281
  Guidance for Industry, 133
  H1N1 flu vaccine approval, 36–37
  misconceptions about, 238
  monitoring of foreign trials, 323–324
  patient selection criteria, 164
  politics of research and, 293–300
  recommendations made to, 233–234
  rejection of trial data, 234
  requirements for compliance with Declaration of Helsinki, 321
  roles of, 8
  Rule on Products to Treat Exposure to Toxic Substances, 354
  Sentinel Initiative, 116
  timeline of acts by, 350–355
  training for inspections by, 182–183
  updates to requirements, 122
  warning letters from, 133, 141, 143, 173, 299
feasibility
  checklist for, 69
  nonrandomized studies, 26
  overview, 67–68
  protocols (*See* protocols/protocol design)
  staff/team members, 73–74
Federal Coordinating Council for Comparative Effectiveness Research, 120
Federal Drug Administration. *See* FDA
federal hormone replacement trial, 17
Federal Investigator Registry of Biomedical Informatics Research Date (FIREBIRD), 233
Federal Policy for the Protection of Human Subjects (Common Rule), 248
fee-for-service structures, 262
feminism, 300
fetal cell use, 310
fialuridine (FIAU), 284, 299
Fiddes, Robert, 280–281
Final Rule, 118
financial disclosures, 130–132, 260–261
financial incentives, 323
financial issues. *See* budget feasibility/costs; funding
financial penalties for violations, 14–15
financial pressures, 258–262
finder's fees, 91

FIREBIRD (Federal Investigator Registry of Biomedical Informatics Research Date), 233
first studies
  approaches to finding, 48–49
  difficulties of attracting, 53–55
  new methods for attracting, 49–51
  requirements for finding, 45–47
flawed designs, 235
flu vaccines, 29, 31, 35, 269–270
folder contents, 188–189
follow-up visits, 193, 194–195, 196
Food and Drug Administration. *See* FDA
food service expenses, 91
for-cause audits, 140–141
foreign clinical trial data, FDA acceptance of, 117–119
foreign research, 237–241
formal training programs, 339–343
Form FDA 483, 140
Form FDA 1572 (Statement of Investigator), 54, 74, 121–122, 130, 136
forms. *See* documentation; worksheets
Frank, Julia Bess, 345–346
fraud, 38, 118, 138–139, 280–281
front-loading costs, 93
funding, 46, 324–325, 332–333
future use research, 269

G

gag orders, 275
Gambia, 319
Gantt charts, 189
GAO (U.S. General Accounting Office), 304, 305
Gates Foundation, 331–332
Gaucher's disease, 327
Gawande, Atul, 163
Gelsinger, Jesse, 106, 246–247, 357
gender issues
  bias, 301
  considerations of, 300
  differences attributable to, 305
  discrimination, 306
  disparities, 293
  gender differences, 305, 323
  gender/race overlap, 313, 314–315
  guidelines for, 304
  inequality, 314
  selection by gender, 124
  study design and, 254, 264
General Accounting Office (GAO), 304, 305
gene sequencing study, 316
gene therapy, 28
Genzyme, 327
Georgetown University, 273, 309–310
Getz, Kenneth, 85, 197
ghostwriters, 275–276
Gilead Sciences, 42
Glass, Harold, 56, 85, 86
GlaxoSmithKline (GSK), 36, 37, 322, 332, 333, 334–335
Global Fund, 332
GMP (good manufacturing practice), 31
Golde, David, 265–266
Goldfarb, Norman, 83, 127, 131, 182, 282, 304
Good Clinical Practice Guidelines (ICH), 321
good clinical practices (GCPs), 59, 113
good manufacturing practice (GMP), 31
Goodyear, Michael, 283, 321
government-sponsored research, 259
grants. *See also* budget feasibility/costs
  for device trials, 27
  for formal training, 343
  payment schedules, 100–102
  per-patient costs, 219
  from sponsors or CROs, 94
  structure of and ethical considerations, 262–263
  vaccine development, 35
Grassley, Charles, 296, 298
Griffith, Linda, 307
growth shifts, 236–237
GSK (GlaxoSmithKline), 36, 37, 322, 332, 333, 334–335
Guerrant, Richard, 329–330
guidance
  Compliance Program Guidance Manual (FDA), 143
  FDA, 14
  Guidance for Industry, 133
  research, 128–129
guidelines
  Belmont Report *(Ethical Principles and Guidelines for the Protection of Human Subjects of Research)*, 246, 247, 248–257, 373–374, 375–384
  developing FDA, 25
  FDA (*See* FDA)
  for gender issues, 304
  Good Clinical Practice Guidelines (ICH), 321
  Guidelines for Human Stem Cell Research (NIH), 121
  ICH (*See* International Conference on Harmonisation (ICH))
  international, 354
  IRB protocol reviews, 69, 79
  Operational Guidelines for Ethics Committees, 354
  practice, 277–278

H

Hager, W. David, 295
Hamburg, Margaret, 133, 139, 297
Hamilton, Kathryn, 356
Harvard Business School, site study, 56
Harvard University, 316
Hatch-Waxman amendments, 353
healthcare expenditures worldwide, 329
Health Insurance Portability and Accountability Act (HIPAA)
  confidentiality, 108
  HIPAA Privacy Rule report, 126
  negative impacts of, 54, 126–129, 240
  procedures for privacy, 184
  rules, 125–128, 268
  and tissue donation, 268
  understanding/misunderstanding of, 126
  withdrawal of informed consent, 152–153
health literacy, 153–156
Heckler, Margaret, 259
helminth infections, 328, 335
Henney, Jane, 295
hepatitis A and B vaccines, 34
Heuser, Stephen, 327
HHS (U.S. Department of Health and Human Services), 263, 278–279
Hierarchy of Needs, Maslow's, 3–4
HIPAA. *See* Health Insurance Portability and Accountability Act (HIPAA)
historical context for ethical issues, 241–247
HIV. *See also* AIDS
  children with, 255
  maternal-fetal transmission, 319
  medications, 268
  racial perceptions and, 312
  vaccine research, 29
HMO Research Network, 161
H1N1 (swine flu), 31, 35–37, 270
H2N2 flu vaccine, 29
Hoofnagle, Jay, 284
hormone replacement therapy trial, 17
Hotez, Peter, 330
Hovde, Mark, 43, 97
How to Lie with Statistics (Huff), 18
HR 2, Drug Abuse Control amendments, 351
Huff, Darryl, 18
human radiation experiments, 248
Hutchinson Cancer Research Center, 356

I

ICH (International Conference on Harmonisation), 113, 118, 148, 149, 151, 206, 214–216
ICH-GCP (Good Clinical Practice Guidelines), 321
ICMJE (International Committee of Medical Journal Editors), 230, 275
IDE (Investigational Device Exemption) applications, 24
IDSA (Infectious Diseases Society of America), 41, 207, 233
illiteracy of participants, 153–156
impropriety, 131, 168
incentives
  to conduct research, 266
  for discoveries, 112
  disincentives, 209, 263, 272
  financial, 42, 317, 323
  finder's fees, 91
  frequency of offers, 262
  for good performance, 228
  institutional, 27
  for investigators, 52, 105
  lack of, 24
  participation, 165–166
  for pediatric testing, 253
  recruitment, 158, 166
  for volunteers, 167, 196
inclusion criteria, 161–162, 239
income allocation, 338–339
indemnification clauses, 105–107, 108–110
independent sites, 68
India, 240, 322
individual research practice, 258
Indonesia, 269–270
IND (investigational new drug)
  safety reports, 123, 137, 159, 207, 212
  testing, 11, 24
infections. *See also* antibiotics; neglected tropical diseases (NTDs)
  antibiotic-resistant, 310
  bacterial, 42, 179, 318, 326
  emerging, 334
  helminthic, 328, 335
  protozoan, 329
Infectious Diseases Society of America (IDSA), 41, 207, 233
influenza-related patents, 269
influenza vaccines, 31, 195, 269–270
informed consent, 125–126. *See also* benefit/risk dilemma; risks
  adequacy of, 106
  audits of forms, 135, 137
  comprehension of, 381
  documentation of obtaining, 151–152
  elements of, 147–153, 364–366
  errors versus fraud, 138–139
  health literacy and, 153–156
  language of, 148, 267
  for medical devices, 27–28
  in overseas trials, 318

informed consent (*continued*)
procedures for process, 183
readability of, 361
regulations, 151
review of, 82
risks,134, 137–138, 149, 178–180
standards for, 380–382
use of drug, 121–122
when to obtain, 150
withdrawal of, 152–153
initiation phase of starting up, 159, 160–161
injured subjects, 34, 107–108, 281–282
innovative trials, 221–224, 225
Institute of Medicine (IOM), 31, 107, 120, 154, 224–225, 284, 285, 299–300, 301, 305
institutional review boards (IRBs)
approval package, 79
approvals from, 19–20
audits by, 142
commercial versus local, 76, 123, 124, 280–281
Communications Checklist, 212
ethical issues, 279–281
for-profit, 281
ICH compliance, 151
IRB registry, 355
nonfinancial ethical conflicts, 280
ongoing reviews, 80
preparation time costs, 88–89
procedures relating to, 183
regulatory issues of, 76–78, 123–125
responsibilities of, 123
roles of, 7
study closure report to, 215
submission process, 78–79
of TeGenero trial, 360
types of, 46, 77
insurance
coverage for catastrophic outcomes, 106–107
mandated coverage, 168
procedures for documenting, 183
for sites, 106, 107
for sponsors, 103
intellectual property rights, 269
interactions, drug, 199
internal audits, 131, 135
international audits, 142
International Code of Medical Ethics, 351
International Committee of Medical Journal Editors (ICMJE), 230, 275
International Conference on Harmonisation (ICH), 113, 118, 148, 149, 206, 214–216, 321
International Ethical Guidelines for Biomedical Research Involving Human Subjects, 107, 247
international guidelines, 354
International Organization of Standardization (ISO), 26
international regulatory agencies, 13
International Serious Adverse Events Consortium (SAEC), 161
interruption of studies, 200–202
inventions and patent clauses, 104
inventories, 193–194
Investigational Device Exemption (IDE) applications, 24
investigational devices, development path of, 25
investigational drugs, development path of, 25
investigational new drug (IND) testing, 11, 24, 28, 75, 118, 123, 207, 221, 222, 236, 237, 286
investigational products (IPs), 183
investigator-initiated studies, 16, 19–20
investigators. *See also* Principal Investigators (PIs)
blacklisted/disqualified, 141
Certified Physician Investigator examination, 341
Federal Investigator Registry of Biomedical Informatics Research Date (FIREBIRD), 233
incentives for, 52, 105, 158
perspectives for starting the study, 158–159
perspectives of, 158–159
risks for, 4–5
sponsor-investigator relationship, 264
Statement of Investigator (Form FDA 1572), 54, 78, 121–122, 130, 136, 281
turnover of, 228
Investigator's Brochure, 74, 78, 122, 124, 206, 207, 209, 211, 288
investigator's meetings, 340
investigator-sponsor relationship, 264
IOM (Institute of Medicine), 31, 107, 120, 154, 224–225, 284, 285, 299–300, 301, 305
IPs (investigational products), 183
ISO (International Organization of Standardization), 26

J

JAMA (Journal of the American Medical Association), 238, 276
Japan, 239, 240
jargon/terminology, 5. *See also* language

Jenner, Edward, 33
John Paul II, Pope, 310
Johns Hopkins, 124, 140, 152, 163, 281
Johnson, Guy, 83–84
Johnson & Johnson, 26, 40, 141, 322, 335
Journal of the American Medical Association (JAMA), 238, 276
The Jungle (Sinclair), 38
justice
  distributive, 250, 253, 315
  principle of, 378–379
  societal needs and, 324–336

K

Kaufman, David G., 341
Kaufman, Leslie, 312
Kefauver, Estes, 39
Kefauver-Harris amendments, 39, 351
Kennedy Institute of Ethics, 273
Kennedy Krieger Institute, 142
Kessler, David, 295
Ketek studies, 138–139, 298
kickbacks, 82
Kirkman-Campbell, Anne, 139
Klein, Daniel B., 16
knowledge-based sourcing, 111

L

labeling, 38, 39
laboratory costs, 87, 88, 191
laboratory regulations and procedures, 183
"Laments of a Clinical Clerk" (poem), 346
  landing a study. *See* acquiring your first study
language
  biased, 361
  of contracts, 92, 105, 110
  exculpatory, 267
  of informed consent, 148
  jargon, 5
  subject's native, 155
Latisse, 327
laws/lawsuits. *See* legal issues; legislation; litigation
Leavitt, Michael, 298
legal issues. *See also* legislation; litigation
  antidiscrimination laws, 154
  Public Law 110-85, 230
  Sarbanes-Oxley laws, 82
  Stark Law (Limitation on Certain Physician Referrals), 82
  U.S. drug laws, 38–40, 350–355
legislation
  Amendments Act, 14, 40, 230
legislation (*continued*)
  American Recovery and Reinvestment Act (ARRA), 119–120, 224–225, 355
  Anti-Tampering Act, 40, 352
  Bayh-Dole Patent and Trademark Laws Amendment Act, 259–260
  Best Pharmaceuticals for Children Act, 253, 354
  Biologics Control Act, 33
  Drug Price Competition and Patent Term Restoration Act, 353
  evolution of U.S. drug law, 38–40
  Food and Drug Administration Act, 294
  Food and Drug Administration Amendments Act (FDAAA), 115, 116–117, 354
  Food and Drug Administration Modernization Act (FDAMA), 248
  Food and Drugs Act of 1906, 38
  Freedom of Information Act (FOIA), 131
  Genetic Information Nondiscrimination Act (GINA), 117, 355
  Health Information Technology for Economic and Clinical Health Act (HITECH Act), 161, 164, 355
  Health Insurance Portability and Accountability Act (HIPAA), 54, 108, 126–129, 152–153, 184, 240, 268
  historical timeline of, 350–355
  Import Drugs Act of 1848, 38
  Medical Devices Amendment Act, 23
  Medical Device and User Fee and Modernization Act, 354
  Medical Device Safety Act of 2009, 24–25
  Modernization Act, 253
  National Childhood Vaccine Injury Act (NcVIA), 34
  National Institutes of Health (NIH), Revitalization Act, 248
  National Research Act, 246
  Orphan Drug Act, 353
  Pediatric Research Equity Act, 253–254, 354
  Pregnancy Discrimination Act, 306
  Prescription Drug User Fee Act (PDUFA), 15, 217–218, 353
  Small Business Patent Procedures Act, 260
  South African Medicines and Related Substance Control Amendment Act, 268–269
  Vaccine Act of 1813, 33, 38
Leo, Jonathan, 277
Leonard, Kate, 102
Levine, Diana, 24

liability, 4–5, 105, 126–127
life cycles of devices/products, 25, 28
lifestyle drugs, 325, 326–327
Lillington, Linda, 165
Limitation on Certain Physician Referrals (Stark Law), 82
Lindhan, John, 26
literacy and informed consent, 153–156
litigation
- *Abney v. Amgen*, 106
- *Gelsinger v. Trustees of University of Pennsylvania*, 142
- *Kathryn Hamilton v. Hutchinson Cancer Research Center*, 356
- *Metabolite v. LabCorp*, 268
- *Riegel v. Medtronic*, 24, 355
- *Suthers v. Amgen*, 106
- *Tummino v. Torti*, 296
- *Washington University v. Catalona*, 266–267
- *Wyeth v. Levine*, 24, 355

local institutional review boards (IRBs), 76, 123, 124, 280–281
long-term follow-up (LTFU) phase of study, 10, 171
long-term studies, 197, 198, 199, 235
Louisiana State University, 201
Lowe, Derek, 223
LTFU (long-term follow-up) phase of study, 10
lupus, 325
lymphatic filariasis, 329

M

Maassab, Hunein, 29
Maheu, Emmanuel, 200
malaria vaccine, 332
male bias, 301
malnutrition, 328, 330
manual of procedures/operations (MOP or MOO), 181
Manufacturer and User Facility Device Experience (MAUDE), 26
marketing, 14
Maslow's Hierarchy of Needs, 3–4
Massachusetts Institute of Technology, 307
material transfer, 269–270
Mathias, Cheryl, 356
Matthews, Anne Wilde, 276
MAUDE (Manufacturer and User Facility Device Experience), 26
McClellan, Mark, 295
meaningful use clause, 119
measles vaccine, 34
Medical Device Innovation Initiative, 25
medical device trials, 22–28
medical evaluations, 89, 93
medical monitors, roles of, 7
medical records, 202–203
medical research associates (MRAs), roles of, 7
Medicare coverage, 27, 89, 119–120, 164
Medicare National Coverage Decision, 80
medications, patients' baseline, 208
medicine administration. *See* administering/dispensing drugs
Medicines and Healthcare products Regulatory Agency (MHRA), 282
Medidata, 84–85
Medtronic, 24, 355
melanoma trial, University or Oklahoma, 356
meningitis, 317–318
mentally disabled subjects, 245–246
mentors, 48
Merck, 224, 275, 276, 297, 329, 334
Merck KGaA, 335
Meyerson, Lisa, 231–232
microdosing approach, 222, 223
middlemen, dealing with, 97–100
mifepristone (RU-486), 295
military personnel as subjects, 250–252
Milstein, Alan C., 106
"minimum necessary" requirements, 128
minority subjects, 248, 257, 267–268, 313–315
Modell, Martin, 189
Moellering, Robert, 41
Moench, Elizabeth, 196
monitoring visits, 97, 194–195, 273
monitors, problems of EMRs for, 163–164
Montgomery, Ron, 47, 53, 72, 174–175
Moore, John, 264
MOP or MOO (manual of procedures/operations), 181
moral obligations, 310
morbidity rates, 274, 302
Morganstern, Julie, *Organizing from the Inside Out*, 193–194
mortality rates, 187, 274, 302
Mosholder, Andrew D., 297
Movahhed, Hassan, 55, 111
MRAs (medical research associates), roles of, 7
MRFIT (Multiple Risk Factor Intervention Trial), 301
"Mrs. G" case study, 285–290
Multiple Risk Factor Intervention Trial (MRFIT), 301
mumps vaccine, 34
Munchausen's syndrome, 271

N

National Bioethics Advisory Committee (NBAC), 248, 353
National Cancer Institute (NCI), 31, 233
National Catholic Bioethics Center, 309–310
National Institute of Allergy and Infectious Diseases (NIAID), 36, 233
National Institute of Child Health and Human Development (NICHD), 253
National Institutes of Health (NIH)
Guidelines for Human Stem Cell Research, 121
NCI Best Practices for Biospecimen Resources, 267–268
Office of Human Subjects Research, 243
Office of Research on Women's Health (ORWH), 304, 305
pediatric drug development authority, 253
Recombinant DNA Advisory Committee, 273
Revitalization Act, 248
standardization of physician training, 341
Therapeutics for Rare and Neglected Diseases (TRND), 222
training grants, 343
National Vaccine Injury Compensation Program (NVICP), 34
NBAC (National Bioethics Advisory Committee), 248, 353
NCI (National Cancer Institute), 31, 233
NDAs (New Drug Applications), 13, 52, 131, 218, 317
neglected tropical diseases (NTDs), 327–329, 330, 331, 333, 334
net present value, 221
networking, 48, 49
New Drug Applications (NDAs), 13, 52, 131, 218, 317
New England Journal of Medicine, 238
NExT (Center for Cancer Research NCI Experimental Therapeutics) program, 222
NIAID (National Institute of Allergy and Infectious Diseases), 233
NIAID, clinical trials sponsored by, 29
niche providers, 99
Nifurtimox-Eflornithine Combination Trial, 334
Nigeria, 312, 318
NOAEL (no observable adverse effect level), 12
no-fault compensation, 107
noncompliance, 107, 118, 183, 195
nondisclosure agreements, 67
noninferiority trials, 225
no observable adverse effect level (NOAEL), 12
Northern California Kaiser Permanente, vaccine trial by, 32
notified bodies, 26
Novartis, 335
novel-device trials, 27–28
NTDs (neglected tropical diseases), 327–329
Nuremberg Code of Ethics, 39, 245, 247, 303, 350, 385–386
Nuremberg trials, 244
NVICP (National Vaccine Injury Compensation Program), 34
Nylen, Ruth Ann, *Ultimate Step-by-Step Guide to Conducting Pharmaceutical Clinical Trials in the USA,* 184

O

obese patients, 257
observational vaccine trials, 32
Occupational Safety and Health Administration (OSHA), 88, 183, 191
Office for Human Research Protections (OHRP), 140, 163, 248, 317
Office of Inspector General (OIG), 14, 124, 176–177, 229, 263
Official Action Indicated (OAI), 140, 142
off-label use of drugs, 278–279
OHRP (Office for Human Research Protections), 140, 248, 317
OHRP, privacy rules, 163
onchocerciasis (river blindness), 329
oncology patients in trials, 288–289
one-time fees, 93–94
on-line site resources, 51
brokers, 49, 51–52
site-listing services, 51
on-treatment phase of study, 10
open label protocol, 21–22
Operation Whitecoat, 252
opportunities in clinical research, 54–55, 338–339
OPTIMO (Oseltamivir Pharmocokinetics in Morbid Obesity), 257
Organizing from the Inside Out (Morganstern), 193–194
orientation of staff, 74–75, 75–76
orphan devices, 25
orphan diseases, 327
orphan drugs, 21, 25, 327
Oseltamivir Pharmocokinetics in Morbid Obesity (OPTIMO), 257
outcome logs, 186
overhead costs, 93

overlapping (competing) studies, 159, 179,
overseas drug manufacturing, 241
overseas trials, 238–241
oversight bodies, 124, 274, 281
ownership of body/tissue, 265–267
ownership rights and patents, 103–104

P

paper trail management, 134, 159, 202
paperwork, 90. *See also* documentation
paperwork management, 186–188
parallel study designs, 20
parasitic infections, 328
participation in studies
  AIDS trial participation in South Africa, 323
  incentives for, 165–166
  rate of participation, 222
  of sponsors, 85–86
  women's, 300–307
partnerships, 333, 334–335
patented versus generic drugs, 278
patent medicine, 39
patent pools, 332
patent protection, 103
patents
  Bayh-Dole Patent and Trademark Laws Amendment Act, 259–260
  clauses for, 110
  Drug Price Competition and Patent Term Restoration Act, 353
  expiration of, 158
  flu-related, 269
  ownership rights and, 103–104, 268–270
  versus public health, 268–270
  Small Business Patent Procedures Act, 260
  time under, 218
patent tools, 332
patient outcome logs, 186
patient-prompted ethics, 270–271
patient-reported outcomes (PROs), 231
patients/subjects/volunteers. *See also* informed consent; Nuremberg Code
  access to, 239
  age-related problems, 304
  approaching potential, 178–180
  assessment of population, 60
  business versus patients, 267–268
  challenging/exposing to infectious agents, 32
  coercion/voluntariness, 381–382
  Common Federal Policy for the Protection of Human Subjects (Common Rule), 7, 353
  compliance/dropout, 69–70, 198

patients/subjects/volunteers (*continued*)
  data mining for, 54
  deaths of, 271, 284, 299
  definition of, 6
  demographics of, 118
  documentation kept by, 203–204
  drop-outs, 95, 195, 231
  dropping from trials, 13, 95, 263
  estimating numbers, 72
  evaluability, 95
  fear of, 148
  identification of, 125
  illiteracy and informed consent, 153–156
  injuries to, 34, 107–108, 281–282
  instructions for, 197–202
  minority, 153, 248, 257
  monitoring visits, 194–195
  noncompliant, 183
  opt-out by, 147
  patient-prompted ethical issues, 270–271
  phases of participation, 10
  pregnant women, 304
  principles and guidelines for research with human subjects, 375–384
  prisoners as, 250–251
  recruitment of (*See* recruiting participants)
  regulations for protection of, 352
  reimbursed expenses/payment, 91
  retention/satisfaction of, 72–73, 195–197, 229
  satisfaction of, 194
  selection of, 384
  special populations, 255–257
  sponsor's requirements for, 68–69
  supportive, 68, 69, 95–96
  time commitments of, 313
  unevaluable, 96
  vulnerable populations, 250–255, 316
  women versus men as, 301–303
Patient Wallet Card, 198, 201
pay for performance clause, 119–120
payment schedules, 100–101, 112, 262
Pediatric Studies Rule, 248, 253
pediatric trials, 245–246, 252–255, 256
penalties, failure to meet timetables, 14
penicillin, 350
personnel. *See* staff/team members
personnel costs, 96–97
PERT—CPM (Program Evaluation and Review Technique—Critical Path Method), 189
Pfizer, 221, 274, 276, 278–279, 280, 316, 318, 319, 333
Pharmaceutical Information Cost Assessment Service (PICAS), 84–85

Pharmaceutical Research and Manufacturers of America (PhRMA), 41, 224, 331
pharmaceuticals companies
antibiotics development by, 41–42
collaboration among, 42–43
investigative sites/databases, 53
site selection by, 55–56
working directly with, 98–99
pharmacists, roles of, 6, 71
pharmacy costs, 87–88
phases of drug development
early development, 11
initiation phase, 159
participation phases, 10
phase 0 trials, 222, 223
phase 1 trials, 11–12, 283, 320, 338–339
phase 2 trials, 12–13
phase 3 trials, 13–14
phase 4 trials, 14–16
preclinical, 12
summary of, 12
time line of, 11
PHI (protected health information), 125
philanthropic companies, 329
PhRMA (Pharmaceutical Research and Manufacturers of America), 41, 224, 331
physician investigators, 237, 341
Physician's Health Study, 301
PICAS (Pharmaceutical Information Cost Assessment Service), 84–85
Pietzshe, Jan, 26
placebo arm of trial, 13, 20–21
placebo-controlled studies, 319, 321–322
placebos, discouragement of use of, 320–321
Plan B, 295
POC (proof of concept), 31
Pocock, Stuart, 221
polio vaccine, 31, 33, 34
politics of research
allocation of resources, 324–325, 338–339
appointments of commissioners, 294–297
censorship, 294
Cuban ransom deal, 39–40
drug approvals (*See* approvals)
FDA, 293–300
funding, 46, 332–333
justice and societal needs, 250, 253, 315, 324–336
race/gender overlap, 314–315
race/minorities, 311–314
religion issues, 267, 294, 307–310
rivalry as, 176
politics of research (*continued*)
shifting studies to developing countries, 315–324
women's participation in research, 300–307
populations
target, 60, 158, 165, 170
vulnerable, 250–255, 316
position, budgeting by, 96–97
postmarket disasters, 304
postmarketing studies, 14–16
practice, clinical. *See* clinical practice
preclinical development, 11, 31, 218
preemption argument, 24
pregnancy/pregnant subjects, 303, 304, 309, 326, 351
preparation time, 88–89
preparedness, 35
prescreening rules, 178
preservatives, 30
President's Emergency Plan for AIDS Relief (PEPFAR), 331
President's National Bioethics Advisory Committee, 124
pressures
cutting corners, 263–264
financial, 258–262
from sponsors, 158
pretreatment (pre-Rx or prestudy drug) phase of study, 10
preventive vaccine trials, 32
price elasticity, 85, 86
PRIM&R (Public Responsibility in Medicine & Research), 124–125
Principal Investigators (PIs)
blacklisted, 141
responsibilities of, 133, 288
roles of, 5–6, 9, 45, 74
Society of Principle Investigators, 78
supervision by, 121, 133
priorities/prioritization
for CER funding, 225
chosen, 330–336
ethical issues of, 315
governmental, 331
IOM's, 120
list of drug priorities, 253
perspectives on, 329–334
quality assurance, 133
society's, 325
WHO's, 35, 334
prisoners as subjects, 250–251
privacy
EMRs and, 162–163
penalties for breaching, 164
procedures for ensuring, 184
Privacy Rule, 129
procedural costs, 93

process mapping, 236
product quality, 19–20
profitability, 56, 261, 325, 330–331, 338–339
Program Evaluation and Review Technique—Critical Path Method (PERT—CPM), 189
Project BioShield, 354
project management techniques, 72, 189, 190–191
project managers, 97
proof of concept (POC), 31
property rights of tissue ownership, 265–267
PROs (patient-reported outcomes), 231
protected health information (PHI), 125
protocols/protocol design
  adherence to, 360–361
  blinding, 22
  changes to, 121
  conflicts with other information in, 192
  exceptions to, 185–186
  feasibility of, 68–72
  focus of, 114
  impossible, 73
  ingredients of, 17–18
  investigator-driven, 16
  miscellaneous concerns, 190–191
  modifications to, 19–20
  of overseas trials, 316
  Part 1: Parts of protocol, 16–18
  Part 2: Patient Mix, 18–19
  Part 3: Mixing Ingredients, 20–22
  product quality, 19–20
  randomization, 20, 25, 26, 27, 136, 156, 157, 277
  regulatory elements of, 151
  review and approval procedures, 183
  TeGenero case study, 359–360
  transparency of, 230
  violations of, 214
protozoan infections, 329
Public Agenda, 324
publication of studies, 103–105, 114, 275–277
public awareness of trials, 167, 175, 197, 229
Public Citizen, 219
public funds allocation, 324–325
public health versus patents, 268–270
Public Law 110-85, 230
Public Responsibility in Medicine & Research (PRIM&R), 124–125

Q

qualification of sites, 57, 58–59
quality assurance, 19–20, 133
query resolutions, 75, 90, 101, 102, 204, 205, 215, 216, 232
quinacrine, 314–315
quinolone study, 212

R

race/racial issues
  disparities, 293
  gender/race overlap, 313
  politics of, 239, 311–314, 323
  race/gender overlap, 314–315, 325
  selection by, 124
  study design and, 254, 264
radiation experiments, 353
radiology, costs, 89
randomization, 20, 25, 26, 27, 136, 156, 157, 277
Rapid Impact packages, 330
Rational Therapeutics for Infants and Children, 253
R&D (research and development), 220, 332, 333
recalls, 31, 40
recombinant DNA vaccines, 30
recordkeeping. *See* documentation
Recruiting Human Subjects, 262–263
recruiting participants. *See also* advertising
  barriers to, 167–168, 256–257, 313
  bonuses for rapid recruitment, 263
  cultural issues/beliefs and, 240
  documenting, 72–73
  ethical issues of, 258
  finder's fees, 91
  identifying potential volunteers, 164–178, 362
  incentives, 158, 166
  inclusion/exclusion criteria, 161–162
  issues to address, 69
  minority subjects, 248, 257, 267–268, 313–315
  for novel devices, 27–28
  reasons for volunteering, 165–166, 285
  referrals to studies, 82
  screening and enrollment, 10, 73, 177–178, 183, 185–186
  third party, 161–162, 168–169
referrals of patients to studies, 82, 168–169
registries for medical devices, 27
regulatory (study) binders, 159–160
regulatory issues
  American Recovery and Reinvestment Act (ARRA), 119–120
  billing for clinical trials, 80–82
  differences among countries, 114
  drug and device development, 25

regulatory issues (*continued*)
Executive Order 13505, 120–121
Food and Drug Administration Amendment Act (FDAAA), 116–117
Genetic Information Nondiscrimination Act, 117
HIPAA rules, 125–128
historical timeline of, 350–355
implementation of, 159–160
informed consent, 151
institutional review boards (IRBs), 76–78, 123–125
international agencies, 13
"minimum necessary" requirements, 128
new regulations, 115
ongoing regulatory requirements, 80
OSHA's, 88
overseas differences in, 240–241
overview, 113–115
process for device development, 26
protection of human subjects, 352
regulatory binder contents checklist, 159
research guidance, 128–129
tracking adverse event reports, 206–211
up-to-date training in, 77
religion issues, 267, 294, 307–310
remote data entry (RDE), 90
Removing Barriers to Responsible Scientific Research Involving Human Stem Cells, 120–122
reporting results
adverse events, 136, 137, 209, 272
case report forms (CRFs), 90, 135, 142, 143, 187, 203–205, 215, 232
Consolidated Standards of Reporting Trials (CONSORT), 276–277
failure to report adverse drug reactions, 142
patient-reported outcomes (PROs), 231
regulatory reports, 206
reporting procedures, 184
safety reports, 207, 212–213
study closure reports, 332
tracking adverse event reports, 206–211
Vaccine Adverse Events Reporting Systems (VAERS), 32–33
WHO standards for, 276–277
Reproductive Health Technologies Project, 314
reproductive studies, 352
research and development (R&D), 220, 332, 333
research barriers, 281
research experience summaries, 58–59
research guidance, 128–129
resistant organisms, antibiotics development for, 41–43, 318
resources
allocation of, 324–325, 338–339
consumption of global, 329–330
for finding/landing studies, 50
respect for persons principle, 248–249, 377
responsibilities
delegating, 121, 133–134, 137, 151, 245, 258
of institutional review boards (IRBs), 123
of Principal Investigators (PIs), 288
Public Responsibility in Medicine & Research (PRIM&R), 124–125
of staff/team members, 5–9, 71, 74–75, 183
results
bias in publishing, 276–277, 301
posting summaries of, 275
WHO standards for reporting, 276–277
retention of subjects, 69, 195–197, 229
review process, 27, 32, 80
rights and patents clauses, 76–77, 81
rights of ownership, 103–104, 269
risk/benefit dilemma, 16, 34, 39, 110, 134, 151, 178–180
risks
active surveillance for, 354
assessment of, 382–383
with biologics, 28
with devices, 28
discussing risks/benefits with patients, 178–180
for investigators, 4–5
mitigation of, 40
proportional, 115
side effects, 15, 32, 33, 40, 104, 120, 211, 212, 254, 259, 271, 273, 287
unanticipated, 281–285
river blindness (onchocerciasis), 329
Roche, Ellen, 281, 358
roles of team members, 5–9, 45, 74–75
Ross, David, 139
Rothman, Kenneth, 276
RU-486 (mifepristone), 295
rubella vaccine, 34
rural sites, 47–48
Rush University, 81–82

S

safety issues
Data Safety Monitoring Boards (DSMBs), 7, 14, 17, 274–275, 279

safety issues (*continued*)
high-profile cases and, 40
IND safety reports, 207
Institute of Medicine safety study, 16
lack of safeguards, 318
Medical Device Safety Act, 24–25
multiple safeguards, 273
Occupational Safety and Health Administration (OSHA), 88, 183, 191
reporting procedures, 184
safety reports, 212–213
trials gone wrong, 356–358
vaccine development trials, 31
Vaccine Safety Datalink (VSD), 33
withdrawals of drugs, 15–16
safety reviews, 115
Sanofi-Aventis, 138–139, 334, 335
Sarbanes-Oxley laws, 82
Satcher, David, 319
SBA (Small Business Association), 46
schistosomiasis, 328–329
Schistosomiasis Control Initiative, 335
Schroeder, Pat, 304
Schuklenk, Udo, 277
scientific bottlenecks, breaking, 225–228
scientific considerations, 67–68
Scott, Janny, 312
screen failures, 70, 72, 84
screening and enrollment logs, 177–178, 185–186
screening phase of study, 10
screening procedures, 183
screen-to-enrollment ratio, 73
seals of approval, 19–20
Sebelius, Kathleen, 35
seed stock, 31
selection criteria, 73
Senak, Mark, 36
send-outs, 46, 61
Sentinel Initiative, 116, 164, 354
sepsis protocols, 235
serious adverse events (SAEs). *See also* adverse events (AEs)
budgeting for, 90
defining, 272
following up on, 211
numbers of, 69, 70, 138, 164–165, 206, 272–273, 320
reporting, 184, 205, 207, 215
time planning for, 89
Sharfstein, Joshua, 297
Shlaes, David, 41
Shulman, Lawrence E., 5
signatures, 79, 122, 138, 139, 156, 163, 164–165, 182, 320
Signs and Symptoms Worksheet, 187
Silverman, Ed, 326
Simian virus 40 contamination, 31
Sinclair, Upton, *The Jungle*, 38
Singapore Economic Development Board, 335
single-blind studies, 21, 22
site-listing services, 51
site management organizations (SMOs), 7, 49, 97–100, 98
site-sponsor relationships, 8, 53, 90–91, 213, 340–341
site-sponsor study documents, 184
sites/site selection
cautions for, 55–56
complaints against, 229
facilities audits, 136
identifying potential, 49, 54
preparing for visits, 61–62
profitability of, 56
promoting your, 63–64
qualification of, 58–59
reasons for choosing, 57–59
relationships with, 111
size and setting, 62–65
small, 77
universities as, 62–63
visits, 59–61
Small Business Association (SBA), 46
smallpox, 33, 34, 38
Smith, James, 38
SMOs (site management organizations), 7, 49, 97–100
Snowe, Olympia, 304
social justice issues, of drug development, 325–329
social networking, 175–176
societal needs, justice and, 324–336
Society for Women's Health Research, 247, 304
Society of Principle Investigators, 106
software programs, 189–190
source documents, 202–203, 230–231
sourcing, knowledge-based, 111
South Africa, 268, 269, 323
special populations, 255–257
special studies, costs, 89
specimen collection/preparation, 61, 74, 88, 183, 191, 195
Specimen Shipping Log, 190
sponsor-investigator relationship, 264
sponsors
audits by, 141
commercial, 68
contact worksheet, 161
cost anticipation, 23, 84
factors in participation of, 85–86
finding, 49
grants from, 94
incentives offered by, 158

sponsors (*continued*)
information required by, 61–62
initiation visits, 160–161
insurance coverage of, 362
payment clauses, 101
pressure from, 158
religious, 307–308
roles of, 6–7
sponsor-site relationships, 8, 213, 340–341
spreadsheets, 84, 85
Srinivasan, Sandhya, 322
staff/team members
base pay, 83–84
budgeting by position, 96–97
cross-cultural training, 313
ER nurses, 170
feasibility issues, 73–74
finder's fees for recruiting patients, 91
key people, 169
orientation of, 70, 75–76
part-time, 76
protocol reviews by, 70
responsibilities of, 71, 183
roles/responsibilities of individuals, 74–75
specialized training, 88
supervision of, 136
technical support personnel, 46
training of (*See* training)
turnover of, 53, 90, 97, 228
standardization, 26, 113, 230–231, 232–235, 320, 343
standard operating procedures (SOPs), 133, 136, 181–184
Stark Law (Limitation on Certain Physician Referrals), 82
starting the study
administrative delays, 236
cross-cultural issues in, 156–157
implementation of regulations, 159–160
informed consent, 147–157
initiation visits, 160–161
investigators' perspectives, 158–159
needed items/people for, 45–47
sponsor pressure, 158
start-up costs, 91, 93–94
terms for start-up contracts, 102–103
volunteer recruitment strategies, 164–178
start-up phase of study, 10
Statement of Investigator (Form FDA 1572), 54, 74, 121–122, 130, 136
stem cell research, 120–121
stem cell therapies, 28
sterilization studies, 313–315
stimulus package, 119–120
storage
of drugs, 192–193
of study records, 92, 201–202
Straus, Stephen, 271, 284, 285
study activities
administration and overhead costs, 93
budget feasibility by, 92–94
at closeout visit, 214–216
cycle of participation activities, 10
delegation of, 110
estimating costs of, 96
grants, 94
medical evaluations, 93
participation in, 10
staffing for, 73
start-up and one-time fees, 93–94
subject compliance, 69–70
worksheets, 92
study binders/folders, 159–160, 188–189
study closings, 212–215
study coordinators. *See* clinical research (or study) coordinators (CRCs)
study tracking, 185–188
subinvestigators, 6, 48
subjects. *See* patients/subjects/volunteers
submission process, 78–79
sub-Saharan Africa, 323
subsidized unprofitable medical projects (SUMPs), 85–86
supplies. *See* equipment/supplies
Supreme Court decisions. *See* legislation
surrogate biomarkers, 224
surrogate markers, 32, 223, 224
surveys, site qualification, 58–59
swine flu (H1N1), 31, 33, 35–37, 270

T

Tabarrok, Alexander, 16
tamper-resistant packaging, 40, 352
target pathogens, 37
target populations, 60, 158, 165, 170
tax credits, 221
team members. *See* staff/team members
technical support personnel, 46
teen subjects, 256
TeGenero study, 106–107, 281–283, 358, 359–366
templates
advertising, 172
budget, 84
contract, 85
CTN Best Practices, 187
HIPAA Consent Template, 126
informed consent, 18
patient instructions, 198
problems of, 83
ready-made, 182

teratogenicity, 39
terminating the study, 212–215
terminology/jargon, 5. *See also* language
thalidomide, 39, 304
therapeutic misconception, 169
Therapeutics for Rare and Neglected Diseases (TRND), 222
thimerosal, 30
third party recruitment, 161–162, 168–169
Tibetan medicine, 157
time management/budgeting
 for adverse events (AEs), 89–90
 for audits, 91
 commitment of patients, 313
 failure to meet timetables, 14
 IRB preparation time, 88–89
time under patent, 218
tissue
 Cooperative Human Tissue Network (CHTN), 268
 donations of, 249, 267, 376
 ownership of, 265–267
tobacco products regulation, 295
Towns, Edolphus, 299
toxicity management, 115, 289
tracking drugs, 129–130
tracking the study, procedures for, 185–188
Trade-Related Aspects of Intellectual Property (TRIPS) Agreement, 268–269
trade secrets, 67
training
 apprenticeships, 48, 342
 for clinical research associates (CRAs), 99
 cross-cultural, 313
 for FDA inspections, 182–183
 formal programs, 339–343
 on-the-job, 342
 opportunities, 337–338
 in regulatory issues, 77
 requirements, 184
 specialized, 88
 standardization of, 341
translational research, 259
transparency, 230, 277
triple-blind studies, 22
TRND (Therapeutics for Rare and Neglected Diseases), 222
tropical diseases, neglected, 327–329
Trovafloxacin (Trovan), 280, 318
trust issues, 311–312, 313
Tufts Center for the Study of Drug Development (CSDD), 217, 218, 219
Tulane University, 201
Tuskegee experiment, 244, 246, 247, 250
Tylenol tampering case, 40

U

Ultimate Step-by-Step Guide to Conducting Pharmaceutical Clinical Trials in the USA (Nylen), 184
unanticipated risks, 281–285
unblinded studies, 21
unethical studies, 244–245, 252
unevaluable patients, 96, 102
unexpected/unanticipated events, 206
Union Pacific, 306
UNITAID, 331–332
United Nations (UN), Universal Declaration of Human Rights, 247
University of California Los Angeles, 265–267
University of Miami, 125
University of Oklahoma, melanoma trial, 356
University of Pennsylvania, 142, 161
University of Rochester, 356–357
University of South Carolina, 161–162
University of Southern California, 150
university versus community sites, 64–65
UN Millennium Development Goals, 335
U.S. Department of Health, Education, and Welfare (HEW), 246
U.S. Department of Health and Human Services (HHS), 263, 278–279
U.S. Department of Justice, 153–154
U.S. drug laws, 38–40, 350–355
U.S. General Accounting Office (GAO), 304, 305
U.S. Indian Health Service, 315
U.S. Public Health Service, Task Force on Women's Health Issues, 247, 301
U.S. Public Health Task Force, 304
U.S. trials, decline in numbers, 237–238

V

vaccines/vaccine development
 administration of vaccines, 30
 decision making, 35–36
 development of vaccines, 28–37
 DNA vaccines, 30
 flu vaccines, 29, 31, 35–37, 269–270
 grants, 35
 historical timeline, 350–355
 HIV/AIDS vaccine, 29
 malaria vaccine, 332
 mandatory vaccinations, 37
 National Institute of Allergy and Infectious Diseases, 36
 observational vaccine trials, 32
 polio vaccine, 31
 preventive vaccine trials, 32
 recalls, 31
 requirements for, 30–31

vaccines/vaccine development (*continued*)
seed strain for H1N1 vaccine, 35
successes, 34
Vaccine Act of 1813, 33, 38
Vaccine Adverse Events Reporting Systems (VAERS), 32–33
Vaccine Safety Datalink (VSD), 33
VAI (Voluntary Action Indicated), 140
Vanderbilt University Ingram Cancer Center, 236
Vaniqa, 331
Varmus, Harold, 5, 260, 319
vendors, 88, 101, 161, 190, 236
Viagra, 326–327, 331
violations, financial penalties for, 14–15
Vioxx, 275, 276, 297
virus seed stocks, 31
visits, site qualification, 59–61
Vogelson, Cullen, 97, 271, 339
voluntariness, 381–382
Voluntary Action Indicated (VAI), 140
volunteers. *See* patients/subjects/volunteers
von Eschenbach, Andrew, 139, 296, 298
VSD (Vaccine Safety Datalink), 33
vulnerable populations, 250–255, 316

W

waiver of authorization, 125, 126, 128, 129, 151
Walters, LeRoy, 273
Wan, Nicole, 356–357
warning letters from FDA, 133, 141, 143, 173, 299
Waxman, Henry, 298, 304
Welsome, Eileen, 252
Willowbrook Study, 244–245, 247
Wilson, James, 271
win-win contracts, 110–111
withdrawal of drugs and devices, 15–16, 25, 274–275
withdrawal of informed consent, 152–153
Witty, Andrew, 332
women
Office of Research on Women's Health (ORWH), 304, 305
participation in studies by, 300–307
pregnant, 304
research on women's health, 248
Women's Health Initiative, 17
Wood, Alastair J. J., 15
Wood, Susan F., 295–296
Woodcock, Janet, 143
Woollen, Stan, 138–139
worksheets
activity budget, 92–94
budget, 84
budget feasibility/costs, 96
budgeting by position, 96–97
designing your own, 187
documentation, 186–189
Signs and Symptoms, 187
sponsor contact, 161
World Health Organization (WHO), 108, 331
Declaration of Helsinki, 247, 351, 362–363, 367–372
Operational Guidelines for Ethics Committees, 354
priority infectious diseases, 334
seed strain for H1N1 vaccine, 35
standards for reporting results, 276–277
World Medical Association, 246
World Trade Organization, 268–269
Wyeth, 24, 355

X

Xigris, 14

Y

young adult subjects, 256

Z

Zinner, Darren, 111
Zithromax, 221

About the Author

Judy Stone, MD, is Board Certified in Internal Medicine and Board Eligible in Infectious Disease. For 25 years, she had a busy solo, 100 percent ID practice in rural Cumberland, Maryland. In addition, Dr. Stone has had considerable experience attracting and successfully conducting numerous phase 2 and 3 clinical trials for a variety of infectious disease indications over more than 20 years. She also is a sought-after speaker on the topics of antibiotics and infectious diseases.

Dr. Stone is a graduate of Washington University in St. Louis, Missouri. She completed medical school at the University of Maryland, residency at Rochester General Hospital (New York), and fellowship at West Virginia University. In addition to her patient practice, Dr. Stone has had 15 years' experience with the Memorial Hospital Infection Control and Pharmacy and Therapeutics Committees and was chair of the their Department of Medicine for 3 years.

In 2004, Dr. Stone volunteered to teach about HIV, STDs, and infections in Dharamsala, India. Subsequently, she attended the Gorgas Expert Course in Tropical Medicine in Lima, Peru, in 2005.

She served on the Clinical Affairs Committee of IDSA (Infectious Diseases Society of America) from 2002 to 2005, particularly enjoying the teaching and mentoring opportunities it has afforded her.

She is the author of the forthcoming book *Volunteering for Clinical Research: A Consumer's Guide.*

Dr. Stone lives in western Maryland with her husband and children. When not working, she can be found tending her nourishing gardens.

Conducting Clinical Research

—ORDER FORM—

PHONE ORDERS	**FAX ORDERS**
(301) 722-2284 Please have your credit card information ready.	Complete this form and fax it to **(301) 722-8344**
MAIL ORDERS	**ONLINE ORDERS**
Complete this form and mail it to **Mountainside MD Press** **725 Park Street, Suite 400** **Cumberland, MD 21502**	Order at **http://ConductingClinicalResearch.com**

Name ______________________________

Address ______________________________

City ____________________ **State**______ **Zip** __________

Telephone ______________________________

E-mail address ______________________________

Payment: ☐ **Check** (Make payable to *Mountainside MD Press*)

☐ **Credit Card:** ___Visa ___MasterCard

Credit Card #______________________________

Name on card ______________________________

Exp. date ______________________________

Signature ______________________________

Description	Qty.	Price	Total
Conducting Clinical Research		$79.95	
Shipping and Handling: Add $12.00 for first book and $7.00 for each additional book. (Allow 1 week for delivery.)			
Sales Tax: Add 5% for books shipped to Maryland addresses.			
TOTAL			

Thank you for your order!